PEDIATRIC
HEART
FAILURE

Fundamental and Clinical Cardiology

Editor-in-Chief
Samuel Z. Goldhaber, M.D.
Harvard Medical School
and Brigham and Women's Hospital
Boston, Massachusetts

1. Drug Treatment of Hyperlipidemia, *edited by Basil M. Rifkind*
2. Cardiotonic Drugs: A Clinical Review, Second Edition, Revised and Expanded, *edited by Carl V. Leier*
3. Complications of Coronary Angioplasty, *edited by Alexander J. R. Black, H. Vernon Anderson, and Stephen G. Ellis*
4. Unstable Angina, *edited by John D. Rutherford*
5. Beta-Blockers and Cardiac Arrhythmias, *edited by Prakash C. Deedwania*
6. Exercise and the Heart in Health and Disease, *edited by Roy J. Shephard and Henry S. Miller, Jr.*
7. Cardiopulmonary Physiology in Critical Care, *edited by Steven M. Scharf*
8. Atherosclerotic Cardiovascular Disease, Hemostasis, and Endothelial Function, *edited by Robert Boyer Francis, Jr.*
9. Coronary Heart Disease Prevention, *edited by Frank G. Yanowitz*
10. Thrombolysis and Adjunctive Therapy for Acute Myocardial Infarction, *edited by Eric R. Bates*
11. Stunned Myocardium: Properties, Mechanisms, and Clinical Manifestations, *edited by Robert A. Kloner and Karin Przyklenk*
12. Prevention of Venous Thromboembolism, *edited by Samuel Z. Goldhaber*
13. Silent Myocardial Ischemia and Infarction: Third Edition, *Peter F. Cohn*
14. Congestive Cardiac Failure: Pathophysiology and Treatment, *edited by David B. Barnett, Hubert Pouleur and Gary S. Francis*
15. Heart Failure: Basic Science and Clinical Aspects, *edited by Judith K. Gwathmey, G. Maurice Briggs, and Paul D. Allen*
16. Coronary Thrombolysis in Perspective: Principles Underlying Conjunctive and Adjunctive Therapy, *edited by Burton E. Sobel and Desire Collen*
17. Cardiovascular Disease in the Elderly Patient, *edited by Donald D. Tresch and Wilbert S. Aronow*
18. Systemic Cardiac Embolism, *edited by Michael D. Ezekowitz*
19. Low-Molecular-Weight Heparins in Prophylaxis and Therapy of Thromboembolic Diseases, *edited by Henri Bounameaux*
20. Valvular Heart Diseases, *edited by Muayed Al Zaibag and Carlos M. G. Duran*
21. Implantable Cardioverter-Defibrillators: A Comprehensive Textbook, *edited by N. A. Mark Estes, Antonis S. Manolis, and Paul J. Wang*

PEDIATRIC HEART FAILURE

edited by

Robert E. Shaddy

University of Utah School of Medicine, Salt Lake City, U.S.A.

Gil Wernovsky

University of Pennsylvania School of Medicine, Philadelphia, U.S.A.
The Cardiac Center at The Children's Hospital of
Philadelphia, Pennsylvania, U.S.A.

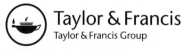

Taylor & Francis
Taylor & Francis Group

Boca Raton   London   New York   Singapore

Published in 2005 by
Taylor & Francis Group
6000 Broken Sound Parkway NW, Suite 300
Boca Raton, FL 33487-2742

© 2005 by Taylor & Francis Group, LLC

No claim to original U.S. Government works
Printed in the United States of America on acid-free paper
10 9 8 7 6 5 4 3 2 1

International Standard Book Number-10: 0-8247-5929-X (Hardcover)
International Standard Book Number-13: 978-0-8247-5929-2 (Hardcover)

Library of Congress Cataloging-in-Publication Data

Catalog record is available from the Library of Congress

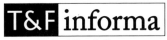

Taylor & Francis Group
is the Academic Division of T&F Informa plc.

**Visit the Taylor & Francis Web site at
http://www.taylorandfrancis.com**

Series Introduction

The Taylor & Francis Group has focused on the development of various series of beautifully produced books in different branches of medicine. These series have facilitated the integration of rapidly advancing information for both the clinical specialist and the researcher.

My goal as editor-in-chief of the Fundamental and Clinical Cardiology Series is to assemble the talents of world-renowned authorities to discuss virtually every area of cardiovascular medicine. In the current monograph, tric Heart Failure, Robert E. Shaddy and Gil Wernovsky have edited a much-needed and timely book. Future contributions to this series will include books on molecular biology, interventional cardiology, and clinical management of such problems as coronary artery disease and ventricular arrhythmias.

Samuel Z. Goldhaber

Preface

Heart failure is a major cause of morbidity and mortality in children. Although there are many similarities between heart failure in children and adults, the etiologies, pathophysiology, and physiologic consequences of heart failure in children are often very different than in adults. We are publishing this book because it is the first book of its kind to specifically focus on heart failure in children and a comprehensive text of this kind is lacking. This text provides a single reference source for pediatric heart failure and is a must-read for all health care professional who care for children with heart disease so they will be able to recognize and treat heart failure in children. The overall objectives of this book are to define the etiologies, pathophysiology, and treatment of heart failure in children from fetal life, childhood, adolesence, and through adult life with congenital heart disease. This book will address both chronic and acute decompensated heart failure, thus providing insights into the diagnosis and management of children from the womb, to the nursery, the intensive care unit, and the outpatient clinic. The target audience for this book includes pediatric cardiologists, pediatric cardiothoracic surgeons, pediatric intensivists, pediatricians, anesthesiologists, nurses, and all health care providers who deal with children with heart failure. This book will have special emphasis on the mechanisms, diagnosis, and management of heart failure that are unique to childern.

Robert E. Shaddy
Gil Wernovsky

Contents

Contributors

M. Jacob Adams   Division of Pediatric Cardiology, University of Rochester Medical Center and Golisano Children's Hospital at Strong, University of Rochester School of Medicine and Dentistry, Rochester, New York, U.S.A.

Michael Artman   Department of Pediatrics, New York University School of Medicine, New York, New York, U.S.A.

Marcelo Auslender   Department of Pediatrics, New York University School of Medicine, New York, New York, U.S.A.

Robyn J. Barst   Columbia University, College of Physicians and Surgeons, New York, New York, U.S.A.

Mark Boucek   Department of Pediatric Cardiology, The Children's Hospital/UCHSC, Denver, Colorado, U.S.A.

N.E. Bowles   Department of Pediatrics (Cardiology), Baylor College of Medicine, Houston, Texas, U.S.A.

Reiner Buchhorn   Department of Pediatric Cardiology, Georg-August-University Göttingen, Göttingen, Germany

Charles E. Canter   Washington University School of Medicine, St. Louis, Missouri, U.S.A.

Dana Connolly   Department of Pediatrics, New York University School of Medicine, New York, New York, U.S.A.

Gul H. Dadlani   Division of Pediatric Cardiology, University of Rochester Medical Center and Golisano Children's Hospital at Strong, University of Rochester School of Medicine and Dentistry, Rochester, New York, U.S.A.

Pedro J. del Nido   Department of Cardiac Surgery, Children's Hospital, Harvard Medical School, Boston, Massachusetts, U.S.A.

Sarah Duffy   Division of Pediatric Cardiology, University of Rochester Medical Center and Golisano Children's Hospital at Strong, University of Rochester School of Medicine and Dentistry, Rochester, New York, U.S.A.

Carol French   Division of Pediatric Cardiology, University of Rochester Medical Center and Golisano Children's Hospital at Strong, University of Rochester School of Medicine and Dentistry, Rochester, New York, U.S.A.

Brian D. Hanna   Department of Pediatrics, Division of Cardiology, Children's Hospital of Philadelphia, University of Pennsylvania School of Medicine, Philadelphia, Pennsylvania, U.S.A.

William G. Harmon   Division of Pediatric Cardiology, University of Rochester Medical Center and Golisano Children's Hospital at Strong, University of Rochester School of Medicine and Dentistry, Rochester, New York, U.S.A.

Larissa Herbowy   Division of Pediatric Cardiology, University of Rochester Medical Center and Golisano Children's Hospital at Strong, University of Rochester School of Medicine and Dentistry, Rochester, New York, U.S.A.

Lisa K. Hornberger Fetal Cardiovascular Program, Department of Pediatrics, Division of Cardiology, University of California, San Francisco, California, U.S.A.

Daphne T. Hsu Columbia University Medical Center, College of Physicians and Surgeons, Children's Hospital of New York, New York, New York, U.S.A.

Amy Kozlowski Division of Pediatric Cardiology, University of Rochester Medical Center and Golisano Children's Hospital at Strong, University of Rochester School of Medicine and Dentistry, Rochester, New York, U.S.A.

Michael J. Landzberg Brigham and Women's Hospital, Boston, Massachusetts, U.S.A..

Catherine A. Leitch Section of Neonatal–Perinatal Medicine, Department of Pediatrics, Indiana University Medical Center, Indianapolis, Indiana, U.S.A.

Steven E. Lipshultz Department of Pediatrics, University of Miami School fof Medicine and Holtz Children Hospital, Miami, Florida, U.S.A.

Katharine McLaughlin Division of Pediatric Cardiology, University of Rochester Medical Center and Golisano Children's Hospital at Strong, University of Rochester School of Medicine and Dentistry, Rochester, New York, U.S.A.

Kathy Mussatto Herma Heart Center, Children's Hospital and Health System, Milwaukee, Wisconsin, U.S.A.

Masaki Nii Department of Pediatrics, Division of Cardiology, The Hospital for Sick Children, Toronto, Canada

Timothy M. Olson Associate Professor of Medicine and Pediatrics, Mayo Clinic College of Medicine, Rochester, Minnesota, U.S.A.

Elfriede Pahl Department of Pediatrics, Children's Memorial Hospital, Northwestern University, Feinberg School of Medicine, Chicago, Illinois, U.S.A.

Stephen G. Pophal Department of Pediatrics, Children's Memorial Hospital, Northwestern University, Feinberg School of Medicine, Chicago, Illinois, U.S.A.

Chitra Ravishankar Department of Pediatrics, Division of Pediatric Cardiology, Children's Hospital of Philadelphia, University of Pennsylvania School of Medicine, Philadelphia, Pennsylvania, U.S.A.

Erika Berman Rosenzweig Columbia University, College of Physicians and Surgeons, New York, New York, U.S.A.

Abraham M. Rudolph Emeritus Professor of Pediatrics and Senior Staff, Cardiovascular Research Institute, University of California, San Francisco, California, U.S.A.

Steven M. Schwartz Division of Cardiology, Children's Hospital Medical Center, Cincinnati, Ohio, U.S.A.

Robert E. Shaddy Division of Pediatric Cardiology, Primary Children's Medical Center, University of Utah School of Medicine, Salt Lake City, Utah, U.S.A.

Michael J. Silka Division of Cardiology, Children's Hospital–Los Angeles, The Keck School of Medicine, University of Southern California, Los Angeles, California, U.S.A.

Jacqueline R. Szmuszkovicz Division of Cardiology, Children's Hospital–Los Angeles, The Keck School of Medicine, University of Southern Los Angeles, California, U.S.A.

Lloyd Y. Tani Division of Pediatric Cardiology, Primary Children's Medical Center, University of Utah School of Medicine, Salt Lake City, Utah, U.S.A.

David F. Teitel Professor of Pediatrics, Division of Pediatric Cardiology, University of California, San Francisco, California, U.S.A.

Svjetlana Tisma-Dupanovic Division of Pediatric Cardiology, University of Rochester Medical Center and Golisano Children's

Hospital at Strong, University of Rochester School of Medicine and Dentistry, Rochester, New York, U.S.A.

J.A. Towbin   Molecular and Human Genetics, and Cardiovascular Sciences, Baylor College of Medicine, Houston, Texas, U.S.A.

Matteo Vatta   Department of Pediatrics (Cardiology), Baylor College of Medicine, Houston, Texas, U.S.A.

Gil Wernovsky   Department of Pediatrics, Division of Pediatric Cardiology, Children's Hospital of Philadelphia, University of Pennsylvania School of Medicine, Philadelphia, Pennsylvania, U.S.A.

Karolina Zareba   Division of Pediatric Cardiology, University of Rochester Medical Center and Golisano Children's Hospital at Strong, University of Rochester School of Medicine and Dentistry, Rochester, New York, U.S.A.

1

Heart Failure—A Historical Perspective

ABRAHAM M. RUDOLPH

Emeritus Professor of Pediatrics and Senior Staff,
Cardiovascular Research Institute,
University of California, San Francisco,
California, U.S.A.

DEFINING HEART FAILURE

Heart failure (HF) is recognized as a leading cause of death in the adult population. Recently, it has been claimed that HF is occurring in adults in epidemic proportions (1,2). The prevalence of HF has been reported to be 3 per 1000 person years (3). In 1913, MacKenzie (4) defined HF as "the condition in which the heart is unable to maintain an efficient circulation when called upon to meet the efforts necessary to the daily life of the individual," whereas Lewis (5) regarded it as "inability of the heart to discharge its contents adequately." Surprisingly, there is still no unanimity of opinion regarding what constitutes HF and a variety of definitions are encountered in current texts.

Based on the experimental and clinical observations of cardiac ventricular function, the concept generally accepted by adult cardiologists is that "the term cardiac failure implies structural heart disease" (6) and that "chronic HF is a syndrome that evolves from damage to the myocardium, resulting in significant reduction in left ventricular function" (7). The definition has, however, been modified to take into consideration the relationship of cardiac function and body requirements. Braunwald (8) states "Heart failure is the pathophysiological state in which an abnormality of cardiac function is responsible for the failure of the heart to pump blood at a rate commensurate with the requirements of the metabolizing tissues and/or allows it to do so only from an elevated diastolic volume. The HF is frequently, but not always, caused by a defect in myocardial contraction, and then the term myocardial failure is appropriate."

Inherent in most definitions is the assumption that myocardial function is disturbed, so that the heart does not adequately eject blood. Based on the clinical features, the term left-sided congestive failure was used to denote the presence of dyspnea, orthopnea, and pulmonary rales, whereas right-sided failure was characterized by hepatomegaly, increased systemic venous pressure, and peripheral edema. To explain these manifestations, the concept of forward and backward HF was proposed. The forward failure hypothesis suggested that impaired left ventricular function reduces cardiac output. Blood flow to the kidneys is decreased, resulting in poor urinary output and fluid retention. The fall in systemic blood flow interferes with tissue oxygen supply that causes increased capillary permeability with edema. The backward failure theory proposed that inadequate output by the left ventricle causes accumulation of blood in the pulmonary veins and left atrium, resulting in an increase in pressure, progressing to pulmonary venous congestion and edema. Reduced ejection by the right ventricle explains the increase in systemic venous pressure, with hepatomegaly and pulmonary edema. A marked increase in systemic venous pressure resulting from back-up of blood by reduced right ventricular ejection was difficult to sustain in view of the large capacitance of the systemic venous system. An increase in circulating blood volume was also proposed, but its origin was not apparent. The concept of forward and backward failure has also been discarded because it was appreciated that reduced cardiac output, pulmonary venous congestion and systemic venous congestion and hepatomegaly are frequently concurrent.

It was not until the mid-1950s that it was appreciated that sodium excretion by the kidneys was impaired with HF. Barger et al. (9,10) showed that urinary excretion of an administered load of sodium was markedly delayed in dogs with experimental congestive cardiac failure. Also, Farber and Soberman (11) demonstrated that total body water and sodium were increased in patients with edema and cardiac disease. The importance of and mechanisms responsible for sodium retention in heart disease are discussed below.

Congestive HF in children was described in association with rheumatic fever and rheumatic heart disease in early texts on pediatrics (12). However, in this text, published in 1897, no mention is made of the occurrence of HF in infants and children with congenital heart disease. In 1936, Abbott (13), in the *Atlas of Congenital Cardiac Disease*, mentioned cardiac insufficiency as one of the causes of death, but did not allude to congestive cardiac failure in the clinical features of the various lesions described. Although, during this era, the development of cardiac failure in association with congenital heart disease was beginning to be recognized, the occurrence of congestive failure in infants was rarely appreciated. The vast majority of infants with respiratory distress, who subsequently were found to have cardiac lesions, were first diagnosed by pediatricians as having respiratory infection. In 1957, Nadas described the occurrence of congestive HF in infants with coarctation of the aorta several months after birth, as well as in babies with large ventricular septal defect. Of interest is the fact that he did not acknowledge the occurrence of cardiac failure in infants with patent ductus arteriosus and mentions that congestive failure does not appear in patients with this lesion until the age of 20–30 years (14).

It is difficult to explain why the presence of congestive HF was for so long either not recognized or not acknowledged in infants. A possible reason is that, as mentioned above, HF was equated with myocardial disease and reduced ejection, especially by the left ventricle. The concept was held that, in infants with congenital heart disease, although communications between the chambers, or inflow or outflow obstructions were present, the heart muscle was normal. In fact, it was recognized that rather than having a reduced output, the left ventricle was capable of ejecting volumes three times or more greater than normal in the presence of a large left-to-right shunt. Although it was recognized that the manifestations of pulmonary congestion and edema (left-sided failure) and systemic venous pressure elevation and hepatomegaly (right-sided failure) were similar in adults and children, the definitions of HF used for adults were not applicable.

In 1957 Nadas, in discussing congestive failure, stated that "since, at present, no precise physiological definition is available, it might well be to regard congestive failure simply as a clinical syndrome associated with heart disease" (14). Despite the current recognition that a complex interplay of mechanical factors influencing the heart and neurohormonal mechanisms are responsible for the manifestations, it still seems appropriate to define HF as a clinical syndrome associated with a multitude of cardiac disorders. Recently, there is a trend for adult cardiologists to apply similar definitions. In a review of HF, Jessup and Brozena state "The clinical syndrome of HF is the final pathway for myriad diseases that affect the heart" (15).

HEART FAILURE SYNDROMES

Recognizing that HF is a clinical syndrome, it is not surprising that noncardiac conditions may present with manifestations of cardiac failure. This also explains the fact that pediatricians frequently failed to recognize cardiac disease as the cause of a variety of clinical presentations.

Cardiac Failure in the Fetus

Heart failure presents in the fetus as generalized edema or hydrops fetalis. Hydrops is associated with many disorders not related to circulatory involvement, including erythroblastosis fetalis, hepatic dysfunction, severe anemia, and genetic conditions such as Turner syndrome. Cardiac lesions as the cause of hydrops had been unusual, because immune hydrops associated with Rh blood incompatibility was by far the commonest etiology. Since the incidence of immune hydrops has decreased dramatically in the United States of America, the relative incidence of cardiac causes of hydrops has increased significantly.

Fetal hydrops is unusual with most congenital cardiac anomalies. The cardiovascular disturbances resulting in the development of hydrops include arrhythmias, decreased myocardial function associated with cardiomyopathy, atrioventricular valve insufficiency, obstructed foramen ovale or ductus arteriosus and high cardiac output states such as sacrococcygeal teratoma and twin-to-twin transfusion syndrome.

The underlying mechanism common to all cardiovascular causes of hydrops is elevated venous pressure. Even small increases of venous pressure in the fetus may induce edema because several factors contribute to tissue fluid accumulation. These are presented in Table 1 (16).

The role of neurohormonal factors in cardiac failure in the fetus has not been evaluated. A fall in arterial pressure induces a rise in arginine vasopressin (AVP) and angiotensin II (A II) concentrations. The AVP decreases urinary output. Angiotensin increases fetal body fluid accumulation. It is likely that these hormones do have a role in affecting extracellular fluid volume in the fetus in cardiac failure.

Fluid accumulation in the lungs resulting from pulmonary venous congestion is commonly associated with

Table 1 Factors Contributing to Tissue Fluid Accumulation in the Fetus

Large capillary filtration coefficient–allows water to pass readily
    into tissues from capillaries
High capillary permeability to protein–reduces the concentration
    difference between blood and tissue and reduces fluid movement
    into the capillary
Low plasma colloidal osmotic pressure–reduces fluid movement from
    tissue space to capillary
High compliance of interstitial space–allows accumulation of
    a large amount of fluid in tissues at low pressure

many cardiac lesions, but it is most unusual prenatally. The well-developed smooth muscle layer in the medial layer of pulmonary arterioles restricts blood flow into the lungs and prevents transmission of the high pulmonary arterial pressure to the pulmonary capillaries and veins. In addition, the presence of the foramen ovale limits the rise in left atrial and thus pulmonary venous pressure associated with left-sided obstructive lesions. Furthermore, the hydrostatic pressure difference between the pulmonary capillaries and the alveoli is less in the fetus, because the positive intra-amniotic pressure is transmitted to the alveoli, whereas postnatally alveolar pressure is negative and thus the capillary–alveolar pressure is greater, thus facilitating fluid movement into the alveoli.

Acute Postnatal Cardiac Failure

Acute cardiac failure after birth is a result of inability of the heart to maintain a cardiac output necessary for providing normal oxygen supply to the tissues. The inadequate left ventricular output is associated with elevation of left atrial and pulmonary venous pressure, leading to pulmonary venous congestion and edema. In most circumstances, cardiac output and systemic blood flow are reduced. Occasionally, cardiac output is normal or increased, whereas peripheral flow is reduced, because a large proportion of the cardiac output is diverted away from the tissues. This association has been termed "high output failure" and occurs with large arteriovenous shunts to the great vein of Galen, in the liver, or in other sites. Similarly, a large proportion of the cardiac output may be directed to a vascular tumor, such as sacrococcygeal teratoma.

Inadequate Systemic Oxygen Delivery

This is usually associated with cardiomyopathy or perinatal myocarditis, left ventricular outflow obstruction due to severe aortic stenosis or coarctation, or with atrial or ventricular tachyarrhythmias. The clinical presentation is similar to that of shock, i.e., pallor, cool extremities, weak pulses, and poor perfusion. Metabolic acidemia due to lactic acid accumulation is the result of increased anaerobic glycolysis and PCO_2 is normal or reduced because CO_2 production is inhibited. It may be difficult to differentiate between acute cardiac failure and other causes of shock, such as severe infection.

Reduced oxygen delivery may be associated with several congenital cardiac anomalies in which myocardial function is considered to be normal. Thus, in infants with aortic atresia or interrupted aortic arch, blood flow to the systemic circulation is derived through a patent ductus arteriosus. Constriction of the ductus will limit systemic blood flow and result in a clinical picture of shock, which cannot be designated as cardiac failure.

Pulmonary Edema

Pulmonary edema, manifesting as increased respiratory effort and tachypnea, results from elevated left atrial and pulmonary venous pressure ventricular pressure. Left ventricular failure may be associated with increased pressure loading, as occurs with severe aortic stenosis or aortic coarctation, myocardial dysfunction, or with volume loading, such as with large left-to-right shunts or high cardiac output states. Pulmonary edema may occur with some congenital cardiac lesions in the absence of left ventricular dysfunction, as with total anomalous pulmonary venous connection with obstruction to pulmonary venous drainage and with cor triatriatum.

Neurohormonal Responses

The neuroendocrine responses to reduced cardiac output and elevated ventricular diastolic and left atrial pressure have been studied extensively in chronic cardiac failure, but little information is available in acute failure in infants and children. The reduced cardiac output is likely to influence aortic and carotid mechanoreceptors to induce sympathetico-adrenal activity and increase vasopressin secretion. Decreased arterial pressure probably increases renin/angiotensin/aldosterone activity, and elevated atrial and ventricular pressures induce release of atrial and brain natriuretic peptide (BNP). These responses are discussed below.

Subacute and Chronic Cardiac Failure

This clinical presentation may follow improvement from acute cardiac failure, or may have an insidious onset due to progressive cardiac dysfunction or changes in loading conditions. The clinical features of chronic cardiac failure include diaphoresis, failure to thrive or actual weight loss, tiring during feeding, and increased respiratory rate and effort. Peripheral edema may occur, but is an unusual feature in early infancy and childhood. The development of cardiac failure is influenced by factors other than the cardiac lesion.

Thus, an increase in cardiac output associated with infection, or with the postnatal decrease in hemoglobin concentration may increase demand on the heart and precipitate the onset of failure. Many of the clinical features of cardiac failure could be explained as direct consequences of disturbed cardiac function. Thus, impaired left ventricular function could result in pulmonary venous congestion and respiratory distress and elevated systemic venous pressure could explain hepatic congestion and enlargement, but the mechanisms for tachycardia, diaphoresis and poor weight gain or weight loss were not apparent until relatively recently, when the important role of neurohormonal responses was recognized.

MECHANISMS OF CARDIAC FAILURE

Mechanical Factors

The ability of heart muscle to increase contraction in response to stretching of its fibers was demonstrated in intact heart preparations by Frank in 1895 (17) and by Starling in 1918 (21). They first described the relationship between ventricular diastolic volume and pressure and stroke output. Subsequently, the concept of the ventricular function curve was developed to define cardiac function (19) and the important role of sympathetic nerve stimulation in increasing cardiac contractility was demonstrated by showing an upward shift of the function curve (20).

When myocardial damage or disease occurs and inotropy is impaired, increasing ventricular filling provides only a limited increase in cardiac output and at relatively high end-diastolic pressure, no further increase in output is achieved. The high end-diastolic pressure results in an increase of atrial and venous pressures. An increase in afterload on the normal ventricle reduces stroke volume, but in the presence of myocardial dysfunction, the reduction of stroke volume with elevation of afterload is greatly exaggerated (21).

In congenital cardiac lesions with left-to-right shunts, an excessive volume load is placed on the ventricle. Depending on the lesion, the output of the left or right or both ventricles is increased. To achieve this increased output, ventricular end-diastolic volume and pressure are increased, based on the Frank–Starling mechanism. Although myocardial performance may be normal, the elevated diastolic pressure may result in pulmonary or systemic venous congestion and may induce neurohormonal responses (see below).

Lesions that obstruct ventricular outflow impose a pressure load on the ventricle. The increased afterload produced by the obstruction reduces ventricular stroke volume. In an attempt to maintain systemic blood flow, based on the Frank–Starling mechanism, ventricular end-diastolic pressure is raised to increase stroke volume.

Although not as common in infants and children as in adults, diastolic filling of the ventricle may be impaired. This altered lusitropy may result from myocardial fibrosis or marked hypertrophy, and from restraint on the ventricle from external factors. Systolic function may be normal, but interference with filling of the ventricle restricts stroke volume. Ventricular diastolic volume enhancement is achieved only by very large increases in diastolic pressure, resulting in atrial distension and venous congestion.

Circulatory Changes at Birth Influencing the Onset of Failure

Many congenital heart lesions do not significantly affect circulatory function during fetal life, but are associated with cardiac failure after birth. The development of failure has generally been explained by alteration in flow patterns, but other postnatal circulatory and metabolic changes may contribute. Fetal and neonatal myocardium develops less tension than adult myocardium with stretch (22) and the relative increase of stroke volume with elevation of ventricular diastolic pressure is less than in the adult heart (23). The stroke volume of the left ventricle is smaller than that of the right ventricle during fetal life, but after birth, associated with the dramatic rise in pulmonary blood flow, left ventricular output increases (24). In the fetus, the afterload on the ventricles is relatively low, because the placental circulation, which has a low vascular resistance, accommodating about 40% of the combined ventricular output, is derived from the aorta via the umbilical arteries. Removal of the placental circulation results in a marked increase in afterload on the left ventricle, particularly after the ductus arteriosus closes. The fetal and neonatal ventricle is very sensitive to the increasing afterload as shown by the marked fall in stroke volume with increases of arterial pressure at the same end-diastolic filling pressure (25,26). This prominent effect of restriction of left ventricular output with increasing afterload is a striking feature of cardiac failure in the adult (21).

In addition to these changes after birth, additional factors may increase demands on the circulation. Oxygen consumption increases after birth in association with the increased metabolism required to maintain body temperature. This stimulates an increase in cardiac output. The presence of a large percentage of fetal hemoglobin in the neonate also tends to maintain cardiac output at high levels, because oxygen extraction from blood in the tissues is limited by the low P_{50} of fetal blood (27).

The possibility that disturbances in myocardial metabolism during the perinatal period may contribute to the development or acceleration of HF should also be considered. During fetal life, glucose is the primary substrate for the myocardium (28) and unlike in the adult, free fatty acids are poorly utilized.

The heart has a high glycogen content at the time of birth, which can provide the substrate for energy if glucose supply is limited (29). However, glycogen is rapidly depleted with stress or hypoxia and energy supply may be limited in the face of increased demand and result in myocardial dysfunction.

The considerable rise in stroke volume and increase in afterload result in a significant increase in the demand on the left ventricle in the normal infant and thus development of failure is likely with additional volume or pressure loading. As mentioned above, unlike in the adult, significant peripheral edema is unusual in infants with HF. The clinical features are predominantly those of left-sided congestion. This difference in presentation can be explained by the relative differences in liver size. In the adult, liver weight averages 1200–1500 g, about 2% of body weight, whereas in the newborn infant, the liver weighs 140–150 g, constituting about 5% of body weight. In the infant, the compliant liver can accommodate a considerably larger proportion of blood volume in the systemic venous reservoir and the venous pressure is thus elevated to a lesser degree than in the adult.

Neurohormonal Responses

Sympathetico-adrenal Responses

The presence of tachycardia, diaphoresis, and peripheral vasoconstriction have suggested that sympathetic nervous

activity is increased in individuals with cardiac failure. This
was proposed by Starling in 1897 (30), and in the early
1960s, it was demonstrated that plasma norepinephrine
levels were increased in adults with HF (31). The concept
was held that the increased sympathetic nervous and norepinephrine response was primarily a compensatory attempt to
increase myocardial contractility. In 1965, the failure to
thrive in some infants with congenital cardiac disease was
ascribed to hypermetabolism (32), suggesting there was
increased sympathetic activity. This was subsequently confirmed by finding increased urinary excretion of products of
catecholamine metabolism in infants with HF (33), as well
as increased plasma levels of norepinephrine (34). The
mechanisms responsible for the increased sympathetic activity have not yet been fully resolved. It was first explained
on the basis of a decrease in cardiac output with a fall in
arterial pressure and pulse pressure that modifies aortic
and carotid baroreceptor discharge and results in reflex
sympathetic stimulation. In patients with cardiac muscle dysfunction or severe ventricular outflow obstruction, the
reduced systemic blood flow could stimulate sympathetic
activity by modifying peripheral baroreceptor activity. However, in many patients with congenital heart lesions with
large left-to-right shunts, there does not appear to be a
decrease in cardiac output or in arterial pressure. Recently,
studies in adults have shown that the cardiac sympathetic
activity may increase before there is any evidence of generalized stimulation of the sympathetic nervous system (35). An
extensive sympathetic nervous network is demonstrable in
heart muscle in the adult, both in the atria and the ventricles,
and norepinephrine is present in high concentrations. Large
amounts of norepinephrine are produced by cardiac muscle;
some of the hormones are liberated into the general circulation (36). The concept is now proposed that distension of the
ventricle, particularly the left ventricle, induces increased
local sympathetic activity and norepinephrine release and
possibly also generalized sympathetic stimulation.

The role of sympathetico-adrenal stimulation in cardiac
failure during the fetal and neonatal period has not been

defined. Studies in fetal sheep have shown that the arterial baroreceptor function increases over gestation, but is well developed at birth (37). However, the responses may be blunted in preterm infants. The degree of sympathetic innervation and the concentration of norepinephrine in the myocardium also increase progressively during fetal development (38). The maturation of the process at the time of birth varies greatly in different species (39), but appears to parallel the state of development of the central nervous system. It is not known what the state of maturation of sympathetic innervation of the human heart is at birth, but it can be assumed that it is less prominent in the adult. It is thus quite likely that in the newborn, and certainly in the premature infant, the heart is not capable of mounting the same magnitude of compensatory response as in the adult.

The general sympathetic stimulation causes peripheral vasoconstriction and diaphoresis, increases metabolism, affects renal function, and activates the renin–angiotensin system, resulting in sodium retention and increased extracellular fluid volume. This compensatory mechanism, in the short term, improves myocardial contractility, but this effect may be lessened by subsequent changes in the cardiac muscle. Studies of cardiac muscle obtained from adult hearts during cardiac transplant procedures showed that the failing hearts had about 50% reduction in beta-adrenergic receptor activity, 50% reduction in adenylate cyclase stimulation by isoproterenol and about 50% decrease in contractility as compared with normal cardiac muscle (40). This downregulation of beta-adrenergic receptor activity has been explained by the continued stimulation of the sympathetic nerve endings and the high circulating plasma norepinephrine concentrations. Cardiac muscle concentrations of norepinephrine are, however, reduced in failing hearts. It was generally believed that the beta-adrenergic blockers were contraindicated in HF patients, because they could interfere with contractility, but these studies prompted trial of beta-adrenergic blockers in adults with chronic cardiac failure. They have consistently shown that chronic administration of the beta-adrenergic blockers bisoprolol, metoprolol, or carvedilol did not depress

myocardial performance but greatly improved symptomatology, decreased incidence of hospitalization, and prolonged
survival (41). The experience with use of beta-blockers in
infants and children is limited.

In a group of eight infants with cardiac failure associated
with congenital heard disease, propranolol administration
reduced plasma norepinephrine concentrations and reduced
left atrial pressure with no depression of ventricular function
(42). Also, chronic administration of carvedilol to children
awaiting cardiac transplant resulted in such symptomatic
improvement in some that they could be removed from the
waiting list (43).

This experience with beta-adrenergic blockers in adults
and limited observations in infants raises important questions regarding the indications for their use in pediatric
patients. During acute cardiac failure beta-blockers are
almost certainly contraindicated, because the sympathetic
nervous and norepinephrine responses represent the acute
adaptation to reduced cardiac output. The time course over
which downregulation of beta-blockers occurs in infants
is, however, not known; it is thus necessary to evaluate
when, after the onset of cardiac failure, beta-blockers may
be indicated.

Beta-adrenergic receptor numbers increase in fetal
myocardium with advancing gestation, but the development
of receptors may be affected by several factors. Thus, removal
of thyroid hormone activity by thyroidectomy in fetal lambs
markedly reduces beta-receptors in myocardium and
decreases the heart rate and left ventricular output response
to isoproterenol after birth (44). Prenatal hypoxia increases
beta-receptor responsiveness postnatally in the rat (45). The
development of myocardial beta-adrenergic receptors in the
presence of cardiac defects in fetal life has not been examined.
Whether they are downregulated in response to increased
pressure or volume loading on either ventricle, or whether
beta-receptors are increased in response to general circulatory stress is still to be resolved, but this could be important
in influencing the development of HF after birth and the
approach to therapy.

In addition to the enhanced myocardial inotropy and effects on metabolism, it has now been recognized that sympathetic stimulation has an important role in the remodeling of the heart following damage and associated with cardiac failure (46). Transgenic overexpression of beta-adrenergic receptors increases myocardial contractility, but also results in progressive loss of myocytes and subsequent fibrosis (47). Increased expression of alpha-adrenergic receptors results in hypertrophy of myocytes and with greater alpha-receptor activity, apoptosis. The long-term administration of beta-adrenergic blockers may inhibit some of these progressive deleterious effects of norepinephrine on the myocardium and may account for the increased survival.

Renin–Angiotensin–Aldosterone System

Renin release from the juxtaglomerular cells in the macula densa in the renal cortex is induced by several stimuli, including decreased pressure in renal arteries, sympathetic nervous stimulation to the kidneys and reduced osmolarity of plasma perfusing the kidney. Renin is an enzyme that acts on angiotensinogen, an alpha$_2$-globulin synthesized in the liver, to produce angiotensin I (AI), a decapeptide. Angiotensin I is cleaved by angiotensin-converting enzyme (ACE) to angiotensin II (AII), an octapeptide. An ACE is present in the vascular system in many organs, but especially in the lung. An important effect of A II is to stimulate receptors in the adrenal cortex to release of aldosterone. Several A II receptors have been identified, but stimulation of A I receptors is responsible for a potent peripheral vasoconstrictor effect and also for the release of aldosterone. Aldosterone increases active reabsorption of sodium in the distal convoluted tubules of the kidney. This system is stimulated to attempt to compensate for the reduced cardiac output and reduced arterial pressure by producing peripheral vasoconstriction and by retaining sodium to increase plasma volume. The activation of this system in patients with cardiac failure has been described in adults (48,49), as well as in infants (50).

The observations indicating that cardiac output is extremely sensitive to the increased afterload in patients with cardiac failure, and that afterload is often markedly increased as a result of the increased sympathetic activity and the effect of A II, introduced the concept that the reducing afterload could decrease loading on the ventricle and possibly improve output. Several vasodilators have been used, but inhibition of production of A II by administering inhibitors of ACE has been favored in recent years. Several studies in adults, using captopril or enalapril, in addition to digitalis and diuretic therapy, have shown symptomatic improvement and prolongation of survival (51,52). The ACE inhibitors have also been administered to infants and children with cardiac failure with beneficial effect (53,54).

Although the reduction of afterload may be responsible for the effects of ACE inhibitors, it is now evident that they may influence the effect of A II on cardiac muscle. A II, which is produced locally in cardiac myocytes in response to stretch, has been shown to induce hypertrophy of myocytes, unrelated to any general hemodynamic effect, as well as apoptosis (55,56). A II directly stimulates fibroblasts and also increases fibrosis in cardiac muscle (57). Restriction of A II production by use of ACE inhibitors, or blockade of A I receptors with losartan limits the development of cardiac hypertrophy, as well as apoptosis and fibrosis.

Furthermore, inhibition of A II effects may not only limit myocardial damage, but may reverse it by inducing regression of fibrosis (58).

Plasma aldosterone concentrations are frequently markedly elevated in patients with cardiac failure. In addition to promoting sodium retention, aldosterone also facilitates potassium excretion. Spironolactone, an aldosterone receptor blocker, has been used as a mild diuretic agent, usually in conjunction with other diuretics, to attempt to limit potassium loss in urine. Recently, however, it has become apparent that, like A II, aldosterone is synthesized in vascular cells and may affect endothelial function, but also induces myocardial fibrosis (59). Administration of spironolactone to hypertensive rats prevents the development of myocardial fibrosis (60).

Inhibition of aldactone effects with spironolactone greatly improved exercise tolerance and ventricular function in adults with severe HF and reduced mortality by 30% (61). Many of these patients were already being treated with ACE inhibitors and it could have been anticipated that, by lowering A II concentrations, aldosterone secretion was reduced. However, after long-term ACE inhibitor treatment, A II and especially aldosterone concentration are elevated. The spironolactone effect appears to be related to the inhibition of the direct effect of aldosterone on myocardium. Recently, eplerenone, a selective aldosterone blocker, has improved ventricular function and reduced mortality following myocardial infarction (62). Eplerenone avoids some of the adverse side effects of spironolactone, because it does not block glucocorticoid and sex hormone receptors.

Although, as mentioned above, ACE inhibitors and spironolactone have been used with benefit in infants and children with HF, it is not known whether they affect ventricular remodeling. Ventricular dysfunction, apparently related to myocardial damage with fibrosis, is not an uncommon development in patients with some types of congenital heart disease, such as various types of single ventricle. It is interesting to speculate whether prolonged treatment with ACE inhibitors or A II receptor blockers, and aldosterone receptor blockers should be considered for prevention of the myocardial deterioration.

Vasopressin

Plasma AVP concentrations are often increased in adults (63), as well as in infants and children with cardiac failure (64). The AVP release into blood is largely regulated by changes in osmolarity of plasma perfusing the brain. It is also released in response to decrease in arterial pressure through baroreceptor mechanisms. Through its action via the V2 receptor in the kidney, it inhibits clearance of free water and thus may contribute to the hyponatremia that is sometimes noted in adults with severe chronic cardiac failure. The AVP antagonists that affect the V2 receptor have been used in adults and have increased plasma sodium concentrations to normal and resulted in clinical improvement (65); there is no report of their use in infants or children. Through the V1 receptors in blood vessels, constriction is induced and thus may contribute to the increased afterload in patients with cardiac failure.

Natriuretic Peptides

Cardiac natriuretic peptides are a group of compounds that are synthesized and stored in myocardium. Atrial natriuretic peptide (ANP) is released from the atrial wall, whereas BNP is stored in the ventricles. Plasma concentrations of ANP, BNP, and clearance natriuretic peptide (CNP) are increased in response to stretch of the atria and ventricles, and have been noted in adults with left ventricular dysfunction (66), as well as in children with HF (67). Unlike the vasoconstrictor hormones described above, these peptides can be considered to be counterregulatory, because they produce peripheral arterial and venous vasodilatation, promote natriuresis and diuresis, and inhibit the renin–angiotensin system. It is difficult to explain why the cardiac failure response should include both the so-called compensatory stimulation of the sympathetico-adrenal and renin–angiotensin–aldosterone systems, and the counterregulatory natriuretic peptide response. The possibility that these peptides could be beneficial in treatment of cardiac failure has been proposed. A recombinant preparation of BNP, nesiritide, has been administered intravenously to adults with severe cardiac failure and poor response to inotropic agents, diuretics, and vasodilators. It has had some beneficial clinical effect and improved hemodynamic parameters, but has not, as yet, appeared to alter mortality (68,69). Nesiritide has not, as yet, to my knowledge, been used in infants or children with acute cardiac failure, but as BNP blood levels are increased in children with HF, it is possible that it may be a useful therapeutic agent.

Other Circulating Factors

A number of other agents such endothelins, prostaglandins and vasointestinal peptide, as will as cytokines, are thought to have a role in the pathophysiology of HF. These are not discussed in this review.

TREATMENT

Digitalis in Adults

Detailed discussions on treatment of cardiac failure are presented in ensuing chapters. In this perspective, I review only the use of digitalis preparations, because the concepts regarding their use have undergone striking changes over the years. Digitalis, administered as foxglove, was first used by Withering (70) in the late 18th century, as treatment for edema in individuals with irregular heart rates; he ascribed its benefit to a diuretic action. It was not until about a century later that digitalis was thought to improve cardiac contraction (71). Various digitalis preparations were subsequently widely used in adults for treatment of cardiac failure.

Digitalis increases myocardial contractility by binding to $Na+$, $K+$, and ATPase in the cell membrane to inhibit the sodium pump, thus increasing intracellular sodium and subsequently, calcium concentration (72). Other effects of digitalis are important in its effect in HF. It has a direct effect on renal tubules to decrease sodium reabsorption and thus increases sodium excretion (73). It also has autonomic nervous system effects, inhibiting sympathetic discharge (74) and decreasing plasma norepinephrine concentrations and renin–angiotensin activity.

After the effect of the drug in modifying arrhythmias became apparent, questions were raised about the effectiveness of digitalis in patients with HF and regular cardiac rhythm. Also, recognition of the importance of the neurohormonal responses prompted the introduction of the newer therapies of vasodilators, beta-adrenergic receptor blockers, and ACE inhibitors. The value of digitalis in addition to these measures in adults with cardiac failure became controversial. During the last decade, several studies have shown that digitalis has a beneficial effect in adults with left ventricular failure. Withdrawal of digoxin therapy from patients receiving both ACE inhibitors and digoxin resulted in clinical deterioration (75), as well as in patients with mild to moderate congestive cardiac failure (76). However, digoxin did not significantly affect mortality (77).

The dose of digoxin recommended for treatment of cardiac failure in adults has been modified recently. It was frequently stated that the correct dose of drug was that which produced clinical improvement without causing toxicity. With the advent of the ability to measure serum digoxin concentrations, it was observed that most patients manifesting clinical response had concentrations of 0.8–2.0 ng/mL. It was therefore tacitly assumed that this was the optimal digoxin level to achieve. Most patients who developed toxicity had digoxin plasma concentrations above 2.0 ng/mL, although toxicity did occur in some with lower levels. Recently the use of higher doses of digoxin for treatment of cardiac failure has been questioned. When serum concentrations exceed 1.0 ng/mL, there is evidence of some improvement of ventricular function, but not in hemodynamic parameters or clinical manifestations (78,79). Furthermore, in a recent study, the mortality was significantly increased with digoxin concentrations above 1.2 ng/mL, and the authors recommend that the optimal dose of digoxin is that which achieves a serum concentration of 0.5–0.8 ng/mL (80).

Digitalis in Infants and Children

Few reports on the use of digitalis in infants and children are available prior to the early 1920s, when McCullough and Rupe (81) suggested that the dose of digitalis required for children was 1.5–2.0 times greater than in adults based on body weight. This was corroborated in a study in which digitoxin was administered and it was stated that "the younger the child, the more digitalis per pound or per square meter of surface area is required, irrespective of the disease causing the congestive HF" (82). In this study, digitalis was most effective in patients with myocardial diseases and was thought to be good in about 10% and fair in about 30% of patients with congenital heart lesions. Despite these relatively poor results, digitalis was routinely administered to all infants and children with congestive HF and Nadas (14) in 1957 stated "As a matter of principle, every child with obvious evidence of HF should be digitalized." The digitalizing dose of digoxin recommended for children was extraordinarily high as compared with adults—80–125 µg/kg body weight for children under 2 years of age and 40–85 µg/kg for older children. The recommendation for this dosage was derived from the concept that "the digitalization of every patient should be an individual experiment" and digitalis dosage was increased until there was clinical improvement or evidence of toxicity. The difference in estimated dosage for infants and adults could relate to the toxic manifestations. In a study in fetal and adult sheep, the adult animals frequently developed arrhythmias at mean plasma digoxin concentrations of 2.3 ng/mL, whereas the fetal lambs rarely developed arrhythmia at mean concentrations of 4.5 ng/mL. Although atrioventricular conduction was prolonged in both fetal and adult animals in relation to the increase in digoxin concentration, it was the onset of arrhythmia that prompted cessation of digoxin administration (83).

The high doses of digoxin were found to cause toxicity frequently in premature infants and lower dosages were recommended (84). Also, doubts were expressed regarding the efficacy of digoxin in improving clinical status in premature infants with patent ductus arteriosus. Arrhythmias were unusual in premature infants receiving digoxin, but heart block was the usual manifestation of toxicity. As in the fetal lambs, serum digoxin concentrations of greater than 3–4 ng/mL could be tolerated, but risks of heart block were considerable. This risk, together with the questionable effect in relieving symptoms, prompted several centers to avoid the use of digitalis in treatment of premature infants with patent ductus arteriosus.

The effectiveness of digoxin in treating HF in mature infants has been examined, with conflicting results. In two studies of infants cardiac failure associated with ventricular septal defect, ventricular function was assessed by ultrasound. Berman et al. (85) noted that ventricular function improved in only six, but clinical improvement was noted in

12 of 21 infants. Kimball et al. (86) found digoxin-enhanced ventricular function in all, but provided clinical benefit in none of 19 infants.

The doses of digoxin currently recommended are considerably lower than those used previously; generally, the digitalizing dose for premature infants is 25 μg/kg, for mature infants to about 2 years it is 50 μg/kg, and for older children 25 μg/kg.

Although digoxin is widely used in treatment of congestive HF in pediatric patients, there is no reliable information documenting its efficacy, nor is there any information regarding optimal serum concentrations of digoxin. There is a crucial need to study these issues.

FUTURE DIRECTIONS

Concepts regarding the mechanisms involved in cardiac failure have changed dramatically in recent years. There is great need to evaluate the use of therapy directed to the various neurohormonal disturbances, such as use of beta-adrenergic receptor blockers, ACE inhibitors, angiotensin receptor blockers, and aldosterone receptor blockers, in infants and children.

Although it has been generally assumed that cardiac muscle development and function are normal in the presence of congenital cardiac lesions, there is increasing evidence that myocardial development may be modified. It is thus important to understand the mechanisms involved in normal myocardial development during fetal and postnatal life and to assess the effects of various congenital cardiac lesions and myocardial diseases. Normal increase in heart weight is produced by hyperplasia prenatally, but almost exclusively by hypertrophy postnatally (87). Abnormal increase in cardiac muscle, as occurs with pulmonary stenosis, also results from increase in cell numbers prenatally, but coronary vascular development may not match myocyte growth (88). It is also important to determine whether factors that influence the myocardium postnatally have similar effects prenatally. Although angiotensin induces hypertrophy, apoptosis, and myocardial fibrosis postnatally, it appears to have different effects in the fetus.

Infusion of A II into fetal lambs did not affect myocytes (unpublished personal observations). Furthermore, angiotensin receptor blockade does not influence the increase in right ventricular muscle mass with experimental pulmonary stenosis (89). It is apparent that the neurohormonal factors may have different effects at different stages of development. These differences need to be resolved to effectively manage cardiac failure.

Loss of myocytes is common in adults in association with myocardial infarct, and as a result of hormonal activity with cardiac failure. Although cardiac regeneration can occur in zebrafish (90), only limited new myocytes can be generated in the adult human. The possibility that damaged heart muscle can be replaced by myocytes generated from embryonic stem cells is being seriously considered (91). Determining the factors that induce the change in growth of cardiac muscle by means of hyperplasia prenatally to hypertophy postanatally could provide a mechanism for replacement of damaged myocytes and grow new cardiac muscle at all ages.

REFERENCES

1. Braunwald E. Shattuck lecture—cardiovascular medicine at the turn of the millennium: triumphs, concerns and opportunities. N Engl J Med 1997; 337:1360–1369.
2. Redfield MM. Heart failure—an epidemic of uncertain proportions. N Engl J Med 2002; 347:1442–1444.
3. Senni M, Tribouilloy CM, Rodeheffer RJ, Jacobsen SJ, Evans JM, Bailey KR, Redfield MM. Congestive heart failure in the community: trends in incidence and survival in a 10-year period. Arch Intern Med 1999; 159:29–34.
4. MacKenzie J. Diseases of the Heart. London: Oxford Medical Publications, 1913.
5. Lewis T. Diseases of the Heart Described for Practitioners and Students. 2nd ed. New York: MacMillan Co., 1937.
6. Francis GS, Gessler JP, Sonnenblick EH. In: Funster V, Alexander RW, O'Rourke RA, Wellens HJ, eds. Hurst's the Heart. 10th ed. New York: McGraw-Hill, 2000.
7. LeJemtel TH, Sonnenblick EH, Frishman WH. Diagnosis and management of heart failure. In: O'Rourke RA, Funster V, Alexander RW, Roberts R, King SB III, Wellens HJJ, eds. Hurst's the Heart— Manual of Cardiology. New York: McGraw-Hill, 2001.

8. Braunwald E. In: Braunwald E, Fauci AS, Kasper DL, Hauser SL, Longo DL, Jameson JL, eds. Harrison's Principle of Internal Medicine. New York: McGraw-Hill, 2001.

9. Barger AC, Ross RS, Price HL. Reduced sodium excretion in dogs with mild valvular lesions of the heart, and in dogs with congestive failure. Am J Physiol 1955; 180:249.

10. Barger AC, Yates FE, Rudolph AM. Renal hemodynamics and sodium excretion in dogs with graded valvular damage, and in congestive failure. Am J Physiol 1961; 200:601–608.

11. Farber SJ, Soberman RJ. Total body water and total exchangeable sodium in edematous states due to cardiac, renal or hepatic disease. Clin Invest 1956; 35:779.

12. Holt LE. The Diseases of Infancy and Childhood. New York: Appleton and Co, 1897.

13. Abbott ME. Atlas of Congenital Cardiac Disease. New York: The American Heart Association, 1936.

14. Nadas AS. Pediatric Cardiology. Philadelphia: WB Saunders Co., 1957.

15. Jessup M, Brozena S. Heart failure. N Engl J Med 2003; 348:2007–2018.

16. Rudolph AM. Congenital Diseases of the Heart. 2nd ed. Armonk: Futura Publishing, 2001.

17. Frank O. Zur Dynamik des Herzmuskels. Z Biol 1895; 27:370–447.

18. Starling EH. The Lineacre Lecture on the Law of the Heart. Delivered at Cambridge. London: Longmans, Green, 1918.

19. Sarnoff SJ, Berglund E. Ventricular function: I. Starling's law of the heart studied by means of simultaneous right and left ventricular function curves in the dog. Circulation 1954; 9:706.

20. Sarnoff SJ, Brockman SK, Giimore JP, Linden RJ, Mitchell JH. Regulation of ventricular contraction: influence of cardiac sympathetic and vagal nerve stimulation on atrial and ventricular dynamics. Circ Res 1960; 8:1108.

21. Ross J Jr. Afterload mismatch and preload reserve: a conceptual framework for the analysis of ventricular function. Prog Cardiovasc Dis 1976; 18:255–264.

22. Friedman WF. The intrinsic properties of the developing heart. In: Sonnenblick E, Leschi M, Friedman WF, eds. Neonatal Heart Disease. New York: Grune and Stratton, 1973:21–50.

23. Klopfenstein HS, Rudolph AM. Postnatal changes in the circulation and responses to volume loading in sheep. Circ Res 1978; 42:839–845.

24. Teitel DF, Iwamoto HS, Rudolph AM. Effects of birth-related events on central blood flow patterns. Pediatr Res 1987; 22:557–566.

25. Hawkins J, Van Hare GF, Schmidt KG, Rudolph AM. Effects of increasing afterload on left ventricular output in fetal lambs. Circ Res 1989; 65:127–134.

26. Van Hare GF, Hawkins JA, Schmidt KG, Rudolph AM. The effects of increasing mean arterial pressure on left ventricular output in newborn lambs. Circ Res 1990; 67:78–83.

27. Lister G, Walter TK, Versmold HT, Dallman PR, Rudolph AM. Oxygen delivery in lambs: cardiovascular and hematologic development. Am J Physiol 1979; 237:H668–H675.

28. Fisher DJ, Rudolph AM, Heymann MA. Myocardial oxygen and carbohydrate consumption in fetal lambs in utero and in adult sheep. Am J Physiol 1980; 238:H399–H405.

29. Shelley HJ. Glycogen reserves and their changes at birth. Brit M Bull 1961; 17:137–143.

30. Starling EH. Points on pathology of heart disease. Lancet 1897; 1: 569–572.

31. Chidsey CA, Harrison DC, Braunwald E. Augmentation of the plasma norepinephrine response to exercise in patients with congestive heart failure. N Engl J Med 1962; 267:650–654.

32. Lees MH, Bristow JD, Griswold HE, et al. Relative hypermetabolism in infants with congenital heart disease and undernutrition. Pediatrics 1965; 36:183..

33. Lees MH. Catecholamine metabolite excretion of infants with heart failure. J Pediatr 1966; 69:259–265.

34. Ross RD, Daniels SR, Schwartz DC, Harrison DW, Skulka R, Kaplan S. Plasma norepinephrine levels in infants and children with congestive heart failure. Am J Cardiol 1987; 59:911–914.

35. Rundqvist B, Elam M, Bergmann-Sverrisodottir Y, et al. Increased cardiac adrenergic drive precedes generalized sympathetic activation in human heart failure. Circulation 1997; 95:169–175.

36. Hasking GJ, Esler MD, Jennings GL, Burton D, Johns JA, Korner PI. Norepinephrine spillover to plasma in patients with congestive heart failure: evidence of increased overall and cardiorenal sympathetic nervous activity. Circulation 1986; 73:615–621.

37. Shinebourne EA, Vapaavuori EK, Williams RL, Heymann MA, Rudolph AM. Development of baroreflex activity in unanesthetized fetal and neonatal lambs. Circ Res 1972; 31:710–718.

38. Lebowitz EA, Novick JS, Rudolph AM. Development of myocardial sympathetic innervation in the fetal lamb. Pediatr Res 1972; 6: 887–893.

39. Lipp JM, Rudolph AM. Sympathetic nerve development in the rat and guinea pig heart. Biol Neonate 1972; 21:76–82.

40. Bristow MR, Ginsburg R, Minobe W, Cubicciotti RS, Sageman WS, Lurie K, Billingham ME, Harrison DC, Stinson EB. Decreased catecholamine sensitivity and beta-adrenergic-receptor density in failing human hearts. N Eng J Med 1982; 307:205–211.

41. Foody MA, Farrell MH, Krumholz HM. Bete-blocker therapy in heart failure: scientific review. JAMA 2002; 287:883–889.

42. Buchhorn R, Hulpke-Wette M, Ruschewski W, Ross RD, Fielitz J, Pregla R, Hetzer R, Regitz-Zagrosek V. Effects of therapeutic beta blockade on myocardial function and cardiac remodelling in congenital cardiac disease. Cardiol Young 2003; 13:36–43.
43. Azeka E, Franchini Ramires JA, Valler C, Alcides Bocchi E. Delisting of infants and children from the heart transplantation waiting list after carvedilol treatment. J Am Coll Cardiol 2002; 40:2034–2038.
44. Birk E, Tyndall MR, Erickson LC, Rudolph AM, Roberts JM. Effects of thyroid hormone on myocardial adrenergic preceptor responsiveness and function during late gestation. Pediatr Res 1992; 31:468–173.
45. Roigas J, Roigas C, Heydeck D, Papies B. Prenatal hypoxia alters the postnatal development of beta-adrenoceptors in the rat myocardium. Biol Neonate 1996; 69:383–388.
46. Hunter JJ, Chien KR. Signaling pathways for cardiac hypertrophy and failure. N Engl J Med 1999; 341:1276–1283.
47. Dorn GW II. Adrenergic pathways and left ventricular remodeling. Card Fail 2002; 8(6 suppl):S370–S373.
48. Brown JJ, Davies DL, Johnson VW, Lever AF, Robertson JL. Renin relationships in congestive heart failure, treated and untreated. Am Heart J 1970; 80:329–342.
49. Dzau VJ, Colucci WS, Hollenberg NK, Williams GH. Relation of the renin–angiotensin–aidosterone system to clinical state in congestive heart failure. Circulation 1981; 63:645–651.
50. Baylen BG, Johnson G, Tsang R, Srivastava L, Kaplan S. The occurrence of hyperaldosteronism in infants with congestive heart failure. Am J Cardiol 1980; 45:305–310.
51. The Captopril Multicenter Research Group. A placebo-controlled trial of captopril in refractory chronic congestive heart failure. J Am Coll Cardiol 1983; 2:755–763.
52. The CONSENSUS Trial Group. Effects of enalapril on mortality in severe congestive failure: results of the cooperative North Scandinavian enalapril study group (CONSENSUS). N Eng J Med 1987; 316: 1429–1435.
53. Friedman WF, George BL. Medical progress—treatment of congestive heart failure by altering loading conditions of the heart. J Pediatr 1985; 106:697–706.
54. Artman M, Graham TP. Guidelines for vasodilator therapy of congestive heart failure in infants and children. Am Heart J 1987; 113: 994–1005.
55. Weber KT, Brilla CG, Campbell SE, Guarda E, Zhou G, Sriram KR. Myocardial fibrosis: role of angiotensin II and aldosterone. Basic Res Cardiol 1993; 88(suppl 1):107–124.
56. Yamazaki T, Shiojima I, Komuro I, Nagai R, Yazaki Y. Involvement of the renin–angiotensin system in the development of left ventricular hypertrophy and dysfunction. J Hypertens (suppl) 1984: 12: S153–S157.

57. Weber KT, Brilla CG. Pathological hypertrophy and cardiac interstitium: fibrosis and renin–angiotensin–aldosterone system. Circulation 1991; 83:1849–1865.
58. Brilla CG, Matsubara L, Weber KT. Advanced hypertensive heart disease in spontaneously hypertensive rats. Lisinopril-mediated regression of myocardial fibrosis. Hypertension 1996; 28:269–275.
59. Burlew BS, Weber KT. Cardiac fibrosis as a cause of diastolic dysfunction. Herz 2002; 27:92–98.
60. Brilla CG, Matsubara LS, Weber KT. Antifibrotic effects of spironolactone in preventing myocardial fibrosis in systemic arterial hypertension. Am J Cardiol 1993; 71:12A–16A.
61. Pitt B, Zannad F, Remme WJ, Cody R, Castaigne A, Perez A, Palensky J, Wittes J. The effect of spironolactone on morbidity and mortality in patients with severe heart failure. Randomized aldactone evaluation study investigators. N Engl J Med 1999; 341:709–717.
62. Pitt B, Remme W, Zannad F, Neaton J, Martinez F, Roniker B, Bittman R, Hurley S, Kleiman J, Gatlin M. Eplerenone post-acute myocardial infarction heart failure efficacy and survival study investigators. Eplerenone, a selective aldosterone blocker, in patients with left ventricular dysfunction after myocardial infarction. N Engl J Med 2003; 348:1309–1323.
63. Goldsmith SR, Francis GS, Cowley AW Jr, Levine TB, Cohn JN. Increased plasma arginine vasopressin levels in patients with congestive heart failure. J Am Coll Cardiol 1983; 1:1385–1390.
64. Stewart JM, Zeballos GA, Woolf PK, Dweck HS, Gewitz MH. Variable arginine vasopressin levels in neonatal congestive heart failure. J Am Coll Cardiol 1988; 11:645–650.
65. Gheorghiade M, Niazi I, Ouyang J, Czerwiec F, Kambayashi J, Zampino M, Orlandi C. Vasopressin v2-receptor blockade with tolvaptan in patients with chronic heart failure: results from a double-blind, randomized trial. Circulation 2003; 107:2690–2696.
66. Stoupakis G, Klapholz M. Natriuretic peptides: biochemistry, physiology, and therapeutic role in heart failure. Heart Dis 2003; 5:215–223.
67. Kikuchi K, Nishioka K, Ueda T, Shiomi M, Takahashi Y, Sugawara A, Nakao K, Imura H, Mori C, Mikawa H. Relationship between plasma atrial natriuretic polypeptide concentration and hemodynamic measurements in children with congenital heart diseases. J Pediatr 1987; 111:335–342.
68. Vichiendilokkul A, Tran A, Racine E. Nesiritide: a novel approach for acute heart failure. Ann Pharmacother 2003; 37:247–258.
69. Keating GM, Goa KL. Nesiritide: a review of its use in acute decompensated heart failure. Drugs 2003; 63:47–70.
70. Withering W. An Account of the Foxglove, and Some of Its Medical Uses: With Practical Remarks on Dropsy and Other Diseases. London: G.G.J. and J. Robinson, 1785.
71. Fothergill JM. Digitalis: Its Mode of Action. London, 1871.

72. Akera T, Brody TM. The role of Na+, K+, and ATPase in the inotropic action of digitalis. Pharmacol Rev 1977; 29:187–220.
73. Rudolph AM, Rokaw SN, Barger AC. Chronic catheterization of the renal artery: technic for studying direct effects of substances on kidney function. Proc Soc Exp Biol Med 1956; 93:323–326.
74. Ferguson DW, Berg WJ, Sanders JS, Roach PJ, Kempf JS, Kienzle MG. Sympathoinhibitory responses to digitalis glycosides in heart failure patients. Direct evidence from sympathetic neural recordings. Circulation 1989; 80:65–77.
75. Packer M, Gheorghiade M, Young JB, et al. Withdrawal of digoxin from patients with chronic heart failure treated with angiotensin-converting-enzyme inhibitors: radiance study. N Engl J Med 1993; 329:1–7.
76. Uretsky BF, Young JB, Shahidi FE, Yellen LG, Harrison MC, Jolly MK. Randomized study assessing the effect of digoxin withdrawal in patients with mild to moderate chronic congestive heart failure: results of the proved trial. Proved investigative group. J Am Coll Cardiol 1993; 22:955–962.
77. The Digitalis Investigation Group. The effect of digoxin on mortality and morbidity in patients with heart failure. N Engl J Med 1997; 336:525–533.
78. Gheorghiade M, Hall VB, Jacobsen G, Alam M, Rosman H, Goldstein S. Effects of increasing maintenance dose of digoxin on left ventricular function and neurohormoncs in patients with chronic heart failure treated with diuretics and angiotensin-converting enzyme inhibitors. Circulation 1995; 92:1801–1807.
79. Slatton ML, Irani WN, Hall SA, Marcoux LG, Page RL, Grayburn PA, Eichhorn EJ. Does digoxin provide additional hemodynamic and autonomic benefit at higher doses in patients with mild to moderate heart failure and normal sinus rhythm?J Am Coll Cardiol 1997; 29: 1206–1213
80. Rathore SS, Curtis JP, Wang Y, Bristow MR, Krumholz HM. Association of serum digoxin concentration and outcomes in patients with heart failure. JAMA 2003; 289:871–878.
81. McCullough H, Rupe WA. Studies of dosage of digitalis in children. South Med J 1922; 15:381–385.
82. Nadas AS, Rudolph AM, Reinhold JDL. The use of digitalis in infants and children. New Engl J Med 1953; 248:98–105.
83. Berman W Jr, Ravenscroft PJ, Sheiner LB, Heymann MA, Melmon KL, Rudolph AM. Differential effects of digoxin at comparable concentrations in tissues of fetal and adult sheep. Circ Res 1977; 41:635–642.
84. Levine OR, Blumenthal S. Digoxin dosage in premature infants. Pediatrics 1962; 29:18.
85. Berman W Jr, Yabek SM, Dillon T, Niland C, Corlew S, Christensen D. Effects of digoxin in infants with congested circulatory state due to a ventricular septal defect. N Engl J Med 1983; 308:363–366.

86. Kimball TR, Daniels SR, Meyer RA, Hannon DW, Tian J, Shukla R, Schwartz DC. Effect of digoxin on contractility and symptoms in infants with a large ventricular septal defect. Am J Cardiol 1991; 68:1377–1382.
87. Oparil S, Bishop SP, Ciubb FJ Jr. Myocardial cell hypertrophy or hyperplasia. Hypertension 1984; (suppl III):III38–III43.
88. Rudolph AM. Myocardial growth before and after birth: clinical implications. Acta Paediatr 2000; 89:1–5.
89. Segar JL, Scholz TD, Bedell KA, Smith OM, Huss DJ, Guillery EN. Angiotensin AT1 receptor blockade fails to attenuate pressure–overload cardiac hypertrophy in fetal sheep. Am J Physiol 1997; 273: R1501–R1508.
90. Poss KD, Wilson LG, Keating MT. Heart regeneration in zebrafish. Science 2002; 298:2188–2141.
91. Sachinidis A, Kolossov E, Fleischmann BK, Hescheler J. Generation of cardiomyocytes forms embryonic stem cells. Herz 2002; 27:589–597.

2

Developmental Aspects of Cardiac Performance

DAVID F. TEITEL

Professor of Pediatrics, Chief, Division of
Pediatric Cardiology, University of California,
San Francisco, California, U.S.A

INTRODUCTION

The effects of heart failure on the infant and child must be considered within the context of the developmental changes of the heart and circulation. Many of the changes occur in the fetus and the newborn, but less dramatic changes occur throughout growth. The cellular and subcellular changes in the myocyte and its surrounding structures are discussed in the following chapter. This section will present information on the development of the heart as a functioning organ within the circulation, with reference to subcellular mechanisms

31

when they are important to an understanding of the developmental differences in function.

Cardiovascular Function in the Pressure–Volume Plane

To consider the function of the heart within the circulation, much of this chapter will present information and concepts within the pressure–volume plane. Although there are many ways in which cardiac and circulatory performance will be described within this chapter and book, the pressure–volume plane is most descriptive of many of the important considerations in the development of the heart and its relationship to the circulation. The main function of the heart is to receive

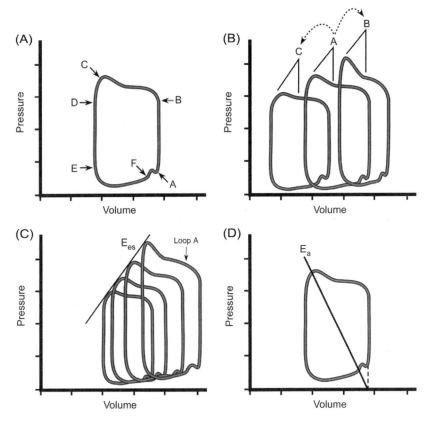

Figure 1 (*Caption on facing page.*)

and eject an adequate amount of blood for hemodynamic stability. This requires that the ventricles contract and relax at an adequate rate, developing characteristic pressure profiles with each beat. The main descriptors of vascular performance are the profile of the volume of blood as it enters the vascular bed and the profile of the pressure generated within the vascular bed as blood passes through it. This interaction of pressure generated and volume ejected within the ventricle, causing pressure to be developed as volume enters the circulation, supports the use of pressure–volume analyses to describe cardiac and vascular function.

Within a single cardiac cycle, the relationship between ventricular pressure and volume is described as a counterclockwise loop, presented in Fig. 1A. Beginning at end-diastole (point A), the myocytes begin to contract, generating

---

Figure 1 (*Facing page*) (A) An idealized representation of the pressure–volume loop, beginning at end-diastole (point A), followed by isovolumic contraction (A–B), the ejection phase of systole (B–D), within which lies "end-systole" (point C), the isovolumic phase of diastole (D–E), and the filling phase of diastole (E–A), with atrial contraction occurring late (point F) during this phase. See text for a full description of the loop. (B) Loop A represents a normal left ventricular pressure–volume loop, with the contour in late ejection (delineated by the lines) showing a modest increase in the rate of pressure rise, caused by the peripheral resistance of the systemic vascular bed. When systemic vascular resistance increases (loop B), the rate and extent of the pressure increase are greater, so that the loop shows a steeper and sharper late ejection contour. When systemic vascular resistance decreases (loop C), the rate and extent of the pressure increase are less, so that the loop shows a relative flat late ejection contour. (C) Loop A represents a resting pressure–volume loop. If preload is decreased (for example, by transient occlusion of the inferior vena cava), a series of pressure–volume loops are generated. Joining the end-systolic points generates a reasonably straight line, the slope of which is end-systolic elastance, or E_{es}. This is a valuable index of ventricular contractility. (D) Vascular elastance can be estimated as the slope of the line (E_a) joining the end-systolic point of the pressure–volume loop with the x-intercept of the end-diastolic volume.

pressure, but volume does not change until ventricular pressure exceeds that in the artery (point B). This phase of systole is called "isovolumic contraction." Because the ventricle is not exposed to the vascular bed, the rate of pressure generation is determined solely by the contractile ability of the myocytes. At point B, ventricular pressure equals that in the aorta, and the aortic valve opens. The ventricle continues to contract, but blood is ejected into the vascular bed, so that the increase in pressure is slower, and occurs as ventricular volume decreases. The contour of this "ejection" phase of systole is determined by the "afterload" against which the muscle contracts. Afterload includes the inertial forces within the ventricular wall and that of the blood, the impedance of the central elastic vessels, and the resistance of the peripheral vessels. The inertial forces are relatively constant and small, so that the ejection contour is determined primarily by the overall compliance of the vascular bed. The more accepting, or compliant, the vascular bed, the less pressure will continue to be generated during ejected. In addition, the central, elastic component of the vascular bed exerts its effects primarily on the earlier part of ejection, as the blood rapidly enters that component, whereas the effects of the resistance vessels of the peripheral vascular bed are exerted later in ejection. The effects of the vascular bed on the ejection pressure contour of the ventricle are presented in Fig. 1B.

Once a myocytes reaches its maximal shortening for an individual beat, the myofilament rapidly discharges calcium and lengthens, or "relaxes." The spatial and temporal sequence of this relaxation is heterogeneous, so that there is no discrete time of "end-systole," when all of the myocytes are maximally shortened. However, the time when the most shortening has occurred will be associated with the shortest overall length of myocytes with the greatest force within the myocardial wall. At this time, the ventricle will be the stiffest, or most elastic (elastance is the *reciprocal* of compliance, and thus describes an object's *resistance* to stretch rather than its stretchability, as commonly thought), so that the least passive change in volume would be associated with the greatest change in pressure. This is accepted as the best approximation of "end-systole," and it occurs at point C on Fig. 1A. This concept of "time-varying elastance" has been used to describe the contractile function of the left (1) and right (2) ventricles. If preload is decreased rapidly and the end-systolic points of each cardiac cycle are linked, they form an approximately straight line, the slope of which is a good descriptor of "end-systolic" elastance (Fig. 1C). This slope, or E_{es}, is a good descriptor of myocardial contractility. As contractility increases, E_{es} increases, because more myofilament crossbridges have occurred, causing the myocardium to be stiffer. Inotropy is the term used to describe this ability of the myocyte to shorten. Thus, the greater the E_{es}, the greater is the inotropic state of the ventricle.

The vascular bed can also be considered in elastic terms. Its elasticity is not time-varying because there is little active contraction of the vascular wall on a beat-to-beat basis. Thus, vascular elastance, or E_a, can be calculated simply as the end-systolic pressure in the vessel (identical to that in the ventricle) divided by the stroke volume (Fig. 1D) (3). There is a close interplay between ventricular and vascular elastance, such that advantageous relationships yield maximal stroke volume, while disadvantageous relationships limit stroke volume (Fig. 2). In the adult dog, there is a relatively large plateau in output, from an E_{es}:E_a ratio of about 0.6 to about 2.0, with a ratio of 1 being associated with the highest output (3). This interaction between ventricular and arterial elastance is critically important to consider when discussing the developmental changes in cardiac performance, because there are dramatic and rapid changes in both during fetal development, and the transition at birth, and slower changes throughout infancy and childhood.

After "end-systole," the myocytes relax rapidly. When ventricular pressure falls below vascular pressure, the semilunar valve closes (point D, occurring at "end-ejection"). The ventricle is once again isolated from the vascular bed, and pressure decreases rapidly, reaching atrial pressure in just a few milliseconds (point E). This phase of the pressure–volume loop is called "isovolumic relaxation," and it is dependent almost entirely on the intrinsic ability of the myocyte to relax. This property is called lusitropy, and can be describe in terms of the rate of pressure loss. As this is defined by an

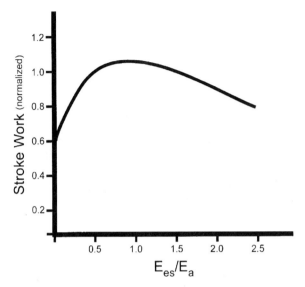

Figure 2 An idealized drawing of the relationship between normalized stroke work of the ventricle and its E_{es}/E_a ratio shows a broad plateau with a peak stroke work occurring around an E_{es}/E_a ratio of approximately 1.

exponential function,

$$P_t = P_0 e^{-t/\tau}$$

the variable used to describe it is τ, the half-life of pressure decay. The more able the ventricle is to relax, the smaller the value for τ, and the greater the lusitropic state of the heart.

Isovolumic relaxation is independent of the passive elements of the ventricular myocardium. Once pressure has fallen below atrial pressure, the atrioventricular valve opens (Fig. 1A, point E). This is followed by rapid filling, as the ventricle continues to relax and thus the pressure difference between atrial and ventricular pressures drives the flow, followed thereafter by the slow filling phase, once relaxation is complete. Later in diastole, the atrium contracts (Fig. 1A, point F), filling the ventricle to end-diastolic volume, immediately before contraction (Fig. 1A, point A). The passive filling phase of diastole is determined by the passive compliance of the ventricle, which is determined primarily by nonmyocytic elements of the myocardium, and by the direct effects of the contralateral ventricle. It can be described by two logarithmic functions (Fig. 3) (4). The positive limb is described by the function

$$P_{\mathrm{p}} = -S_{\mathrm{p}}\ln\left[\frac{(V_m - V)}{(V_m - V_0)}\right]$$

and the negative limb is described as

$$P_{\mathrm{n}} = -S_{\mathrm{n}}\ln\left[\frac{(V - V_n)}{(V_0 - V_n)}\right]$$

the former of which can be used at end-diastole to determine the stiffness constant S_{p}, which is a sensitive index of the passive compliance of the ventricle. It is important to appreciate

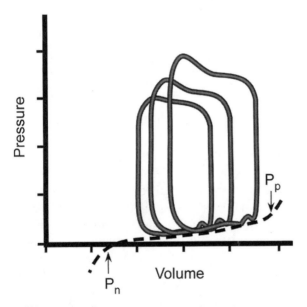

Figure 3 The end-diastolic pressure–volume relationship generated from a series of loops is much more complex than the end-systolic pressure–volume relationship. Rather than being linear, it can be defined by two logarithmic functions representing the positive limb (P_{p}) and the negative limb (P_{n}). See the text for the formulae.

that indices of diastolic function often mix properties of isovolumic relaxation, which is determined primarily by myocytic function, with those of passive compliance, determined primarily by nonmyocytic elements. Thus, they must be considered with skepticism and care, particularly as they relate to diastolic dysfunction. Heart failure is frequently described as causing diastolic dysfunction initially and primarily, but it is important to separate its effects on the myocyte, or lusitropy, from those on the supporting structures, or passive compliance, if one is to understand and develop treatment strategies which address that dysfunction.

Determinants of Ventricular Performance

The primary determinants of ventricular performance are contractility, afterload, preload, and heart rate. These are interdependent, not independent, determinants, as was believed for many years. Their interdependence is exemplified by the mechanisms which mediate much of their effect. Moreover, those mechanisms may be limited in the developing heart, explaining many of its differences in its response to stress.

Contractility can be defined as a change in myocyte function induced by a change in calcium availability to the myofilament, or the sensitivity of the myofilament to that activator calcium. As the myofilament produces more force when it shortens, there is an increase in the work of the ventricle. Within that definition of contractility, the effects of each of the other three determinants are in large part transduced by a change in either calcium availability or sensitivity, and thus contractility, particularly in the mature heart.

As afterload increases, if all other determinants remain constant, stroke volume should decrease, because the same force of contraction should lead to lesser shortening. Yet, over a wide range of increases in afterload in the mature heart, stroke volume is maintained constant. This has been termed "homeometric autoregulation." It has been demonstrated in the adult (5) and newborn lamb heart (6). The mechanism behind homeometric autoregulation has been shown to be calcium-based (7). As afterload increases, the myofilament increases its sensitivity to calcium on a beat-to-beat basis. This is associated with an increase in cross-bridge formation, an increase in force generation, and thus a maintenance of output in the presence of increased afterload.

The Frank–Starling relationship defines the increase in cardiac output or work in response to an increase in preload, or initial myofilament length. This had long been thought to be an intrinsic property of the myofilament, independent of changes in contractility, but it has been shown to be transduced by an increase in the sensitivity of troponin C to activator calcium (8).

Lastly, the force–frequency relationship describes the increase in force generation of a myocyte as its rate of contraction increases. Several mechanisms have been implicated in its genesis, but all are mediated by an increase in activator calcium availability to the myofilament. Part of the increase in activator calcium is thought to be secondary to activation of the L-type calcium channels in the sarcolemma, with higher heart rates leading to a greater percentage of time that the sarcolemma is not fully repolarized, which in turn leads to a greater duration of opening of these channels, since they are voltage gated. However, most studies suggest that alterations in calcium flux across the sarcoplasmic reticulum lead to greater calcium availability. Recently, much of the force–frequency relationship has been shown to be related to changes in phospholamban activity (9). Phospholamban is a pentamer closely associated with the calcium pumps of the sarcoplasmic reticulum (SERCA2). In its non-phosphorylated state, phospholamban impairs calcium reuptake by SERCA2, maintaining high cytosolic calcium activity. When phosphorylated, it allows rapid reuptake of calcium during diastole. The phospholamban knockout mouse demonstrated the abolition of the force–frequency relationship (9), suggesting that increased phosphorylation of phospholamban at high heart rates may be causal to the increase in contractility. Phospholamban has also been shown to be critical to the maintenance of low resting contractility and beta-adrenergic responsiveness, as the phospholamban knockout mouse has also been shown to have a very high resting contractility and is unresponsive to beta-adrenergic stimulation (10). Lastly, the Na^+–Ca^{2+} exchanger recently has been implicated in the genesis of the force–frequency relationship (11). Calcium efflux via the exchanger has been shown to decrease significantly as rate increases, due to a shorter diastolic interval.

Thus, when considering the benefits of interventions on the failing heart that are directed at altering any of the four primary determinants, it is important to understand their interdependency, the mechanism which modulate these effects, and differences in the activity of these mechanisms over development. It is particularly instructive to understand the developmental difference in these mechanisms, because the heart that is failing has been shown to mirror many of the findings which are seen in the immature heart.

FETAL CARDIOVASCULAR PERFORMANCE

Fetal Circulation

Over the past 40 years, many studies in animal models and humans have advanced our understanding of the fetal circulation, since the pioneering work in fetal sheep in the laboratories of Abraham Rudolph and Geoffrey Dawes. The postnatal circulation consists of two distinct vascular beds without communication, each receiving identical amounts of blood. The pulmonary vascular bed has very low resistance in the normal mature circulation, in the range of 1–3 Resistance (Wood) Units, with minimal resting vasoconstrictor tone and only a modest ability to increase its resistance. Control over resistance is primarily exerted locally to match perfusion to ventilation in the presence of parenchymal lung disease. The systemic vascular bed has moderate and quite variable resistance in the mature circulation, in the range of 20–50 Resistance Units, and has a great ability to vary its resistance via a variety of neurohormonal, local metabolic, and autoregulatory mechanisms, depending on the particular vascular bed. Vascular beds that serve organs of high oxygen consumption, such as the cerebral and myocardial beds, are predominantly under local control; beds that require relatively low flow, such as the skin and muscle vessels, are predominantly under neurohormonal control; and beds that require high flow but consume relatively little oxygen, such as the renal vascular bed, are predominantly under pressure autoregulation.

Because both ventricles eject the same stroke volume, the left ventricle sees a much greater afterload than the right throughout ejection, and must generate far greater pressure (Fig. 4). The right ventricle thus has very little direct effect on left ventricular mechanics in systole, whereas the left has large effects on the right. Thus, this circulation is considered left-dominant, due to the pressure differences. The right ventricle can affect left ventricular function only in diastole, by a direct effect on ventricular filling, and in systole, by a "series" effect, whereby left ventricular filling is determined

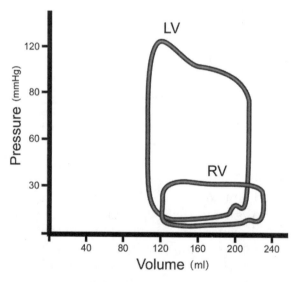

Figure 4 Representative pressure–volume loops of the adult left and right ventricles. Each ejects the same stroke volume, but the left ventricle does so at a much higher pressure because it sees a greater afterload, and despite this, ejects a greater fraction of its end-diastolic volume. It is also less compliant than the right ventricle in diastole, and thus has a greater end-diastolic pressure despite a lesser end-diastolic volume.

by right ventricular output. And because the ventricles eject identical stroke volumes, each ejects the same minute output, which is termed "cardiac output." When indexed to surface area, it is termed "cardiac index."

The fetal circulation is very different than the mature circulation, and thus impacts ventricular function very differently. Pulmonary vascular resistance is very high, allowing the right ventricle to eject the majority of its output down the ductus arteriosus to the placenta, for oxygen uptake. Systemic vascular resistance is low, because there is a large placental vascular bed of very low resistance arising from the bilateral iliac arteries. There are also communications between the two sides of the heart, both internally, at the foramen ovale, and externally, at the ductus arteriosus (Fig. 5). The internal communication allows the ventricles to fill differently, and thus eject different stroke volumes, and the external communication allows the ventricles to eject into overlapping vascular beds. Because of the differential filling and ejecting, one cannot talk of "cardiac output" but rather of "combined ventricular output" (CVO), which is equivalent to two cardiac outputs of the mature circulation. Because of the communications between the vascular beds, the afterload against which each ventricle ejects is very difficult to determine. The circulation is not truly "parallel," because the small fetal aortic arch acts as a resistor between the upper and lower bodies. The left ventricle sees a very small vascular bed of the upper body, ejecting only a very small amount of blood across the aortic arch (Fig. 6), while the right ventricle sees a large vascular bed, ejecting its output into the lungs, the lower body, and the placenta. Both ventricles eject to the same peak systolic pressure, but, because the right ventricle ejects a greater proportion of CVO, the fetal circulation is considered right-dominant. Because of this, the fetal right ventricle has a far greater direct effect on left ventricular systolic function as compare to the postnatal right ventricle. This is confirmed by two-dimensional echocardiography, which shows a flattening of the ventricular septum by the right ventricle into the left ventricle, so that the shape of the left ventricle in the short axis view is almost semicircular in the fetal state, rather than circular, as it is in the postnatal state.

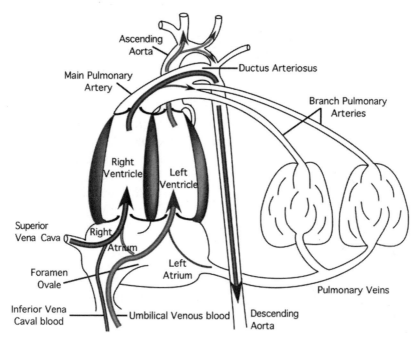

Figure 5 Schematic representation of the fetal circulation. Umbilical venous blood is preferentially shunted across the foramen ovale to the left heart, and right ventricular blood is preferentially shunted across the ductus arteriosus to the lower body and placenta.

Fetal Systolic Mechanics

Within the context of our understanding of the determinants of systolic performance and their interdependence, the changes in performance over development are logical. In the fetus, resting CVO is somewhat higher than that of the adult (i.e., higher than two "cardiac outputs") (12), and indices of muscle performance, such as ventricular elastance (E_{es}), or dP/dt_{max} are similar or higher. The systolic performance of the heart is clearly not stressed in the fetus, as evidenced by the fact that the fractional extraction of oxygen is approximately 30%, similar to the postnatal state (13). Despite the difficulty in accurately assessing the specific vascular resistance that each fetal ventricle is exposed to, the

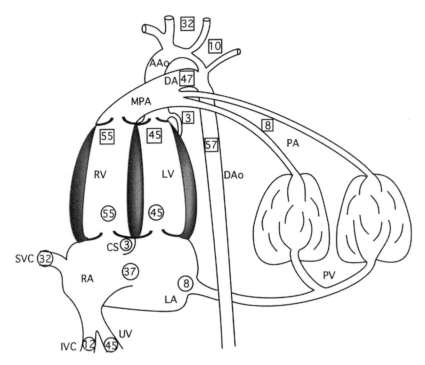

Figure 6 Percentages of blood flow through the fetal circulation. The numbers in circles represent percentage of combined venous return and the numbers in squares represent percentage of combined ventricular output. On the input (venous) side, the abbreviations are: UV, umbilical venous blood; IVC, inferior vena caval blood; SVC, superior vena caval blood; PV, pulmonary venous blood; CS, coronary sinus blood; RA, right atrium; LA, left atrium. On the output (ventricular) side, the abbreviations are: AAO, ascending aortic blood; MPA, main pulmonary arterial blood; DAO, descending aortic blood; DA, ductus arteriosus blood; PA, branch pulmonary arterial blood; LV, left ventricle; RV, right ventricle.

overall afterload of each is quite low as compared to the mature left ventricle. In late gestation, stroke volume is relatively high, yet peak systolic pressure is quite low, in the range of 60–70 mmHg. A representation of the pressure volume loops of the two fetal ventricles, and of the ventricles after birth, is presented in Fig. 7A–B. The fetal left ventricle

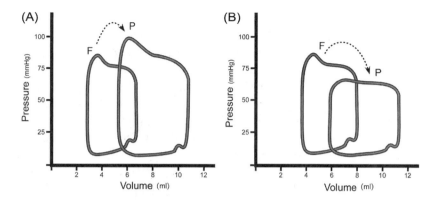

Figure 7 Representation of left and right ventricular pressure–volume loops in the fetus and after birth. (A) The fetal left ventricle (F) ejects a relatively small stroke volume under relatively low systolic pressure, and has a low diastolic compliance. At birth, compliance of the ventricle (P) improves, allowing the ventricle to fill much more, but at the same pressure, and allowing its stroke volume to increase substantially. Peak systolic pressure increases modestly. (B) The fetal right ventricle (F) ejects somewhat more blood than that of the left but at the same systolic pressure. At birth, the ventricle (P) ejects more blood at a lower pressure, because of the marked decrease in the vascular elastance of the pulmonary vascular bed (secondary to a decrease in pulmonary vascular resistance).

fills to a lesser volume than the right and ejects a lesser stroke volume than the right and at the same peak pressure, so that its arterial elastance is greater. The ventricular elastance, or contractility, are probably quite similar, although right ventricular elastance has not been evaluated in the fetus.

High resting indices of fetal systolic performance can be explained by the fact that, although the sarcoplasmic reticulum is underdeveloped (14), the myocyte has a large surface area to volume ratio, so that the myofilaments are in close proximity to the sarcolemma. Activity of sarcolemmal calcium channels can supply a far greater proportion of activator calcium to the myofilament than the 10% that they contribute in the mature heart (15). Moreover, it is thought that mechanisms such as reverse activity of the Na^+–Ca^{2+} exchanger may be active in the fetal heart, contributing to trans-sarcolemmal calcium influx (16,17), which does not occur in the normal mature heart.

Despite maintenance of resting systolic performance, the fetal heart is very limited in its ability to increase output in response to alterations in the major determinants of performance, thus severely limiting the fetus' ability to respond to stress. Inotropic stimulation with p-adrenergic agents (13), and increases in preload (18) have limited effects on output, and increases in afterload severely impair output (19,20), unlike in the postnatal state. Maximal recruitment of all of these determinants yields an increase in CVO in the fetus of only about 30–40%, as compared to 300–400% in the mature heart. Much of the limitation in output reserve is likely due to the immaturity of the myocyte. The immaturity occurs both at the level of the sarcoplasmic reticulum, which is underdeveloped (21), and in the myofilament itself. An immature sarcoplasmic reticulum limits the ability of the myocyte to increase activator calcium on a beat-to-beat basis, and the myofilament may also be less sensitive to any increase. Developmental differences in troponin I and T isoforms exist, the degree of phosphorlyation of tropomyosin is increased, and nonmuscle isoforms of tropomyosin are present (22–24). The expression of alpha- and beta-myosin heavy chain genes is also developmentally regulated and is associated with alterations in their products, with alpha heavy chains much more ubiquitous in the fetus (25). All of these differences would decrease the maximum availability of activator calcium and may decrease the sensitivity of the myofilament to that calcium. Taken together, these development differences in the myocyte may allow the heart to maintain adequate output at rest, but be unable to respond normally to alterations in contractility, preload, or afterload.

In addition to immaturity of the myocyte limiting the ability of the fetal heart to increase its output in response to volume loading, the relationship between the ventricles and with the circulation significantly limits output reserve as well. In utero ventilation alone significantly increases output, and does so concomitantly with a marked change in the circulation of the fetus (26). In the normal fetus, the right ventricle is dominant in utero, and can impair left ventricular filling by a direct effect. In addition, there is no series effect of the right ventricle on left ventricular filling because right ventricular output is predominantly directed down the ductus arteriosus to the descending aorta rather than to the lungs. Thus, a volume load administered to the fetus is less likely to cause an increase in preload, or end-diastolic volume, of the left ventricle. Not only is the left ventricle constrained by the right ventricle to limit its filling, but also the myocardium is less compliant (27). This limits the ability of the pericardium to modulate filling in the fetus (28). Lastly, the venous capacitance of the fetal circulation is quite large, with a large placental venous bed in continuity with the hepatic and lower body venous beds. Thus, the immature myocyte, constraint and restraint of ventricular filling, and a large venous capacitor together greatly limit the ability of the fetal heart to increase its output in response to an increase in circulating blood volume.

The fetal heart is also severely limited in its ability to increase or even maintain its output in response to heart rate increases, which can have severely deleterious effects on fetal well being. The immature myocyte and the inability to maintain preload at fast rates leads to rapid deterioration of systolic performance with increasing heart rate, with hydrops rapidly developing (29). The immaturity of the myocyte is evidenced by its inability to recruit mechanisms intrinsic to the sarcoplasmic reticulum to increase calcium availability as rate of contraction increases.

Thus, the fetal heart is remarkably able to function similarly to the mature heart at rest, but mechanisms which can be recruited to improve output during stress, or to maintain output in a failing heart, are not available to the fetus. Manipulation of any of the major determinants of ventricular performance in the fetal heart is unlikely to improve output significantly, so that maintenance of the normal status of each of these determinants is critical to fetal well being.

Fetal Diastolic Mechanics

Although resting systolic function of the fetal heart is quite similar to that of the adult, diastolic function is not. As discussed above, diastolic function can be divided into the myocytic component, relaxation, and the nonmyocytic component, passive compliance. During the isovolumic relaxation phase of the pressure volume loop (Fig. 1A), cross-bridge detachment determines the rate of pressure fall. The relaxation constant τ is normal, suggesting that, at rest, calcium efflux is normal. Although it has not been investigated in depth, it is likely that positive lusitropic agents (lusitropy is the term used to describe relaxation) such as β-adrenergic stimulation have limited effects, since their action is transduced by increasing the rate of calcium sequestration into the sarcoplasmic reticulum, through increasing SERCA2 activity. This is likely mediated by phosphorylation of phospholamban. Although phosphorylation of troponin I also occurs in response to positive lusitropic agents, causing more rapid ejection of calcium from the troponin complex, it is not known whether fetal isoforms of troponin I are affected differently than mature isoforms.

Rapid filling is determined both by myocyte relaxation and by the passive components of the myocardium. Diastasis, or slow filling, and atrial contraction follow rapid filling. During this time, relaxation is complete and the end-diastolic state of the ventricle is determined by passive, nonmyocytic characteristics alone (Fig. 1A). The fetal heart has been shown to be quite stiff, with a high stiffness constant (27,28). This is thought to be secondary to structural differences in the myocardium, including a higher water content and more disorganized structure, and to the direct interactive forces between the ventricles, which are of similar mass. As mentioned above, this relative stiffness limits the ability of the heart to recruit the Frank–Starling mechanism to increase output in response to an increase in volume. Thus, limitations in diastolic performance secondary to increased passive stiffness do not have significant effects on resting diastolic performance, but can manifest when stresses are imposed. Tachycardia and increased circulating volume, which can increase output in response to stress in the postnatal heart, have limited positive, and even deleterious effects, in the fetus. Thus, heart failure, manifesting as hydrops fetalis, develops in many pathophysiolgic processes which compromise fetal cardiac performance.

POSTNATAL CARDIOVASCULAR PERFORMANCE

Circulatory Changes After Birth

Dramatic changes in the circulation occur at birth and less dramatic changes occur over the next several weeks of postnatal life. The tasks of oxygen uptake and delivery become separated immediately after birth, as oxygen uptake moves from the placental to the pulmonary circulation. This is achieved primarily by vasodilation of the pulmonary vascular bed, which decreases its resistance by about 2/3 of the complete fall immediately after birth (30). Most of this decrease is secondary to gaseous distension of the lung, with a lesser effect induced by oxygenation. The mechanisms transducing this effect are complex and not fully understood, but direct effects of changes in surface tension at the alveolar air–liquid interface, alterations in the concentration of various prostaglandin and leukotriene metabolites, and changes in concentrations of bradykinin, angiotensin II, and histamine may all play a role. Over the next several weeks of life, there is remodeling of the pulmonary vascular bed, with thinning of the more proximal arteriolar muscle and extension of the muscle distally. This leads to a further fall in pulmonary vascular resistance to mature levels, of approximately 1–3 Resistance Units, and transfers primary control of pulmonary vascular resistance to local segments and away from central mechanisms. This allows for matching of perfusion to ventilation when local parenchymal pulmonary disease occurs.

The large decrease in pulmonary vascular resistance at birth decreases peak right ventricular pressure and redirects all of its output to the pulmonary vascular bed. Pulmonary blood flow increases even further, as a small amount of left ventricular output passes through the ductus arteriosus, until it closes within the next 24–48 hr. At the same time that pulmonary vascular resistance falls precipitously, placental vascular resistance increases to a similar extent, also in response to the increase in oxygen levels. Thus, the placental circulation is effectively removed from the circulation even prior to separation of the umbilical cord. Overall, the right ventricle sees a marked reduction in its afterload because of pulmonary vasodilation.

The effects of the changes in the circulation have more complex effects on the left ventricle. Vasoconstriction of some systemic vascular beds in response to oxygenation, particularly of the brain and heart, leads to an increase in afterload, but at the same time, the left ventricle can now eject to the lower body without competition of flow from the right ventricle, which had supplied most of the blood to the lower body prior to birth (Fig. 6). The cumulative effects lead to a moderate decrease in the afterload seen by the left ventricle (31,32).

The dramatic alteration in the distribution of arterial output leads to a marked alteration in venous return and thus right and left ventricular preload. In the fetus, about 90% of combined venous return arrives via the systemic venous system to the right atrium (Fig. 6), with only the small amount of blood passing directly to the left atrium via the pulmonary veins. This large difference in systemic and pulmonary venous return allows for a large right-to-left shunt across the foramen ovale. However, because combined resistance to flow from the right atrium to the left ventricle (via the foramen ovale, left atrium, and mitral valve) is greater than that to the right, most (about 60%) right atrial blood passes to the right ventricle. Thus, the right ventricle has a greater end-diastolic volume and output than the left. Because both ventricles eject at the same pressure, the right ventricle has a significant direct effect on the left ventricle during ejection as well as during filling in the fetus.

Immediately after birth, the changes in blood flow distribution decrease right atrial venous return and markedly increase left atrial return, via the pulmonary veins, above right atrial levels. This causes abrupt closure of the foramen ovale, or permits only a small left-to-right shunt because the foramen ovale functions as a windsock into the left atrium, closing when the pressure in that atrium exceeds that in the right. The increase in left ventricular venous return increases its end-diastolic volume to levels at least equal to that seen in the right, and at somewhat higher filling pressures. That increase in end-diastolic volume and pressure, in conjunction with a greater left ventricular ejection pressure, causes septal configuration to change, oriented and moving in conjunction with the free wall of the left ventricle. Thus, the direct effects of the right ventricle on left ventricular filling and ejection are dramatically reduced immediately following birth.

Circulatory changes after the immediate newborn period are much more gradual and limited. Pulmonary vascular resistance continues to decrease over the next two to three months after birth, when they reach their minimum. Thereafter, parenchymal lung growth matches vascular development, so that growth is not associated with a significant change in pulmonary vascular resistance. Conversely, the systemic vascular bed shows a slow increase in resistance over the years after birth, and a redistribution of flow from the upper to the lower body. This increase in left ventricular afterload is well tolerated, as demonstrated by the presence of homeometric autoregulation in the mature heart (5).

Postnatal Changes in Cardiac Mechanics

Not only are there dramatic changes in the circulatory environment to which the heart is exposed at birth, but the demands on the heart increase greatly. Prior to birth, the fetus is in a very accommodating environment, with minimal demands. The primary work of the fetus is directed toward growth, as it rests in a neutral thermal environment, breathes little, and receives substrates and oxygen via the placental circulation. Immediately after birth, the infant must use energy for thermoregulation, breathe to take up oxygen, and eat and process nutrients. Because of these increased demands, oxygen consumption triples at birth (33). To do so while maintaining fractional extraction relatively constant, ventricular output must increase greatly. Left ventricular output increases about threefold at birth, while right ventricular output increases somewhat less (34). It has been a matter of great interest to researchers that, in the fetal state, the heart is only able to increase its output modestly despite maximal load, heart rate, and inotropic manipulations; at birth, however, output can triple almost instantaneously.

To understand how this is possible, it is useful to turn again to the pressure–volume loop (Fig. 7A–B). The interaction of changes in systolic and diastolic mechanics is intertwined and together cause this dramatic increase in output. This will be discussed together in this section rather than separately.

Immediately at birth, pulmonary venous return increases far in excess of systemic venous return, leading to an increase in left atrial volume above that of the right. This causes increased filling of the left ventricle as compared to the right. That increased filling, along with a much higher left ventricular afterload relative to the right, shifts the ventricular septum into the right ventricle, allowing the left ventricle to fill more, under much less pressure. That is, the left ventricle becomes more compliant, and its filling characteristics become much more dependent on the pericardium. Increased left ventricular compliance and filling allows the sarcomeres to stretch far more than in fetal life, and thus preload increases greatly. The increase in preload far exceeds that possible in fetal life and is associated with a greater increase in stroke volume. Heart rate increases simultaneously, so that there is a large increase in left ventricular output. The greater compliance of the left ventricle is still less than that of the mature left ventricle (27), and thus the maintenance of an adequate heart rate within a relatively narrow range remains important, as in the fetus.

Two other mechanisms have been considered as causal to the large increase in left ventricular output at birth—an increase in contractility and better matching of ventricular and arterial elastance (contractility and afterload, respectively). There is a thyroid surge at birth, leading to increased beta-adrenergic receptor numbers and function. The increased beta-adrenergic stimulation associated with birth, induced by the increased oxygen requirements of thermoregulation and breathing, would logically thus has been thought to increase left ventricular contractility. It is also logical to assume that left ventricular contractility is relatively low in the fetus, and left ventricular afterload relatively high. This might lead to an adverse $E_{es}{:}E_a$ ratio in the fetus. An increase in contractility associated with a decrease in afterload could significantly increase that ratio and improve output.

However, studies of fetal sheep acutely delivered demonstrate that no such mechanisms are causal to the increase in output (31,32). The large increase in left-ventricular end-diastolic volume is associated with an increase in dP/dt_{max}, which may lead one to assume that contractility does indeed increase. However, that increase in dP/dt_{max} is secondary solely to the increase in preload (the Starling phenomenon), as E_{es} did not change in either study. $E_{es}{:}E_a$ ratio also did not change substantially.

The ability of the left ventricle of the newborn to increase its output greatly is not limited to the full term infant. The preterm infant has been shown to have similar contractile function as the newborn using the fiber shortening–end systolic wall stress relationship and greater than that of the older child (35). In situations where the newborn left ventricle is not capable of maintaining systemic output, either because it is obstructed (e.g., critical aortic stenosis) or myopathic, the right ventricle is recruited to perform left ventricular work. At this stage of development, it is very capable of performing that work. Studies of the isolated right and left ventricles of the pig heart have shown that maximal E_{es} (or E_{max}, as presented in the study) of the two ventricles is similar, and that both can generate greater pressure at an increased rate of development up to a filling pressure of 18 mmHg (36). Despite the reorientation of the ventricular septum, the right ventricle remains somewhat more compliant than the left and relaxation of the two ventricles is the same. Thus, the right ventricle is capable of filling adequately under low pressures and eject at a similar contractile force as the left.

Developmental Changes in Cardiac Mechanics
After Birth

The myocyte of the newborn mammalian heart is structurally immature. It is much thinner, with a far greater surface area to volume ratio, and, except in the ferret (37), the sarcoplasmic reticulum is underdeveloped. Fiber orientation and extracellular matrix composition may also be immature, leading to less well developed contractile pattern and a stiffer heart in diastole. The differences in myocyte and cardiac structure in the newborn are associated with differences in sensitivity to various stresses to which the healthy and failing neonatal heart may be exposed and its ability to invoke various mechanisms to increase output. This is particularly important when heart failure occurs, since the mechanisms available to the physician to improve heart function are different. An understanding of the developmental differences in myocyte mechanics is thus critical to the treating physician.

Despite the immaturity of the newborn myocyte, the normal newborn left ventricle is capable of generating outputs far exceeding those of the adult left ventricle (38–40). In the sheep, the output of the newborn left ventricle is more than three times greater than that of the adult (38). Over the first month of life, resting cardiac output indexed to surface area decreases fairly rapidly, and then decreases much more slowly over the next several months. This high resting cardiac output is associated with a high resting contractile state, as there is a very limited contractile response to inotropic stimulation in the newborn heart (40,41). Similar to the differences in output, the resting newborn contractile state far exceeds that of the adult (38,40).

These findings are not, on the surface, congruent with the presence of myocyte immaturity, particularly of the sarcoplasmic reticulum, which is the source of up to 85% of activator calcium to the sarcomere in the mature heart. However, the immature myocyte has a much greater surface area to volume ratio, as myocardial growth, sometime around birth becomes solely based upon hypertrophy. Depending on the species, hyperplasia is no longer evident either in fetal life, in the larger mammals, or soon after birth, in the smaller mammals. Thus, the heart grows by increasing the volume of the myocytes, removing the contractile elements from their proximity to the sarcolemma. It can be postulated that the immature myocyte, with the proximity of the contractile elements to the sarcolemma, is much less dependent than the mature myocyte on a well-developed sarcoplasmic reticulum to generate a similar force of contraction. This hypothesis is supported by a variety of studies on the immature myocyte, which have shown the fetal and neonatal myocyte to have a greater dependence on sarcolemmal calcium flux (42–45). To support the greater need for trans-sarcolemmal calcium flux in the immature myocyte, there is evidence that L-type calcium channels are far more active (45) and that there is increased activity and reversal of the Na^+–Ca^{2+} exchanger (17), leading to calcium influx early in systole, when subsarcolemmal concentrations of sodium are high.

Because of the high resting contractile state, the normal newborn has a very limited contractile reserve, so that mechanisms to improve output based upon contractile stimulation may be met with limited success. Of course, the failing ventricle with abnormal myocyte mechanics can be stimulated to improve its contractility, but mechanisms that are directed toward increasing sarcolemmal calcium flux rather than flux across the sarcoplasmic reticulum are likely to be met with greater success. The positive inotropic effects of phosphodiesterase inhibitors are uncertain in the young heart (but their beneficial effects on afterload may still be extremely important, as discussed below). Cardiac glycosides, however, are not of much use in the "high output failure" of the newborn heart with a large left-to-right shunt because of its limited contractile reserve, but may be beneficial in the failing newborn heart, which has a larger percentage of high affinity ouabain $(Na^+$–$K^+)$ -ATPase isoforms as compared to the adult (46).

An increase in left ventricular preload is likely causal to much of the increase in left ventricular output at birth. The newborn is capable of responding well to this increase in preload, being able to increase indices of muscle performance to a similar extent as the adult (47). However, diastolic performance is still not at the same level as that in the adult. The newborn lamb heart has been shown to be less compliant than that of the adult (27) and relaxation of the newborn guinea pig heart is slower, in association with reduced function of the sarcoplasmic reticulum (48). Thus, despite a far greater response to volume loading than that of the fetus, the newborn is still less capable than the adult of responding to further volume loading because of relative diastolic dysfunction. This is corroborated by studies in the lamb, which show a limited response to volume loading as compared to adult sheep (49). In addition, it is important to note that, after birth, the pericardium may have a major effect on ventricular function. Unlike the fetus and even more so than the adult, direct ventricular interaction is pronounced in the newborn, because the pericardium is capable of transferring pressure from one ventricle to the other due to the relative compliances of the ventricular free walls, the septum, and the pericardium (28). Although the normal right ventricle has only modest effects on left ventricular function in the normal newborn heart, increases in right ventricular filling and pressure can have more serious effects. This is extremely important to remember when treating heart failure in the newborn, when left atrial hypertension is often associated with pronounced increases in pulmonary arterial pressure. Without treating the elevated pulmonary arterial pressures, therapy toward improving left ventricular output may be compromised.

Unlike the relatively normal ability of the newborn heart to respond to changes in preload, it is very sensitive to increases in afterload. Van Hare et al. (50) showed that any limitation in preload response in the young lamb was due to the concomitant increase in afterload. Even at one month of age, the lamb cannot respond normally to an afterload stress (39). Although the newborn heart does demonstrate some degree of homeometric autoregulation (6), the range of an ideal $E_{es}{:}E_a$ ratio is likely much more limited. In addition, the newborn operates at a much lower arterial elastance (afterload) and a higher ventricular elastance (contractility), so that the resting ratio is already quite high, and the limited plateau means that output can drop precipitously with even a modest increase in afterload. As heart failure is associated with ventricular dilation and systemic vasoconstriction, even modest failure can be associated with a dramatic decrease in output, leading to rapid deterioration. Thus, a mainstay of therapy in the newborn with heart failure should be afterload reduction. Because the newborn heart has a normal Frank–Starling relationship, maintenance of a relatively high preload during afterload reduction is possible, and will maximize output.

The newborn heart is operating not only near its maximal stroke volume but also near its maximal heart rate. Increasing heart rate above resting levels by atrial pacing in the newborn lamb was not associated with an increase in cardiac output, but decreasing it was associated with a significant decline (51). The lack of an increase in output occurs despite an increase in contractility (52), suggesting that the limitation is likely related to impaired filling at rapid heart rates. This supports the finding that normal atrial function is critical to normal ventricular performance in the immature heart. Klautz et al. (53) found that atrial contraction contributed nearly 30% to ventricular output, which is significantly in excess of what occurs in the mature heart. With maturation, the range of heart rates over which output is maintained is far greater, and increasing heart rate above baseline has a significant beneficial effect. Therefore, it is very important in the failing newborn heart that heart rate is maintained in the optimal range and that synchronous atrial and ventricular contraction occurs. Because of this, it is possible that β-adrenergic blockade in the young patient with chronic heart failure may not be as advantageous as a strategy. Particularly in the postoperative patient, pacing may be required to achieve the most advantageous heart rates to maximize output in the presence of ventricular dysfunction.

Developmental Differences in the Response to Metabolic Derangements

Metabolic stresses particular to the neonate are especially important to consider when treating heart failure, because the immature neonatal myocyte may respond differently to them. Two of the most common additional stresses a newborn sees are asphyxia and hypocalcemia, and the response of the newborn heart to these two stresses is quite different. Birth asphyxia is common and is associated with arterial acidemia and tissue hypoxia. The adult heart is very sensitive to acidemia, showing a marked decrease in function even with a modest decrease in pH. However, the neonatal myocardium is particularly insensitive to this stress. This is likely due to two factors peculiar to the neonatal myocyte. A decrease in extracellular pH from 7.3 to 6.3 caused only a modest decrease in contraction force of the isolated newborn myocyte of about 15%, whereas a comparable decrease in pH cause a decrease of contraction force of about 45% in the adult myocyte (54). This appeared to be caused by a lesser inhibition of the calcium current, associated with a lesser change in the membrane potential at which maximum flux occurred. In addition, there was a lesser decrease in calcium current conductance. In addition, intracellular pH decreases less in the neonatal myocyte due to better buffering capacity (55). Since protons directly impair sarcomeric function, these mechanisms all cause a far greater tolerance of acidemia by the young heart. This is not to imply that acidemia is benign to the newborn heart. A reduction in pH to 7.11 by infusion of HCl was associated with a significant reduction in cardiac output, by 49% (56). However, hypoxemia to oxygen levels below 30 mmHg was not associated with any such reduction. Interestingly, acidemia caused significant vasoconstriction whereas hypoxemia caused vasodilation, so that the much of the reduction in output during the former stress may have been caused by the afterload stress rather than an impairment in intrinsic contractility. Thus, it is important to not only maintain as normal an acid–base status as possible in the newborn with the failing heart, but also to ensure that afterload is not excessively elevated secondary to the metabolic stress.

Conversely to its relative insensitivity to an increase in extracellular hydrogen ions, the newborn heart is more sensitive to levels of extracellular calcium. Because it is so dependent of trans-sarcolemmal flux of calcium, adequate extracellular calcium levels are critical for normal myocyte function. As discussed above, this increased flux is transduced by increased L-type calcium channel currents (15) and by reversal of the Na^+–Ca^{2+} exchanger (17), and these changes are associated with a dramatic increase in sensitivity to calcium channel blockade. When neonatal mouse ventricular muscle was exposed to nicarpidine or verapamil, there was a 70% decrease in contractile force generated, as compared to a 30% decrease in the adult mouse muscle (44). Thus, it is important to maintain normal levels of ionized calcium to maintain normal cardiac function in the neonate, and calcium channel blockade may be associated with severe compromise of that function.

Lastly, glucose homeostasis is very important to the neonatal myocardium, but no more so than to the adult. Although the fetal myocardium consumes only glucose, lactate, and pyruvate, and is not able to metabolize free fatty acids, changes in the metabolic function of the organism occur immediately at birth, so that the heart is able to use free fatty acids almost immediately. In fact, despite the large increase in myocardial oxygen consumption that occurs at birth concomitant with the increase in cardiac output and myocardial work, the amount of glucose consumed does not change (57). Hypoglycemia does, however, significantly impair myocardial performance and the ill newborn, with limited glycogen stores, is more prone to hypoglycemia than the older child. Thus, despite the absence of developmental differences in myocardial glucose homeostasis after birth, it is important to ensure adequate circulating glucose levels in the infant and child with heart failure.

REFERENCES

1. Sagawa K. The ventricular pressure–volume diagram revisited. Circ Res 1978; 43:677–687.
2. Karunanithi MK, Michniewicz J, Copeland SE, Feneley MP. Right ventricular preload recruitable stroke work, end-systolic pressure–volume, and dp/dt_{max}-end-diastolic volume relations compared as

indexes of right ventricular contractile performance in conscious dogs. Circ Res 1992; 70:1169–1179.
3. Little WC, Cheng CP. Left ventricular-arterial coupling in conscious dogs. Am J Physiol 1991; 261:H70–H76.
4. Nikolic S, Yellin EL, Tamura K, Vetter H, Tamura T, Meisner JS, Frater RW. Passive properties of canine left ventricle: diastolic stiffness and restoring forces [published erratum appears in Circ Res 1988 jun;62[6]:Preceding 1059]. Circ Res 1988; 62:1210–1222.
5. Sarnoff SJ, Mitchell JH, Gilmore MS, Remensnyder JP. Homeometric autoregulation in the heart. Circ Res 1960; 8:1077–1091.
6. Klautz RJ, Teitel DF, Steendijk P, van Bel F, Baan J. Interaction between afterload and contractility in the newborn heart: evidence of homeometric autoregulation in the intact circulation. J Am Coll Cardiol 1995; 25:1428–1435.
7. Leach JK, Priola DV, Grimes LA, Skipper BJ. Shortening deactivation of cardiac muscle: physiological mechanisms and clinical implications. J Investig Med 1999; 47:369–377.
8. Lakatta EG. Starling's law of the heart is explained by an intimate interaction of muscle length and myofilament calcium activation. J Am Coll Card 1987; 10:1157–1164.
9. Bluhm WF, Kranias EG, Dillmann WH, Meyer M. Phospholamban: a major determinant of the cardiac force–frequency relationship. AmJ Physiol Heart Circ Physiol 2000; 278:H249–H255.
10. Luo W, Grupp IL, Harrer J, Ponniah S, Grupp G, Duffy JJ, Doetschman T, Kranias EG. Targeted ablation of the phospholamban gene is associated with markedly enhanced myocardial contractility and loss of beta-agonist stimulation. Circ Res 1994; 75:401–409.
11. Vila Petroff MG, Palomeque J, Mattiazzi AR. Na(+)–Ca^{2+} exchange function underlying contraction frequency inotropy in the cat myocardium. J Physiol 2003; 550:801–817.
12. Rudolph AM, Heymann MA. The circulation of the fetus in utero. Methods for studying distribution of blood flow, cardiac output and organ blood flow. Circ Res 1967; 21:163–184.
13. Teitel D, Rudolph AM. Perinatal oxygen delivery and cardiac function. Adv Pediatr 1985; 32:321–347.
14. Mahony L, Jones LR. Developmental changes in cardiac sarcoplasmic reticulum in sheep. J Biol Chem 1986; 261:15257–15265.
15. Liu W, Yasui K, Opthof T, Ishiki R, Lee JK, Kamiya K, Yokota M, Kodama I. Developmental changes of Ca$^{[2+]}$ handling in mouseventricular cells from early embryo to adulthood. Life Sci 2002; 71:1279–1292.
16. Artman M, Ichikawa H, Avkiran M, Coetzee WA. Na$^+$/Ca^{2+} exchange current density in cardiac myocytes from rabbits and guinea pigsduring postnatal development. Am J Physiol 1995; 268:H1714–H1722.
17. Chin TK, Christiansen GA, Galdwell JG, Thorbum J. Contribution of the sodium–calcium exchanger to contractions in immature rabbit ventricular myocytes. Pediatr Res 1997; 41:480–485.

18. Gilbert RD. Control of fetal cardiac output during changes in blood volume. Am J Physiol 1980; 238:H80–H86.
19. Hawkins J, Van Hare GF, Schmidt KG, Rudolph AM. Effects of increasing afterload on left ventricular output in fetal lambs. Circ Res 1989; 65:127–134.
20. Gilbert RD. Effects of afterload and baroreceptors on cardiac function in fetal sheep. J Dev Physiol 1982; 4:299–309.
21. Agata N, Tanaka H, Shigenobu K. Inotropic effects of ryanodine and nicardipine on fetal, neonatal and adult guinea-pig myocardium. Eur J Pharmacol 1994; 260:47–55.
22. Saggin L, Ausoni S, Gorza L, Sartore S, Schiaffino S. Troponin t switching in the developing rat heart. J Biol Chem 1988; 263:18488–18492.
23. Saggin L, Gorza L, Ausoni S, Schiaffino S. Troponin i switching in the developing heart. J Biol Chem 1989; 264:16299–16302.
24. L'Ecuyer TJ, Schulte D, Lin JJ. Thin filament changes during in vivo rat heart development. Pediatr Res 1991; 30:232–238.
25. Lompré AM, Nadal GB, Mahdavi V. Expression of the cardiac ventricular alpha- and beta-myosin heavy chain genes is developmentally and hormonally regulated. J Biol Chem 1984; 259:6437–6446.
26. Teitel DF, Dalinghaus M, Cassidy SC, Payne BD, Rudolph AM. In utero ventilation augments the left ventricular response to isoproterenol and volume loading in fetal sheep. Pediatr Res 1991; 29:466–472.
27. Romero T, Covell J, Friedman WF. A comparison of pressure–volume relations of the fetal, newborn, and adult heart. Am J Physiol 1972; 222:1285–1290.
28. Minczak BM, Wolfson MR, Santamore WP, Shaffer TH. Developmental changes in diastolic ventricular interaction. Pediatr Res 1988; 23:466–469.
29. Gest AL, Hansen TN, Moise AA, Hartley CJ. Atrial tachycardia causes hydrops in fetal lambs. Am J Physiol 1990; 258:H1159–H1163.
30. Teitel DF, Iwamoto HS, Rudolph AM. Effects of birth-related events on central blood flow patterns. Pediatr Res 1987; 22:557–566.
31. Lewinsky RM, Szwarc RS, Benson LN, Ritchie JW. Determinants of increased left ventricular output during in utero ventilation in fetal sheep. Pediatr Res 1994; 36:373–379.
32. Berning RA, Klautz RJ, Teitel DF. Perinatal left ventricular performance in fetal sheep: Interaction between oxygen ventilation and contractility. Pediatr Res 1997; 41:57–64.
33. Lister G, Walter TK, Versmold HT, Dallman PR, Rudolph AM. Oxygen delivery in lambs: cardiovascular and hematologic development. Am J Physiol 1979; 237:H668–H675.
34. Teitel DF, Iwamoto HS, Rudolph AM. Changes in the pulmonary circulation during birth-related events. Pediatr Res 1990; 27:372–378.
35. Toyono M, Harada K, Takahashi Y, Takada G. Maturational changes in left ventricular contractile state. Int J Cardiol 1998; 64:247–252.

36. Joyce JJ, Ross-Ascuitto NT, Ascuitto RJ. A direct comparison of right and left ventricular performance in the isolated neonatal pig heart. Pediatr Cardiol 2000; 21:216–222.
37. Bonnet V, Leoty C. An estimate of the participation of the sarcoplasmic reticulum in the intracellular Ca^{2+} regulation in adult and newborn ferret hearts. Comp Biochem A Physiol Physiol 1996; 115: 341–348.
38. Berman W Jr, Musselman J. Myocardial performance in the newborn lamb. Am J Physiol 1979; 237:H66–H70.
39. Minoura S, Gilbert RD. Postnatal change of cardiac function inlambs: effects of ganglionic block and afterload. J Dev Physiol 1987; 9: 123–135.
40. Teitel DF, Sidi D, Chin T, Brett C, Heymann MA, Rudolph AM. Developmental changes in myocardial contractile reserve in the lamb. Pediatr Res 1985; 19:948–955.
41. Cassidy SC, Chan DP, Allen HD. Left ventricular systolic function, arterial elastance, and ventricular–vascular coupling: a developmental study in piglets. Pediatr Res 1997; 42:273–281.
42. Mahony L. Maturation of calcium transport in cardiac sarcoplasmic reticulum. Pediatr Res 1988; 24:639–643.
43. Nakanishi T, Jarmakani JM. Developmental changes in myocardial mechanical function and subcellular organelles. Am J Physiol 1984; 246:H615–H625.
44. Tanaka H, Sekine T, Nishimaru K, Shigenobu K. Role of sarcoplasmic reticulum in myocardial contraction of neonatal and adult mice. Comp Biochem Physiol A Mol Integr Physiol 1998; 120:431–438.
45. Vornanen M. Contribution of sarcolemmal calcium current tototal cellular calcium in postnatally developing rat heart. Cardiovasc Res 1996; 32:400–410.
46. Alves CM, Silva CL, Moura GM, Noel F. Decrease in the ratio ofhigh-to low-affinity isozymes of $(Na^+ + K^+)$-ATPase during thedevelopment of rat cardiac ventricles. Braz J Med Biol Res 1995; 28:363–367.
47. Berman W, Christensen D. Effects of acute preload and afterload stress on myocardial function in newborn and adult sheep. Biol Neonate 1983; 43:61–66.
48. Kaufman TM, Horton JW, White DJ, Mahony L. Age-related changes in myocardial relaxation and sarcoplasmic reticulum function. Am J Physiol 1990; 259:H309–H316.
49. Klopfenstein HS, Rudolph AM. Postnatal changes in the circulation and responses to volume loading in sheep. Circ Res 1978; 42:839–845.
50. Van Hare GF, Hawkins JA, Schmidt KG, Rudolph AM. The effects of increasing mean arterial pressure on left ventricular output in newborn lambs. Circ Res 1990; 67:78–83.
51. Shaddy RE, Tyndall MR, Teitel DF, Li C, Rudolph AM. Regulation of cardiac output with controlled heart rate in newborn lambs. Pediatr Res 1988; 24:577–582.

52. Fisher DJ, Gross DM. The effect of atrial pacing-induced tachycardia on left ventricular contractile function in conscious newborn and adult sheep. Pediatr Res 1983; 17:651–656.

53. Klautz RJ, Baan J, Teitel DF. Contribution of synchronized atrialsystole to left ventricular contraction in the newborn pig heart. Pediatr Res 1998; 43:331–337.

54. Chen F, Wetzel GT, Friedman WF, Klitzner TS. Developmental changes in the effects of pH on contraction and Ca^{2+} current in rabbit heart. J Mol Cell Cardiol 1996; 28:635–642.

55. Nakanishi T, Seguchi M, Tsuchiya T, Yasukouchi S, Takao A. Effect of acidosis on intracellular pH and calcium concentration in the newborn and adult rabbit myocardium. Circ Res 1990; 67:111–123.

56. Fisher DJ. Comparative effects of metabolic acidemia and hypoxemia on cardiac output and regional blood flows in unanesthetized newborn lambs. Pediatr Res 1986; 20:756–760.

57. Fisher DJ, Heymann MA, Rudolph AM. Myocardial consumption of oxygen and carbohydrates in newborn sheep. Pediatr Res 1981; 15: 843–846.

3

Cellular and Molecular Aspects of Myocardial Dysfunction

STEVEN M. SCHWARTZ

Division of Cardiology,
Children's Hospital Medical Center,
Cincinnati, Ohio, U.S.A.

Pediatric cardiology is often the practice of applied cardiovascular physiology. For many, the logical, engineering-like interplay of the predominant forces that influence cardiovascular function become almost intuitive and form the basis for the appeal of cardiology as a clinical practice. We are well aware of the importance of systemic vascular resistance, pulmonary vascular resistance, preload, afterload, and contractility and how they affect cardiac output, chamber remodeling, tissue oxygen delivery, and response to various drugs. The cellular and molecular processes that underlie normal and altered cardiovascular physiology often seem less accessible and more remote from clinical practice. Nevertheless, complex and highly integrated pathways of signal transduction and protein synthesis underlie the physiology that is so apparent to the clinician. New elements of these processes are constantly being elucidated and indicate the importance of structural elements, contractile proteins, ion channels, and even nonmyocyte cardiac cells as vital components in the process of myocardial adaptation and the clinical syndrome of heart failure. New therapeutic targets are emerging from this research, and advanced understanding of conventional drugs like angiotensin-converting enzyme (ACE) inhibitors and β-adrenergic agonists, and antagonists is helping to refine their uses. It is thus becoming progressively important for the clinician to understand the multiple mechanisms by which myocardial dysfunction can occur.

Primary myocardial dysfunction in neonates and children is generally observed following surgery involving cardiopulmonary bypass (CPB) associated with cardioplegia and myocardial ischemia, or as the consequence of either a genetic or acquired (e.g. postmyocarditis) cardiomyopathy. Studies of numerous models of genetic cardiomyopathy, pressure overload hypertrophy, and ischemic heart disease have yielded significant insight into many of the cellular and molecular pathways involved in the progression of myocardial dysfunction. The challenge for the pediatric cardiologist is to apply information from these types of studies to the care of pediatric patients while recognizing ways in which the pediatric heart differs from the adult heart. The purpose of this chapter is to review the key elements involved in generating cardiac contraction and relaxation and the cellular and molecular alterations that occur when the heart is faced with intrinsic changes in loading or function. It is these changes that underlie both the compensatory and decompensatory aspects of heart failure.

CELLULAR AND MOLECULAR BASIS
OF CARDIAC CONTRACTILITY

To understand myocardial dysfunction, it is first necessary to be familiar with the basic molecular and cellular biology of the cardiomyocyte and the cardiac cycle. Myocardial contraction is initiated by a large increase in available intracellular calcium, which, in turn, leads to movement of the contractile elements of the sarcomere. A sharp decrease in calcium availability then brings about diastolic relaxation.

Contractile Elements

The primary contractile elements of the sarcomere (Fig. 1) are the thin filament, comprised primarily of monomers of α-actin arranged into two long, intertwined strands that are anchored at the Z-discs, and the thick filament, consisting of myosin molecules joined together at the tail with the globular heads protruding from this central axis. In most mammalian species including humans, both actin and myosin exist in several isoforms the expression of which is regulated in both a

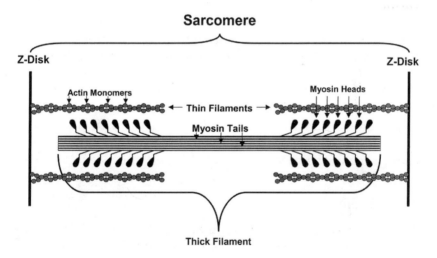

Figure 1 *Organization of the sarcomere.* The sarcomere is composed of thin filaments made up of two intertwined strands of repeating actin monomers, and thick filaments made up the tails of myosin molecules. The heads of the myosin molecules protrude from the thick filament and are poised to attach to the actin strands. The actin strands are anchored at the z-disks that form the lateral edges of the sarcomere.

tissue- and developmentally specific manner. Actin isoforms include both cardiac and skeletal α-actin. In the fetal and neo-natal human ventricle, the majority of actin is cardiac α-actin, but as the heart matures, a progressively greater proportion of skeletal α-actin is incorporated into the sarcomere (1). Myosin similarly exists in different isoforms, although the regulation of myosin is somewhat more complex than actin. The myosin molecule is constructed from two heavy and four light chains. The heavy chains form the rod of the molecule that comprises the thick filament. The cardiac myosin heavy chain exists as either the α- or β-myosin heavy chain. Because each myosin molecule contains two heavy chains, there are three isoforms of myosin. The V1 isoform contains two α chains, the V2 isoform contains one α and one β chain and the V3 isoform contains two β chains. The V3 isoform is the predominant myosin isoform present in human ventricle during development and throughout maturation (2). In rodents, the V3 isoform predominates in the fetal heart but the adult ventricle is virtually all V1 (3), a fact that may limit the applicability of some rodent models of heart failure. The myosin head is composed of the light chains and generates the movement of the actin filament along the length of the thick filament. The myosin head binds to actin and undergoes a conformational change driven by the hydrolysis of ATP (Fig. 2). The cycle of attachment of the myosin head to actin and hydrolysis of ATP with pivoting of the myosin head causes movement of the actin filament and shortening of the sarcomere.

Troponin and Tropomyosin

Troponin and tropomyosin regulate the binding of myosin to actin (Fig. 3). Tropomyosin winds around the thin filament in the groove between the two strands of actin monomers. Tropomyosin strengthens the actin filament and increases myosin binding. The troponin complex consists of three elements: troponin I (TnI), troponin C (TnC), and troponin T (TnT). The troponin complex makes the binding of actin and myosin a calcium-dependent process. TnI inhibits the interaction of actin and myosin. There are two isoforms of

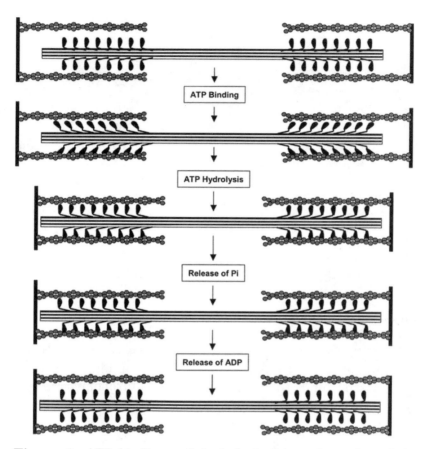

Figure 2 *ATP binding and hydrolysis drives shortening of the sarcomere.* Contraction of the sarcomere occurs when myosin binds adenosine triphosphate (ATP). The myosin head undergoes a conformational change and binds to actin. Hydrolysis of ATP drives pivoting of the myosin head causing shortening of the sarcomere. Pyrophosphate (Pi) and adenosine diphosphate (ADP) are then released by myosin allowing release of actin from myosin. The cycle repeats throughout systole.

TnI: cardiac and skeletal muscle isoforms. The neonatal heart contains mostly the skeletal isoform, but the cardiac isoform predominates as the heart matures (4). TnI is affected by numerous stimuli, including β-adrenergic receptor activation and ischemia–reperfusion injury (5–8) and the appearance of

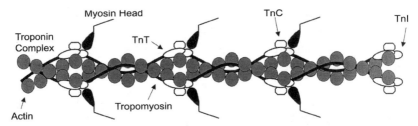

Figure 3 *Tropomyosin and the troponin complex.* Troponin and tropomyosin regulate the binding of myosin to actin. Tropomyosin winds around the thin filament in the groove between the two strands of actin monomers to strengthen the actin filament and increase myosin binding. The troponin complex consists of three elements: troponin I (TnI), troponin C (TnC), and troponin T (TnT). TnI inhibits the interaction of actin and myosin. TnC binds calcium and initiates a conformational shift that releases inhibition of actin–myosin binding caused by TnI. TnT binds the troponin complex to tropomyosin.

cardiac TnI in serum is a highly specific marker of myocardial injury (9). TnC binds calcium and initiates a conformational shift that releases inhibition of actin–myosin binding caused by TnI. TnT binds the troponin complex to tropomyosin.

Anchoring Proteins

The contractile apparatus within the cardiomyocyte must be able to communicate with the extracellular matrix. This communication can translate external biomechanical stress, such as pressure overload, to the cytoplasm and can also signal intracellular events to neighboring cells. Some of the most important proteins responsible for this function are the integrins, a family of heterodimeric transmembrane receptors composed of α and β subunits. Because of the large number of different subunits and splice variants, there are numerous potential α/β heterodimers, but only a subset has been detected in the heart. Seven of the at least 18 α subunits and the β_1 isoform have been reliably detected in myocardial tissue, although there is some suggestion that the β_3 and β_5 isoforms may also be present (10). Like many other structural elements, there is developmental regulation of integrin expression, and isoform expression may change in response to a variety of stimuli (11). In addition to structural anchoring proteins, it is important to realize that other signaling molecules may also be anchored to either the cell membrane or other membranous structures within the cell. Ion channels and protein kinases may be anchored in place so as to effectively compartmentalize their effects. For example, protein kinase A (PKA), a major signaling molecule in adrenergic receptor signaling, can have numerous effects depending on the target molecules. The specific substrates for PKA depend largely on their proximity to the activated receptor and PKA, a relationship maintained by A-kinase anchoring proteins (AKAP) (12,13). Other proteins can be regulated in similar fashion, and thus compartmentalization is an essential principle to understand the means by which cardiac function can be manipulated by various agents and/or diseases.

Calcium Cycling

The binding and release of actin and myosin, and therefore cardiac contraction and relaxation, are mediated by cyclic fluctuations in cytoplasmic calcium concentration. The cardiomyocyte is highly specialized to allow rapid release and resequestration of calcium. The degree to which these calcium fluxes are dependent on intracellular vs. extracellular sources of calcium is subject to maturational forces and may explain some differences between neonatal and adult heart responses to various stimuli.

Calcium influx into the cardiomyocyte is initiated during phase 2 of the action potential with the slow inward calcium current generated by the L-type calcium channels (Fig. 4). These channels consist of multiple subunits with the α_{1c} subunit forming the core of the channel. The other subunits modify the function of the α-subunit and potentially allow modification of channel activity in response to stimuli such as β-AR activation (14–16). The channel is voltage-gated, which means when a certain level of depolarization is achieved, the channel opens and calcium flows into the cell.

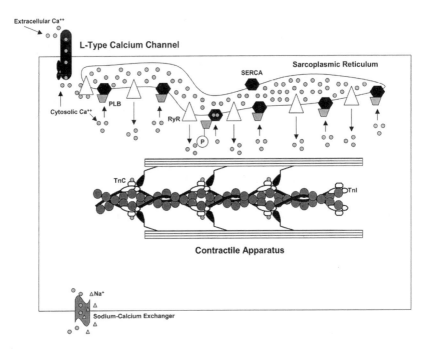

Figure 4 *Myocardial calcium cycling.* Extracellular calcium enters the cell through voltage-gated (L-type) calcium channels on the cell membrane. The influx of extracellular calcium initiates massive calcium release from the sarcoplasmic reticulum via the ryanodine receptor (RyR). Cytosolic calcium binds to troponin C (TnC) causing a conformational change in troponin I (TnI) and allowing myosin to bind to actin and initiate sarcomere shortening. In diastole, calcium is resequestered in the sarcoplasmic reticulum by the sarcoplasmic reticulum calcium ATPase (serca). Serca itself is gated by phospholamban, which in its dephosphorylated state inhibits reuptake of calcium by serca. A small amount of calcium is pumped out of the cell by sodium–calcium exchanger on the cell surface.

In the neonatal heart, the increase in cytosolic calcium from the L-type calcium channels contributes directly and significantly to the calcium that binds to TnC and causes cardiac contraction (excitation–contraction coupling) (17,18). The increase in intracellular calcium caused by the slow inward calcium current activates the ryanodine receptor and causes further calcium release from the primary intracellular store of calcium, the sarcoplasmic reticulum (SR) (Fig. 4). In the adult heart, the calcium released from the SR accounts for the overwhelming majority of calcium that is bound by TnC, minimizing the direct effect of the L-type channels on contractility.

The switch from systolic contraction to diastolic relaxation is initiated by resequestration of the calcium from the cytosol back into the SR and/or the extracellular space. The majority of calcium removal is via the SR calcium ATPase (SERCA) (Fig. 4). This pump is present on the membrane of the SR and actively transports calcium back into the SR. The pump is regulated by the multimeric protein phospholamban, which in the dephosphorylated state inhibits reuptake of calcium by SERCA (19,20). Phospholamban can be phosphorylated by any of three protein kinases including PKA (also known as cAMP-dependent protein kinase). A much smaller amount of calcium is removed from the cell by the sodium–calcium exchanger. The sodium–calcium exchanger may have increased importance in the neonatal heart trans-sarcolemmal calcium fluxes because of the relative immaturity of the SR system (21–23).

Nonmyocytes

In addition to contractile cells, the myocardium contains fibroblasts, vascular cells including endothelium, and noncellular elements such as collagen. These cells and proteins participate both actively and passively in determining systolic and diastolic properties of the myocardium and in signaling cascades that result in functional and structural responses to various stressors.

In the healthy heart, collagen exists as a fine latticework surrounding myocytes and blood vessels. Collagen fibers and the cytoskeleton of the cellular components of the myocardium impart a passive elastic quality to the myocardium as a whole, which has important implications for diastolic function. As the ventricle begins to fill in early diastole, active relaxation due to calcium sequestration is the primary determinant of myocardial compliance (24). At high filling volumes, as can occur in volume overload lesions and myocardial dysfunction, a greater portion of the axial stress is borne by collagenous elements of the myocardium (25,26). Many of the signals that inform cardiomyocytes of increased load may be channeled through the extracellular matrix via connections between this matrix and the myocyte. There is evidence of signaling between myocytes, fibroblasts, and endothelial cells both through biomechanical transduction as well as paracrine release of such potent growth stimuli as angiotensin II (27–30). The end result is that increases in loading stimulate not only cardiomyocyte hypertrophy, but also fibroblast proliferation and collagen production. This is important from a clinical standpoint because cardiac dysfunction is associated with significant fibrosis, and loss of myocytes is likely to have only a limited response to therapy primarily targeted to improve myocyte function such as inotropic or lusitropic agents.

ACUTE MYOCARDIAL DYSFUNCTION

Ischemia–reperfusion injury associated with cardiopulmonary bypass (CPB) and aortic cross-clamping is the most common cause of acute myocardial dysfunction in the pediatric population. Much of the work detailing the effects of ischemia and reperfusion on the myocardium has been performed with models more applicable to myocardial infarction, the most common adult cause of ischemia–reperfusion injury. Nevertheless, there is great potential to develop effective treatment and prevention strategies for pediatric patients. Compared to the situation with myocardial infarction, surgically related ischemia–reperfusion injury occurs at a predetermined, planned time and is not associated with significant necrosis or scarring. However, the differences between the immature and mature myocardium, in terms of contractile proteins, troponins, and calcium handling, suggest the need to study these processes in the immature heart.

Inflammatory Reaction

Cardiopulmonary bypass is associated with alterations in cytokines and endothelial function characteristic of an inflammatory response (31). Peripheral blood leukocytes become activated and attach to endothelial surfaces by means of adhesion molecules that are upregulated during CPB (32). Leukocytes then roll on the endothelial surface and migrate into the extravascular space through separations in endothelial cell junctions. The stimulus for the inflammatory response may have several components including endotoxin release and/or activation of complement caused by exposure of blood to air or the artificial surfaces of the bypass circuit (33–35). Although much work has been done to define the nature of the inflammatory response to CPB, a clear understanding of the exact cytokines involved, the cause and source of their release, the mechanisms by which they alter myocardial function and potential preventive strategies remain elusive.

The proinflammatory cytokines most commonly implicated in CBP-related myocardial ischemia–reperfusion injury are IL-6 and IL-8 (36–39). Generation of TNF-α by the heart upon release of the aortic cross-clamp is a possible stimulus for IL-6 and IL-8 release (39–41), but other data suggest that TNF-α may not be necessary to induce IL-6 and IL-8 production by the myocardium (36). The anti-inflammatory cytokine IL-10 may also increase after surgery and correlates with the duration of CPB (42) and may offer some protection against inflammatory injury. The exact mechanisms by which inflammatory mediators depress myocardial function is unknown, but TNF-α decreases phosphorylation levels of both phospholamban and TnI in isolated cardiomyocytes (43). Neutrophil adhesion molecules and chemoattractant proteins that are stimulated by the inflammatory process have also been shown to be associated with cardiomyocyte apoptosis (44).

Further information regarding the relationship of a systemic inflammatory response to myocardial function can be gained from studies of sepsis. The systemic inflammatory response accompanying sepsis is generally associated with significantly greater production of inflammatory mediators than is CPB. It has been observed that sepsis is associated with decreased inotropy, although cardiac index may rise as a consequence of decreased systemic vascular resistance (45). Similar to CPB, septic shock is associated with increased TNF-α and IL-6 among other cytokines (46). Myocardial depression can result from increased nitric oxide production induced by IL-6 or alterations in calcium fluxes caused directly by TNF-α (47).

Protease Activation

Despite emphasis on inflammatory mediators in studies of CPB related to myocardial depression, there are also data that suggest inflammation may not be the only cause of post-CPB myocardial dysfunction. Studies of isolated, ischemic, buffer-reperfused hearts have shown that TnI is degraded by the calcium-dependent cysteine protease calpain I upon myocardial reperfusion (7,8). Buffer reperfusion inherently lacks leukocytes, which are thought to be crucial in maintaining the inflammatory response, but these experiments have shown that TnI is degraded after reperfusion with calcium-containing buffer. The proteolysis of TnI is not the consequence of ischemia alone, as ischemic, nonreperfused hearts do not exhibit TnI degradation (8). The appearance of degraded TnI is associated with decreased contractile function (5), and other studies have shown that myocardial trabeculae exposed to calpain I in vitro exhibit the decreased calcium responsiveness characteristic of stunned myocardium (48). Furthermore, transgenic mice that overexpress the truncated form of TnI develop a cardiomyopathy, strongly suggesting that TnI degradation is sufficient to induce myocardial dysfunction in the absence of other CPB-related stimuli (49).

Calpain is normally bound to its inhibitor, calpastatin. Upon activation by calcium, calpain is released by calpastatin and cleaves TnI at the C-terminus to produce the degradation fragment TnI (1–193). In studies of dysfunctional myocardium in humans and other species, several smaller degradation products have also been demonstrated (7,50). A recent analysis of TnI degradation in humans undergoing coronary artery bypass grafting showed several patients had TnI fragments present in the myocardium even before CPB (50). Interestingly, some patients developed further degradation after CPB, while others had less fragmentation. Evidence of TnI fragmentation can also be detected in the serum of patients with acute myocardial infarction (51). The issue of calpain and calpastatin activities after CPB may be of even more importance in children, particularly neonates, as calpastatin has been shown to ameliorate inactivation of L-type calcium channels in cell-free patch systems (52). Neonatal pigs are much more prone to TnI degradation and loss of calpastatin in association with CPB-related myocardial ischemia than are more mature pigs (5), implying this mechanism may be particularly relevant to the myocardial dysfunction that can occur after neonatal surgery. These findings suggest that inhibition of calpain and/or enhancement of calpastatin may be useful targets for treatment or prevention of CBP-related ischemia–reperfusion injury. Clearly, much work remains to be done regarding this potentially important cause of myocardial dysfunction.

Treatment

Although targeted anti-inflammatory and/or anti-protease strategies remain elusive, several commonly used agents have important cellular and molecular mechanisms of action that may be particularly important in children. Steroids can inhibit TNF-α and IL-8 production and enhance IL-10 generation and are associated with improved ventricular function after CPB (40,53). Decreased inflammation induced by steroid pretreatment has been associated with a reduction in apoptotic myocytes after CPB-related ischemia in neonatal piglets (44), and with improved indices of oxygen delivery during the first 2 hr after CPB in children (54).

In addition to their known anti-inflammatory properties, steroids are a potent stimulus for myosin synthesis and may enhance L-type calcium channel function (55,56). Steroids have also been shown to preserve calpastatin and prevent TnI degradation in neonatal piglets subjected to CPB and

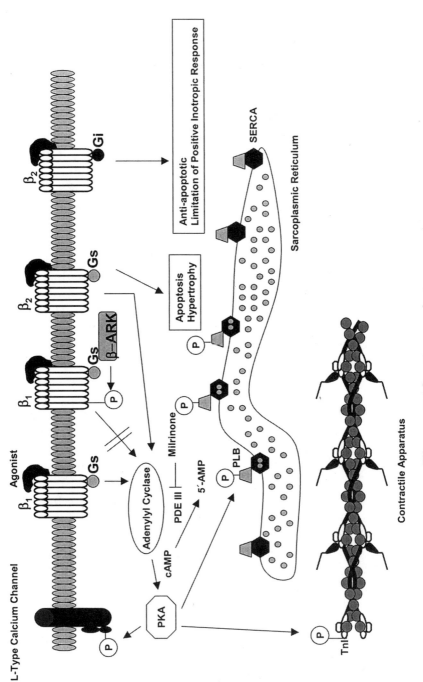

Figure 5 (*Caption on facing page.*)

myocardial ischemia (5). Interestingly, steroids were able to limit TnI degradation induced by exogenous calpain in cultured cardiomyocytes, suggesting this property of steroids is unrelated to any anti-inflammatory properties. Ultrafiltration has been speculated to remove TNF-α, IL-6, and other cytokines, but the clinical importance of this is unproven (57,58). Targeted interference with the inflammatory process by blocking leukocyte adhesion to sialyl Lewis[x], a neutrophil-bound oligosaccharide ligand, has been effective in animal models but has yet to prove useful in clinical practice (59).

The use of β-adrenergic agonists and phosphodiesterase (PDE) inhibitors after CPB also affects contractile function at several levels. β-Adrenergic agonists bind to the G_s coupled β-adrenergic receptor and activate adenylyl cyclase (Fig. 5). Protein kinase A then phosphorylates TnI, phospholamban, and L-type calcium channels (60,61). Consequently, the L-type calcium channels increase calcium transport, the troponin complex becomes more calcium responsive and calcium is resequestered into the SR more rapidly (19,61–63). Both systolic and diastolic ventricular functions are enhanced.

Myocardial cAMP is degraded by PDE III. This enzyme can be inhibited by specific PDE inhibitors such as milrinone and amrinone. This provides a receptor-independent mechanism to bring about the same salutary effects as β-adrenergic agonists, even in the presence of decreased β-adrenergic

---

Figure 5 *(Facing page) β-Adrenergic signaling. $β_1$-* and *$β_2$-* Adrenergic receptors couple to stimulatory G-proteins (Gs). Agonist binding activates adenylyl cyclase, which increases cyclic AMP (cAMP) and activates protein kinase A (PKA). PKA phosphorylates L-type calcium channels, phospholamban (PLB), and troponin I (TnI) among other proteins. cAMP is degraded to 5'-AMP by phosphodiesterase III (PDE III) which is inhibited by milrinone. Activation of Gs also promotes apoptosis and hypertrophy, whereas activation of the inhibitory G protein, Gi by $β_2$ receptors has anti-apoptotic effects and may limit the positive inotropic response to β-adrenergic agonists. Increased levels of the β-adrenergic receptor kinase (β-ARK) phosphorylate the receptors and render them less responsive to agonist.

receptor responsiveness or downregulation, which can occur after CPB (64). PDE inhibitors may also enhance calcium flux via reverse activity of the sodium–calcium exchanger and improve ventricular function by a mechanism unrelated to increases in cAMP (65,66). As noted previously, increased influx of extracellular calcium may be particularly significant in neonates.

MYOCARDIAL COMPENSATION AND CHRONIC HEART FAILURE

In the presence of chronic pressure and/or volume overload ventricular adaptation occurs, generally in the form of hypertrophy and/or dilation. It has long been accepted that this type of myocardial hypertrophy is compensatory, enabling the heart to meet the increased workload while minimizing wall stress. In the presence of structural congenital heart disease, the development of hypertrophy and/or dilation is often regarded as an indication for intervention, but is not generally recognized as being a pathologic process in and of itself. Hypertrophy and chamber enlargement in the absence of increased workload are generally referred to as cardiomyopathies, with an inherent implication that this type of cardiac enlargement is decompensatory. Over the last decade, it has become increasingly clear that many of the cellular and molecular processes that result in "compensatory" hypertrophy are quite similar to the processes that occur in "decompensatory" cardiac enlargement. Myocardial pressure and/or volume overload initiate a complex series of signaling cascades that transmit the chemical or mechanical stimulus for cell growth and protein synthesis to the nucleus where DNA transcription takes place. Protein synthesis, however, is not limited to structural and contractile elements. Collagen production (25,67), alteration of receptors (68,69), and calcium handling proteins (70–73) and apoptosis (74) may all be initiated during this process of apparent compensation, thus planting the seeds of myocardial decompensation and failure firmly within the ground of "compensatory" hypertrophy.

This interplay between molecular signals that initiate hypertrophy and those that cause the transition to heart failure has left open the question of whether or not hypertrophy really bestows any compensatory benefit. The complexities of this issue are demonstrated by an experiment in which transgenic mice with deficient β-adrenergic signaling that were incapable of mounting a hypertrophic response to pressure overload were nevertheless able to maintain ventricular function better than wild-type controls after the imposition of a significant increase in wall-stress (75). Since mice that have altered β-adrenergic signaling may also be unable to activate many of the underlying initiators of ventricular dysfunction, the animals may have been protected from failure, rather than simply deficient in hypertrophy. Even though interpretation of these data is limited because of the interplay between the mechanisms of hypertrophy and failure, the compensatory role of myocardial hypertrophy remains open to debate.

Information regarding biomechanical stress must be sensed by the cell directly, or communicated to the cardiomyocyte by activation of neurohormonal pathways. Activation of specific pathways then enables intracellular messenger molecules to enter the nucleus and promote protein synthesis. A complete review of all known signaling molecules that can generate cardiac hypertrophy in response to pressure overload would be a confusing "alphabet soup" of terms and would no doubt be out of date quickly. Conceptually, however, it is important to understand that hypertrophic signaling is essentially a web-like cascade. Extracellular signals trigger one or two proteins, generally kinases that phosphorylate other kinases. This type of reaction proceeds for several generations with each kinase phosphorylating other kinases so that by the time the signals are ready to be transmitted to the nucleus and alter protein synthesis, multiple cellular functions can be affected and there is a significant overlap in the end result regardless of the specific initiating stimulus. Furthermore, blocking one step in the process is often insufficient to completely prevent or reverse the entire spectrum of cellular processes activated by altered loading. As a result, extrapolation of data from studies of clearly defined disease entities or populations should be done cautiously.

Although the precise nature by which biomechanical stress results in protein synthesis and cardiac hypertrophy is not yet known, certain aspects of the ways in which signals associated with increased load can be transmitted through the extracellular matrix or sensed within the cell have been well delineated. This probably occurs via anchoring proteins and other elements of the cytoskeleton (76). The elucidation of integrin function is instructive as a model for how such signaling occurs. Binding of ligand, such as laminin, to the extracellular integrin domain brings the integrin into communication with the extracellular matrix. The cytoplasmic domain of the integrins communicates with elements of the cytoskeleton via α-actinin which binds actin directly, and talin which is connected to the thin filament via vinculin (Fig. 6) (11). Furthermore, and perhaps more importantly, integrins are bound to numerous molecules that are part of comprehensive enzymatic cascades. For example, integrin signaling can activate focal adhesion kinase (FAK), which may help mediate the hypertrophic response to adrenergic agonists and endothelin (77–80). Focal adhesion kinase also offers a potential link between the integrins and the process of apoptosis (81).

A detailed understanding of the molecular biology of hypertrophic signaling remains more essential for the basic scientist than the clinician. Nevertheless, there are certain pathways and molecules that are currently therapeutic targets or may become targets in the near future. Angiotensin II and endothelin-1 are both potent stimuli for myocardial hypertrophy in pressure overload (29,82,83). Inhibition of angiotensin signaling, either by inhibition of angiotensin-converting enzyme (ACE) or angiotensin receptor antagonism, has become standard of care for heart failure patients. Large clinical studies have shown ACE inhibition in congestive heart failure is associated with decreased hospitalization and improved survival (84). Animal studies indicate that ACE inhibitors can prevent or reverse pressure overload hypertrophy and ventricular fibrosis (83,85). Endothelin

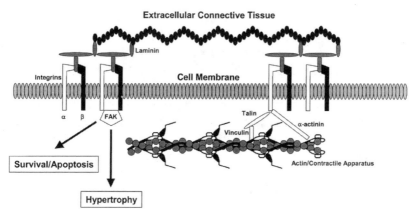

Figure 6 *Integrin signaling of biomechanical stress.* The extracellular domain of integrins can bind ligands such as laminin that communicate directly with the extracellular matrix. Signals about stress can then be transmitted to the contractile apparatus via proteins such as α-actinin (which binds directly to actin) or talin (which binds to actin via vinculin). Integrins can also transmit extracellular signals to signaling molecules such as focal adhesion kinase (FAK) that leads to downstream effects on cell survival and hypertrophy.

receptor antagonists such as bosentan have more recently become available, and although data supporting their use in pulmonary hypertension continue to accumulate, results in congestive heart failure are mixed (86–88).

The role of the renin–angiotensin system in the development of myocardial hypertrophy and failure has been appreciated for many years. Early studies of ACE inhibition for patients with congestive heart failure revealed increased survival compared to other afterload reducing agents (84,89). Numerous subsequent studies have shown that the myocardium is capable of synthesizing angiotensinogen, ACE, and angiotensin receptors (29,90,91). The heart may also be capable of generating renin, but this has been more controversial (92,93). Failing hearts have increased ACE activity, and exposure of the myocardium to angiotensin II in experimental models causes hypertrophy independent of pressure load (90,94). Upregulation of the renin–angiotensin system has also been associated with myocardial fibrosis (91,95). Furthermore, stretching of cardiomyocytes may cause the local release of angiotensin II from the myocyte (28). Subsequent activation of the angiotensin II type 1 receptor on the cardiomyocyte results in a cascade of phosphorylation reactions that leads to transcription of several genes involved in cell growth and hypertrophy (96). Activation of the angiotensin II type 1 receptor on the surface of myocardial fibroblasts induces cell growth and collagen production (91).

Despite overwhelming evidence of the importance of the local myocardial renin–angiotensin system in the development of myocardial dysfunction, it has been demonstrated that hypertrophy can be induced even in the presence of ACE inhibition or angiotensin receptor blockade (97). In all likelihood, the renin–angiotensin system interacts with other important pathways involved in cardiomyocyte growth and function to compensate for increased loading conditions or genetically abnormal contractile proteins. Endothelin-1 is a potent positive inotrope and may have a compensatory role in the face of increased loading conditions (98). Unlike healthy cardiomyocytes, failing myocytes no longer synthesize endothelin-1 in response to angiotensin II (99). Therefore, it appears that disruption of myocyte architecture, loading, or molecular function (or even abnormalities of nonmyocyte cardiac cells) can lead to decompensatory consequences of what initially were compensatory responses. The renin–angiotensin system provides a potential pharmacologic target to intervene in this cascade of detrimental events.

Both angiotensin and endothelin, as well as several other mediators of cardiac hypertrophy, bind to G-protein coupled receptors (GPCR) on the cardiomyocyte membrane and then activate the mitogen-activated protein kinase (MAPK) pathway (Fig. 7). The MAPK pathway is well established as a model of signal amplification and crosstalk and is a particularly important signaling cascade because of the large number of stimuli that result in its activation. Understanding of this type of signaling is thus helpful in providing a framework for understanding how biomechanical and biochemical

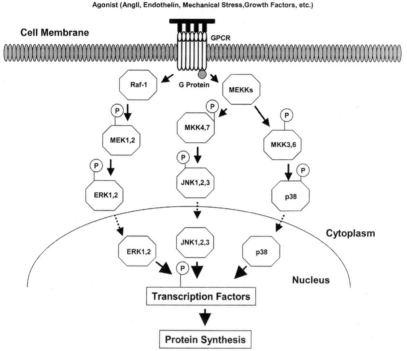

Figure 7 *Mitogen-activated protein kinase (MAPK) signaling.* Binding of agonist to any one of a number of G-protein coupled receptors (GPCR) can initiate the MAPK signaling cascades. Initial activation of the MAPK pathway leads to signal amplification and eventual phosphorylation of ERK1,2, JNK1,2,3, and p38, which are then able to translocate from the cytoplasm to the nucleus and phosphorylate transcription factors and other mediators of protein synthesis.

signals stimulate protein synthesis and the actual processes of hypertrophy, remodeling, and alterations in myocardial function. In the MAPK pathway, extracellular signals such as angiotensin (100,101), endothelin (102,103), growth factors (100,104), and stress stimuli (105) among others activate protein kinases that phosphorylate other protein kinases. Phosphorylation induces conformational changes converting these kinases to their active state and rendering them capable of phosphorylating the next set of protein kinases. This sequence eventually leads to phosphorylation of proteins such as ERK, JNK, and p38 that are able to translocate to the nucleus upon phosphorylation in the cytoplasm (106,107). Once in the nucleus these proteins phosphorylate numerous transcription factors that directly induce transcription of a variety of genes including those that regulate myocardial function via membrane receptors, calcium handling, and intracellular signaling. Transcription of sarcomeric proteins such as actin and myosin is also induced by these activated transcription factors and thus cardiac hypertrophy is able to occur in response to this wide variety of stimuli.

The new proteins added to the sarcomere may be different isoforms of myosin or actin than are present in the mature heart. Rodent models of cardiac hypertrophy show the isoforms of actin and myosin present in the fetal heart, β-myosin heavy chain, and α-skeletal actin, re-emerge during the development of cardiac hypertrophy (108). The β-myosin heavy chain has a slower velocity of shortening, but better energetics and calcium response than does α-myosin (109,110), which predominates in the normal adult ventricle. Therefore, one component of functional alterations that occur during cardiac remodeling may be the altered composition of the sarcomere in terms of actin and myosin isoforms. An important caveat however is that although there is some evidence that hypertrophied human ventricles have a relative increase in β-myosin compared to α-myosin, the human ventricle is composed of greater than 90% β-myosin starting in early fetal life and persisting through adulthood. The importance of isoform switching in human hypertrophy therefore remains unclear.

Hypertrophy and failure also involve important alterations of calcium handling. During hypertrophy, there tends to be an increased phospholamban to SERCA ratio (111,112). Several studies have demonstrated significant changes in calcium handling proteins such as SERCA and phospholamban, which alter calcium availability to the failing myocardium. Although the exact nature of the abnormalities may be model or disease specific as both increases and decreases in phospholamban phosphorylation have been reported (113,114), alteration of calcium handling proteins is likely to be crucial in chronic myocardial dysfunction. For example, mice with a particular form of cardiomyopathy show significant functional improvement with either ablation of the phospholamban gene or overexpression of a mutant (nonactive) phospholamban (115).

Cardiac hypertrophy and failure increase the diastolic availability of calcium (76,116), via these changes in SERCA and phospholamban, as well as other calcium handling proteins. This can directly depress diastolic relaxation, but it also is a key component of multiple mechanisms by which cardiomyocyte structure and function are altered. Sustained elevation of intracelluiar calcium is sensed by calmodulin (Fig. 8). Binding of calcium to calmodulin activates calcium/calmodulin-dependent protein kinase (CaMK) that subsequently activates an important downstream effector,

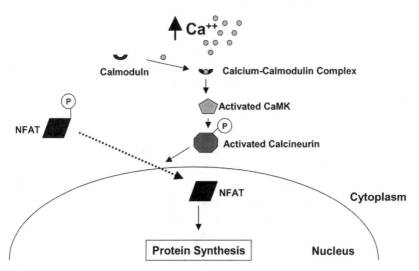

Figure 8 *Calcium-mediated hypertrophic signaling.* Persistently elevated intracellular calcium levels lead to binding of calcium to calmodulin and activation of calcium/calmodulin-dependent protein kinase (CaMK). Activated CaMK phosphorylates calcineurin, which then dephosphorylates nuclear factor of activated T-cells (NFAT). In its dephosphorylated state, NFAT can translocate from the cytoplasm to the nucleus and initiate protein synthesis.

calcineurin (117–119). Activated calcineurin dephosphorylates nuclear factor of activated T cells (NFAT), a DNA transcription factor, that is then able to translocate from the
cytoplasm to the nucleus and initiate protein synthesis much
in the same way MAPK activation leads to structural and
functional changes in the myocyte. In addition to the changes
that occur in diastolic calcium levels, there is also evidence
that systolic peak calcium is decreased (120). This might be
because of impaired L-type calcium channel function (121)
or because of changes in the ryanodine receptor (122,123).
Interestingly, these changes in calcium cycling appear to be
recoverable in hypertrophied hearts that function well, but
may become permanent once the myocyte begins to fail.

Another important GPCR system in the processes of
myocardial compensation and failure is the β-adrenergic
system (Fig. 5). β-Adrenergic agonists improve myocardial
contractility acutely. However, long-term stimulation of the
β-adrenergic system in chronic heart failure appears to be
associated with a worse outcome, potentially caused by a feedback mechanism whereby increased β-adrenergic stimulation
leads to desensitization (124). One particularly important
mechanism by which desensitization occurs is through activation of the β-adrenergic receptor kinase (β-ARK) (125) which
phosphorylates the β-receptor and renders it less sensitive
to stimulation by agonist. Overexpression of β-ARK has been
associated with diminished ventricular function (126), and a
β-ARK inhibitor has been shown to preserve ventricular function in certain models of heart failure (127,128). This may
explain observations in patients with chronic congestive heart
failure, where an increase in β-adrenergic stimulation from
increased sympathetic nervous system activity leads to downregulation and decreased sensitivity of β-adrenergic receptors
along with progressive myocardial dysfunction (129). The use
of β-AR blocking agents may therefore paradoxically maintain
β-AR sensitivity and improve myocardial function.

Both β_1 and β_2-adrenergic receptors couple to adenylyl
cyclase by means of the stimulatory G-protein, Gs. Acutely,
the predominant effect of Gs activation is therefore increased
inotropic and chronotropic response of the myocardium.

Chronic exposure to adrenergic agonists results in more complex and comprehensive effects on the cardiomyocyte. In mice, overexpression of β_1 receptors is associated with increased contractility both at baseline and in response to adrenergic stimulation over the first 15 weeks of life (130). Longer exposure and higher levels of β_1 expression, however, have resulted in depression of contractile function and myocyte hypertrophy, fibrosis, and apoptosis (130). Similar deleterious effects have occurred in mice overexpressing a Gs protein (131,132) suggesting that this is a potential mechanism for the adverse consequences of prolonged β-adrenergic stimulation.

β_2-Adrenergic receptors appear to couple to inhibitory G proteins (Gi) in addition to Gs (133). Gi is thought to oppose the effects of Gs to some degree, including limitation of the acute positive inotropic response to adrenergic stimulation and offering some protection from apoptosis (134–136). Transgenic mice with cardiac-specific overexpression of β_2-AR show increased contractility, similar to that observed early in β_1 overexpression but without the long-term decompensation (137). At very high levels of overexpression though, these mice develop a dilated cardiomyopathy (138), perhaps because of relative amounts of Gs and Gi signaling.

Another intriguing area regarding β-adrenergic signaling and heart failure is that of single nucleotide polymorphisms (SNPs). SNPs are normal variants in genetic sequences in the population. Although they do not, by definition, cause disease, they may alter the course of a specific disease by conferring variable responsiveness to therapeutic drugs or modifying the natural progression of the disease. Polymorphic variants of both β_1 and β_2-adrenergic receptors have been identified in the adult population and although they are not associated with altered exercise performance or increased risk of cardiomyopathy in healthy subjects, it appears increasingly clear that they are important modifying factors for individuals with either asthma or cardiomyopathy. β_1-Adrenergic receptor polymorphisms have been identified at two loci that are likely to be important in either receptor downregulation or G protein coupling (139,140). Heart failure patients with one of these SNPs have decreased exercise tolerance (141–143) and this SNP has also been associated with an increased risk of systemic hypertension (144). There are three potentially important SNPs that have been identified in the β_2 receptor, also associated with either receptor downregulation or coupling to G-proteins. One of these SNPs, a threonine/isoleucine (Thr/Ile) polymorphism at position 164 shows significantly reduced adenylyl cyclase activity in the Ile 164, both at baseline and in response to epinephrine than the Thr 164 when expressed in recombinant cells (145). Population studies have shown that 95% of the adult population is homozygous Thr and 5% heterozygous Thr/Ile. To date, no reports of individuals homozygous for Ile have been published although the number of subjects examined should have been sufficient to identify more than one such individual (146). Transgenic mice that express the Ile form of the receptor in the myocardium show decreased receptor coupling to adenylyl cyclase and decreased physiologic responsiveness to the β-adrenergic agonist isoproteronol (147). Studies in humans likewise suggest that this particular polymorphism is an important modifier of cardiovascular disease. Heterozygous heart failure patients have decreased exercise tolerance (148), and 1-year survival for adults with heart failure who are homozygous for 164 Thr is 76% compared to 42% for heterozygous individuals (145). Even healthy subjects heterozygous at the 164 locus show a blunted cardiovascular response to intravenous terbutaline (149). These findings clearly imply that the β_2-adrenergic receptor polymorphism at position 164 can have a major effect on outcome in individuals with cardiovascular disease and that variable response of the receptor to β-adrenergic agonists may be a key underlying mechanism.

Compared to the vast amount of data regarding the molecular biology of cardiac hypertrophy in pressure overload, relatively little is known about volume overload. This is particularly pertinent to the pediatric population in that many patients at high-risk for ventricular dysfunction have a significant component of volume overload. Single ventricle lesions, for example, are associated with volume overload for at least the first several months of life and these patients seem to remain at higher than normal risk of systemic ventricular dysfunction as they age. Left-to-right shunts in two-ventricle patients are also volume overload lesions, although they are usually repaired before there is any evidence of permanent functional changes. Likewise, atrio-ventricular or semi-lunar valve insufficiency also imposes a volume overload, often for an extended period because of the reluctance to perform valve replacements in infants and children.

Clearly, volume overload can lead to ventricular dysfunction just as does pressure overload. Nevertheless, recent data regarding the role of the renin–angiotensin system in chronic volume overload induced by mitral regurgitation in dogs suggest that the interaction of mast cells with bradykinin may play a role in cardiac remodeling with volume overload (150–152). In these studies, the combination of an ACE inhibitor and bradykinin receptor blockade was associated with the least amount of ventricular dilation. Since volume overload lesions are often treated with ACE inhibitors, and since ACE is important for the breakdown of bradykinin, such a finding could have therapeutic implications for many pediatric lesions. Although these results need to be duplicated in other models and in clinical studies, they raise the possibility that it is unwise to consider all types of increased ventricular workload as identical and remind us that treatment of pediatric heart failure is not simply a matter of extrapolating data from adult studies.

SUMMARY

Myocardial dysfunction can result from disruption of any one of a number of balanced systems that maintain cardiomyocyte structure and function. Such disruption can occur either in response to acute stresses such as cardiac surgery with CPB and cross-clamping of the aorta or because of more chronic stresses resulting from genetic abnormalities, infection, chronic ischemia, etc. Although the exact mechanisms of myocardial dysfunction are constantly being elucidated, it is clear that myocardial structure and physiology are intimately related by molecular conversation between the extracellular matrix, cytoskeleton, contractile elements, calcium handling apparatus, and cell survival signals. This is all modified by neurohormonal input from receptors such as the renin–angiotensin and β-adrenergic systems that report back to the heart information regarding the rest of the body. Several currently available therapies such as β-adrenergic receptor agonists and antagonists, PDE inhibitors, ACE inhibitors, angiotensin receptor blockers, and other agents have effects on the cardiomyocyte that are more far reaching than initially appreciated when these agents were first introduced, thus underscoring the importance of appreciating the cellular and molecular aspects of myocardial dysfunction in clinical practice. As our knowledge and understanding of myocardial dysfunction increases and we begin to understand how these mechanisms differ in the neonatal and pediatric patient, we will be able to further target interventions to highly specific perturbations of cellular function and individual genetic variability.

REFERENCES

1. Boheler KR, Carrier L, de la Bastie D, Allen PD, Komajda M, Mercadier JJ, Schwartz K. Skeletal actin mRNA increases in the human heart during ontogenic development and is the major isoform of control and failing adult hearts. J Clin Invest 1991; 88:323–330.
2. Bouvagnet P, Neveu S, Montoya M, Leger JJ. Development changes in the human cardiac isomyosin distribution: an immunohistochemical study using monoclonal antibodies. Circ Res 1987; 61:329–336.
3. Mercadier JJ, Lompre AM, Wisnewsky C, Samuel JL, Bercovici J, Swynghedauw B, Schwartz K. Myosin isoenzyme changes in several models of rat cardiac hypertrophy. Circ Res 1981; 49:525–532.
4. Sasse S, Brand NJ, Kyprianou P, Dhoot GK, Wade R, Arai M, Periasamy M, Yacoub MH, Barton PJ. Troponin I gene expression during human cardiac development and in end-stage heart failure. Circ Res 1993; 72:932–938.
5. Schwartz SM, Duffy JY, Pearl JM, Goins S, Wagner CJ, Nelson DP. Glucocorticoids preserve calpastatin and troponin I during cardiopulmonary bypass in immature pigs. Pediatr Res 2003; 54:91–97.

6. Rapundalo ST, Solaro RJ, Kranias EG. Inotropic responses to isoproterenol and phosphodiesterase inhibitors in intact guinea pig hearts: comparison of cyclic AMP levels and phosphorylation of sarcoplasmic reticulum and myofibrillar proteins. Circ Res 1989; 64:104–111.

7. McDonough JL, Arrell DK, Van Eyk JE. Troponin I degradation and covalent complex formation accompanies myocardial ischemia/reperfusion injury. Circ Res 1999; 84:9-20.

8. Gao WD, Atar D, Liu Y, Perez NG, Murphy AM, Marban E. Role of troponin I proteolysis in the pathogenesis of stunned myocardium. Circ Res 1997; 80:393–399.

9. Antman EM, Tanasijevic MJ, Thompson B, Schactman M, McCabe CH, Cannon CP, Fischer GA, Fung AY, Thompson C, Wybenga D, Braunwald E. Cardiac-specific troponin I levels to predict the risk of mortality in patients with acute coronary syndromes. N Engl J Med 1996; 335:1342–1349.

10. Nagai T, Laser M, Baicu CF, Zile MR, Cooper Gt, Kuppuswamy D. Beta 3-integrin-mediated focal adhesion complex formation: adult cardiocytes embedded in three-dimensional polymer matrices. Am J Cardiol 1999; 83:38H–43H.

11. Ross RS, Borg TK. Integrins and the myocardium. Circ Res 2001; 88: 1112–1119.

12. Colledge M, Scott JD. AKAPs: from structure to function. Trends Cell Biol 1999; 9:216–221.

13. Fink MA, Zakhary DR, Mackey JA, Desnoyer RW, Apperson-Hansen C, Damron DS, Bond M. AKAP-medtated targeting of protein kinase a regulates contractility in cardiac myocytes. Circ Res 2001; 88: 291–297.

14. Haase H, Karczewski P, Beckert R, Krause EG. Phosphorylation of the L-type calcium channel beta subunit is involved in beta-adrenergic signal transduction in canine myocardium. FEBS Lett 1993; 335: 217–222.

15. Gerhardstein BL, Puri TS, Chien AJ, Hosey MM. Identification of the sites phosphorylated by cyclic AMP-dependent protein kinase on the beta 2 subunit of L-type voltage-dependent calcium channels. Biochemistry 1999; 38:10361–10370.

16. Skeberdis VA, Jurevicius J, Fischmeister R. a. Beta-2 adrenergic activation of L-type Ca^{++} current in cardiac myocytes. J Pharmacol Exp Ther 1997; 283:452–461.

17. Osaka T, Joyner RW. Developmental changes in calcium currents of rabbit ventricular cells. Circ Res 1991; 68:788–796.

18. Katsube Y, Yokoshiki H, Nguyen L, Yamamoto M, Spereiakis N. L-type Ca^{2+} currents in ventricular myocytes from neonatal and adult rats. Can J Physiol Pharmacol 1998; 76:873–881.

19. James P, Inui M, Tada M, Chiesi M, Carafoli E. Nature andsite of phospholamban regulation of the Ca^{2+} pump of sarcoplasmic reticulum. Nature 1989; 342:90–92.

20. Kranias EG, Mandel F, Wang T, Schwartz A. Mechanism of the stimulation of calcium ion dependent adenosine triphosphatase of cardiac sarcoplasmic reticulum by adenosine 3', 5'-monophosphate dependent protein kinase. Biochemistry 1980; 19:5434–5439.

21. Hanson GL, Schilling WP, Michael LH. Sodium-potassium pump and sodium-calcium exchange in adult and neonatal canine cardiac sarcolemma. Am J Physiol 1993; 264:H320–H326.

22. Boucek RJ Jr, Shelton M, Artman M, Mushlin PS, Starnes VA, Olson RD. Comparative effects of verapamil, nifedipine, and diltiazem on contractile function in the isolated immature and adult rabbit heart. Pediatr Res 1984; 18:948–952.

23. Klitzner TS, Friedman WF. A diminished role for the sarcoplasmic reticulum in newborn myocardial contraction: effects of ryanodine. Pediatr Res 1989; 26:98–101.

24. Swynghedauw B. Remodelling of the heart in response to chronic mechanical overload. Eur Heart J 1989; 10:935–943.

25. Jalil JE, Doering CW, Janicki JS, Pick R, Shroff SG, Weber KT. Fibrillar collagen and myocardial stiffness in the intact hypertrophied rat left ventricle. Circ Res 1989; 64:1041–1050.

26. Brutsaert DL, Sys SU. Relaxation and diastole of the heart. Physiol Rev 1989; 69:1228–1315.

27. Matsusaka T, Katori H, Inagami T, Fogo A, Ichikawa I. Communication between myocytes and fibroblasts in cardiac remodeling in angiotensin chimeric mice. J Clin Invest 1999; 103:1451–1458.

28. Sadoshima J, Xu Y, Slayter HS, Izumo S. Autocrine release ofangiotensin II mediates stretch-induced hypertrophy of cardiac myocytes in vitro. Cell 1993; 75:977–984.

29. Schunkert H, Dzau VJ, Tang SS, Hirsch AT, Apstein CS, Lorell BH. Increased rat cardiac angiotensin converting enzyme activity and mRNA expression in pressure overload left ventricular hypertrophy. Effects on coronary resistance, contractility, and relaxation. J Clin Invest 1990; 86:1913–1920.

30. Schwartz SM, Hewett TE, Klevitsky R, Goins S, Liggett S, Robbins J. Increased myocardial angiotensin converting enzyme activity potentiates responsiveness to β-adrenergic agonists in transgenic mice. Circulation 2000; 102(suppl II):198.

31. Hall RI, Smith MS, Rocker G. The systemic inflammatory response to cardiopulmonary bypass: pathophysiological, therapeutic, and pharmacological considerations. Anesth Analg 1997; 85:766–782.

32. Kilbridge PM, Mayer JE, Newburger JW, Hickey PR, Walsh AZ, Neufeld EJ. Induction of intercellular adhesion molecule-1 and E-selectin mRNA in heart and skeletal muscle of pediatric patients undergoing cardiopulmonary bypass. J Thorac Cardiovasc Surg 1994; 107:1183–1192.

33. Jansen NJ, van Oeveren W, Gu YJ, van Vliet MH, Eijsman L, Wildevuur CR. Endotoxin release and tumor necrosis factor

formation during cardiopulmonary bypass. Ann Thorac Surg 1992; 54:744–747. Discussion 747–748.

34. Rocke DA, Gaffin SL, Welis MT, Koen Y, Brock-Utine JG. Endotoxemia associated with cardiopulmonary bypass. J Thorac Cardiovasc Surg 1987; 93:832–837.

35. Steinberg JB, Kapelanski DP, Olson JD, Weiler JM. Cytokine and complement levels in patients undergoing cardiopulmonary bypass. J Thorac Cardiovasc Surg 1993; 106:1008–1016.

36. Wan S, LeClerc JL, Vincent JL. Cytokine responses to cardiopulmonary bypass: lessons learned from cardiac transplantation. Ann Thorac Surg 1997; 63:269–276.

37. Burns SA, Newburger JW, Xiao M, Mayer JE Jr, Walsh AZ, Neufeld EJ. Induction of interleukin-8 messenger RNA in heart and skeletal muscle during pediatric cardiopulmonary bypass. Circulation 1995; 92:II315–II321.

38. Kawamura T, Wakusawa R, Okada K, Inada S. Elevation of cytokines during open heart surgery with cardiopulmonary bypass: participation of interleukin 8 and 6 in reperfusion injury. Can J Anaesth 1993; 40:1016–1021.

39. Hennein HA, Ebba H, Rodriguez JL, Merrick SH, Keith FM, Bronstein MH, Leung JM, Mangano DT, Greenfield LJ, Rankin JS. Relationship of the proinflammatory cytokines to myocardial ischemia and dysfunction after uncomplicated coronary revascularization. J Thorac Cardiovasc Surg 1994; 108:626–635.

40. Jansen NJ, van Oeveren W, van den Broek L, Oudemans-van Straaten HM, Stoutenbeek CP, Joen MC, Roozendaal KJ, Eysman L, Wildevuur CR. Inhibition by dexamethasone ofthe reperfusion phenomena in cardiopulmonary bypass. J Thorac Cardiovasc Surg 1991; 102:515–525.

41. Wan S, Marchant A, DeSmet JM, Antoine M, Zhang H, Vachiery JL, Goldman M, Vincent JL, LeClerc JL. Human cytokine responses to cardiac transplantation and coronary artery bypass grafting. J Thorac Cardiovasc Surg 1996; 111:469–477.

42. Seghaye M, Duchateau J, Bruniaux J, Demontoux S, Bosson C, Serraf A, Lecronier G, Mokhfi E, Planche C. Interleukin-10 release related to cardiopulmonary bypass in infants undergoing cardiac operations. J Thorac Cardiovasc Surg 1996; 111:545–553.

43. Yokoyama T, Arai M, Sekiguchi K, Tanaka T, Kanda T, Suzuki T, Nagai R. Tumor necrosis factor-alpha decreases the phosphorylation levels of phospholamban and troponin I in spontaneously beating rat neonatal cardiac myocytes. J Mol Cell Cardiol 1999; 31:261–273.

44. Pearl JM, Nelson DP, Schwartz SM, Wagner CJ, Bauer SM, Setser EA, Duffy JY. Giucocorticoids reduce ischemia-reperfusion-induced myocardial apoptosis in immature hearts. Ann Thorac Surg 2002; 74:830–836. Discussion 836–837.

45. Parker MM, Shelhamer JH, Bacharach SL, Green MV, Natanson C, Frederick TM, Damske BA, Parrillo JE. Profound but reversible myocardial depression in patients with septic shock. Ann Intern Med 1984; 100:483–490.

46. Selberg O, Hecker H, Martin M, Klos A, Bautsch W, Kohl J. Discrimination of sepsis and systemic inflammatory response syndrome by determination of circulating plasma concentrations of procalcitonin, protein complement 3a, and interleukin-6. Crit Care Med 2000; 28:2793–2798.

47. Finkel MS, Oddis CV, Jacob TD, Watkins SC, Hattler BG, Simmons RL. Negative inotropic effects of cytokines on theheart mediated by nitric oxide. Science 1992; 257:387–389.

48. Gao WD, Liu Y, Mellgren R, Marban E. Intrinsic myofilament alterations underlying the decreased contractility of stunned myocardium. A consequence of Ca^{2+}-dependent proteolysis? Circ Res 1996; 78: 455–465.

49. Murphy AM, Kogler H, Georgakopouios D, McDonough JL, Kass DA, Van Eyk JE, Marban E. Transgenic mouse model of stunned myocardium. Science 2000; 287:488–491.

50. McDonough JL, Labugger R, Pickett W, Tse MY, Mackenzie S, Pang SC, Atar D, Ropchan G, Van Eyk JE. Cardiac troponin I is modified in the myocardium of bypass patients. Circulation 2001; 103:58–64.

51. Labugger R, Organ L, Collier C, Atar D, Van Eyk JE. Extensive troponin I and T modification detected in serum from patients with acute myocardial infarction. Circulation 2000; 102:1221–1226.

52. Kameyama M, Kameyama A, Takano E, Maki M. Run-down of the cardiac L-type Ca^{2+} channel: partial restoration of channel activity in cell-free patches by calpastatin. Pflugers Arch 1998; 435:344–349.

53. Tabardel Y, Duchateau J, Schmartz D, Marecaux G, Shahla M, Barvais L, Leclerc JL, Vincent JL. Corticosteroids increase blood interleukin-10 levels during cardiopulmonary bypass in men. Surgery 1996; 119:76–80.

54. Schroeder VA, Pearl JM, Schwartz SM, Shanley TP, Manning PB, Nelson DP. Combined steroid treatment for congenital heart surgery improves oxygen delivery and reduces postbypass inflammatory mediator expression. Circulation 2003; 107:2823–2828.

55. Whitehurst RM Jr, Zhang M, Bhattacharjee A, Li M. Dexamethasone-induced hypertrophy in rat neonatal cardiac myocytes involves an elevated L-type Ca(2+) current. J Mol Cell Cardiol 1999; 31:1551–1558.

56. Wang L, Feng ZP, Duff HJ. Glucocorticoid regulation of cardiac K+ currents and L-type Ca^{2+} current in neonatal mice. Circ Res 1999; 85:168–173.

57. Saatvedt K, Lindberg H, Geiran OR, Michelsen S, Pedersen T, Seem E, Mollnes TE. Ultrafiltration after cardiopulmonary bypass

in children: effects on hemodynamics, cytokines and complement. Cardiovasc Res 1996; 31:596–602.

58. Grunenfelder J, Zund G, Schoeberlein A, Maly FE, Schurr U, Guntli S, Fischer K, Turina M. Modified ultrafiltration lowers adhesion molecule and cytokine levels after cardiopulmonary bypass without clinical relevance in adults. Eur J Cardiothorac Surg 2000; 17:77–83.

59. Schermerhorn ML, Tofukuji M, Khoury PR, Phillips L, Hickey PR, Sellke FW, Mayer JE Jr, Nelson DP. Sialyl lewis oligosaccharide preserves cardiopulmonary and endothelial function after hypothermic circulatory arrest in lambs. J Thorac Cardiovasc Surg 2000; 120:230–237.

60. Kranias EG, Solaro RJ. Phosphorylation of troponin I and phospholamban during catecholamine stimulation of rabbit heart. Nature 1982; 298:182–184.

61. Puri TS, Gerhardstein BL, Zhao XL, Ladner MB, Hosey MM. Differential effects of subunit interactions on protein kinase A- and C-mediated phosphorylation of L-type calcium channels. Biochemistry 1997; 36:9605–9615.

62. Sculptoreanu A, Scheuer T, Catterall WA. Voltage-dependent potentiation of L-type Ca^{2+} channels due to phosphorylation by cAMP-dependent protein kinase. Nature 1993; 364:240–243.

63. Tobacman LS. Thin filament-mediated regulation of cardiac contraction. Annu Rev Physiol 1996; 58:447–481.

64. Schwinn DA, Leone BJ, Spahn DR, Chesnut LC, Page SO, McRae RL, Liggett SB. Desensitization of myocardial beta-adrenergic receptors during cardiopulmonary bypass. Evidence for early uncoupling and late downregulation. Circulation 1991; 84:2559–2567.

65. Sutko JL, Kenyon JL, Reeves JP. Effects of amrinone and milrinone on calcium influx into the myocardium. Circulation 1986; 73:MI52–MI58.

66. Alousi AA, Johnson DC. Pharmacology of the bipyridines: amrinone and milrinone. Circulation 1986; 73:IM10–IM24.

67. Weber KT, Brilla CG. Pathological hypertrophy and cardiac interstitium. Fibrosis and rennin-angiotensin-aldosterone system. Circulation 1991; 83:1849–1865.

68. Chevalier B, Mansier P, Callens-el Amrani F, Swynghedauw B. Beta-adrenergic system is modified in compensatory pressure cardiac overload in rats: physiological and biochemical evidence. J Cardiovasc Pharmacol 1989; 13:412–420.

69. Eschenhagen T, Mende U, Nose M, Schmitz W, Scholz H, Haverich A, Hirt S, Doring V, Kalmar P, Hoppner W, et al. Increased messenger RNA level of the inhibitory G protein alpha subunit Gi alpha-2 in human end-stage heart failure. Circ Res 1992; 70:688–696.

70. Arai M, Alpert NR, MacLennan DH, Barton P, Periasamy M. Alterations in sarcoplasmic reticulum gene expression in human heart

failure. A possible mechanism for alterations in systolic and diastolic properties of the failing myocardium. Circ Res 1993; 72:463–469.

71. Arai M, Matsui H, Periasamy M. Sarcoplasmic reticulum gene expression in cardiac hypertrophy and heart failure. Circ Res 1994; 74:555–564.

72. Ito Y, Suko J, Chidsey CA. Intracellular calcium and myocardial contractility. V. Calcium uptake of sarcoplasmic reticulum fractions in hypertrophied and failing rabbit hearts. J Mol Cell Cardiol 1974; 6:237–247.

73. Suko J, Vogel JH, Chidsey CA. Intracellular calcium and myocardial contractility. 3. Reduced calcium uptake and ATPase of the sarcoplasmic reticular fraction prepared from chronically failing calf hearts. Circ Res 1970; 27:235–247.

74. Cheng W, Li B, Kajstura J, Li P, Wolin MS, Sonnenblick EH, Hintze TH, Olivetti G, Anversa P. Stretch-induced programmed myocyte cell death. J Clin Invest 1995; 96:2247–2259.

75. Esposito G, Rapacciuolo A, Naga Prasad SV, Takaoka H, Thomas SA, Koch WJ, Rockman HA. Genetic alterations that inhibit in vivo pressure-overload hypertrophy prevent cardiac dysfunction despite increased wall stress. Circulation 2002; 105:85–92.

76. Sussman MA, McCulloch A, Borg TK. Dance band on the Titanic: biomechanical signaling in cardiac hypertrophy. Circ Res 2002; 91:888–898.

77. Pham CG, Harpf AE, Keller RS, Vu HT, Shai SY, Loftus JC, Ross RS. Striated muscle-specific beta(1D)-integrin and FAKare involved in cardiac myocyte hypertrophic response pathway. Am J Physiol Heart Circ Physiol 2000; 279:H2916–H2926.

78. Ross RS, Pham C, Shai SY, Goldhaber JI, Fenczik C, Glembotski CC, Ginsberg MH, Loftus JC. Beta 1 integrins participate in the hypertrophic response of rat ventricular myocytes. Circ Res 1998; 82:1160–1172.

79. Taylor JM, Rovin JD, Parsons JT. A role for focal adhesion kinase in phenylephrine-induced hypertrophy of rat ventricular cardiomyocytes. J Biol Chem 2000; 275:19250–19257.

80. Eble DM, Strait JB, Govindarajan G, Lou J, Byron KL, Samarel AM. Endothelin-induced cardiac myocyte hypertrophy: role for focal adhesion kinase. Am J Physiol Heart Circ Physiol 2000; 278:H1695–H1707.

81. Franchini KG, Torsoni AS, Soares PH, Saad MJ. Early activation of the multicomponent signaling complex associated with focal adhesion kinase induced by pressure overload in the rat heart. Circ Res 2000; 87:558–565.

82. Ito H, Hirata Y, Adachi S, Tanaka M, Tsujino M, Koike A, Nogami A, Murumo F, Hiroe M. Endothelin-1 is an autocrine/paracrine factor in the mechanism of angiotensin II-induced hypertrophy in cultured rat cardiomyocytes. J Clin Invest 1993; 92:398–403.

83. Baker KM, Chernin MI, Wixson SK, Aceto JF. Renin-angiotensin system involvement in pressure-overload cardiac hypertrophy in rats. Am J Physiol 1990; 259:H324–H332.

84. Pfeffer MA, Braunwald E, Moye LA, Basta L, Brown EJ Jr, Cuddy TE, Davis BR, Geltman EM, Goldman S, Flaker GC, et al. Effect of captopril on mortality and morbidity in patients with left ventricular dysfunction after myocardial infarction. Results of the survival and ventricular enlargement trial. The SAVE Investigators. N Engl J Med 1992; 327:669–677.

85. Ruzicka M, Yuan B, Leenen FH. Effects of enalapril versus losartan on regression of volume overload-induced cardiac hypertrophy in rats. Circulation 1994; 90:484–491.

86. Williamson DJ, Wallman LL, Jones R, Keogh AM, Scroope F, Penny R, Weber C, Macdonald PS. Hemodynamic effects of Bosentan, an endotheiin receptor antagonist, in patients with pulmonary hypertension. Circulation 2000; 102:411–418.

87. Rich S, McLaughlin W. Endothelin receptor blockers in cardiovascular disease. Circulation 2003; 108:2184–2190.

88. Kalra PR, Moon JC, Coats AJ. Do results of the ENABLE (Endothelin Antagonist Bosentan for Lowering Cardiac Events in Heart Failure) study spell the end for non-selective endothelin antagonism in heart failure? Int J Cardiol 2002; 85:195–197.

89. Cohn JN, Johnson G, Ziesche S, Cobb F, Francis G, Tristani F, Smith R, Dunkman WB, Loeb H, Wong M, et al. A comparison of enalapril with hydralazine-isosorbide dinitrate in the treatment of chronic congestive heart failure. N Engl J Med 1991; 325:303–310.

90. Hirsch AT, Talsness CE, Schunkert H, Paul M, Dzau VJ. Tissue-specific activation of cardiac angiotensin converting enzyme in experimental heart failure. Circ Res 1991; 69:475–482.

91. Hafizi S, Wharton J, Morgan K, Allen SP, Chester AH, Catravas JD, Polak JM, Yacoub MH. Expression of functional angiotensin-converting enzyme and AT1 receptors in cultured human cardiac fibroblasts. Circulation 1998; 98:2553–2559.

92. Paul M, Wagner D, Metzger R, Ganten D, Lang RE, Suzuki F, Murakami K, Burbach JH, Ludwig G. Quantification of renin mRNA in various mouse tissues by a novel solution hybridization assay. J Hypertens 1988; 6:247–252.

93. Muller DN, Fischli W, Clozel JP, Hilgers KF, Bohlender J, Menard J, Busjahn A, Ganten D, Luft FC. Local angiotensin II generation in the rat heart: role of renin uptake. Circ Res 1998; 82:13–20.

94. Mazzolai L, Nussberger J, Aubert JF, Brunner DB, Gabbiani G, Brunner HR, Pedrazzini T. Blood pressure-independent cardiac hypertrophy induced by locally activated rennin-angiotensin system. Hypertension 1998; 31:1324–1330.

95. Lee AA, Dillmann WH, McCulloch AD, Villarreal FJ. Angiotensin II stimulates the autocrine production of transforming growth

factor-beta 1 in adult rat cardiac fibroblasts. J Mol Cell Cardiol 1995; 27:2347–2357.

96. Sadoshima J, Qiu Z, Morgan JP, Izumo S. Angiotensin II and other hypertrophic stimuli mediated by G protein-coupled receptors activate tyrosine kinase, mitogen-activated protein kinase, and 90-kD S6 kinase in cardiac myocytes. The critical role of Ca(2+)-dependent signaling. Circ Res 1995; 76:1–15.

97. Koide M, Carabello BA, Conrad CC, Buckley JM, DeFreyte G, Barnes M, Tomanek RJ, Wei CC, Dell'Italia LJ, Cooper Gt, Zile MR. Hypertrophic response to hemodynamic overload: role of load vs. renninangiotensin system activation. Am J Physiol 1999; 276:H350–H358.

98. Sakai S, Miyauchi T, Sakurai T, Kasuya Y, Ihara M, Yamaguchi I, Goto K, Sugishita Y. Endogenous endothelin-1 participates in the maintenance of cardiac function in rats with congestive heart failure. Marked increase in endothelin-1 production in the failing heart. Circulation 1996; 93:1214–1222.

99. Serneri GGN, Boddi M, Cecioni I, Vanni S, Coppo M, Papa ML, Bandinelli B, Bertolozzi I, Polidori G, Toscano T, Maccherini M, Modesti PA. Cardiac angiotensin II formation in the clinical course of heart failure and its relationship with left ventricular function. Circ Res 2001; 88:961–968.

100. Ruwhof C, van der Laarse A. Mechanical stress-induced cardiac hypertrophy: mechanisms and signal transduction pathways. Cardiovasc Res 2000; 47:23–37.

101. Yamazaki T, Komuro I, Kudoh S, Zou Y, Shiojima I, Mizuno T, Takano H, Hiroi Y, Ueki K, Tobe K. et al. Mechanical stress activates protein kinase cascade of phosphorylation in neonatal rat cardiac myocytes. J Clin Invest 1995; 96:438–446.

102. Bogoyevitch MA, Glennon PE, Andersson MB, Clerk A, Lazou A, Marshall CJ, Parker PJ, Sugden PH. Endothelin-1 and fibroblast growth factors stimulate the mitogen-activated protein kinase signaling cascade in cardiac myocytes. The potential role of the cascade in the integration of two signaling pathways leading to myocyte hypertrophy. J Biol Chem 1994; 269:1110–1119.

103. Jiang T, Pak E, Zhang HL, Kline RP, Steinberg SF. Endothelin-dependent actions in cultured AT-1 cardiac myocytes. The role of the epsilon isoform of protein kinase C. Circ Res 1996; 78:724–736.

104. Takahashi T, Fukuda K, Pan J, Kodama H, Sano M, Makino S, Kato T, Manabe T, Ogawa S. Characterization of insulin-like growth factor-1-induced activation of the JAK/STAT pathway in rat cardiomyocytes. Circ Res 1999; 85:884–891.

105. Takeishi Y, Huang Q, Abe J, Glassman M, Che W, Lee JD, Kawakatsu H, Lawrence EG, Hoit BD, Berk BC, Walsh RA. Src and multiple MAP kinase activation in cardiac hypertrophy and congestive heart failure under chronic pressure-overload: comparison with acute mechanical stretch. J Mol Cell Cardiol 2001; 33:1637–1648.

106. Sugden PH, Clerk A. "Stress-responsive" mitogen-activated protein kinases (c-Jun N-terminal kinases p38 mitogen-activated protein kinases) in the myocardium. Circ Res 1998; 83:345–352.
107. Garrington TP, Johnson GL. Organization and regulation of mitogen-activated protein kinase signaling pathways. Curr Opin Cell Biol 1999; 11:211–218.
108. Izumo S, Nadal-Ginard B, Mahdavi V. Protooncogene induction and reprogramming of cardiac gene expression produced by pressure overload. Proc Natl Acad Sci USA 1988; 85:339–343.
109. Tardiff JC, Hewett TE, Factor SM, Vikstrom KL, Robbins J, Leinwand LA. Expression of the beta (slow)-isoform of MHC in the adult mouse heart causes dominant-negative functional effects. Am J Physiol Heart Circ Physiol 2000; 278:H412–H419.
110. Morano I, Bletz C, Wojciechowski R, Ruegg JC. Modulation of cross-bridge kinetics by myosin isoenzymes in skinned human heart fibers. Circ Res 1991; 68:614–618.
111. Hasenfuss G, Meyer M, Schillinger W, Preuss M, Pieske B, Just H. Calcium handling proteins in the failing human heart. Basic Res Cardiol 1997; 92(suppl 1):87–93.
112. Frank KF, Bolck B, Brixius K, Kranias EG, Schwinger RH. Modulation of SERCA: implications for the failing human heart. Basic Res Cardiol 2002; 97(suppl 11):172–178.
113. Schmidt U, Hajjar RJ, Kim CS, Lebeche D, Doye AA, Gwathmey JK. Human heart failure: cAMP stimulation of SR Ca(2+)-ATPase activity and phosphorylation level of phospholamban. Am J Physiol 1999; 277:H474–H480.
114. Currie S, Smith GL. Enhanced phosphorylation of phospholamban and downregulation of sarco/endoplasmic reticulum Ca^{2+} ATPase type 2 (SERCA 2) in cardiac sarcoplasmic reticulum from rabbits with heart failure. Cardiovasc Res 1999; 41:135–146.
115. Minamisawa S, Hoshijima M, Chu G, Ward CA, Frank K, Gu Y, Martone ME, Wang Y, Ross J Jr, Kranias EG, Giles WR, Chien KR. Chronic phospholamban-sarcoplasmic reticulum calcium ATPase interaction is the critical calcium cycling defect in dilated cardiomyopathy. Cell 1999; 99:313–322.
116. Maisel AS, Phillips C, Michel MC, Ziegler MG, Carter SM. Regulation of cardiac beta-adrenergic receptors by captopril. Implications for congestive heart failure. Circulation 1989; 80:669–675.
117. Molkentin JD. Calcineurin and beyond: cardiac hypertrophic signaling. Circ Res 2000; 87:731–738.
118. Lim SK, Ali A, Law HY, Ng I, Ming Chung MC, Lee SH. An anemic patient with phenotypical beta-thalassemic trait has elevated level of structurally normal beta-globin mRNA in reticulocytes. Am J Hematol 2000; 65:243–250.
119. Zhu W, Zou Y, Shiojima I, Kudoh S, Aikawa R, Hayashi D, Mizukami M, Toko M, Shibasaki F, Yazaki Y, Nagai R, Komuro I.

Ca^{2+}/calmodulin-dependent kinase II and calcineurin play critical roles in endothelin-1-induced cardiomyocyte hypertrophy. J Biol Chem 2000; 275:15239–15245.

120. Beuckelmann DJ, Nabauer M, Erdmann E. Intracellular calcium handling in isolated ventricular myocytes from patients with terminal heart failure. Circulation 1992; 85:1046–1055.

121. Takahashi T, Schunkert H, Isoyama S, Wei JY, Nadal-Ginard B, Grossman W, Izumo S. Age-related differences in the expression of proto-oncogene and contractile protein genes in response to pressure overload in the rat myocardium. J Clin Invest 1992; 89:939–946.

122. Hittinger L, Ghaleh B, Chen J, Edwards JG, Kudej RK, Iwase M, Kim SJ, Vatner SF, Vatner DE. Reduced subendocardial ryanodine receptors and consequent effects on cardiac function in conscious dogs with left ventricular hypertrophy. Circ Res 1999; 84:999–1006.

123. Milnes JT, MacLeod KT. Reduced ryanodine receptor to dihydropyridine receptor ratio may underlie slowed contraction in a rabbit model of left ventricular cardiachypertrophy. J Mol Cell Cardiol 2001; 33:473–485.

124. Kaye DM, Lefkovits J, Jennings GL, Bergin P, Broughton A, Esier MD. Adverse consequences of high sympathetic nervous activity in the failing human heart. J Am Coll Cardiol 1995; 26:1257–1263.

125. Choi DJ, Koch WJ, Hunter JJ, Rockman HA. Mechanism of beta-adrenergic receptor desensitization in cardiac hypertrophy is increased beta-adrenergic receptor kinase. J Biol Chem 1997; 272:17223–17229.

126. Koch WJ, Rockman HA, Samama P, Hamilton RA, Bond RA, Milano CA, Lefkowitz RJ. Cardiac function in mice overexpressing the beta-adrenergic receptor kinase or a beta ARK inhibitor. Science 1995; 268:1350–1353.

127. Rockman HA, Chien KR, Choi DJ, Laccarino G, Hunter JJ, Ross J Jr, Lefkowitz RJ, Koch WJ. Expression of a beta-adrenergic receptor kinase 1 inhibitor prevents the development of myocardial failure in gene-targeted mice. Proc Natl Acad Sci USA 1998; 95:7000–7005.

128. Harding VB, Jones LR, Lefkowitz RJ, Koch WJ, Rockman HA. Cardiac beta ARK1 inhibition prolongs survival and augments beta blocker therapy in a mouse model of severe heart failure. Proc Natl Acad Sci USA 2001; 98:5809–5814.

129. Choi DJ, Rockman HA. Beta-adrenergic receptor desensitization in cardiac hypertrophy and heart failure. Cell Biochem Biophys 1999; 31:321–329.

130. Engelhardt S, Hein L, Wiesmann F, Lohse MJ. Progressive hypertrophy and heart failure in beta 1-adrenergic receptor transgenic mice. Proc Natl Acad Sci USA 1999; 96:7059–7064.

131. Geng YJ, Ishikawa Y, Vatner DE, Wagner TE, Bishop SP, Vatner SF, Homey CJ. Apoptosis of cardiac myocytes in Gs alpha transgenic mice. Circ Res 1999; 84:34–42.

132. Iwase M, Uechi M, Vatner DE, Asai K, Shannon RP, Kudej RK, Wagner TE, Wight DC, Patrick TA, Ishikawa Y, Homcy CJ, Vatner SF. Cardiomyopathy induced by cardiac Gs alpha overexpression. Am J Physiol 1997; 272:H585–H589.

133. Xiao RP, Avdonin P, Zhou YY, Cheng H, Akhter SA, Eschenhagen T, Lefkowitz RJ, Koch WJ, Lakatta EG. Coupling of beta 2-adrenocep-tor to Gi proteins and its physiological relevance in murine cardiac myocytes. Circ Res 1999; 84:43–52.

134. Communal C, Singh K, Sawyer DB, Colucci WS. Opposing effects of beta(1)- and beta(2)-adrenergic receptors on cardiac myocyte apopto-sis: role of a pertussis toxin-sensitive G protein. Circulation 1999; 100:2210–2212.

135. Chesley A, Lundberg MS, Asai T, Xiao RP, Ohtani S, Lakatta EG, Crow MT. The beta(2)-adrenergic receptor delivers an antiapoptotic signal to cardiac myocytes through G(i)-dependent coupling to phos-phatidylinositol 3'-kinase. Circ Res 2000; 87:1172–1179.

136. Zaugg M, Xu W, Lucchinetti E, Shafiq SA, Jamali NZ, Siddiqui MA. Beta-adrenergic receptor subtypes differentially affect apoptosis in adult rat ventricular myocytes. Circulation 2000; 102:344–350.

137. Bittner HB, Chen EP, Milano CA, Lefkowitz RJ, Van Trigt P. Func-tional analysis of myocardial performance in murine hearts overex-pressing the human beta 2-adrenergic receptor. J Mol Cell Cardiol 1997; 29:961–967.

138. Liggett SB, Tepe NM, Lorenz JN, Canning AM, Jantz TD, Mitarai S, Yatani A, Dorn GW II. Early and delayed consequences of beta(2)-adrenergic receptor overexpression in mouse hearts: critical role for expression level. Circulation 2000; 101:1707–1714.

139. Moore JD, Mason DA, Green SA, Hsu J, Liggett SB. Racial differences in the frequencies of cardiac beta(1)-adrenergic receptor polymorph-isms: analysis of c145A > G and c1165G > C. Hum Mutat 1999; 14:271.

140. Mason DA, Moore JD, Green SA, Liggett SB. A gain-of-function poly-morphism in a G-protein coupling domain of the human beta 1-adre-nergic receptor. J Biol Chem 1999; 274:12670–12674.

141. Mason DA, Moore JD, Green SA, Liggett SB. A gain-of-function poly-morphism in a G-protein coupling domain of the human beta 1-adre-nergic receptor. J Biol Chem 1999; 274:12670–12674.

142. Wagoner LE, Lamba S, Craft LL, Zengel PW, McGuire N, Abraham WT, Rathz DA, Dorn GWn, Liggett SB. Polymorphic Gly 389 beta-1 adrenergic receptors depress exercise capacity in heart failure (abstract). Circulation 2000; 102:11–378.

143. Rathz DA, Liggett SB. Heirarchy of genotype and desensitization permutations on b1-adrenergic receptor signaling (abstract). Circula-tion 2000; 102:11–102.

144. Bengtsson K, Meiander O, Orho-Melander M, Lindblad U, Ranstam J, Rastam L, Groop L. Polymorphism in the beta(1)-adrenergic recep-tor gene and hypertension. Circulation 2001; 104:187–190.

145. Liggett SB, Wagoner LE, Craft LL, Hornung RW, Hoit BD, McIntosh TC, Walsh RA. The lle164 beta 2-adrenergic receptor polymorphism adversely affects the outcome of congestive heart failure. J Clin Invest 1998; 102:1534–1539.

146. Liggett SB. Pharmacogenetics of beta-1- and beta-2-adrenergic receptors. Pharmacology 2000; 61:167–173.

147. Turki J, Lorenz JN, Green SA, Donnelly ET, Jacinto M, Liggett SB. Myocardial signaling defects and impaired cardiac function of a human beta 2-adrenergic receptor polymorphism expressed in transgenic mice. Proc Natl Acad Sci USA 1996; 93:10483–10488.

148. Wagoner LE, Craft LL, Singh B, Suresh DP, Zengel PW, McGuire N, Abraham WT, Chenier TC, Dom GW II, Liggett SB. Polymorphisms of the beta(2)-adrenergic receptor determine exercise capacity in patients with heart failure. Circ Res 2000; 86:834–840.

149. Bodde OE, Buscher R, Tellkamp R, Radke J, Dhein S, Insel PA. Blunted cardiac responses to receptor activation in subjects with Thr164lle beta(2)-adrenoceptors. Circulation 2001; 103:1048–1050.

150. Dell'Italia LJ, Meng QC, Balcells E, Straeter-Knowlen IM, Hankes GH, Dillon R, Cartee RE, Orr R, Bishop SP, Oparil S, et al. Increased ACE and chymase-like activity in cardiac tissue of dogs with chronic mitral regurgitation. Am J Physiol 1995; 269:H2065–H2073.

151. Perry GJ, Wei CC, Hankes GH, Dillon SR, Rynders P, Mukherjee R, Spinale FG, Dell'Italia LJ. Angiotensin II receptor blockade does not improve left ventricular function and remodeling in subacute mitral regurgitation in the dog. J Am Coll Cardiol 2002; 39:1374–1379.

152. Stewart JA, Wei CC, Brower GL, Rynders PE, Hankes GH, Dillon AR, Lucchesi PA, Janicki JS, Dell'Italia LJ. Cardiac mast cell- and chymase-mediated matrix metalloproteinase activity and left ventricular remodeling in mitral regurgitation in the dog. J Mol Cell Cardiol 2003; 35:311–319.

4

Neurohormonal and Immunologic Aspects of Pediatric Heart Failure

REINER BUCHHORN

Department of Pediatric Cardiology,
Georg-August-University Göttingen,
Göttingen, Germany

INTRODUCTION

The conceptual model for heart failure has changed radically over the past 20 years. No longer a simple hemodynamic paradigm of pump dysfunction, heart failure is now characterized as a complex clinical syndrome with release of many neurohormones (1) and cytokines (2), which are believed to be most responsible for progression of the disease (3). This change in the understanding of the pathophysiology of heart failure has important therapeutic implications. Interventions aimed solely at correcting low cardiac output or reduced blood flow do not necessarily slow heart failure progression or reduce

105

mortality. Neurohormonal activation and cardiac remodeling (4) are now recognized as important aspects of cardiovascular disease progression and are, therefore, emerging as therapeutic targets in heart failure. Many data confirm that the neurohormonal and possibly the cytokine hypothesis of heart failure in adults may be valid in children with heart failure as well. Neurohormonal activation seems to be the final common pathway of different cardiovascular disorders caused by myocardial insufficiency, valvular or congenital heart disease; that may explain comparable clinical symptoms despite differences in the hemodynamic trigger. However, nearly 20 years after Cohn's finding that neurohormonal activation predicts prognosis in chronic heart failure (5), we have no comparable

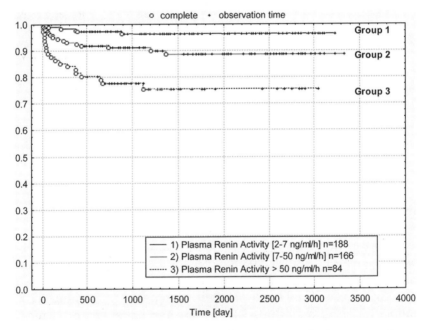

Figure 1 Kaplan–Meier analysis showing cumulative rates of survival in 438 children with congenital heart disease stratified into three groups according to their plasma renin activities. The probability of survival decreases with increasing activation of renin–angiotensin–aldosterone system. The mean observation time was 46 months. Individual observation times are characterized by the +sign

data in pediatric cardiology. A retrospective life-table analysis of 438 children based on initial measurements of renin activity confirm the high impact of neurohormonal activation on prognosis in children with congenital heart disease (Fig. 1) and should be a challenge to transfer this "new" model of adult heart failure to pediatric heart failure. Pediatric cardiologists have to realize that the most promising drugs in clinical heart failure trials—angiotensin-converting enzyme (ACE) inhibitors, angiotensin receptor blockers, beta-blockers, and aldosterone antagonists—are inhibitors of the neurohormonal system (Fig. 2). New drugs under investigation in current clinical trials—recombinant b-type natriuretic peptide, endothelin receptor, and vasopressin antagonists—are also based on the neurohormonal model of heart failure. Hemodynamic medical interventions in chronic heart failure with inotropes like phosphodiesterase inhibitors or vasodilators like calcium antagonists have shown disappointing results in clinical trials and an increased mortality. These results in adult patients should be a warning for any further "off label" use of these drugs in children with heart failure.

CLINICAL ASPECTS OF NEUROHORMONAL ACTIVATION IN PEDIATRIC HEART FAILURE

The pathophysiology of pediatric heart failure predominantly depends on the underlying disease. An analysis of diagnoses from 5324 patients from our institution showed four main groups of patients who potentially suffer from heart failure (Fig. 3):

1. Children with cardiomyopathies
2. Children with cardiac defects before cardiac surgery
3. Children and young adults with cardiac defects after cardiac surgery
4. Children with pulmonary hypertension and right heart failure

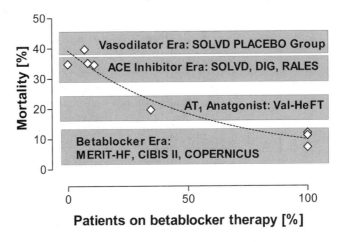

Patients on betablocker therapy [%]

Clinical Trial [§]	PLACEBO*	SOLVD	DIG	RALES	MERIT-HF	CIBIS II	COPERNICUS	Val-HeFT
Mortality [%]	39.7	35.2	34.8	34.6	7.3	12.0	11.2	19.7
Betablocker [% of pts]	7.0	8.3		11	100	100	100	34.5
ACE-Inhibitor [% of pts]		100	94.8	95	89	96	97	92.6
AT$_1$-Antagonist [% of pts]					7			100
Digitalis [% of pts]	68.2	65.7	100	75	63	53	67	67.1
Diuretics [% of pts]	85.3	85.6	82.2	100	91	98	99	85.8
Spironolactone [% of pts]				100				
Calcium Antagonist [% of pts]	32.4	29.4				2		
Vasodilator [% of pts]	52.4	49.7	1.5					
Antiarrhythmics [% of pts]	20.8	22.8				14	18	

§The data show the mortality and the percentage of patients on a drug in the verum group of the clinical trial or the * Placebo group of the SOLVD Study; # Amiodarone

Figure 2 Study mortality and percentage of patients receiving indicated medications in the group of the heart failure trials between 1991 and 2001 (SOLVD, DIG, RALES, MERIT-HF, CIBIS II, COPERNICUS, Val-HEFT). There is a trend to lower mortality (Y-axis) according to a more complete neurohormonal inhibition with ACE inhibitors, aldosterone antagonists, AT$_1$ antagonists, and most of all with the percentage of patients on beta-blocker therapy (X-axis).

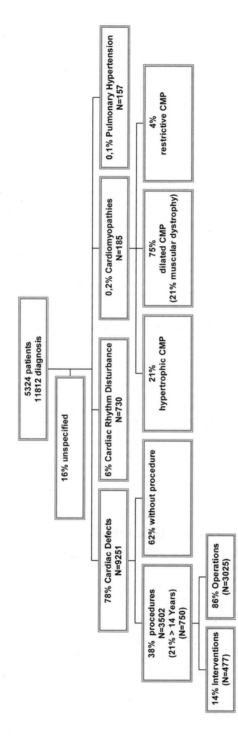

Figure 3 Distribution of diagnoses in 5324 patients from our institution (University Göttingen, Germany) with respect to the etiology of heart failure. Cardiomyopathies, the main cause of heart failure in adults, are relatively rare in children. Patients with congenital cardiac defects represent the main group who are threatened by heart failure, pre- or postoperatively.

There are many differences in the pathophysiology of heart failure in these four groups that should be considered in terms of neurohormonal and immunologic aspects of pediatric heart failure.

Cardiomyopathies

The neurohormonal and cytokine hypotheses of heart failure have been developed for patients with cardiomyopathies as one of the main causes of myocardial dysfunction in adults. There are a small number of studies in children with cardiomyopathies investigating neurohormonal activation or immune activation (6). There is no evidence that the pathophysiology of heart failure due to dilated cardiomyopathies is significantly different between children and adults. However, cardiomyopathies in children are occasionally related to muscular dystrophy, hemosiderosis or metabolic disorders; for example, neurohormonal activation with respect to medical treatment was investigated by Ishikawa et al. in children with Duchenne's muscular dystrophy (7).

Children with Cardiac Defects Before Cardiac Surgery

Congestive heart failure in children with congenital heart disease is usually not caused by pump dysfunction (8) but is characterized by hemodynamic disturbances due to left-to-right shunts, pulmonary overcirculation, and volume overload. Recently published data in infants with congenital heart disease suggest that the "neurohormonal hypothesis" (9) as well as the "cytokine hypothesis" (10) of heart failure may be valid in this population as well. Tachypnea and failure to thrive are well-recognized symptoms of heart failure in infants with congenital cardiac malformations, a phenomenon that is thought to be explained by the well-known hemodynamic disturbances of pulmonary hypertension and overcirculation. The anticipated correlations between the hemodynamic and clinical parameters, however, have yet to be demonstrated (11). Our own data, demonstrated in Table 1, showed that tachypnea

Table 1   Univariate and Multiple Regression Correlations of Hemodynamic and Neurohormonal Parameters as Potential Determinants of Tachypnea in 63 Infants with Congenital Heart Disease. R-value for Multiple Regression Analysis: $r^2 = 0.60$; $r = 0.78$

	Univariate regression		Multiple regression	
	Coefficient of correlation	p-Value	Coefficient of regression	p-Value
Heart rate	0.62***	< 0.001	0.41	0.002
Norepinephrine	0.47***	< 0.001	0.18	0.16
Mean arterial pressure	−0.42**	0.001	−0.23	0.08
Ejection fraction	0.3*	0.03	0.27	0.25
Q_p/Q_s	0.27*	0.03	0.27	0.04
Q_s	−0.32*	0.01	0.15	0.30

Q_p/Q_s: ratio of pulmonary-to-systemic flow; Q_s: systemic cardiac index; *** $p < 0.01$; ** $p < 0.01$; * $p < 0.05$.

in infants with congenital cardiac malformations is associated not only with conventional measures of the severity of hemodynamic disturbance, like the ratio of pulmonary-to-systemic blood flows, but also to neurohormonal changes. Interestingly, we found a significant but paradoxical correlation between the ejection fraction and respiratory rate showing the positive inotropic effects of neurohormonal activation on the intact myocardium of these infants. These results were confirmed by both univariate and multiple regression analysis (12). In chronic heart failure, an augmented peripheral chemosensitivity due to autonomic imbalance has provided a pathophysiological explanation of tachypnea. Such autonomic imbalance due to elevated sympathetic activity is manifested by elevated norepinephrine levels and reduced variability in heart rate (13).

Corrective cardiac surgery in early infancy seems to be the most effective therapy to reverse neurohormonal activation in patients with congenital heart disease (14). However, infants with complex cardiac anomalies frequently may not undergo a complete repair in infancy or may need palliative surgery like pulmonary artery banding or aortic-pulmonary shunts which may have a negative impact on their prognosis (15). In these patients, cardiac hypertrophy seems to be the most important risk factor for a poor outcome of after a Fontan operation (16) and seems to be a marker of cardiac remodeling induced by volume overload and neurohormonal activation (17). Moreover, β-adrenergic receptor downregulation due to neurohormonal activation has an impact on the postoperative course in children with congenital disease and at least partly depends on preoperative medical treatment (18).

Children and Young Adults with Cardiac Defects After Cardiac Surgery

As a result of successful cardiac operations and interventions in patients with congenital heart defects, there is a growing group of children and young adults with congenital heart disease. Preoperative cardiac remodeling and residual lesions contribute to the cause of heart failure in this group of patients with an increased late postoperative morbidity and mortality (19). The incidence of heart failure in this patient group increases with patient age and is paralleled by neurohormonal activation (20,21). Heart failure in these patients with congenital heart disease is frequently related to right heart failure or failure of a systemic right ventricle (22). Figure 4 shows significant correlations between plasma N-terminal pro-b-type natriuretic peptide and physical performance, measured by maximal oxygen uptake during spiroergometry in patients with tetralogy of Fallot during long term follow up after corrective surgery (23). A further group of children with cavopulmonary anastomosis as long term palliation for univentricular hearts showed a significant neurohormonal activation (24) and severely impaired cardiac autonomic nervous activity (25) late after operation. As previously demonstrated in adults with heart failure, neurohormonal parameters like b-type natriuretic peptide (26) or measurements of heart rate variability (27) may be important surrogate end points (28) for evidence-based management and

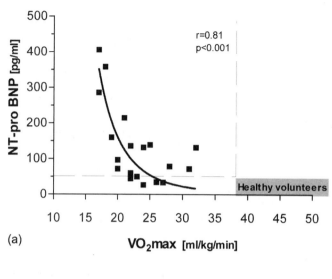

(a)

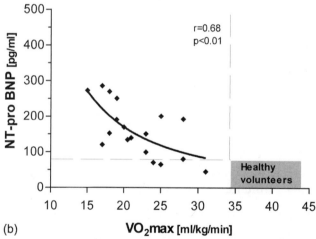

(b)

Figure 4 (a) NT-pro BNP level vs. maximal oxygen uptake during spiroergometry in 19 men with tetralogy of Fallot late after corrective surgery. (b) NT-pro BNP level vs. maximal oxygen uptake during spiroergometry in 18 women with tetralogy of Fallot late after corrective surgery.

risk stratification in this group of older children and adults with congenital heart disease (29).

Children with Pulmonary Hypertension and Right Heart Failure

Secondary pulmonary hypertension due to a left-to-right shunt is one of the most important prognostic factors in congenital heart disease. Despite intensive investigations, the pathophysiology of primary and secondary pulmonary hypertension remains uncertain and most therapies have shown disappointing results. Investigation with respect to neurohormonal activation seems to be one of the most promising tools for a better understanding of this disease. Again, the first step has been to show that neurohormonal activation (norepinephrine, endothelin) more than hemodynamic factors (pulmonary artery pressure, pulmonary vascular resistance) predict prognosis in pulmonary hypertension (30). However, the link between elevated endothelin levels (31) and an over-expression of nitric oxide synthase in humans (32) and animal models (33) remains uncertain. Elevated nitric oxide levels in children with left-to-right shunts (34) may be related to immune activation (35) as a possible cause of pulmonary vascular remodeling.

METHODOLOGICAL ASPECTS OF NEUROHORMONAL ACTIVATION IN PEDIATRIC HEART FAILURE

Renin–Angiotensin–Aldosterone System

Theoretically, the plasma level of angiotensin II would seem to offer the best index of the activity of the renin–angiotensin–aldosterone system, but for practical purposes angiotensin II measurements are difficult, in part because of the very short half life. Since angiotensin I levels are a direct representation of plasma renin activity (PRA), its determination has been widely adopted to evaluate the renin–angiotensin system in disease states by an angiotensin I radio immunoassay. Age specific normal values for angiotensin I and II, angiotensin-converting enzyme, and aldosterone in infancy and childhood are available (36). More recently, an immunoradiometric assay for the measurement of active renin protein has been used and normal values determined in 281 healthy children (37).

Myocardial gene expression has become a new target for the evaluation of neurohormonal activation in the heart itself. Absolute quantification of mRNA using real-time reverse transcription polymerase chain reaction assays in specimens obtained during cardiac surgery seems to be a good method for investigations in children with congenital heart disease (38). However, the lack of normal values and the quantification related to different target genes is a limitation of this method at present.

Sympathetic Nervous System

Many methods have been used for measurements of sympathetic nervous system activation but a gold standard is not clearly defined. Plasma norepinephrine levels, measured by radio enzymatic assays or by high-performance liquid chromatography with fluorescence detection have frequently been used. However, there is a wide range of normal values in healthy infants and children that probably depends at least partially on the level of stress associated with the blood specimen collection itself (39). Alternatively, catecholamine excretion in the urine has been assessed in children with congenital heart disease but, in one study, sympathetic activation was not clearly detected in children with heart failure (40). Analysis of heart rate variability is another noninvasive screening method for the detection of an autonomic imbalance caused by high sympathetic and concomitant low parasympathetic activity, but age specific normal values have to be taken into account (41). β-Adrenergic receptor density measured by binding assays or more recently myocardial gene expression using real-time reverse transcription polymerase chain reaction assays gives new insights into alterations of the β-adrenergic receptor-G protein-adenylyl cyclase pathway in children with heart failure. Measurement of muscle sympathetic nerve activity (MSNA) in the peroneal nerve or impaired cardiac adrenergic innervation assessed by metaiodobenzylguanidine (MIBG) imaging (42) have also been used for the evaluation of the sympathetic nervous system during heart failure in children and adults.

Endothelin, Natriuretic Peptides, Antidiuretic Hormone, Cytokines

Plasma levels of endothelin, natriuretic peptides, antidiuretic hormone, and cytokines have been measured in children by radioimmuno- and enzyme-linked immunosorbent assays. Age specific normal values are available for N-terminal pro-b-type natriuretic peptide (43) and several cytokines (44). Gene expression of endothelin, b-type natriuretic peptide, tumor necrosis factor (TNF)-α, interleukin-6, and several chemokines have been measured in myocardial tissue and lung specimens from children with congenital heart disease (38).

PATHOPHYSIOLOGY OF NEUROHORMONAL ACTIVATION IN PEDIATRIC HEART FAILURE

Renin–Angiotensin–Aldosterone System

Stimulation of the renin–angiotensin–aldosterone system leads to increased concentrations of renin, plasma angiotensin II, and aldosterone. Angiotensin II is a potent vasoconstrictor of the renal efferent arterioles and systemic circulation, where it stimulates release of norepinephrine from sympathetic nerve terminals. This leads to the retention of sodium and water and the increased excretion of potassium. In addition, angiotensin II and aldosterone have important effects on cardiac remodeling and may contribute to endothelial dysfunction.

In infants with heart failure due to left-to-right shunts, PRA is markedly enhanced (45). As previously demonstrated in adults with congestive heart failure (46), arterial hypotension is the most important hemodynamic trigger of renin

Table 2 Correlation Coefficients of Hemodynamic, Neurohormonal, and Clinical Signs of Heart Failure in Infants with Congenital Heart Disease

	PRA ($N = 47$)	Aldosterone ($N = 43$)	Norepinephrine ($N = 34$)	HF score ($N = 47$)
MAP	−0.72***	−0.62***	−0.57***	−0.67***
HF score	0.71***	0.72***	0.43**	—
PAP	0.15	0.18	−0.12	0.27
CI	−0.43**	−0.27	−0.21	−0.41**
$Q_p{:}Q_s$	0.33*	0.32*	−0.13	0.39**
RAP	0.15	−0.16	−0.15	0.11
EF	0.12	0.27	−0.19	0.26

PRA: plasma renin activity; MAP: mean arterial pressure; HF score: Ross's heart failure score; PAP: mean pulmonary artery pressure; CI: systemic cardiac index; Q_p/Q_s: ratio of pulmonary-to-systemic flow; RAP: mean right atrial pressure; EF: ejection fraction. Results of Spearman correlation: *** $p < 0.001$; ** $p < 0.01$; * $p < 0.05$.

release in infants with congenital heart disease (Table 2). A sympathetically mediated shift of threshold pressure in congestive heart failure on the pressure-dependent renin release curve (47) may explain the interrelationship between the renin–angiotensin–aldosterone and sympathetic nervous system (Fig. 5a) that is important for a better understanding of medical treatment. The decrease of mean arterial pressure from 60 to 50 mmHg during ACE inhibitor therapy with captopril in infants with large left-to-right shunts (48) appears to be at least partially responsible for a reactive renin release during this therapy (49) (Fig. 5b). This so-called escape phenomenon may be the reason that 20 years after introduction of angiotensin-converting enzyme inhibitor therapy in children with congenital heart disease, no study has yet to show a beneficial effect on clinical endpoints (50). In contrast, captopril in children with dilated cardiomyopathy effectively reduces neurohormonal activation and has a beneficial effect on prolonging survival in infants and children (51).

Beta-blocker therapy in infants with congenital heart disease may significantly reduce renin release (52) by preventing the sympathetically mediated shift of threshold pressure on the pressure-dependent renin release curve (Fig. 5b). In

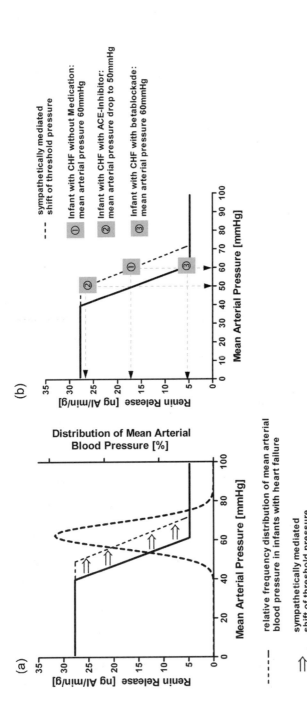

Figure 5 (a) Schematic diagram showing the effect of a sympathetically mediated shift of threshold pressure (dashed line) in congestive heart failure on the pressure-dependent renin release. (b) The effect of ACE inhibition (2) or beta blockade (3) on pressure dependent renin release in infants with left-to-right shunts. Renin release increases during ACE inhibition due to the mean aterial pressure drop from 60 to 50 mmHg (1 ⇉ 2). Renin release decreases during beta blockade due to the prevention of the sympathetically mediated shift of threshold pressure (dashed line) (1 ⇉ 3).

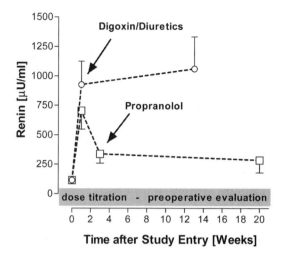

Figure 6 Renin levels in the digoxin/diuretics group and propranolol group in infants with left-to-right shunts during the prospective randomized CHF-PRO-INFANT trial. Renin levels steeply increase after the use of digoxin/diuretics and decrease only after beta blockade treatment with propranolol.

the prospective randomized clinical trial CHF-PRO-INFANT, renin release in these infants was initiated by treatment with loop diuretics (Fig. 6).

With respect to elevated aldosterone levels in children with heart failure, spironolactone given in infants with left-to-right shunts has been shown to have a beneficial effect in a randomized trial (53).

Sympathetic Nervous System

The sympathetic nervous system is activated in heart failure, via low- and high-pressure baroreceptors, as an early compensatory mechanism that provides inotropic support and maintains cardiac output. Chronic sympathetic activation, however, has deleterious effects, causing a further deterioration in cardiac function.

Sustained sympathetic stimulation activates the renin–angiotensin–aldosterone system and increased plasma norepinephrine concentrations. Excessive sympathetic activity is also associated with cardiac myocyte apoptosis, hypertrophy, and focal myocardial necrosis that may contribute to cardiac remodeling.

Elevated levels of norepinephrine (54) and a reduced heart rate variability (55) are evidence for sympathetic activation in pediatric heart failure. This recently published data showed significant correlations of heart rate variability and norepinephrine levels with the clinical severity of heart failure measured by a previously described heart failure score for children. However, despite evidence of a highly activated sympathetic system, the mean heart rate in infants with congestive heart failure (135 beats/min) was not significantly different than a "healthy control" group (137 beats/min). The pathophysiological explanation of this discrepancy may be that, in conditions characterized by a marked and unopposed persistent sympathetic excitation, the sinus node is able to diminish its responsiveness to neural inputs, possibly through downregulation of β-adrenergic receptors and a post-receptor defect of adenylyl cyclase (56). In children with congenital heart disease, the degree of the left-to-right shunt and pulmonary artery systolic pressure correlate directly with plasma norepinephrine levels and inversely with lymphocyte β-adrenergic receptor density (57). In addition, β-adrenergic receptor density is significantly lower in patients with heart failure than in those without. In most cases, β-adrenergic receptor downregulation is β_1-subtype selective, but in children with left-to-right shunts downregulation seems not to be β_1 selective (58). In these infants, myocardial β-adrenergic receptor downregulation seems to be a risk factor for postoperative complications after cardiac surgery (18). These results are in accordance with previously published data that showed β-adrenergic receptor downregulation in donor hearts as a predictor of early graft heart failure in the first month after orthotopic cardiac transplantation (59). β-Adrenergic receptor downregulation in infants with left-to-right shunts correlates not only with preoperative heart failure but also to preoperative medical therapy, which usually includes digoxin and diuretics. This standard medical treatment is unable to prevent downregulation. In contrast, the β-antagonist propranolol may significantly increase β-adrenergic receptor gene expression in infants with left-to-right shunts (18) and β-adrenergic receptor number in children with tetralogy of Fallot (60). These results are similar to the effect of metoprolol treatment of adults with heart failure in which there is an increase in myocardial β-adrenergic receptor density.

Endothelin

Activation of the endothelin system seems to be involved in the pathogenesis of chronic heart failure by elevating systemic vascular resistance (61) and possibly by the changes of the myocardial endothelin receptor gene expression in human end-stage heart failure (62). Moreover, pulmonary artery hypertension due to any cause is associated with an activation of the endothelin system (30). Activation of the endothelin system has been described in children with congenital heart disease (63), pulmonary artery hypertension (64), and after cardiopulmonary bypass (65). Endothelin A receptors are upregulated in the lungs of children with pulmonary artery hypertension (66). These results have been confirmed in a well-established animal model with increased pulmonary blood flow (67).

Studies in adults with heart failure have shown acute beneficial hemodynamic effects in patients treated with the selective endothelin A receptor antagonist sitaxsentan (68). However, in a phase III trial (ENABLE-1) bosentan, a dual endothelin receptor antagonist, showed no benefit in the incidence of mortality, death, and heart failure hospitalization.

Evidence-based clinical data are now available for the use of bosentan in patients with pulmonary artery hypertension. Two double-bind, placebo-controlled studies (69,70) showed significantly improved 6-min walking distances, cardiopulmonary hemodynamics, Borg dyspnea index, and World Health Organization functional class. Side effects like hepatic toxicity seem to be dose dependent and relatively rare at a dose of 125 mg twice daily. Endothelin antagonists have been evaluated in three animal models of heart failure due to

pulmonary artery hypertension: (1) left-to-right shunt model
(71); (2) hyaline membrane disease (72); (3) meconium aspiration (73). All these studies showed hemodynamic benefits.
However, there has been only one clinical study that has
assessed the effect of the endothelin A receptor antagonist
BQ-123 in three infants with postoperative pulmonary
hypertension (74). In this study, a reduction in the ratio
of pulmonary-to-systemic artery pressures and a tendency
for the cardiac index to rise were associated with an unwanted
fall in mean arterial pressure.

Natriuretic Peptides

There are three natriuretic peptides of similar structure and
with a wide range of effects on the heart, kidneys, and central
nervous system. Atrial natriuretic peptide (ANP) is released
from the atria in response to stretch, leading to natriuresis
and vasodilatation. Brain or b-type natriuretic peptide
(BNP) is also released from the heart and its actions are similar to those of atrial natriuretic peptide. C-type natriuretic
peptide is limited to the vascular endothelium and central
nervous system and has only limited effects on natriuresis
and vasodilatation.

The atrial and b-type natriuretic peptide levels increase
in response to volume expansion and pressure overload of
the heart and act as a physiological antagonists to vasoconstriction and renal-tubule sodium reabsorption caused by
the sympathetic nervous and renin–angiotensin–aldosterone
systems. Due to these beneficial effects, substantial interest
has emerged regarding the therapeutic potential of natriuretic peptides. Nesiritide, a recombinant b-type natriuretic peptide, is the first in a new drug class for the treatment of
decompensated heart failure (75).

Since circulating concentrations of natriuretic peptides
are increased in patients with heart failure, special interest
has developed as to the prognostic potential of these peptides.
BNP and N-terminal b-type natriuretic peptide (NT-BNP) has
become an important prognostic marker in human heart failure (26,76) and a surrogate end point in recent heart failure

trials (77). b-Type natriuretic peptide has been used for risk stratification in children and young adults with right ventricular dysfunction after surgery for congenital heart disease (29), doxorubicin-induced left ventricular diastolic dysfunction (78), and heart failure in children with Duchenne's progressive muscular dystrophy (79).

Antidiuretic Hormone

Antidiuretic hormone or arginine vasopressin concentrations are increased in severe chronic heart failure. High concentrations of this hormone are common in patients receiving diuretic treatment and are related to the development of hyponatraemia.

Arginine vasopressin, through its receptor-mediated effects, could theoretically also contribute to progression of left ventricular dysfunction and heart failure by aggravating systolic and diastolic wall stress, and by directly stimulating myocardial hypertrophy. A randomized, double-blind, placebo-controlled study of tolvaptan, a vasopressin antagonist, is in progress to determine the effects of this new treatment on the acute and chronic outcomes of patients with worsening heart failure (80).

IMMUNOLOGIC ASPECTS OF PEDIATRIC HEART FAILURE

Pathophysiology of Immune Activation in Heart Failure

Although several cytokines appear to be involved in heart failure (81), particular interest has been directed toward the role of TNF-α in heart failure. It has been shown in vitro that TNF can act on the cardiovascular system by reducing the contractility of myocardial cells. In animals, TNF causes dilatation and remodeling of the left ventricle, and transgenic mice over-expressing TNF develop left ventricular dilatation and dysfunction. Despite this paradigm of TNF being harmful, some studies revealed that TNF has a protective inotropic action on the failing heart and stimulates the production of heat shock proteins, which enables cells to resist transient stress such as ischemia. Furthermore, injection of TNF improves survival of $TNF^{-/-}$ knockout mice infected with encephalomyocarditis virus in a dose-dependent manner by increasing viral clearance. Further interest has been focused on interleukin-6 (IL-6) in heart failure. IL-6 may exert endocrine effects such as a decrease of left ventricular contractility by nitric oxide production. The IL-6/IL-6 receptor complex, including gp-130, may play an important role in ventricular hypertrophy and ventricular remodeling. IL-6 is produced not only in leukocytes, but also in endothelial cells, vascular smooth muscle cells, cardiomyocytes, and fibroblasts in various cardiovascular organs and the lung.

The response of the immune system to initial hemodynamic disturbances, possibly caused by myocardial dysfunction or congenital heart defects, may include secretion of various cytokines that promote inflammation, resulting in necrotic cardiomyocyte damage and endothelial activation, thereby triggering production of secondary inflammatory mediators. Simultaneously, counteracting mechanisms are stimulated that promote secretion of anti-inflammatory cytokines and peptides. Among them, interleukin-10 (IL-10) inhibits the respiratory burst in phagocytes and prevents the induction of monocyte coagulant activity. The secretion of the various cytokines depends on the normal function of the traditional immune cells. After acute myocardial damage, patients show significantly increased IL-10 plasma levels that are negatively correlated to the TNF release of monocytes. Thus, during heart failure, the function of the immune cells seems to be disturbed resulting in an imbalance between pro- and anti-inflammatory cytokines. At present, there are three main theories as to why there are high cytokine levels in patients with congestive heart failure.

One hypothesis is that the heart is the main source of cytokines, as it has been shown that the failing myocardium is capable of producing TNF-α (82). The second hypothesis is that altered gut permeability with bacterial translocation and endotoxemia would be increased in patients with edema secondary to heart failure (83). The third hypothesis is based on the relationship between the activated sympathetic nervous system and the immune axis in congestive heart failure with concomitant lymphocyte β_2-adrenergic receptor desensitization (84,85).

Cytokines in Pediatric Heart Failure

Immune activation measured by cytokine levels and endogenous nitric oxide production occurs in children with heart failure due to left-to-right shunts (Table 3) (10). There is no evidence of elevated cytokine levels and endogenous oxide production in children with cyanotic heart defects who usually do not suffer from congestive heart failure (34). Little is known, however, about the pathophysiological role of this immune activation in infants with heart failure due to left-to-right shunts. As previously demonstrated in adults with heart failure (86), increased nitric oxide synthesis in

Table 3 Myocardial Gene Expression, Endogenous Nitric Oxide, and Cytokine Release in Patient Groups[a]

	Healthy control	Left-to-right shunts	Cyanotic defects	*p*-Value[b]
Myocardial biopsies (*N*)[c]		11	9	
TNF-α expression	?	0.63 ± 0.21	0.85 ± 0.5	0.52
IL-6 expression	?	0.43 ± 0.33	1.15 ± 1.0	0.22
RANTES expression	?	0.87 ± 0.7	0.63 ± 0.31	0.3
MCP-1 expression	?	0.58 ± 0.32	1.0 ± 0.95	0.54
Plasma samples (*N*)	8	15	11	
Nitrate/nitrite (μM)	11 ± 5	40 ± 24	23 ± 7	0.028
TNF-R1 (ng/mL)	1.0 ± 0.2	1.7 ± 0.5	0.8 ± 0.3	< 0.001
TNF-R2 (ng/mL)	3.4 ± 0.4	8.1 ± 4.0	5.1 ± 3.3	0.048

IL-6 = Interleukin-6; MCP = monocyte chemoattractant protein-1; RANTES = regulated upon activation, normal T-cell expressed, and presumably secreted; TNF-α = tumor necrosis factor-α; TNF-R1 = tumor necrosis factor-α receptor 1; TNF-R2 = tumor necrosis factor-α receptor 2.
[a]Plus or minus values are means ± SD.
[b]*t*-Test left-to-right shunts versus cyanotic defects.
[c]The target gene expression was normalized to the expression of glyceralaldehyde-3-phosphate dehydrogenase.

infants with heart failure and pulmonary artery hypertension is related to the activation of the TNF-α system (10). There is a link between expression patterns of inducible and endothelial nitric oxide synthase and pulmonary plexogenic arteriopathy in children with congenital heart disease (32).

As shown in Table 3, increased plasma levels of TNF-α receptors 1 and 2 in children with left-to-right shunts when compared to children with cyanotic heart disease are not due to a higher expression of myocardial TNF-α gene. Cardiac myocyte injury in human heart failure may be associated with inflammatory lesions possibly due to myocardial chemokine release (87). However, there is no significantly different myocardial gene expression of the chemokines monocyte chemoattractant protein-1 and RANTES (regulated upon activation, normal T-cell expressed, and presumably secreted) in children with congenital heart disease with or without heart failure. Based on these results, there is no evidence to support the hypothesis that a higher cytokine release in children with left-to-right shunts compared to children with cyanosis is caused by the myocardium itself. These results arc in accordance with recently published data that demonstrate that cytokines are expressed in the myocardium in end-stage heart failure to a much greater degree than in patients with recent onset of symptoms (88). This suggests that induction of cytokines in the myocardium is a relatively late event in the pathogenesis of heart failure.

In terms of elevated peripheral levels of proinflammatory cytokines in children with congenital heart disease, several important questions remain unanswered. Recently published data demonstrate that endotoxemia in children with congenital heart disease, measured by lipopolysaccharide-binding protein is more common than previously suspected, and correlates with clinical outcomes (89) after cardiac surgery. One explanation is that altered gut permeability with bacterial translocation and endotoxemia seems to be increased in patients with edema secondary to heart failure. Further clinical trials targeting endotoxin and an impaired β-adrenergic control of immune function in children with congenital heart disease will be necessary to determine if immune activation is a causal etiologic agent in the disease process and a target of new therapeutic approaches. For example, growth failure in children with congenital heart disease is not well explained by a reduced uptake of nutrition or an elevated basal metabolic rate (12). Growth failure in infants with heart failure is not necessarily related to hemodynamic abnormalities or caloric intake but may be associated with neurohormonal activation and a reduced heart rate variability due to autonomic imbalance (Table 4). There is no doubt that cardiac cachexia in adults with severe heart failure is more closely associated with elevated cytokine levels than with conventional measures of heart failure (90) but comparable data are unfortunately missing in pediatric cardiology.

Table 4 Effects of Caloric Intake, Hemodynamics, Neurohormonal Activation, and Heart Rate Variability on Weight Gain in Infants with Left-to-Right Shunts

Weight gain (g/month)	> 400	200–400	< 200	p-Value[a]
Age (month)	4.5 ± 1.9	4.9 ± 2.5	3.6 ± 2.4	0.23
Caloric intake (kcal/kg/day)	93 ± 16	107 ± 24	90 ± 25	0.13
VO_2 (mL/min/m^2)	130 ± 25	132 ± 21	128 ± 26.9	0.92
Q_p/Q_s	3.4 ± 1.7	4.3 ± 3.2	3.0 ± 1.0	0.17
PAP (mmHg)	33.8 ± 12.9	33.2 ± 11.9	35.4 ± 14.6	0.88
MAP (mmHg)	59.4 ± 6.9	62.3 ± 11.2	56.7 ± 9.5	0.17
SaO_2	94.5 ± 4.8	92.6 ± 7.4	92.5 ± 6.2	0.45
PRA (ng/mL/h)	20 ± 18	67 ± 65	61 ± 68	0.14
Aldosterone (pg/mL)	604 ± 634	1508 ± 1742	852 ± 721	0.05
Norepinephrine (ng/L)	410 ± 257	610 ± 449	800 ± 752	0.07
SDRR (ms)	55.7 ± 18.5	48.0 ± 17.2	37.1 ± 12.3	0.1
VLF (ms)	14.5 ± 5.0	12.5 ± 5.7	7.3 ± 2.5	0.004

VO_2, oxygen consumption; Q_p/Q_s, ratio of pulmonary-to-systemic flow; PAP, mean pulmonary artery pressure; MAP, mean arterial pressure; SaO_2, systemic oxygen saturation.
Heart rate variability: SDRR, standard deviation of all RR intervals; VLF, very low frequency power spectrum between 0.003 and 0.04 Hz.
[a]Results of one-way-ANOVA.

Cytokines as a Target of Medical Treatment

In some studies, the hypothesis that anticytokine therapy in heart failure may be of clinical benefit has been addressed. However, in one prospective randomized trial, vesnarinone, a phoshodiesterase inhibitor that reduces the level of TNF in heart failure patients, increased mortality (91). More recently, a specific anticytokine therapy using a TNF receptor fusion protein (etanercept) showed disappointing clinical results in a large clinical trial and had to be stopped prematurely because of futility (92).

On the other hand, recently published studies have shown that the beneficial effect of β-blocker therapy in patients with heart failure is paralleled by altered levels of inflammatory and anti-inflammatory cytokines. Gullestad et al. (93) measured an increase of soluble IL-2 receptor in patients with heart failure, an increase that was reversed after treatment with the selective β-blocker metoprolol after 3 months of therapy. In contrast, the elevated plasma levels of IL-6, IL-8, and TNF are not reversed in metoprolol-treated patients. On the other hand, Ohtsuka et al. (94) described enhanced levels of TNF, sTNF-R2, and IL-10 in patients with heart failure. After selective blockade of the β-adrenergic receptors with metoprolol they found a reduction of these cytokine levels. Reduction of IL-6 levels in patients with heart failure treated with diverse β-blockers has been observed in other clinical studies (95). Increased soluble TNF receptor and IL-10 plasma levels observed in heart failure patients treated with standard medication are reversed in patients additionally treated with metoprolol (96). Accordingly, elevated TNF receptor levels decrease during propranolol therapy in infants with heart failure (10).

Taken together, treatment of patients with heart failure with β-blockers appears to result in alterations within the cytokine system. The resulting "normalization" of the cytokine system, or parts thereof, as indicated by the reversal of cytokine, cytokine antagonist, or soluble cytokine receptor levels toward levels in healthy controls, may contribute to the beneficial effects of β-blockers in treatment of CHF. It is tempting to speculate that the observed changes of plasma cytokine, cytokine antagonist, or cytokine receptor levels in patients with heart failure treated with β-blocker therapy may result from an unbalanced interaction of the neurohormonal and the cytokine systems, possibly caused by altered cAMP levels in certain cells, in particular leukocytes. As a consequence of altered cellular cAMP, an unbalanced production and/or release of cytokines, cytokine antagonists, or soluble cytokine receptors occurs that may be reversed by β-blocker therapy.

REFERENCES

1. Packer M. The neurohormonal hypothesis: a theory to explain the mechanism of disease progression in heart failure. J Am Coll Cardiol 1992; 20:248–254.
2. Dibbs Z, Kurrelmeyer K, Kalra D, Seta Y, Wang F, Bozkurt B, Baumgarten G, Sivasubramanian N, Mann DL. Cytokines in heart failure: pathogenetic mechanisms and potential treatment. Proc Assoc Am Phys 1999; 111:423–428.
3. Cohn JN, Ferrari R, Sharpe N. Cardiac remodeling—concepts and clinical implication: a consensus paper from an international forum on cardiac remodeling. J Am Coll Cardiol 2000; 35:569–582.
4. Mann DL. Mechanisms and models of heart failure. Circulation 1999; 100:999–1008.
5. Cohn JN, Levine TB, Olivari MT, Garberg V, Lura D, Francis GS, Simon AB, Rector T. Plasma norepinephrine as a guide to prognosis in patients with chronic congestive heart failure. NEngl J Med 1984; 311:819–823.
6. Stern H, Weil J, Genz T, Vogt W, Bühlmeyer K. Captopril in children with dilated cardiomyopathy: acute and long-term effects in a prospective study of hemodynamic and hormonal effects. Pediatr Cardiol 1990; 11:22–28.
7. Ishikawa Y, Bach JR, Minami R. Cardioprotection for Duchenne's muscular dystrophy. Am Heart J 1999; 137:895–902.
8. Kimball TR, Daniels SR, Hannon DW, Khoury P, Schwartz DC. Relation of symptoms to contractility and defect size in infants with ventricular septal defect. Am J Cardiol 1991; 67:1097–1102.
9. Buchhorn R, Ross RD, Wessel A, Hulpke-Wette M, Bürsch J. Activity of the renin–angiotensin–aldosterone and sympathetic nervous system and their relation to hemodynamic and clinical abnormalities in infants with left-to-right shunts. Int J Cardiol 2001; 78:225–230.
10. Buchhorn R, Wessel A, Hulpke-Wette M, Bürsch J, Werdan K, Loppnow H. Endogenous nitric oxide production and soluble tumor necrosis

factor-receptor levels are enhanced in infants with congenital heart disease. Crit Care Med 2001; 29:2208–2210.

11. Gidding SS, Bessel M. Hemodynamic correlates of clinical severity in isolated ventricular septal defect. Pediatr Cardiol 1993; 14:135–139.

12. Buchhorn R, Hammersen A, Bürsch J. The pathogenesis of heart failure in infants with congenital heart disease. Cardiol Young 2001; 11:498–504.

13. Ponikowski P, Chua TP, Piepoli M, Ondusova D, Webb-Peploe K, Harrington D, Anker SD, Volterrani M, Colombo R, Mazzuero G, Giordano A, Coats AJ. Augmented peripheral chemosensitivity as a potential input to baroreflex impairment and autonomic imbalance in chronic heart failure. Circulation 1997; 96:2586–2594.

14. Ross RD, Danniels SR, Schwartz DC, Hannnon DW, Kaplan S. Return of plasma norepinephrine to normal after resolution of congestive heart failure in congenital heart disease. Am J Cardiol 1987; 60:1411–1413.

15. Jenkins KJ, Gauvreau K, Newburger JW, Spray TL, Moller JH, Iezzoni LI. Consensus-based method for risk adjustment for surgery for congenital heart disease. J Thorac Cardiovasc Surg 2002; 101:110–118.

16. Seliem M, Muster AJ, Paul MH, Benson DW. Relation between preoperative left ventricular muscle mass and outcome of the Fontan procedure in patients with tricuspid atresia. J Am Coll Cardiol 1989; 14:750–755.

17. Hunter JJ, Chien KR. Signaling pathways for cardiac hypertrophy and failure. N Engl J Med 1999; 341:1276–1283.

18. Buchhorn R, Hulpke-Wette M, Ruschewski W, Pregla R, Fielitz J, Regitz-Zagrosek V. Beta-receptor downregulation in congenital heart disease: a risk factor for complications after surgical repair? Ann Thorac Surg 2002; 73:610–613.

19. Silka MJ, Hardy BG, Menashe VD, Morris CD. A population-based prospective evaluation of risk of sudden cardiac death after operation for common congenital heart defects. J Am Coll Cardiol 1998; 32: 245–251.

20. Bolger AP, Sharma R, Li W, Leenarts M, Kalra PR, Kemp M, Coats AJS, Anker SD, Gatzoulis MA. Neurohormonal activation and the chronic heart failure syndrome in adults with congenital heart disease. Circulation 2002; 106:92–99.

21. Ohuchi H, Suzuki H, Toyohara K, Tatsumi K, Ono Y, Arakaki Y, Echigo S. Abnormal cardiac autonomic nervous activity after right ventricular outflow tract reconstruction. Circulation 2002; 104:2732–2738.

22. Piran S, Veldtman G, Siu S, Webb GD, Liu PP. Heart failure and ventricular dysfunction in patients with single or systemic right ventricles. Circulation 2002; 105:1189–1194.

23. Norozi K, Buchhorn R, Bartmus D, Hagen A, Kaiser Ch, Hess G, Binder L, Wessel A. Serum Pro-BNP: Ein Marker derRV-Funktions-

störung bei operierter Fallot'scher Tetralogie (abstract) Z Kardiol 2002; 91:773.

24. Hjordal VE, Stenbog EV, Ravn HB, Emmertsen K, Jensen KT, Pedersen EB, Olsen KH, Hansen OK, Sorensen KE. Neurohormonal activation late after cavopulmonary connection. Heart 2000; 83: 439–443.

25. Ohuchi H, Hasegawa S, Yasuda K, Yamada O, Ono Y, Echigo S. Severely impaired cardiac autonomic nervous activity after the Fontan operation. Circulation 2001; 104:1513–1518.

26. Troughton RW, Frampton CM, Yandle TG, Espiner EA, Nicholls MG, Richards AM. Treatment of heart failure guided by plasma aminoterminal brain natriuretic peptide (N-BNP) concentrations. Lancet 2000; 355:1126–1130.

27. Nolan J, Batin PD, Andrews R, et al. Prospective study of heart rate variability and mortality in chronic heart failure: results of the United Kingdom heart failure evaluation and assessment of risk trial (UK-heart). Circulation 1998; 98:1510–1516.

28. Anand IS, Florea VG, Fisher L. Surrogate end points in heart failure. J Am Coll Cardiol 2002; 39:1414–1421.

29. Tulevski II, Groenink M, van Der Wall EE, van Veldhuisen DJ, Boomsma F, Stoker J, Hirsch A, Lemkes JS, Mulder BJ. Increased brain and atrial natriuretic peptides in patients with right ventricular pressure overload: correlation between plasma neurohormones and right ventricular dysfunction. Heart 2001; 86:27–30.

30. Nootens M, Kaufmann E, Rector T, Toher C, Judd D, Francis GS, Rich S. Neurohormonal activation in patients with right ventricular failure from pulmonary hypertension: Relation of hemodynamic variables and endothelin levels. J Am Coll Cardiol 1995; 26:1581–1585.

31. Gorenflo M, Gross P, Bodey A, Schmitz L, Brockmeier K, Berger F, Bein G, Lange PE. Plasma endothelin-1 in patients with left-to-right shunt. Am Heart J 1995; 130:537–542.

32. Berger RM, Geiger R, Hess J, Bogers AJ, Mooi WJ. Altered arterial expression patterns of inducible and endothelial nitric oxide synthase in pulmonary plexogenic arteriopathy caused by congenital heart disease. Am J Respir Crit Care 2001; 163:1493–1499.

33. Black SM, Fineman JR, Steinhorn RH, Bristow J, Soifer SJ. Increased endothelial NOS in lambs with increased pulmonary blood flow and pulmonary hypertension. Am J Physiol 1998; 275:H1643–H1651.

34. Seghaye MC, Duchateau J, Bruniaux J, Demontoux S, Detruit H, Bosson C, Lecoronier G, Mokhfi E, Planche C. Endogenous nitric oxide production and atrial natriuretic peptide biological activity in infants undergoing cardiac operations. Crit Care Med 1997; 25: 1063–1070.

35. Takaya J, Ikemoto Y, Teraguchi S, Nogi S, Kobayashi Y. Plasma nitric oxide products correlate with cardiac index of congenital heart disease. Pediatr Cardiol 2000; 21:378–381.

36. Fiselier TJW, Lijnen P, Monnens L, van Munster P, Jansen M, Peer P. Levels of renin, angiotensin I and II, angiotensin-converting enzyme and aldosterone in infancy and childhood. Eur J Pediatr 1993; 141:3–7.

37. Krüger C, Rauh M, Dorr HG. Immunoreactive renin concentrations in healthy children from birth to adolescence. Clin Chem Acta 1998; 274:15–27.

38. Buchhorn R, Hulpke-Wette M, Ruschewski W, Ross RD, Fielitz J, Pregla R, Hetzer R, Regitz-Zagrosek V. Effects of therapeutic beta blockade on myocardial function and cardiac remodeling in congenital cardiac disease. Cardiol Young 2003; 13:36–43.

39. Eichler I, Eichler HG, Rotter M, Kyrle PA, Gasic S, Korn A. Plasma concentrations of free and sulfoconjugated dopamine, epinephrine, and norepinephrine in healthy infants and children. Klin Wochenschr 1989; 67:672–675.

40. Folger GM Jr, Hollowell JG. Excretion of catecholamine in urine by infants and children with cyanotic congenital heart disease. Pediatr Res 1972; 6:151–157.

41. Massin M, von Bernuth G. Normal ranges of heart rate variability during infancy and childhood. Pediatr Cardiol 1997; 18:297–302.

42. Acar P, Merlet P, Iserin L, Bonnet D, Sidi D, Syrota A, Kachaner J. Impaired cardiac adrenergic innervation assessed by MIBG imaging as a predictor of treatment in childhood dilated cardiomyopathy. Heart 2001; 85:692–696.

43. Mir TS, Marohn S, Laer S, Eiselt M, Grollmus O, Weil J. Plasma concentrations of N-terminal pro-brain natriuretic peptide in control children from the neonatal to adolescent period and in children with congestive heart failure. Pediatrics 2002; 110:e76.

44. Sack U, Burhardt U, Borte M, Schädlich H, Berg K, Emmrich F. Age-dependent levels of select immunological mediators in sera of healthy children. Clin Diagn Lab Immunol 1998; 5:28–32.

45. Scammell AM, Diver MJ. Plasma renin activity in infants with congenital heart disease. Arch Dis Child 1987; 62:1136–1138.

46. Harris P. Congestive cardiac failure: central role of the arterial blood pressure. Br Heart J 1987; 57:190–203.

47. Kirchheim HR, Ehmke H, Persson P. Physiology of the renal baroreceptor-mechanism of renin release and its role in congestive heart failure. Am J Cardiol 1988; 62:68E–71E.

48. Shaddy RE, Teitel DF, Brett C. Short-term hemodynamic effects of captopril in infants with congestive heart failure. Am J Dis Child 1988; 142:100–105.

49. Buchhorn R, Ross RD, Hulpke-Wette M, Bartmus D, Wessel A, Schulz R, Bürsch J. Effectiveness of low dose captopril versus propranolol therapy in infants with severe congestive failure due to left-to-right shunts. Int J Cardiol 2000; 76:227–233.

50. Leversha ML, Wilson NJ, Clarkson PM, Calder AL, Ramage MC, Neutze JM. Efficacy and dosage of enalapril in congenital and acquired heart disease. Arch Dis Child 1994; 70:35–39.

51. Lewis AB, Chabot M. The effect of treatment with angiotensin-converting enzyme inhibitors on survival of pediatric patients with dilated cardiomyopathy. Pediatr Cardiol 1993; 14:9–12.

52. Buchhorn R, Hulpke-Wette M, Hilgers R, Bartmus D, Wessel A, Bürsch J. Propranolol treatment of congestive heart failure in infants with congenital heart disease: the CHF-PRO-INFANT trial. Int J Cardiol 2001; 79:167–173.

53. Hobbins SM, Fowler RS, Rowe RD, Korey AG. Spironolactone therapy in infants with congestive heart failure secondary to congenital heart disease. Arch Dis Child 1981; 56:934–938.

54. Ross RD, Daniels RD, Schwartz DC, Hannon DW, Shukla R, Kaplan S. Plasma norepinephrine levels in infants and children with congestive heart failure. Am J Cardiol 1987; 59:911–914.

55. Buchhorn R, Hulpke-Wette M, Nothroff J, Paul T. Heart rate variability in infants with heart failure due to congenital heart disease: reversal of depressed heart rate variability by propranolol. Med Sci Monit 2002; 8:CR661–CR666.

56. Reithmann C, Reber D, Kozlik-Feldmann R, Netz H, Pilz G, Welz A, Werdan K. A post-receptor defect of adenylyl cyclase in severely failing myocardium from children with congenital heart disease. Eur J Pharmacol 1997; 330:79–86.

57. Wu JR, Chang HR, Huang TY, Chiang CH, Chen SS. Reduction in lymphocyte beta-adrenergic receptor density in infants and children with heart failure secondary to congenital heart disease. Am J Cardiol 1996; 77:170–174.

58. Kozlik R, Kramer HH, Wicht H, Krian A, Ostermeyer J, Reinhardt D. Myocardial β-adrenoreceptor density and the distribution of $\beta 1$–$\beta 2$-adrenoreceptor subpopulations in children with congenital heart disease. Eur J Pediatr 1991; 150:388–394.

59. Chester MR, Amadi AA, Barnett DB. Beta adrenoceptor density in the donor heart: a guide to prognosis? Br Heart J 1995; 73:540–543.

60. Kozlik-Feldmann R, Kramer HH, Feldmann R, Netz H, Reinhardt D. Distribution of myocardial β-adrenoreceptor subtypes and coupling to the adenylyl cyclase in children with congenital heart disease and implications for treatment. J Clin Pharmacol 1993; 33:588–595.

61. Tsutamoto T, Wada A, Hisanaga T, Maeda K, Ohnishi M, Mabuchi N, Sawaki M, Hayashi M, Fujii M, Kinoshita M. Relationship between endothelin-1 extraction in the peripheral circulation and systemic vascular resistance in patients with severe congestive heart failure. J Am Coll Cardiol 1999; 33:530–537.

62. Zolk O, Quattek J, Sitzler G, Schrader T, Nickenig G, Schnabel P, Shimada K, Takashashi M, Bohm M. Expression of endothelin-1,

endothelin-converting enzyme, and endothelin receptors in chronic heart failure. Circulation 1999; 99:2118–2123.

63. Vincent JA, Ross RD, Kassab J, Hsu JM, Pinsky WW. Relation of elevated plasma endothelin in congenital heart disease to increased pulmonary blood flow. Am J Cardiol 1993; 71:1204–1207.

64. Yoshibayashi M, Nishioka K, Nakao K, Saito Y, Matsumura M, Ueda T, Temma S, Shirakami G, Imura H, Mikawa H. Plasma endothelin concentrations in patients with pulmonary hypertension associated with congenital heart defects. Circulation 1991; 84:2280–2285.

65. Komai H, Adatia IT, Elliott MJ, de Leval MR, Haworth SG. Increased plasma levels of endothelin-1 after cardiopulmonary bypass in patients with pulmonary hypertension. J Thorac Cardiovasc Surg 1993; 106:473–478.

66. Lutz J, Gorenflo M, Habighorst M, Vogel M, Lange PE, Hocher B. Endothelin-1- and endothelin-receptors in lung biopsies of patients with pulmonary hypertension due to congenital heart disease. Clin Chem Lab Med 1999; 37:423–428.

67. Black SM, Bekker JM, Johengen MJ, Parry AJ, Soifer SJ, Fineman JR. Altered regulation of the ET-1 cascade in lambs with increased pulmonary blood flow and pulmonary hypertension. Pediatr Res 2000; 47:97–106.

68. Givertz MM, Colucci WS, LeJemtel TH, Gottlieb SS, Hare JM, Slawsky MT, Leier CV, Loh E, Nicklas JM, Lewis BE. Acute endothelin A receptor blockade causes selective pulmonary vasodilation in patients with chronic heart failure. Circulation 2000; 101:2922–2927.

69. Channick RN, Simonneau G, Sitbon O, Robbins IM, Frost A, Tapson VF, Badesch DB, Roux S, Rainisio M, Bodin F, Rubin LJ. Effects of the dual endothelin-receptor antagonist bosentan in patients with pulmonary hypertension: a randomised placebo-controlled study. Lancet 2001; 358:1119–1123.

70. Rubin LJ, Badesch DB, Barst RJ, Galie N, Black CM, Keogh A, Pulido T, Frost A, Roux S, Leconte I, Landsberg M, Simonneau G. Bosentan therapy for pulmonary arterial hypertension. NEngl J Med 2002; 346:896–903.

71. Reddy VM, Hendricks-Munoz KD, Rajasinghe HA, Petrossian E, Hanley FL, Fineman JR. Post-cardiopulmonary bypass pulmonary hypertension in lambs with increased pulmonary blood flow. Circulation 1997; 95:1054–1061.

72. Ivy DD, Parker TA, Kinsella JP, Abman SH. Endothelin A receptor blockade decreases pulmonary vascular resistance in premature lambs with hyaline membrane disease. Pediatr Res 1998; 44:175–180.

73. Kuo CY. Endothelin-A receptor antagonist prevents neonatal pulmonary hypertension in meconium aspiration in piglets. JFormos Med Assoc 2001; 100:420–423.

74. Prendergast B, Newby DE, Wilson LE, Webb DJ, Mankad PS. Early therapeutic experience with the endothelin antagonist BQ-123 in pul-

monary hypertension after congenital heart surgery. Heart 1999; 82:505–508.

75. Elkayam U, Akhter MW, Tummala P, Khan S, Singh H. Nesiritide: a new drug for the treatment of decompensated heart failure. J Cardiovasc Pharmacol Ther 2002; 7:181–194.

76. Maisel AS, Krishnaswamy P, Nowak RM, McCord J, Hollander JE, Duc P, Omland T, Storrow AB, Abraham WT, Wu AH, Clopton P, Steg PG, Westheim A, Knudsen CW, Perez A, Kazanegra R, Herrmann HC, McCullough PA. Rapid measurement of B-type natriuretic peptide in the emergency diagnosis of heart failure. N Engl J Med 2002; 347:161–167.

77. Stanek B, Frey B, Hülsmann M, Berger R, Sturm B, Strametz-Juranek J, Bergler-Klein J, Moser P, Bojic A, Hartter E, Pacher R. Prognostic evaluation of neurohumoral plasma levels before and during beta-blocker therapy in advanced leftventricular dysfunction. J Am Coll Cardiol 2001; 38:436–442.

78. Nousiainen T, Vanninen E, Jantunen E, Puustinen J, Remes J, Rantala A, Vuolteenaho O, Hartikainen J. Natriuretic peptides during the development of doxorubicin-induced left ventricular diastolic dysfunction. J Intern Med 2002; 251:228–234.

79. Mori K, Manabe T, Nii M, Hayabuchi Y, Kuroda Y, Tatara K. Plasma levels of natriuretic peptide and echocardiographic parameters in patients with doxorubicin-induced left ventricular diastolic dysfunction. Pediatr Cardiol 2002; 23:160–166.

80. Gheorghiade M, Gattis WA, Barbagelata A, Adams KF Jr, Elkayam U, Orlandi C, O'Connor CM. Rationale and study design for a multicenter, randomized, double-blind, placebo-controlled study of the effects of tolvaptan on the acute and chronic outcomes of patients hospitalized with worsening congestive heart failure. Am Heart J 2003; 145(suppl 2):S51–S54.

81. Sharma RB, Coats AJS, Anker SD. The role of inflammatory mediators in chronic heart failure: cytokine, nitric oxide, and endothelin-1. Int J Cardiol 2000; 72:175–186.

82. Torre-Amione G, Kapadia S, Lee J, Durand JB, Bies RD, Young JB, Mann DL. Tumor necrosis factor-alpha and tumor necrosis factor receptors in the failing human heart. Circulation 1996; 93:704–711.

83. Niebauer J, Volk HD, Kemp M, Dominguez M, Schuman RR, Rauchhaus M, Poole-Wilson PA, Coats AJS, Anker SD. Endotoxin and immune activation in chronic heart failure: a prospective cohort study. Lancet 1999; 353:1838–1842.

84. Maisel AS. Beneficial effects of metoprolol treatment in congestive heart failure. Reversal of sympathetic-induced alterations of immunologic function. Circulation 1994; 90:1774–1780.

85. Werner C, Werdan K, Pönicke K, Brodde OE. Impaired beta-adrenergic control of immune function in patients with chronic heart failure: reversal by beta 1-blocker treatment. Basic Res Cardiol 2001; 96:290–298.

86. Comini L, Bachetti T, Agnoletti L, Gaia G, Curello S, Milanesi B, Volterrani M, Parrinello G, Ceconi C, Giordano A, Corti A, Ferrari R. Induction of functional inducible nitric oxide synthase in monocytes of patients with congestive heart failure. Link with tumor necrosis factor-alpha. Eur Heart J 1999; 20:1503–1513.

87. Aukrust P, Ueland T, Muller F, Andreassen AK, Nordoy I, Aas H, Kjekhus J, Simonsen S, Froland SS, Gullestad L. Elevated circulating levels of C–C chemokines in patients with congestive heart failure. Circulation 1998; 97:1136–1143.

88. Kubota T, Miyagishima M, Alvarez RJ, Kormos R, Rosenblum WD, Demetris AJ, Semigran MJ, Dec GW, Holubkov R, McTierman CF, Mann DL, Feldman AM, McNamara DM. Expression of proinflammatory cytokines in the failing human heart: comparison of recent-onset and end-stage congestive heart failure. J Heart Lung Transplant 2000; 19:819–824.

89. Lequier LL, Nikaidoh H, Leonard SR, Bokovoy JL, White ML, Scannon PJ, Giroir BP. Preoperative and postoperative endotoxemia in children with congenital heart disease. Chest 2000; 117:1706–1712.

90. Anker SD, Rauchhaus M. Insights into the pathogenesis of chronic heart failure: immune activation and cachexia. Curr Opin Cardiol 1999; 14:211–216.

91. Cohn JN, Goldstein SO, Greenberg BH, Lorell BH, Bourge RC, Jaski BE, Gottlieb SO, McGrew F III, DeMets DL, White BG. A dose-dependent increase in mortality with vesnarinone among patients with severe heart failure. N Engl J Med 1998; 339:1810–1816.

92. Louis A, Cleland J G, Crabbe S, Ford S, Thackray S, Houghton T, Clark A. Clinical trials update: CAPRICORN, COPERNICUS, MIRACLE, STAF, RITZ-2, RECOVER and RENAISSANCE and cachexia and cholesterol in heart failure. Eur J Heart Fail 2001; 3:381–387.

93. Gullestad L, Ueland T, Brunsvig A, Kjekshus J, Simonsen S, Froland SS, Aukrust P. Effect of metoprolol on cytokine levels in chronic heart failure—a substudy in the Metoprolol Controlled-Release Randomised Intervention Trial in Heart Failure (MERIT-HF). Am Heart J 2001; 141:418–421.

94. Ohtsuka T, Hamada M, Hiasa G, Sasaki O, Suzuki M, Hara Y, Shigematsu Y, Hiwada K. Effect of b-blockers on circulating levels of inflammatory and anti-inflammatory cytokines in patients with dilated cardiomyopathy. J Am Coll Cardiol 2001; 37:412–417.

95. Matsumura T, Tsushima K, Ohtaki E, Misu K, Tohbaru T, Asano R, Nagayama M, Kitahara K, Umemura J, Sumiyoshi T, Hosoda S. Effects of carvedilol on plasma levels of interleukin-6 and tumor necrosis factor-α in nine patients with dilated cardiomyopathy. J Cardiol 2002; 39:253–257.

96. Loppnow H, Werdan K, Werner C. The enhanced plasma levels of soluble tumor necrosis factor receptors and interleukin-10 in patients suffering from chronic heart failure are reversed in patients treated with β-adrenoceptor antagonist. Auton Autacoid Pharmacol 2002; 22:83–92.

5

Genetics of Pediatric Heart Failure

TIMOTHY M. OLSON

Associate Professor of Medicine and Pediatrics,
Mayo Clinic College of Medicine, Rochester,
Minnesota, U.S.A.

INTRODUCTION

Heart failure, in the absence of underlying metabolic or structural defects, remains a multifactorial disorder whose pathogenesis and progression are attributable to both genes and environment. Inherited and acquired risk factors impact cardiac structure and function throughout prenatal and postnatal development, yet cardiovascular decompensation and onset of clinical heart failure in ischemic or idiopathic myocardial disease are often delayed until adulthood. Recognition of pathogenic mechanisms and identification of risk factors for coronary artery disease have focused public health policy on preventative measures, beginning in childhood. In heart failure due to primary myocardial disease, by contrast, limited understanding of etiology and years of presymptomatic but progressive cardiac dysfunction have hampered early diagnosis, effective treatment, and prevention. Similarly, when cardiomyopathic heart failure occurs in children, typically in the first year of life, the etiology is usually idiopathic and traditional medical therapy has not appeared to alter the natural history (1,2). Indeed, advanced myocardial disease with substantial remodeling is often present in adults who present with symptomatic congestive cardiomyopathy, and the 5-year mortality rate was 20–60% in an era when beta-adrenergic receptor blockers were investigational drugs (3). Outcome in the current era is no different in children, nearly 40% of who die or require cardiac transplantation (2). The prognosis in individual patients, nevertheless, is often unpredictable, ranging from intractable heart failure to occasional spontaneous recovery (4,5). Idiopathic dilated cardiomyopathy is the most common basis for cardiomyopathy in children (2,6,7), for congestive heart failure in adult referral populations (8), and for cardiac transplantation, despite a much higher prevalence of coronary artery disease (5).

Inherent in their design, most case-control studies investigating molecular alterations in advanced cardiomyopathy cannot distinguish primary causes from adaptive or maladaptive effects. Over the past decade, however, clinical research, ongoing advances in DNA-based technologies, and the Human Genome Project have provided an unprecedented opportunity to unravel fundamental molecular mechanisms for idiopathic cardiomyopathy (9–12). In this chapter, new insights into the pathobiology of heart failure will be presented, based on molecular genetic studies in patients and families with idiopathic dilated cardiomyopathy.

DILATED CARDIOMYOPATHY, A HERITABLE FORM OF HEART FAILURE

Prior to 1992, the importance of hereditary factors in the pathogenesis of idiopathic dilated cardiomyopathy (DCM) was not fully recognized. Even a focused family history identified a hereditary form of DCM in only 6–8% of cases (13). Moreover, when familial and nonfamilial cases of idiopathic DCM were compared, no differences in baseline clinical, serological, or histopathological characteristics or in long-term outcome were observed to help distinguish familial cases (13–15). Conventional wisdom viewed DCM as primarily a sporadic, multifactorial disorder. The concept of DCM as a genetic disorder received major impetus from a 1992 study in which first-degree relatives of index patients were screened by echocardiography (13). DCM, defined as left ventricular ejection fraction < 50% and left ventricular dimensions > 95th percentile for body surface area and age (16), was identified in presymptomatic members of several families, accounting for a 20% frequency of familial disease in this patient cohort. A similar study in the United Kingdom identified familial disease in 25% of cases (17). In both studies, the average age at diagnosis in probands and their relatives was in the fourth to fifth decade, yet children in their first decade of life were also diagnosed with either symptomatic or clinically silent DCM. In children younger than 10 years of age presenting with dilated cardiomyopathy, recent epidemiological studies report a 15–20% frequency of familial disease despite lack of systematically applied family screening (6,7). In studies that have performed screening echocardiograms on relatives of the index cases, 9–18% of asymptomatic individuals had left ventricular enlargement with normal ejection fraction, suggesting that cardiac dilation is a precursor of DCM (13,17). Indeed, progression to DCM was confirmed in subsequent longitudinal follow-up studies (18,19). If less stringent criteria, such as isolated left ventricular enlargement or sudden unexplained death, are used to diagnosis DCM in relatives, the frequency of familial disease may be as high as 35–48% (18,20). The importance of genetics in the pathogenesis of DCM, in fact, may be even greater than suggested by these studies. For example, sporadic cases can be caused by *de novo* mutations (21), inheritance of two copies of a recessive mutation due to parental consanguinity (22), or the combined effects of two or more distinct mutations, which are clinically silent in isolation (23). Furthermore, inheritance of a common genetic polymorphism may not cause DCM, yet have a favorable (24) or unfavorable (25) modifying effect on disease progression.

Familial DCM is most commonly inherited as an autosomal dominant trait, conferring a 50% risk of DCM on offspring of an individual with DCM (13,17,18,20,26,27). Less commonly, DCM is an X-linked disorder in males who have inherited a mutation from their mothers who exhibit mild or no cardiac disease. Barth syndrome, characterized by cardiac and skeletal myopathy, short stature, 3-methylglutaconic aciduria, and neutropenia, is an X-linked disorder caused by mutations in the *G4.5* gene that encodes tafazzin (28). Left ventricular noncompaction can also be caused by defects in this gene (29). Males with Barth syndrome usually develop fatal infantile DCM (30). DCM alone, however, in the absence of noncardiac features of Barth syndrome, has not been clearly documented. Autosomal recessive and maternally inherited cardiomyopathy due to defects in fatty acid oxidation and mitochondrial oxidative phosphorylation, respectively, may present as DCM (26,31). Patients with disorders of cardiac energy metabolism, however, usually have hypertrophic cardiomyopathy, neuromuscular disease, and metabolic derangements.

Traits such as subtle skeletal myopathy, cardiac conduction system disease, and atrial arrhythmia segregate with DCM in certain families with autosomal dominant or X-linked disease (20,27,32,33). These phenotypic subtypes may suggest specific gene defects and predict progression of DCM (34). Most reports of familial DCM as an isolated disorder or as part of a syndrome, however, have shown age-dependent penetrance and variable expression of disease among members of the same family. In other words, some carriers of a gene mutation may not have DCM or may have a partial cardiomyopathy phenotype, such as isolated left ventricular enlargement or conduction system disease. Consequently, interpretation of a normal or nondiagnostic screening echocardiogram and electrocardiogram in a child or adolescent at risk for familial DCM should take into account disease penetrance as low as 5–20% in this age group (35).

Conversely, when a child presents in congestive heart failure, familial DCM may not be suspected because of variable expression in a parent with asymptomatic DCM (36,37). Collectively, family-based studies of DCM provide the rationale for clinical screening in first-degree relatives, regardless of family history or age of the index case (2,13,19,38).

IDENTIFYING GENES FOR DILATED CARDIOMYOPATHY

Dramatic technological advances in DNA and genomic analysis have evolved over the last half-century, beginning with Watson and Crick's discovery of the double helical structure of DNA and culminating in the decoding of the entire human genome through the Human Genome Project (39). Key advances include: (1) conceptualization of genetic linkage analysis to identify genes causing familial disease; (2) discovery of the polymerase chain reaction (PCR) for rapid DNA "cloning"; (3) identification of PCR-based polymorphic DNA markers and high-resolution maps of the human genome; and (4) development of methods and high throughput systems for genotyping, mutation scanning, and DNA sequencing. In 1990, the year the Human Genome Project officially began, the first report of a gene for hypertrophic cardiomyopathy (HCM) was published (40). Using genetic linkage analysis in a large family, the disease-causing gene was mapped to chromosome 14 and a mutation in the gene encoding the beta-myosin heavy chain was identified. Over the next 5 years, the application of human molecular genetics led to discovery of several additional genes for familial HCM, providing new insight into the molecular pathogenesis of maladaptive cardiac hypertrophy (41). Coincident with the era of HCM gene discovery, recognition of DCM as potentially a monogenic disorder was emerging. The same strategies used to identify HCM genes soon would be employed in DCM gene discovery (35,42).

In the field of DCM genetics, two general approaches have been used to discover disease-causing gene defects—gene

localization by genetic linkage analysis and mutation identification by DNA sequence analysis of candidate genes (42).
Genetic linkage analysis is the strategy used to identify
familial disease-causing genes based on chromosomal position. Linkage is established by identifying a polymorphic
DNA marker of known location within the genome that is
inherited by all family members with disease. Cosegregation
of a specific genotype and disease phenotype thus indicates
the gene locus responsible for the disorder. Candidate genes
located within this chromosomal region are then investigated
by mutation analysis. The power of linkage analysis is its ability to narrow the list of potential candidate genes to a defined
region of the genome, without prior knowledge of the disease
mechanism. Indeed, several familial DCM genes identified
by linkage analysis have provided new, even unexpected,
insights into the molecular basis of disease.

In its application to DCM, however, genome-wide linkage
analysis has important limitations. Large multigenerational
families with many living, unambiguously affected individuals, critical for detecting linkage, are relatively rare. Children and young adults with a mutation may have normal
cardiac size and function due to incomplete, age-dependent
penetrance. Consequently, mutation status cannot be
inferred in young, phenotypically normal individuals, necessitating "uncertain" classification and decreasing power to
detect linkage. At the other extreme, high mortality rates
limit the number of living family members with DCM and
DNA samples available for analysis. Even in families suitably
large to identify a chromosome locus for DCM, family size
may nevertheless impede refined mapping to demarcate
a region harboring a relatively small number of positional
candidate genes. As a result, several studies that have
mapped DCM loci have not yet led to identification of the
disease-causing gene.

Since cardiac dilation may be an early marker for DCM,
accurate phenotypic classification, especially in children,
requires knowledge of normal values for left ventricular
dimensions, indexed for age and body surface area (16). Erro-
neous classification may also occur when heart failure caused

by prior myocarditis or coronary artery disease is mistakenly attributed to the inherited idiopathic DCM. Misclassification due to such phenocopies within a family can result in failure to identify linkage. Potential pitfalls of genetic linkage analysis may be minimized by quantitative scoring systems that account for age-dependent penetrance and partial DCM phenotypes (43), acquisition of autopsy tissue for DNA extraction and genotyping, and strict phenotypic classification criteria.

An alternative strategy to linkage analysis in large families is direct mutation analysis of candidate genes in small families and sporadic cases in which chromosome position information is unobtainable (42). Rationales for this approach include: (1) the rarity of large families in which DCM segregates as a Mendelian disorder; (2) the possibility that DCM genes in such families do not represent the full spectrum of genetic causes for DCM; and (3) the potential to discover *de novo* or recessive mutations in genes unique to sporadic DCM. A nonpositional candidate gene approach necessitates a mechanistic hypothesis for DCM and previous identification of genes for specific cellular structures or pathways in the heart. This strategy may appear daunting since a very large number of genes are expressed in the heart and, by definition, the molecular bases for idiopathic DCM are unknown. Moreover, once a putative mutation in a candidate gene is discovered, cosegregation with DCM cannot be statistically "proven" without a large, extended family. Distinguishing a disease-causing or disease-modifying mutation from a benign DNA polymorphism thus requires a high level of scrutiny. Data in support of a mutation include: (1) its absence in a large number of control individuals; (2) its disruption of a highly conserved domain critical to protein structure and function; (3) demonstration that the encoded mutant protein is dysfunctional *in vitro* or *in vivo*; and (4) identification of additional mutations in the same gene in other patients with DCM. Despite its limitations, the candidate gene approach has proven complementary to positional cloning in defining genetic defects in DCM. Genetic, biochemical, and physiological studies of human cardiomyopathy, together with genetic models of cardiomyopathy in mice, have defined molecular pathways for myocardial failure (9–12,44), facilitating focused candidate gene selection in DCM. Moreover, a nonpositional candidate gene approach has become increasingly feasible as the identity, structure, and tissue expression pattern of most human genes are now known, and as high throughput systems for mutation scanning have been developed.

In other heritable cardiac disorders, like hypertrophic cardiomyopathy or long QT syndrome, a spectrum of mutations in relatively few functionally related genes appear to account for a large fraction of prototypical phenotypes. By contrast, DCM has proven to be markedly heterogeneous in both phenotype and genotype. Over the past decade, a substantial number of DCM genes have been discovered, yet no common gene (genetic heterogeneity) or mutation (allelic heterogeneity) for isolated DCM has emerged. In the following sections, key discoveries will be presented in a historical context to emphasize conceptual advances in human DCM genetics. A comprehensive catalog of loci and genes for monogenic, nonsyndromic DCM, identified by linkage analysis and/or candidate gene approaches, is displayed in Tables 1 and 2.

X-LINKED DCM AND DUCHENNE MUSCULAR DYSTROPHY—A COMMON ETIOLOGY

Dystrophin is a large structural protein localized to the inner cell membrane in myocytes (45). Its amino-terminus binds to actin, whereas its carboxy-terminus binds to the dystrophin–glycoprotein complex, a cluster of proteins spanning the cell membrane. Dystrophin, therefore, links the sarcomere to the extracellular basement membrane. Its function has been viewed as both passive and active, conferring stability to the sarcolemma during myocyte contraction, and transducing force from the intracellular contractile apparatus to noncontractile proteins of the extracellular matrix, respectively. Dystrophin in cardiac muscle also localizes to Z-discs, structures that anchor thin filaments, suggesting an additional role in the structural integrity of the sarcomere (46).

Table 1 Dilated Cardiomyopathy Loci Identified by Genetic Linkage Analysis

Chromosome	Locus size	Associated phenotypes	Age of individuals with DCM	References
2q14–q22	11 cM	Conduction defects	17–55 years	Ref. 58
3p22–p25	30 cM	Automaticity and conduction defects; atrial arrhythmia	6–88 years	Ref. 43
6q12–q16	16 cM	None	17–66 years	Ref. 67
6q23	3 cM	Conduction defects, skeletal myopathy	Unknown	Ref. 59
6q23–q24	3 cM	Sensorineural hearing loss	27–61 years	Ref. 60
9q13–q22	15 cM	None	Unknown	Ref. 66
10q21–q23	4 cM	Mitral valve prolapse	14–78 years	Refs. 64 and 65

Mutations in the genes encoding dystrophin and other proteins of the dystrophin–glycoprotein complex cause muscular dystrophies (47). While skeletal myopathy is the primary feature of these disorders, later-onset cardiac myopathy often develops. Patients with mutations in *dystrophin* are clinically classified into two groups. In Duchenne muscular dystrophy, skeletal manifestations begin at 3–6 years of age and cardiomyopathy is invariably present by 18 years of age, albeit cardiac symptoms may be masked by physical inactivity (45). Conversely, in Becker muscular dystrophy, skeletal myopathy is milder and cardiac myopathy may be the primary reason for morbidity and mortality. On the most extreme end of this phenotypic spectrum are families with X-linked dominant DCM where males develop a rapidly progressive dilated cardiomyopathy in adolescence or early adulthood and females have a milder, more indolent form of disease (48). Skeletal muscle involvement is subclinical, evident only by elevated serum muscle creatine kinase (CK). A positive family history may be less obvious than in autosomal dominant DCM or even absent in the case of a

Table 2 Dilated Cardiomyopathy Genes

Locus	Gene symbol, protein	Inheritance	Age of individuals with DCM	Variably associated phenotypes	Allelic disorders	Primary strategy	Protein class	References
1q32	*TNNT2*, cardiac troponin T2	Autosomal dominant	1–84 and 1–53 years	None	HCM	Both	Thin filament of sarcomere	Refs. 61 and 62
1q21.2–q21.3	*LMNA*, lamin A/C	Autosomal dominant	19–53 years	Conduction defects, myopathy, increased CK	Six distinct disorders (see text)	Linkage analysis	Nuclear membrane	Refs. 55 and 56
2q31	*TTN*, titin	Autosomal dominant	9–53 years	None	HCM, 1° myopathy	Linkage analysis	Sarcomere	Refs. 57 and 63
2q35	*DES*, desmin	Autosomal dominant	Unknown	None	1° myopathy	Candidate gene	Cytoskeleton	Ref. 82
5q33–q34	*SGCD*, delta sarcoglycan	Autosomal dominant, sporadic	9 months–38 years	None	1° myopathy	Candidate gene	Dystrophin complex	Ref. 87
6q22.1	*PLN*, phospholamban	Autosomal dominant	20–30 years	None	HCM	Candidate gene	Sarcoplasmic reticulum	Ref. 114
10q22.1–q23	*VCL*, vinculin	Autosomal dominant	29–70 years	None	None	Candidate gene	Intercalated disc	Ref. 90

Locus	Gene	Inheritance	Age			Method	Location	Ref.
11p15.1	*CSRP3*, cardiac LIM protein (MLP)	Autosomal dominant	32–70 years	None	HCM	Candidate gene	Z-disc	Ref. 98
14q12	*MYH7*, cardiac beta myosin heavy chain	Autosomal dominant	1 day-57 years	None	HCM	Linkage analysis	Thick filament of sarcomere	Ref. 62
15q11–q14	*ACTC*, cardiac actin	Autosomal dominant	2–41 years	None	HCM	Candidate gene	Thin filament of sarcomere	Ref. 36
15q22.1	*TPM1*, alpha-tropomyosin 1	Autosomal dominant	3 months–33 years	None	HCM	Candidate gene	Thin filament of sarcomere	Ref. 37
Xp21.2	*DMD*, dystrophin	X-linked	15–22 years (M) 45–53 years (F); 13–36 years (M)	Subclinical myopathy increased CK	1° myopathy	Linkage analysis	Dystrophin complex	Ref. 49 Ref. 50

spontaneous mutation. Consequently, serum CK measurement is critical in evaluation of children presenting with DCM. An elevated CK level may be the only clue of X-linked DCM, a DCM subtype that may portend a worse prognosis. While serum CK is a sensitive marker for subclinical skeletal muscle disease in patients with DCM, CK elevation is not necessarily specific for mutations in *dystrophin* (34).

In 1993, the first gene for DCM was identified in families with X-linked DCM (49,50). Focusing genotype and linkage analysis on the X chromosome, a gene defect was mapped to the proximal region of the *dystrophin* gene (49). Consistent with the clinical phenotype, dystrophin was significantly decreased or absent in cardiac muscle but normally abundant in skeletal muscle. Later that year, a deletion that removed the muscle-specific promoter and first exon of *dystrophin* was identified in another family with X-linked DCM (50). It was postulated that compensatory upregulation of gene expression in skeletal muscle mediated by the "brain" promoter, but not cardiac muscle, accounted for the cardiac-specific phenotype. Indeed, later identification of a point mutation affecting proximal gene splicing suggested a similar mechanism (51). Alternative mechanisms for cardio-selective effects of *dystrophin* mutations in X-linked DCM, however, are implicated by mutations discovered in nonregulatory domains (52).

Identification of *dystrophin* as a DCM gene had several implications. It demonstrated the value of linkage analysis as a tool for DCM gene discovery. Without positional information implicating a mutation in dystrophin, mutation scanning of genes on the X chromosome would have been a formidable task, given the large number of potential candidate genes expressed in the heart and the very large size of *dystrophin* itself. Indeed, *dystrophin* is one of the largest human genes, impeding genotype–phenotype correlative studies and routine mutation testing on a clinical basis. Recently, however, technologies for comprehensive high throughput mutation scanning have been applied (53).

Dystrophin mutations highlighted the importance of "gene dosage" in the pathogenesis of DCM, namely age at onset and rate of progression. Males with a *dystrophin* mutation, carrying only a single X chromosome, are hemizygous, i.e., a defect is present in their one and only gene. Female mutation-carriers, with two copies of the *dystrophin* gene, are heterozygous, i.e., only one gene is mutated. In this way, females in X-linked families are similar to both females and males in families with autosomal dominant DCM caused by heterozygous mutations, in whom onset of symptomatic disease may be delayed until 30–50 years of age (13,27).

Identification of *dystrophin* mutations in X-linked DCM suggested that other genes for skeletal myopathies were candidates for DCM. Moreover, discovering that genetic defects in dystrophin cause DCM led to further investigations to determine if dystrophin had a broader role in the pathobiology of heart failure. Indeed, disruption of dystrophin by enteroviral proteases was identified in myocarditis, establishing a common mechanism for both inherited and acquired forms of heart failure (54).

AUTOSOMAL DOMINANT DCM—A GENETICALLY HETEROGENEOUS DISORDER

In 1994, the first locus for autosomal dominant DCM was mapped to chromosome 1 (55). The success of linkage analysis can be attributed to several factors. First, a very large, multigenerational family was studied, comprised of 23 individuals classified as "affected." Second, the cardiac phenotype segregating in the family included both early-onset atrial arrhythmia and conduction system disease with later-onset DCM. Consequently, rhythm disturbances, observed in several family members without diagnostic criteria for DCM, were considered an early marker for DCM. Classifying such individuals as "affected" increased the likelihood that linkage to a DCM locus would be identified. Third, innovative statistical analyses were employed since all individuals in the four oldest generations were deceased and could not be genotyped. The Human Genome Project would not be completed for several years, so DNA marker and gene maps of the chromosome 1 locus were relatively crude by today's standards. As a result,

5 years transpired before the disease-causing gene was localized to this region and mutations within it were ultimately identified (56). Notwithstanding, a critical first step toward gaining new insights into the pathogenesis of heart failure had been achieved by linkage analysis.

Over the next 7 years, 10 additional unique loci for autosomal DCM were identified by genome-wide linkage analysis, establishing DCM as a genetically heterogeneous disorder. These studies also emphasized the phenotypic heterogeneity of DCM among and within families due to incomplete penetrance, variable expression, and associated noncardiac phenotypes. Indeed, the ability of some studies to localize and refine mapping of DCM loci was based on use of less stringent diagnostic criteria for DCM. For example, left ventricular dilation in systole or diastole with normal ejection fraction (57), reduced ejection fraction with normal cardiac dimensions (58), and sudden death without an echocardiographic or pathological diagnosis of DCM (59), were sufficient to classify individuals as "affected" in some studies. Early-onset arrhythmias and/or conduction system disease preceding DCM were observed in four families (43,55,58,59). In isolation, rhythm disturbances were considered either diagnostic of the familial cardiac syndrome in dichotomous classification schemes (55,59), or suggestive of the inherited disease in schemes that assigned point values to specific phenotypic traits (43,58). Similarly, individuals with noncardiac traits variably expressed with DCM, like skeletal myopathy (59) and sensorineural hearing loss (60), were classified as "affected" in some studies. Linkage studies that capitalized on early-onset cardiac and noncardiac phenotypes, coinherited with DCM, increased the number of family members classified as "affected" and the power to detect linkage.

The disease-causing genes at four mapped DCM loci have ultimately been discovered (56,61–63). Linkage studies led to identification of DCM genes that may not have been considered prime candidates without positional information placing them within a mapped DCM locus. Among the loci at which DCM genes have not yet been identified, only three are relatively small (59,60,64,65). Because essentially all human genes are now characterized and mapped to specific regions of the genome (39), it is conceivable that DCM genes at these loci will be identified in the near future. Four mapped loci, however, are very large with > 100 potential candidate genes (43,58,66,67). Refined mapping will require identification of genetic recombination events within these loci, either in family members with DCM who were not previously studied, or in those who have now developed DCM or a phenotypic trait that portends DCM. Alternatively, a previously unsuspected positional candidate gene may come to light based on its functional similarity to a newly discovered DCM gene. In addition, new technologies for high throughput mutation scanning and DNA sequencing have made analysis of a large number of candidate genes increasingly feasible.

Collectively, the many DCM loci mapped by linkage analysis have brought to light the extraordinary genetic heterogeneity of familial DCM. If the genes at these loci are representative of the spectrum of DCM genes in smaller families and sporadic cases, it appears that a common genetic basis for DCM may not exist. In this regard, future prospects for routine, comprehensive genetic testing appear challenging. Nevertheless, clinically relevant observations have emerged from the detailed phenotypic evaluation of extended families. Age at onset for familial DCM may be highly variable among related family members who carry the same mutation. Moreover, cardiac and noncardiac phenotypes may be associated with DCM and these traits may serve as early markers for disease. Consequently, serial evaluation of at-risk children by complete physical examination, echocardiography, and electrocardiography is warranted.

INHERITED DEFECTS IN ACTIN—DCM GENE DISCOVERY USING A CANDIDATE GENE APPROACH

In 1998, the first gene for autosomal dominant DCM was identified by a nonpositional candidate gene strategy (36). Previous advances in cardiomyopathy genetics provided a conceptual framework supporting the hypothesis that defects in cardiac actin could lead to DCM. First, it had been established that mutations in genes encoding sarcomeric proteins could cause hypertrophic cardiomyopathy (HCM) (68). Since these proteins were involved in myocellular contraction, the proposed mechanism for maladaptive hypertrophy was chronic reduction of force generation (69,70). Second, discovery of *dystrophin* as a gene for X-linked DCM showed that dysfunction of a protein transmitting force from the contractile apparatus to the extracellular matrix caused DCM. In this context, *cardiac actin* was a plausible candidate gene for DCM because: (1) it is highly, almost exclusively, expressed in the heart; and (2) it forms sarcomeric thin filaments whose ends opposite to myosin cross-bridge domains are anchored to Z-discs and intercalated discs, sites of contractile force transmission between sarcomeres and adjacent myocytes, respectively (71,72). Conceivably, mutations that disrupted force transmission within and between cardiac myocytes could cause DCM, rather than HCM. Mutation scanning of the *cardiac actin* gene identified two missense mutations in small DCM families with 3–4 affected individuals. Mutations were absent in 435 controls and resulted in substitution of amino acids that are invariant in other human actin isoforms and in actins found in other species (73). Age at diagnosis in these families was highly variable, ranging from 1 to 41 years, and two mutation-carriers had dilated left ventricles with preserved systolic function. Haplo-insufficiency of cardiac actin in mice created by heterozygous disruption of cardiac actin does not cause DCM (74). Consequently, the heterozygous mutations identified in humans are likely to alter actin function by incorporation of mutant proteins into actin filaments, i.e., a dominant-negative effect. This is the proposed mechanism for most mutations subsequently identified in other DCM genes, although some may cause loss of protein function. Consistent with the mechanistic hypothesis of defective force transmission, atomic modeling placed these amino acid substitutions in domains that do not interface with myosin to generate contractile force (21). Subsequent *in vitro* studies confirmed that these mutations compromised actin function (75). One of the mutations did not affect *in vitro* actomyosin motility, yet it caused a threefold reduction in alpha-actinin binding affinity. Notably, alpha-actinin is localized to Z-discs and intercalated discs, principal sites of actin filament anchoring and contractile force transmission.

The families with identified *cardiac actin* mutations were too small for genome-wide linkage analysis and mapping studies in larger DCM families have not implicated the *cardiac actin* locus on chromosome 15q14. Thus, the candidate gene approach has complemented traditional linkage analysis in the discovery of DCM genes. Indeed, this approach has become increasingly attractive, as the Human Genome Project comes to its completion. Like linkage studies, candidate gene studies have demonstrated the profound genetic heterogeneity of DCM. In fact, eight DCM genes have been identified by a hypothesis-based candidate gene approach, more than the number of genes identified by linkage analysis. Most of these investigations have focused on genes encoding cytoskeletal and sarcomeric proteins that confer structural integrity and/or mediate contractile force dynamics in the myocardium.

MUTATIONS IN GENES ENCODING CYTOSKELETAL PROTEINS—A UNIFYING ETIOLOGY FOR DCM

The cytoskeleton is an intracellular scaffold comprised of many proteins that link, anchor, or tether other cellular components (76,77). In cardiac myocytes, the cytoskeleton plays a critical role both in maintaining cellular integrity in the face of ongoing mechanical stress and in mechanical force transduction. In this regard, both contractile proteins of the sarcomere, such as actin and myosin, and proteins of the cytoskeleton are important in contractile force dynamics. Cytoskeletal alterations occur in idiopathic, ischemic, and tachycardia-induced cardiomyopathic remodeling (78–80), yet molecular genetic studies were needed to establish a cause–effect relationship. For improved clarity, the following classification scheme for cytoskeletal proteins has been proposed, based on their structural and functional properties: membrane-associated proteins, e.g., dystrophin; "true" cytoskeletal proteins, e.g., desmin; intercalated disc proteins, e.g., vinculin; and proteins of the sarcomeric skeleton, e.g., titin (77). Mutations in genes for each of these components have been identified in DCM, establishing heritable defects in the cytoskeleton as a primary mechanism for heart failure (81).

In 1999, the first mutation in a "true" cytoskeletal protein gene, *desmin*, was reported in a small family with DCM (82). Like the discovery of *cardiac actin* as a DCM gene, a candidate-gene approach was employed. The rationale for selecting *desmin* as a candidate included high cardiac expression, reports that *desmin* mutations in mice and humans cause cardioskeletal myopathy (83,84), and knowledge that certain mutations in the same gene could cause either skeletal myopathy with cardiac involvement, or isolated DCM with no clinically apparent skeletal muscle disease (49,50). An incompletely penetrant missense mutation was identified in four family members, two of whom had DCM. It was speculated that location of the defect in the tail domain of desmin accounted for its heart-specific effects, since previously reported mutations in skeletal myopathy occurred in the central rod domain. However, the identical mutation was subsequently reported in a family with skeletal myopathy but no cardiac involvement (85). These findings demonstrated that the same mutation could have different phenotypic manifestations, presumably determined by other genetic and/or environmental factors. The mechanism by which the mutation causes desmin dysfunction remains unknown, since *in vitro* studies were uninformative (85).

By 2002, four additional DCM genes that encode cyto–skeletal proteins were identified by either linkage analysis or candidate gene strategies—*delta-sarcoglycan, vinculin, titin,* and *CSRP3* (encoding muscle LIM protein, MLP). Sarcoglycan, like dystrophin, is a component of the dystrophin–glycoprotein complex expressed in both cardiac and skeletal muscle. Mutations in *delta-sarcoglycan* cause autosomal recessive limb–girdle muscular dystrophy, i.e., affected individuals have two copies of the same mutation (homozygosity) or two different mutations in the same gene (compound heterozygosity) (86). By contrast, mutation scans of *delta-sarcoglycan* in patients with DCM identified two dominant mutations, i.e., a mutation in one of two genes (heterozygosity), sufficient to cause DCM (87). A missense mutation was found to segregate with DCM in a small family, and the same *de novo* 3-bp deletion was found in two unrelated individuals with sporadic DCM. The majority of mutation-carriers presented as children with congestive heart failure and rapidly progressive DCM; one was only 9 months of age. Muscle CK was mildly elevated in one patient, but none had clinically apparent skeletal muscle disease.

Vinculin and its isoform metavinculin are protein components of intercalated discs, structures that anchor actin filaments and transmit contractile force between adjacent cardiac myocytes (72). Based on a mechanistic hypothesis of altered force transmission (36) and other studies potentially implicating vinculin in the pathogenesis of DCM (88,89), *vinculin* was investigated as a candidate gene (90). *Vinculin* encodes a smaller, ubiquitously expressed protein and a larger protein isoform expressed exclusively in cardiac and smooth muscle. Mutation analyses were confined to a single alternatively spliced exon that is expressed only in the muscle-specific isoform, called metavinculin. An incompletely penetrant missense mutation was identified in a small family and a 3-bp deletion was found in a sporadic case, both associated with adult-onset DCM. A rare polymorphism was also reported, postulated to confer risk for DCM. Mutant proteins significantly altered metavinculin-mediated cross-linking of actin filaments in an established *in vitro* assay (91). Ultrastructural examination of cardiac tissue, performed in one patient, revealed disruption of intercalated discs.

Titin is a huge muscle protein that spans sarcomeres from M-lines, the myosin-binding midportions of thick filaments, to Z-discs, the anchoring sites for actin-containing thin filaments (92). Thus it is a cytoskeletal protein with intimate apposition to contractile proteins, critical for muscle assembly and for conferring structural stability and resting tension to the sarcomere (93). An initial link between titin defects and myocardial disease was made when a missense mutation, altering alpha-actinin binding, was identified in a patient with hypertrophic cardiomyopathy (94). *Titin* was first investigated as a candidate gene for DCM based on its colocalization with a DCM locus mapped to chromosome 2 by linkage analysis (57). Analogous to the strategy used for mutation scanning of *vinculin*, exons encoding a cardiac-specific region of *titin* were initially targeted but no mutations were identified. Subsequent comprehensive scans of 313 *titin* exons expressed in the heart revealed a missense mutation (63). In another family with autosomal dominant DCM, a 2-bp insertion/frameshift mutation, predicted to truncate the translated protein, was also identified. Since each mutation in *titin* involved exons expressed in both cardiac and noncardiac isoforms, it remained unclear why there was lack of skeletal muscle disease. Notably, a recessive *titin* mutation in zebra fish with a DCM phenotype was reported at the same time (95). Consistent with the emerging paradigm for genes encoding cytoskeletal proteins, *titin* mutations were reported in patients with a form of muscular dystrophy soon after *titin* was identified as a DCM gene (96). Titin is the largest protein known and, like dystrophin, routine mutation screening in patients with DCM would be an enormous undertaking.

The most recent discovery of a cytoskeletal gene for DCM followed insights derived from a mouse model (44). Targeted disruption of the murine gene encoding the Z-disc protein muscle LIM protein (MLP) caused a DCM phenotype (97). Like humans with DCM, *MLP* knockout mice have age-dependent onset of DCM and heart failure. Biochemical and biophysical analyses of cardiac muscle before DCM developed identified defective sensing of passive mechanical stretch as the primary defect (98). *MLP* knockout mice were rescued from DCM by concomitant knockout of the *phospholamban* gene, postulated to remove the mechanical stress stimulus (99). Remarkably, later it would be discovered that *phospholamban* mutations *cause* DCM in humans, opposite the effect observed in *MLP* knockout mice.

Phenotypic characterization of the *MLP* knockout mouse prompted investigation of *CSRP3*, the gene encoding MLP in humans, as a candidate for human DCM (98), The same missense mutation in *CSRP3* was identified in 10 patients with DCM from a cohort of 536 European patients, but this mutation was not found in a cohort of 285 Japanese patients nor in > 500 normal controls from both populations. Haplotype analyses suggested a common founder as the most likely explanation for these findings. Family segregation data were limited, yet mutant MLP was shown to cause an *in vitro* defect in interaction and localization with TCAP, another Z-disc protein that binds to titin. In a subsequent study, distinct mutations in *CSRP3* were identified in patients with hypertrophic cardiomyopathy (100). This extended the paradigm, previously established for contractile proteins of the sarcomere, that defective proteins encoded by the same gene can cause either DCM or HCM (discussed below).

DCM WITH CONDUCTION DISEASE—NOVEL DISEASE GENE DISCOVERY BY LINKAGE ANALYSIS

In 1999, the first gene for autosomal dominant DCM to be identified by genetic linkage analysis, *lamin A/C*, was reported (56). *Lamin A/C* encodes an intermediate filament protein of the inner nuclear membrane (101). The specific functions of the alternatively spliced gene products, Lamin A and Lamin C, are unknown but they are thought to confer structural integrity to the nuclear envelope and may influence gene expression. Notwithstanding, discovery of *lamin A/C* as a DCM gene expanded the list of myocellular structures implicated in the pathogenesis of myopathic heart failure beyond the cytoskeleton and sarcomere. Like other DCM genes that encode cytoskeletal proteins, *lamin A/C* was previously identified as a gene for a skeletal myopathy—autosomal dominant Emery–Dreifuss muscular dystrophy (102). As discussed above, the DCM locus previously mapped to the centromeric region of chromosome

1 was identified in a family whose phenotype included atrial arrhythmias and conduction system disease with absence of overt skeletal muscle disease (55). Accordingly, 11 families with similar phenotypes were scanned for mutations in *lamin A/C*, a positional candidate gene on chromosome 1 (56). Distinct missense mutations that segregated with DCM, atrial fibrillation, and/or conduction system disease (age at onset 19–53 years) were identified in five of the families. Most mutation-carriers younger than 30 years of age did not have cardiac disease, yet sudden death occurred frequently, typically in the fourth to sixth decades of life.

Remarkably, *lamin A/C* mutations have been identified in five other, very distinct human diseases: limb–girdle muscular dystrophy type IB, Dunnigan partial lipodystrophy, mandibuloacral dysplasia, Charcot–Marie–Tooth neuropathy type 2 Bl, and Hutchinson–Gilford progeria (101). The pleiotropic manifestations of *lamin A/C* mutations emphasize both the critical importance of the nuclear membrane and its diverse but poorly understood functions. Unlike mutations in *cardiac actin*, which appear to cause DCM or HCM depending on the functional domain they disrupt (21,36), genotype–phenotype correlations in the laminopathies are generally inapparent. Indeed, a frameshift mutation in *lamin A/C* was reported to cause either isolated DCM with conduction defects, DCM with Emery–Dreifuss-like skeletal muscle disease, or DCM with limb–girdle muscular dystrophy-like myopathy among members of the same family (103). Findings in a recent study and review of *lamin A/C* mutations in DCM provide a rationale for targeted mutation screening in a subset of patients (34). The presence of skeletal muscle involvement, atrial arrhythmia, conduction defects, and DCM with mild left ventricular dilation was predictive of *lamin A/C* mutations. Moreover, patients with *lamin A/C* mutations had more progressive disease and worse outcome than patients without *lamin A/C* mutations, albeit penetrance and expression were quite variable.

DCM AND HCM—SHARED DISEASE GENES, DIVERGENT CARDIAC REMODELING PATHWAYS

Coordinated, synchronous contraction of the heart requires mechanical coupling of individual myocytes to the rest of the myocardium. Contractile force is generated by actin–myosin interaction within cardiac sarcomeres and transmitted to adjacent sarcomeres via Z-discs (71), to neighboring myocytes via intercalated discs (72), and to the extracellular matrix via costameres (104) and the dystrophin–glycoprotein complex. Actin, the main protein of thin filaments, plays a dual role in force dynamics by regulating contractile force generation through thick filament (myosin) interaction and transmitting force through filament ends anchored to Z-discs and intercalated discs. At the time mutations in *cardiac actin* were identified and hypothesized to cause DCM by defective transmission of contractile force (36), it had been well established that molecular defects in force-generating proteins of the sarcomere caused HCM (41). Subsequently, missense mutations in myosin-binding domains of *cardiac actin* were identified in familial and sporadic HCM (21,105). Thus, distinct defects in the same sarcomeric protein were shown to cause either maladaptive hypertrophy or congestive heart failure. Mapping of the identified *cardiac actin* mutations in an atomic model of the actin–myosin complex (21), coupled with *in vitro* analysis (75), indicated that HCM-associated mutations were in myosin-binding domains. By contrast, DCM-associated mutations were in domains important for anchoring the thin filament.

A candidate gene strategy further validated the hypothesis that defects in a sarcomeric protein could cause either HCM or DCM. Mutational analyses were carried out in the gene encoding alpha-tropomyosin (37), previously implicated in the pathogenesis of HCM (106). The thin filament is comprised of both actin and tropomyosin. Tropomyosin lies within a groove along the surface of the actin filament, providing stability to the thin filament and regulating actin–myosin interaction. The electrostatic surface charge of tropomyosin is predominantly negative whereas domains in the actin groove interfacing with tropomyosin are positively charged, supporting an electrostatic basis for protein interaction (107). Missense mutations in the *alpha-tropomyosin* gene were identified in two small families with DCM. One individual had developed DCM and congestive heart failure at 3 months of age, while her 33-year-old mother was first diagnosed with DCM by a screening echocardiogram, prompted by her daughter's diagnosis. Protein modeling predicted these mutations would cause electrostatic charge reversal on the surface of tropomyosin, compromising thin filament stability. In fact, electron microscopy demonstrated an irregular, fragmented appearance of sarcomeres in cardiac tissue from one of the patients.

Genetic studies of the thin filament proteins actin and tropomyosin suggest that differential effects of mutations on contractile force generation and transmission determine the cardiac remodeling pathway. Yet, a specific mutation is unlikely to exclusively alter the generation or transmission of force in myocytes and alone may not completely account for the resultant phenotype. In a hamster model of cardiomyopathy caused by mutation of the *delta-sarcoglycan* gene, either HCM or DCM developed, depending on the strain of animal (108). The modifying effects of other genes are clearly important in cardiac remodeling pathways (10), even in cardiomyopathies attributable to single gene defects.

Further evidence that DCM and HCM are allelic disorders came from linkage and candidate gene studies in families with autosomal dominant DCM (62). Mutations in the genes encoding the beta-myosin heavy chain and troponin T, previously implicated in HCM, were discovered. Initially, a DCM locus was identified on chromosome 14 where the *beta-myosin heavy chain* gene is located, prompting its investigation as a positional candidate. A missense mutation was identified that segregated with relatively early-onset DCM, yet variable penetrance was observed in the family, as a 2-year-old presented in heart failure and an asymptomatic 42-year-old had a mild form of DCM. A different missense mutation was found in another family who also had early onset of DCM. In fact, left ventricular dilation was recognized prenatally in one case. Mutation analyses of other genes encoding sarcomeric proteins identified the same 3-bp deletion in the *troponin T* gene in two small, unrelated families in whom sudden death was prominent, even in infancy. These mutations were predicted to cause a deficit in force generation, yet it remains unclear why they would cause DCM, since a similar effect on force dynamics has been implicated in most HCM-associated mutations (109).

In a genetically engineered mouse model, heterozygosity for a myosin mutation causes HCM whereas homozygosity causes neonatal DCM with myocardial necrosis (110), suggesting that the amount of defective protein determines the cardiomyopathy phenotype. By analogy, human mutations that have a more extreme effect on sarcomere function may cause DCM. Such mutations could compromise structural integrity of sarcomeres and render the cardiac myocyte more vulnerable to injury and death under physiological hemodynamic stress (111). Because myocytes lack the capacity to regenerate, hypertrophy of viable myocytes may be inadequate compensation for cumulative cell loss, leading to dilation and pump failure rather than cardiac hypertrophy.

A NEW MECHANISM FOR FAMILIAL DCM—DEFECTIVE MYOCELLULAR CALCIUM REGULATION

High-fidelity regulation of intracellular calcium flux, orchestrated by the coordinated actions of many proteins, is critical for excitation–contraction coupling in the heart (112). Indeed, defective myocellular calcium cycling is central to the pathobiology of heart failure (113). Phospholamban is a small protein of the sarcoplasmic reticulum (SR) that regulates the calcium ATPase SERCA2a pump, critical for calcium reuptake by the SR and for cardiac relaxation. Accordingly, *phospholamban* was investigated as a candidate gene and a missense mutation that segregated with DCM was identified in a familial case (114). Affected family members developed cardiomyopathy at age 20–30 years, which rapidly progressed to clinical heart failure. The DCM phenotype was replicated in a transgenic mouse model, while cellular and biochemical studies determined that mutant phospholamban exerted a dominant-negative effect on wild-type phospholamban by sequestering protein kinase A. In a separate study, heterozygosity and homozygosity for a truncation mutation, causing functional deletion of *phospholamban*, was identified in two families (115). Heterozygotes developed either left ventricular hypertrophy or DCM, while homozygotes developed a malignant form of DCM necessitating cardiac-transplantation at a young age. Collectively, these studies defined intracellular calcium dysregulation as a new mechanism for DCM.

CONCLUSIONS

Little more than 10 years ago, the importance of genetics in the pathogenesis of DCM was unrecognized. We now know that DCM is familial in 20–30% of cases and attributable to single gene defects. Given the profound genetic heterogeneity of DCM and lack of evidence for a common DCM gene, routine genetic testing is not currently feasible. Targeted *lamin A/C* screening in patients with associated skeletal muscle or conduction system disease, however, is a possible exception. Because DCM is often clinically silent until advanced myocardial disease has developed, the importance of screening echocardiography in family members cannot be over-emphasized. Penetrance may be highly variable, and a family member at risk for DCM is probably never too young or too old for clinical screening. Early diagnosis and treatment of asymptomatic DCM may clearly prevent or attenuate development of heart failure (116).

The Human Genome Project, together with technological advances in DNA and whole genome analysis, has provided new and powerful tools with which to uncover the molecular basis of heart failure in DCM. Through the application of complementary genetic linkage and candidate gene approaches, seven DCM loci have been mapped and mutations in 12 genes causing DCM have been discovered. The genetic heterogeneity of DCM is matched by the diverse structure and function of proteins these genes encode. Heritable defects in proteins of the cytoskeleton (sarcomeric, extra-sarcomeric, submembranous, intercalated disc), sarcomere (thin and thick filament, Z-disc), nuclear membrane, and sarcoplasmic reticulum have been identified. The implicated mechanisms for heart failure include defective transmission of contractile force, decreased generation of contractile force, and dysregulation of intracellular calcium. Biochemical, cellular, and animal studies of mutant proteins promise to provide additional mechanistic insight. Discovery of novel genes for DCM is ongoing and will continue to advance our understanding of the pathobiology of heart failure.

REFERENCES

1. Schwartz M, Cox G, Lin A. Clinical approach to genetic cardiomyopathy in children. Circulation 1996; 94:2021–2038.
2. Strauss A, Lock J. Pediatric cardiomyopathy—a long way to go. N Engl J Med 2003; 348:1703–1705.
3. Dec G, Fuster V. Idiopathic dilated cardiomyopathy. N Engl J Med 1994; 331:1564–1575.
4. Wiles H, et al. Prognostic features of children with idiopathic dilated cardiomyopathy. Am J Cardiol 1991; 68:1372–1376.
5. Manolio T, et al. Prevalence and etiology of idiopathic dilated cardiomyopathy (summary of a National Heart, Lung, and Blood Institute workshop). Am J Cardiol 1992; 69:1458–1466.
6. Lipshultz S, et al. The incidence of pediatric cardiomyopathy in two regions of the United States. N Engl J Med 2003; 348:1647–1655.
7. Nugent A, et al. The epidemiology of childhood cardiomyopathy in Australia. N Engl J Med 2003; 348:1639–1646.
8. Kasper E, et al. The causes of dilated cardiomyopathy: a clinicopathologic review of 673 consecutive patients. J Am Coll Cardiol 1994; 23:586–590.
9. Chien, K. Stress pathways and heart failure. Cell 1999; 98:555–558.
10. Seidman J, Seidman C. The genetic basis for cardiomyopathy: from mutation identification to mechanistic paradigms. Cell 2001; 104:557–567.

11. Schonberger J, Seidman C. Many roads lead to a broken heart: the genetics of dilated cardiomyopathy. Am J Hum Genet 2001; 69:249–260.

12. Towbin J, Bowles N. The failing heart. Nature 2002; 415:227–233.

13. Michels V, et al. The frequency of familial dilated cardiomyopathy in a series of patients with idiopathic dilated cardiomyopathy. N Engl J Med 1992; 326:77–82.

14. Michels V. Genetics of idiopathic dilated cardiomyopathy. Heart Failure 1993; 9:87–94.

15. Michels V, et al. Progression of familial and non-familial dilated cardiomyopathy: long term follow up. Heart 2003; 89:757–761.

16. Henry W, Gardin J, Ware J. Echocardiographic measurements in normal subjects from infancy to old age. Circulation 1980; 100: 461–464.

17. Keeling P, et al. Familial dilated cardiomyopathy in the United Kingdom. Br Heart J 1995; 73:417–421.

18. Baig M, et al. Familial dilated cardiomyopathy: cardiac abnormalities are common in asymptomatic relatives and may represent early disease. J Am Coll Cardiol 1998; 31:195–201.

19. Michels V, et al. Frequency of development of idiopathic dilated cardiomyopathy among relatives of patients with idiopathic dilated cardiomyopathy. Am J Cardiol 2003; 91:1389–1392.

20. Grunig E, et al. Frequency and phenotypes of familial dilated cardiomyopathy. J Am Coll Cardiol 1998; 31:186–194.

21. Olson T, et al. Inherited and de novo mutations in cardiac actin cause hypertrophic cardiomyopathy. J Mol Cell Cardiol 2000; 32: 1687–1694.

22. Olson T, et al. Myosin light chain mutation causes autosomal recessive cardiomyopathy with mid-cavitary hypertrophy and restrictive physiology. Circulation 2002; 105:2337–2340.

23. Bezzina C, et al. Compound heterozygosity for mutations (W156X and R225W) in SCN5A associated with severe cardiac conduction disturbances and degenerative changes in the conduction system. Circ Res 2003; 92:159–168.

24. Loh E, et al. Common variant in AMPD1 gene predicts improved clinical outcome in patients with heart failure. Circulation 1999; 99:1422–1425.

25. Liggett S, Wagoner L, Craft L. The Ile164 beta2-adrenergic receptor polymorphism adversely affects the outcome of congestive heart failure. J Clin Invest 1998; 102:1534–1539.

26. McMinn T, Ross J. Hereditary dilated cardiomyopathy. Clin Cardiol 1995; 18:7–15.

27. Mestroni L, et al. Familial dilated cardiomyopathy: evidence for genetic and phenotypic heterogeneity. J Am Coll Cardiol 1999; 34: 181–190.

28. Bione S, et al. A novel X-linked gene, G4.5. is responsible for Barth syndrome. Nat Genet 1996; 12:385–389.
29. Bleyl S, et al. Neonatal, lethal noncompaction of the left ventricular myocardium is allelic with Barth syndrome. Am J Hum Genet 1997; 61:868–872.
30. D'Adamo P, et al. The X-linked gene G4.5 is responsible for different infantile dilated cardiomyopathies. Am J Hum Genet 1997; 61: 862–867.
31. Kelly D, Strauss A. Inherited cardiomyopathies. N Engl J Med 1994; 330:913–919.
32. Graber H, et al. Evolution of a hereditary cardiac conduction and muscle disorder: a study involving a family with six generations affected. Circulation 1986; 74:21–35.
33. Greenlee P, et al. Familial automaticity-conduction disorder with associated cardiomyopathy. West J Med 1986; 144:33–41.
34. Taylor M, et al. Natural history of dilated cardiomyopathy due to lamin A/C gene mutations. J Am Coll Cardiol 2003; 41:771–780.
35. Mestroni L, et al. Familial dilated cardiomyopathy. Br Heart J 1994; 72:S35–S41.
36. Olson T, et al. Actin mutations in dilated cardiomyopathy, a heritable form of heart failure. Science 1998; 280:750–752.
37. Olson T, et al. Mutations that alter the surface charge of alpha-tropomyosin are associated with dilated cardiomyopathy. J Mol Cell Cardiol 2001; 33:723–732.
38. Crispell K, et al. Clinical profiles of four large pedigrees with familial dilated cardiomyopathy. Preliminary recommendations for clinical practice. J Am Coll Cardiol 1999; 34:837–847.
39. Consortium T.G.I.S. Initial sequencing and analysis of the human genome. Nature 2001; 409:860–921.
40. Geisterfer-Lowrance A, et al. A molecular basis for familial hypertrophic cardiomyopathy: a beta cardiac myosin heavy chain gene missense mutation. Cell 1990; 62:999–1006.
41. Watkins H, Seidman J, Seidman C, Familial hypertrophic cardiomyopathy: a genetic model of cardiac hypertrophy. Hum Mol Genet 1995; 4:1721–1727.
42. Olson T, Keating M. Defining the molecular genetic basis of idiopathic dilated cardiomyopathy. Trends Cardiovasc Med 1997; 7: 60–63.
43. Olson T, Keating M. Mapping a cardiomyopathy locus to chromosome 3p22–p25. J Clin Invest 1996; 97:528–532.
44. Ross J. Dilated cardiomyopathy. Concepts derived from gene deficient and transgenic animal models. Circ J 2002; 66:219–224.
45. Beggs A. Dystrophinopathy, the expanding phenotype. Dystrophin abnormalities in X-linked dilated cardiomyopathy. Circulation 1997; 95:2344–2347.

46. Meng H, et al. The association of cardiac dystrophin with myofibrils/Z-disc regions in cardiac muscle suggests a novel role in the contractile apparatus. J Biol Chem 1996; 271:12364–12371.

47. Campbell K. Three muscular dystrophies: loss of cytoskeleton-extracellular matrix linkage. Cell 1995; 80:675–679.

48. Berko B, Swift M. X-linked dilated cardiomyopathy. N Engl J Med 1987; 316:1186–1191.

49. Towbin J, et al. X-linked dilated cardiomyopathy: molecular genetic evidence of linkage to the Duchenne muscular dystrophy (dystrophin) gene at the Xp21 locus. Circulation 1993; 87:1854–1865.

50. Muntoni F, et al. Deletion of the dystrophin muscle-promoter region associated with x-linked dilated cardiomyopathy. New Engl J Med 1993; 329:921–925.

51. Milasin J, et al. A point mutation in the 5′ splice site of the dystrophin gene first intron responsible for X-linked dilated cardiomyopathy. Hum Mol Genet 1996; 5:73–79.

52. Ortiz-Lopez R, et al. Evidence for a dystrophin missense mutation as a cause of X-linked dilated cardiomyopathy. Circulation 1997; 95:2434–2440.

53. Feng J, et al. Comprehensive mutation scanning of the dystrophin gene in patients with nonsyndromic X-linked dilated cardiomyopathy. J Am Coll Cardiol 2002; 40:1120–1124.

54. Badorff C, Lee G, Lamphear B. Enteroviral protease 2A cleaves dystrophin: evidence of cytoskeletal disruption in an acquired cardiomyopathy. Nat Med 1999; 5:320–326.

55. Kass S, et al. A gene defect that causes conduction system disease and dilated cardiomyopathy maps to chromosome 1p1–1q1. Nat Genet 1994; 7:546–551.

56. Fatkin D, et al. Missense mutations in the rod domain of the lamin A/C gene as causes of dilated cardiomyopathy and conduction-system disease. N Engl J Med 1999; 341(23):1715–1724.

57. Siu B, et al. Familial dilated cardiomyopathy locus maps to chromosome 2q31. Circulation 1999; 99(8):1022–1026.

58. Jung M, et al. Investigation of a family with autosomal dominant dilated cardiomyopathy defines a novel locus on chromosome 2q14–q22. Am J Hum Genet 1999; 65(4):1068–1077.

59. Messina D, et al. Linkage of familial dilated cardiomyopathy with conduction defect and muscular dystrophy to chromosome 6q23. Am J Hum Genet 1997; 61:909–917.

60. Schonberger J, et al. Dilated cardiomyopathy and sensorineural hearing loss: a heritable syndrome that maps to 6q23–24. Circulation 2000; 101(15):1812–1818.

61. Durand J-B, et al. Localization of a gene responsible for familial dilated cardiomyopathy to chromosome 1q32. Circulation 1995; 92:3387–3389.

62. Kamisago M, et al. Mutations in sarcomere protein genes as a cause of dilated cardiomyopathy. N Engl J Med 2000; 343:1688–1696.
63. Gerull B, et al. Mutations of TTN, encoding the giant muscle filament titin, cause familial dilated cardiomyopathy. Nat Genet 2002; 30:201–204.
64. Bowles K, et al. Gene mapping of familial autosomal dominant dilated cardiomyopathy to chromosome 10q21–23. J Clin Invest 1996; 98:1355–1360.
65. Bowles K, et al. Construction of a high-resolution physical map of the chromosome 10q22–q23 dilated cardiomyopathy locus and analysis of candidate genes. Genomics 2000; 67:109–127.
66. Krajinovic M, et al. Linkage of familial dilated cardiomyopathy to chromosome P. Am J Hum Genet 1995; 57:846–852.
67. Sylvius N, et al. A new locus for autosomal dominant dilated cardio-myopathy identified on chromosome 6q12–q16. Am J Hum Genet 2001; 68:241–246.
68. Spirito P, et al. The management of hypertrophic cardiomyopathy. N Engl J Med 1997; 336:775–785.
69. Lankford E, et al. Abnormal contractile properties of muscle fibers expressing mutations in beta-myosin in patients with hypertrophic cardiomyopathy. J Clin Invest 1995; 95:1409–1414.
70. Watkins H, et al. Expression and functional assessment of a trun-cated cardiac troponin T that causes hypertrophic cardiomyopathy. Evidence for a dominant negative action. J Clin Invest 1996; 98:2456–2461.
71. Goldstein M, Schroeter J, Michael L. Role of the Z band in the mechanical properties of the heart. FASEB J 1991; 5:2167–2174.
72. Severs N. The cardiac gap junction and intercalated disc. Int J Cardiol 1990; 26:137–173.
73. Sheterline P, Clayton J, Sparrow J. Appendix: protein sequence align-ments. Actin. New York: Oxford University Press, 1998:243–272.
74. Kumar A, et al. Rescue of cardiac alpha-actin-deficient mice by enteric smooth muscle gamma-actin. Proc Natl Acad Sci USA 1997; 94:4406–4411.
75. Wong W, et al. Functional studies of yeast actin mutants correspond-ing to human cardiomyopathy mutations. J Muscle Res Cell Motil 2001; 22:665–674.
76. Stromer M. The cytoskeleton in skeletal, cardiac and smooth muscle cells. Histol Histopathol 1998; 13:283–291.
77. Hein S, et al. The role of the cytoskeleton in heart failure. Cardiovasc Res 2000; 45:273–278.
78. Schaper J, et al. Impairment of the myocardial ultrastructure and changes of the cytoskeleton in dilated cardiomyopathy. Circulation 1991; 83:504–514.
79. Ganote C, Armstrong S. Ischaemia and the myocyte cytoskeleton: review and speculation. Cardiovasc Res 1993; 27:1387–1403.

80. Eble D, Spinale F. Contractile and cytoskeletal content, structure, and mRNA levels with tachycardia-induced cardiomyopathy. Am J Physiol 1995; 268:H2426–H2439.

81. Towbin J. The role of cytoskeletal proteins in cardiomyopathies. Curr Opin Cell Biol 1998; 10:131–139.

82. Li D, et al. Desmin mutation responsible for idiopathic dilated cardiomyopathy. Circulation 1999; 100:461–464.

83. Milner D, et al. Disruption of muscle architecture and myocardial degeneration in mice lacking desmin. J Cell Biol 1996; 134:1255–1270.

84. Goldfarb L, et al. Missense mutations in desmin associated with familial cardiac and skeletal myopathy. Nat Genet 1998; 19:402–403.

85. Dalakas M, et al. Progressive skeletal myopathy, a phenotypic variant of desmin myopathy associated with desmin mutations. Neuromuscul Disord 2003; 13:252–258.

86. Nigro V, et al. Autosomal recessive limb–girdle muscular dystrophy, *LGMD2F*, is caused by a mutation in the delta-sarcoglycan gene. Nat Genet 1996; 14:195–198.

87. Tsubata S, et al. Mutations in the human δ-sarcoglycan gene in familial and sporadic dilated cardiomyopathy. J Clin Invest 2000; 106:655–662.

88. Maeda M, et al. Dilated cardiomyopathy associated with deficiency of the cytoskeletal protein metavinculin. Circulation 1997; 95(1):17–20.

89. Xu W, Baribault H, Adamson E. Vinculin knockout results in heart and brain defects during embryonic development. Development 1998; 125(2):327–337.

90. Olson T, et al. Metavinculin mutations alter actin interaction in dilated cardiomyopathy. Circulation 2002; 105:431–437.

91. Rudiger M, et al. Differential actin organization by vinculin isoforms: implications for cell type-specific microfilament anchorage. FEBS Lett 1998; 431(1):49–54.

92. Gregorio C, et al. Muscle assembly: a titanic achievement? Curr Opin Cell Biol 1999; 11:18–25.

93. Labeit S, Kolmerer B. Titins: giant proteins in charge of muscle ultrastructure and elasticity. Science 1995; 270:293–296.

94. Satoh M, et al. Structural analysis of the titin gene in hypertrophic cardiomyopathy: identification of a novel disease gene. Biochem Biophys Res Commun 1999; 262:411–417.

95. Xu X, et al. Cardiomyopathy in zebra fish due to mutation in an alternatively spliced exon of titin. Nat Genet 2002; 30:205–209.

96. Hackman P, et al. Tibial muscular dystrophy is a titinopathy caused by mutations in TTN, the gene encoding the giant skeletal-muscle protein titin. Am J Hum Genet 2002; 71:492–500.

97. Arber S, et al. MLP-deficient mice exhibit a disruption of cardiac cytoarchitectural organization, dilated cardiomyopathy, and heart failure. Cell 1997; 88:393–403.

98. Knoll R, et al. The cardiac mechanical stretch sensor machinery involves a Z disc complex that is defective in a subset of human dilated cardiomyopathy. Cell 2002; 111:943–955.
99. Minamisawa S, et al. Chronic phospholamban-sarcoplasmic reticulum calcium atpase interaction is the critical calcium cycling defect in dilated cardiomyopathy. Cell 1999; 99:313–322.
100. Geier C, et al. Mutations in the human muscle LIM protein gene in families with hypertrophic cardiomyopathy. Circulation 2003; 107:1390–1395.
101. Mounkes L, et al. The laminopathies: nuclear structure meets disease. Curr Opin Genet Dev 2003; 13:223–230.
102. Bonne G, et al. Mutations in the gene encoding lamin A/C cause autosomal dominant Emery–Dreifuss muscular dystrophy. Nat Genet, 1999; 21: 285–288.
103. Brodsky G. et al. Lamin A/C gene mutation associated with dilated cardiomyopathy with variable skeletal muscle involvement. Circulation 2000; 101(5): 473–476.
104. Danowski B, et al. Costameres are sites of force transmission to the substratum in adult rat cardiomyocytes. J Cell Biol 1992; 118: 1411–1420.
105. Mogensen J, et al. Alpha-cardiac actin is a novel disease gene in familial hypertrophic cardiomyopathy. J Clin Invest 1999; 103: R39–R43.
106. Thierfelder L, et al. Alpha tropomyosin and cardiac troponin T mutations cause familial hypertrophic cardiomyopathy: a disease of the sarcomere. Cell 1994; 77: 701–712.
107. Lorenz M, et al. An atomic model of the unregulated thin filament obtained by x-ray fiber diffraction on oriented actin–tropomyosin gels. J Mol Biol 1995; 246: 108–119.
108. Sakamoto A, et al. Both hypertrophic and dilated cardiomyopathies are caused by mutation of the same gene, delta-sarcoglycan, in hamster: an animal model of disrupted dystrophin-associated glycoprotein complex. Proc Natl Acad Sci USA 1997; 94: 13873–13878.
109. Redwood C, Moolman-Smook J, Watkins H. Properties of mutant contractile proteins that cause hypertrophic cardiomyopathy. Cardiovasc Res 1999; 44:20–36.
110. Fatkin D, Christe M, Aristizabal O. Neonatal cardiomyopathy in mice homozygous for the Arg403Gln mutation in the alpha cardiac myosin heavy chain gene. J Clin Invest 1999; 103:147–153.
111. Olson T, Chan D. Dilated congestive cardiomyopathy. In: Allen H, et al., eds. Heart Disease in Infants, Children, and Adolescents. Philadelphia: Lippincott Williams & Wilkins, 2001:1187–1196.
112. Bers D. Cardiac excitation–contraction coupling. Nature 2002; 145: 198–205.
113. Chien K, Ross J, Hoshijima M. Calcium and heart failure: the cycle game. Nat Med 2003; 9:508–509.

114. Schmitt J, et al. Dilated cardiomyopathy and heart failure caused by a mutation in phospholamban. Science 2003; 299:1410–1413.

115. Haghighi K, et al. Human phospholamban null results in lethal dilated cardiomyopathy revealing a critical difference between mouse and human. J Clin Invest 2003; 111:869–876.

116. Eichhorn E, Bristow M. Medical therapy can improve the biological properties of the chronically failing heart. A new era in the treatment of heart failure. Circulation 1996; 94:2285–2296.

6

Heart Failure in the Fetus

LISA K. HORNBERGER

Fetal Cardiovascular Program, Department of Pediatrics, Division of Cardiology, University of California, San Francisco, California, U.S.A.

MASAKI NII

Department of Pediatrics, Division of Cardiology, The Hospital for Sick Children, Toronto, Canada

BACKGROUND

The task of the heart both before and after birth is to sustain the circulation to the peripheral tissue by developing pressure, ejecting and receiving blood. As is true after birth, heart failure in the fetus occurs when there is inadequate tissue perfusion. It may be caused by primary cardiac pathologies, but may also evolve secondary to extracardiac pathologies that influence myocardial function and output through increased workload or reduced atrial and ventricular filling. Congestive heart failure (CHF) in utero is manifested as right heart failure with the development of pericardial and pleural effusions, ascites and peripheral, including

171

placental, edema (Fig. 1). Our understanding of fetal heart failure has largely been derived from early fetal animal models and, more recently, noninvasive observations made at fetal echocardiography.

Although the definition of heart failure in the fetus is similar to that observed in postnatal life, an appreciation of the evolution of fetal heart failure requires an understanding of the many unique aspects of the fetal circulation. In the newborn, child, and adult, gas exchange is accomplished by the lungs, which must restore venous blood gases to acceptable levels for arterial blood and ultimately the organs by eliminating carbon dioxide and replenishing oxygen. In the fetus, gas exchange occurs in the placenta, which receives less oxygenated blood from the fetal descending aorta and passively provides oxygenated blood to the systemic venous circulation. The fetal circulation is dependent on intracardiac and extracardiac shunts, which include the ductus venosus, the ductus arteriosus, and the foramen ovale. These shunts permit a more "parallel" rather than an in-series circulation. Highly oxygenated placental blood which courses through the ductus venosus preferentially streams through the foramen ovale to the left side of the heart resulting in little mixing with the less oxygenated blood of the inferior and superior vena cava (1). With minimal contribution of blood from the pulmonary circulation, the left ventricle ejects approximately 70% of the more highly oxygenated blood to the upper body, including the myocardial and cerebral vascular beds. The right ventricular preload is comprised of the less oxygenated blood of the venae cavae which is primarily ejected via the ductus arteriosus to the descending aorta and to the low resistance placental circulation. As a result of the parallel circulation, the combined ventricular output in the human fetus as determined by Doppler interrogation, approximately 450 ml/kg/min (2), is dramatically less than the combined output observed after birth in which both ventricles must eject 400 ml/kg/min. In addition to the differences in the circulation, there are also unique properties of the fetal myocardium relative to the postnatal myocardium, which result in a reduced ability of the fetal heart to

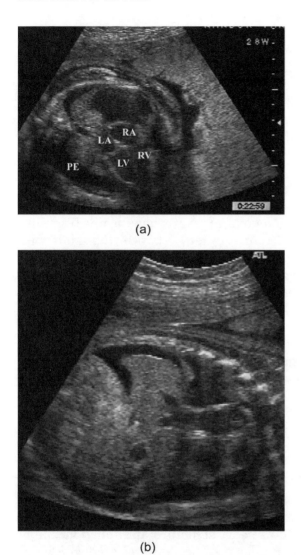

Figure 1 Images obtained at fetal echocardiography in a 28-week gestational age fetus with supraventricular tachycardia. (a) In addition to cardiomegaly, there is placental edema, bilateral pleural effusions (PE) and skin edema. (b) Rotating into a long-axis projection with the fetal head to the right of the image and the feet to the left, the inferior vena cava and hepatic veins appear dilated and there is a moderate degree of ascites. LA—left atrium; LV—left ventricle; RA—right atrium; RV—right ventricle; PE—pleural effusion.

compensate in response to stress, at least acute stress. These are outlined in Chapter 2.

Fetal heart failure is consistently associated with elevated central venous pressures irrespective of the underlying etiology. Fetal lamb models of acute ductus arteriosus constriction (3) and rapid atrial pacing (4) have demonstrated increases in central venous pressure. In the human fetus, heart failure is typically associated with abnormal venous Dopplers, which have been shown to reflect elevated central venous and downstream atrial pressures (5–7). Fetal lymphatic flow is up to five times greater than in the adult (8,9). Changes in systemic venous pressure have a much greater effect on lymphatic flow in the fetus than in the adult with cessation of flow at pressures of 15 vs. 25 mmHg in the adult. As such small changes in ventricular and atrial filling pressures and consequent systemic venous pressures can result in the clinical manifestation of fetal heart failure. Additional factors that contribute to edema formation in the fetus as compared to the postnatal circulation include: (1) a higher compliance of the interstitial space which can accommodate a large volume at low tissue pressures, (2) higher capillary filtration coefficient which permits a large water flux at low venous pressures, and (3) lower colloidal osmotic pressure and higher capillary permeability to protein, which reduce movement from the extracellular space back into the capillary (10).

While very little change in systemic venous pressures is believed to easily compromise the fetus, it is interesting how infrequently fetal heart failure is observed even with significant alterations in fetal heart structure and function. Major structural heart disease, for instance, is associated with heart failure in less than 10% of cases. In single ventricle lesions, the single ventricle must produce an equivalent of the combined cardiac output. In certain high-output conditions, as well, the fetal heart may tolerate outputs of twice or more greater than that observed in the normal fetal heart without developing hydrops (11). We have also observed fetal hydrops in less than 13% of fetuses with primary myocardial disease, including dilated and hypertrophic cardiomyopathies (12).

This clinical experience suggests there is still much to be understood about the adaptive potential of the fetal circulation to chronic cardiovascular disease.

CLINICAL FINDINGS ASSOCIATED WITH FETAL CHF

Fetal hydrops is a nonspecific term used when there are two or more fluid collections identified in the fetus. When evaluating a fetus with hydrops, the fetal cardiologist must determine if there is evidence for a primary cardiac origin. Fetal heart failure accounts for 26–40% of all causes of nonimmune hydrops fetalis (13–16). Other causes include primary lymphatic pathology, metabolic abnormalities, and inflammation. Occasionally more than one abnormality contributes to the clinical picture. When myocardial dysfunction leads to the development of hydrops, or CHF, the echocardiographic findings are fairly constant with an abnormality in cardiac size, altered myocardial function and most consistently changes in systemic venous flow patterns. Atrioventricular and semilunar valve regurgitation may be present secondary to myocardial dysfunction, or may be the primary causative lesion. In contrast to clinical heart failure after birth, in the absence of a dysrhythmia, the fetal heart rate is usually normal. Bradycardia may be the only significant change in heart rate, which typically occurs late in the disease in response to hypoxemia.

One of the most obvious signs of a primary cardiac origin of fetal hydrops is the presence of cardiomegaly (Fig. 2). The normal cardio-thoracic area ratio is < 0.3 and the cardio-thoracic circumference ratio < 0.5 (17). Cardiomegaly may occur as a result of reduced ejection, myocardial hypertrophy, which may be associated with altered ventricular diastolic function, or a high-output state. In most noncardiac etiologies of fetal hydrops, the heart remains normal in size. When cardiomegaly is identified in the setting of fetal hydrops, an assessment of systolic and diastolic function parameters is necessary to better define the hemodynamic problem.

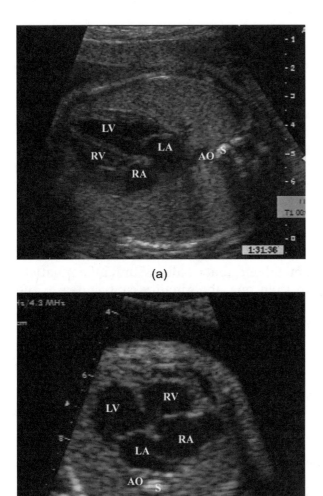

(a)

(b)

Figure 2 These images demonstrate a normal cardio-thoracic ration vs. the cardiomegaly identified typically in a primary cardiac cause of fetal hydrops. (a) The normal cardiothoracic area ratio as shown is < 0.3 and the circumference ratio 0.5. (b) In contrast, in this 25-week fetus with a dilated cardiomyopathy, the cardio-thoracic area ratio is 76% and the circumference ratio 48%. LA—left atrium; LV—left ventricle; RA—right atrium; RV—right ventricle; Ao—descending aorta; S—spine.

Estimates of systolic function in the fetus are largely determined by measures of fractional shortening. The normal fractional shortening of the left and right ventricle is 28–40% with no significant change in the mid and third trimesters (18). Frequently, reduced systolic function is evident in the hydropic fetus with structural, functional, or rhythm-related heart disease.

Assessment of diastolic inflow velocities may also be useful in defining the cause of the heart failure. The normal left and right ventricular inflow in the fetus consists of an E wave during early ventricular diastole and A wave during atrial systole (Fig. 3a) (19–21). Normally the A wave is dominant throughout gestation. The E wave, however, increases with increasing gestation, which has been thought to reflect changes in the ability of the immature myocardium to relax. When there is abnormal ventricular filling, the E wave decreases in velocity or may even be absent with ventricular filling only occurring during a very short period of atrial systole (Fig. 3b) (12). In contrast to a primary myocardial disorder, when fetal hydrops evolves secondary to restricted atrial and ventricular preload from a thoracic mass, or primary pleural or pericardial effusions, the E wave of the left and right ventricular inflow is typically dominant.

Given their reflection of central venous pressures and thus atrial and ventricular filling pathology, systemic venous flow pattern abnormalities are the most conclusive findings in the confirmation of a primary cardiac etiology for fetal hydrops. Inferior vena caval and hepatic venous flow patterns in the human fetus consist of three phases (Fig. 4) (22). The first phase of forward flow occurs late in diastole during atrial relaxation and continues throughout ventricular systole. The second phase of forward flow occurs during early ventricular diastole when the atrioventricular valves passively open and the ventricles begin to fill. In the third phase, the A wave, which occurs during atrial contraction, consists of a reversal of flow in the systemic veins. An A wave is seen in 87% of normal human fetus and time–velocity integral ratio of A wave to total forward flow is 4.7% in normal fetus. With gestational age, the ratio of the area of the A wave reversal to the entire

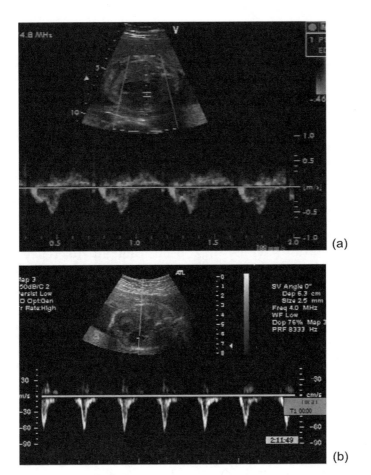

(a)

(b)

Figure 3 Doppler interrogation of the left ventricular inflow in a normal 27-week gestational age fetus without heart failure reveals (a) a biphasic flow pattern with a taller A wave during atrial contraction. There is still a significant amount of ventricular filling that occurs during early ventricular diastole. In contrast in a 25-week fetus with a dilated cardiomyopathy (b) there is only a very short period of ventricular filling during atrial systole, consistent with abnormal diastolic function.

forward flow decreases from 17% to 5% in the second and third trimesters (6,23,24). In the failing heart, as ventricular and thus atrial pressures rise, the A wave velocity slowly increases and ultimately lengthens in time. Concomitantly, the forward flow during early ventricular diastole slowly decreases, and eventually only a to and fro pattern is demonstrated with forward flow during ventricular systole and reversed flow in atrial systole (25). Increased A wave reversal in the inferior vena cava has been demonstrated in pregnancies associated with placental insufficiency which is believed to be evidence of myocardial dysfunction in this state (26).

As central venous pressures increase, flow in the ductus venosus is influenced. Normally the ductus venosus flow consists of two similar but higher velocity forward flow phases with a reduced but forward flow velocity in atrial systole (Fig. 5). With increasing central venous pressures, the forward flow velocities decrease, and there is eventually retrograde flow during atrial contraction. At this stage, the normally continuous, low velocity flow in the umbilical vein begins to develop pulsations, which occur during atrial systole (Fig. 6) (25). It is at this time that placental flow to the fetus is most critically compromised. The normal function of the ductus venosus at least in part is to limit the return of blood from the placenta to the fetus preventing a clinical picture of over-circulation as suggested from observations in fetuses without a functional ductus venosus (11). When there is elevation of the central venous pressures, the ductus venosus may in fact limit the flow reversal during atrial systole that is encountered in the umbilical vein until a critical pressure is reached. Umbilical venous pulsations have been found to be most predictive of a poor prognosis in fetal hydrops as compared to other cardiac parameters (27).

On review of 50 cases of fetal cardiomyopathy, Fontes-Pedra et al. (12) found ventricular filling and systemic venous Doppler abnormalities to be most predictive of perinatal mortality, suggesting that diastolic dysfunction and elevated central venous pressures are less tolerated by the fetal circulation than systolic dysfunction in and of itself (12). In this way, the fetal circulation is much like that of the Fontan circulation. Systemic venous blood including oxygenated blood from the placenta must passively reach the fetal heart. Elevated downstream ventricular and atrial filling pressures when a critical point is reached results in compromised systemic and thus umbilical

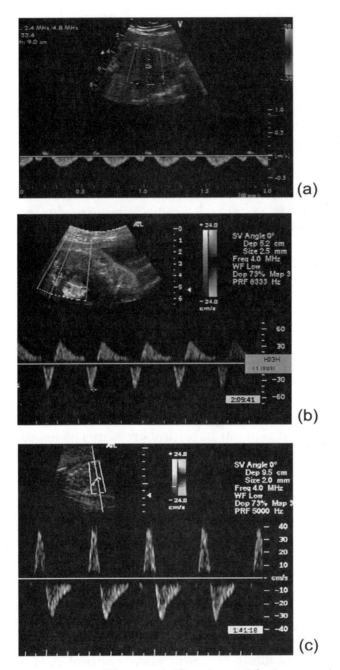

(a)

(b)

(c)

Figure 4 (*Caption on facing page*)

venous return. This in turn results in altered placental function, further compromising the fetus.

ETIOLOGIES ASSOCIATED WITH FETAL HEART FAILURE

Primary cardiac entities associated with fetal heart failure can be divided into three categories: structural pathology, intrinsic myocardial disease, and dysrhythmias. While structural heart disease has remained a dominant etiology in fetal heart failure over the past two decades, dysrhythmias have become less frequently associated with heart failure largely due to the routine use of maternal/transplacental pharmacological therapy. In contrast, myocardial disease has become a more recognized cause in part due to improved evaluation of fetal heart function (14,28,29). Table 1 lists the primary cardiovascular disorders associated with fetal heart failure.

Most structural heart disease is well tolerated in fetal life. For hemodynamic stability, the fetus has to have a well-functioning placenta, an unobstructed ventricular inflow, a ventricle with sufficient diastolic and systolic function, and an unobstructed outflow with reasonable competency of the AV and semilunar valve. Biventricular dysfunction and dysfunction of the ventricle in single ventricle

---

Figure 4 (*Facing page*) Doppler interrogation of the fetal inferior vena cava flow in (a) a fetus without cardiac pathology or placental insufficiency. The normal inferior vena caval flow is triphasic with biphasic forward flow and only a very short period of flow reversal in atrial systole. (b) In contrast, this Doppler pattern suggests elevated central venous pressures with a higher velocity and longer period of reversal during atrial systole (+) and decreasing antegrade flow in early ventricular diastole. (c) Finally, in the most compromised fetus with severely elevated atrial filling and central venous pressures, the flow is only to and fro with antegrade flow during ventricular systole and significant A wave reversal which may be of only slightly less volume than the forward flow.

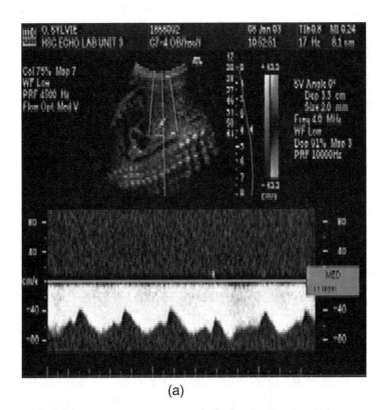

(a)

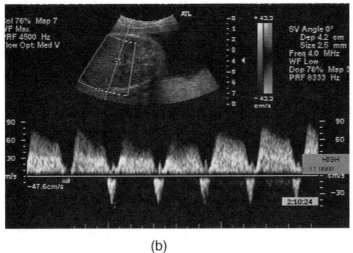

(b)

Figure 5 (*Caption on facing page*)

physiology are not well tolerated. That severe left or right heart obstruction is usually well tolerated despite significant ventricular dysfunction on the ipsilateral side of the obstruction, is likely due to their gradual development of the obstruction and dysfunction with an equally gradual redistribution of the preload and output towards the ventricle contralateral to the obstruction (30,31). As long as the "unaffected" ventricle can tolerate the increased work through an increase in preload and stroke volume, without change in heart rate, the fetus continues to thrive and is not hemodynamically compromised before birth. In contrast, however, significant atrioventricular valve regurgitation such as occurs in fetal Ebstein's anomaly of the tricuspid valve or critical aortic stenosis with severe mitral insufficiency, is poorly tolerated and more frequently associated with heart failure (Fig. 7) (32–36). This may be due to the influence of the volume load on the contralateral ventricle. Inamura et al. (34) recently demonstrated abnormal global left ventricular function as assessed using the Tei index in fetuses with severe tricuspid valve disease, with more abnormal left ventricular function observed among nonsurvivors. Further investigation revealed that the isovolumic relaxation time of the left ventricle is prolonged in severe tricuspid insufficiency suggesting that the right ventricular volume load may most influence left ventricular filling. Compromised left ventricular filling leads to an inability to redistribute flow towards the left heart, ultimately resulting in elevated central venous pressures. This is further confirmed by observations of small foramen ovale in this population of fetuses and reduced left ventricular outputs (35). Preliminary

---

Figure 5 (*Facing page*) The ductus venosus flow in the normal fetus (a) consists of two peak forward velocity phases that correspond to the same forward phases observed in the inferior vena cava with a reduction in the velocity during atrial systole. (b) When the filling pressures and systemic venous pressures reach a critical point, the peak forward velocities decrease in magnitude and ultimately there is a reversal during atrial contraction as demonstrated in this 25-week fetus with a dilated cardiomyopathy.

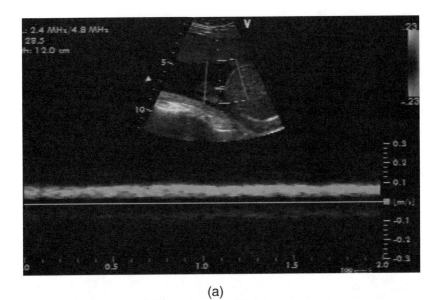

(a)

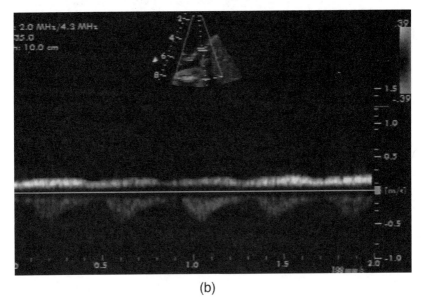

(b)

Figure 6 Finally, umbilical venous flow that is (a) normally characterized by continuous low velocity flow with mild undulations in velocity during fetal breathing, (b) develops pulsations with a phasic reduction in the velocity or absence of flow during atrial systole when there is a critically high central venous pressure.

Table 1 Primary Cardiovascular Etiologies of Fetal Congestive Heart Failure

---

Structural heart disease
  With significant AV valve regurgitation
  Functional single ventricle with dysfunction
  Bilateral inflow obstruction
  Bilateral outflow obstruction
  With severe semilunar valve regurgitation
  Associated with dysrhythmias
    Left atrial isomerism/polysplenia (AV block)
    Tricuspid valve dysplasias (SVT and atrial flutter)
    Cardiac tumors
  Ductus arteriosus constriction
  Premature restriction of the foramen ovale
Dysrhythmias
  Supraventricular tachycardias
    Atrial flutter
    Ectopic atrial tachycardia
    Chaotic atrial rhythm
    Accessory AV pathway
    Junctional ectopic tachycardia
  Ventricular tachycardias
  Atrioventricular block
    Autoimmune-mediated
    Isolated nonautoimmune-mediated
Primary myocardial disease
  Instrinsic causes
    Single gene disorders
    Mitochondrial disorders
    Chromosome abnormalities
  Extrinsic causes
    Maternal–fetal infections
    Maternal diabetes
    Maternal autoantibodies
    Twin–twin transfusion syndrome

---

work of Inamura and colleagues suggests similar pathophysiology in the setting of severe semilunar valve regurgitation such as found in tetralogy of Fallot with absent pulmonary valve (Inamura and Hornberger, unpublished observations). Other structural heart defects associated with fetal heart failure include lesions with bilateral outflow tract obstruction,

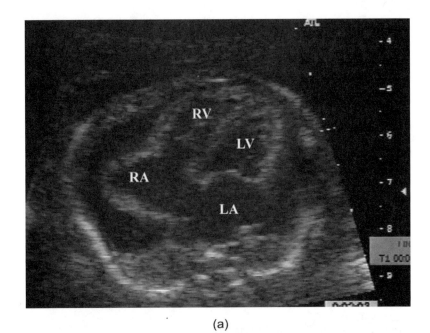

(a)

(b)

Figure 7 (*Caption on facing page*)

bilateral inflow obstruction (including restriction of the foramen ovale in right heart obstructive lesions), and more acute obstructive lesions such as ductus arteriosus constriction, which may occur spontaneously or with cyclo-oxygenase inhibitors (14,28,29).

Structural heart defects may be identified in fetuses with hydrops of a noncardiovascular origin. Structural heart defects that do not have ventricular dysfunction, bilateral inflow or outflow tract obstruction, or dysrhythmias to explain the hydrops should prompt a thorough search for another etiology. Aneuploidy (37,38), for example, may be present in a fetus with atrioventricular septal defect or complex structural heart disease, presumably from lymphatic pathology (39). Furthermore, first and early mid-trimester resolution of a hydropic state in structural heart disease which may occur in conditions such as Turner syndrome (Hornberger, unpublished observation) should also prompt a search for another etiology of hydrops as CHF due to structural heart disease in utero is not known to resolve before birth and may even progress after birth if there is no intervention (Table 2).

Fetal bradycardias and tachycardias are occasionally poorly tolerated and may result in the development of fetal heart failure. Of fetal supraventricular tachycardias, those associated with a unidirectional or bidirectional accessory AV pathway, atrial flutter, and junctional ectopic tachycardia may all be associated with the development of fetal heart failure (40–44) (Fig. 8). Fetal hydrops has been observed in up to 41% of cases of fetal supraventricular tachyarrhythmias

---

Figure 7 (*Facing page*) Ebstein's anomaly of the tricuspid valve is demonstrated in this 20-week gestational age fetus. (a) This is a two-dimensional image obtained which demonstrates displacement of the tricuspid valve towards the right ventricular apex. There is also notable cardiomegaly and a pericardial effusion with the left and right lungs compressed to the back of the thorax. (b) Confirmation of the diagnosis is made using color flow mapping, which demonstrates severe tricuspid regurgitation that originates within the body of the right ventricle. LA–left atrium; LV—left ventricle; RA—right atrium; RV—right ventricle.

Table 2 Noncardiac Etiologies of Myocardial Dysfunction and
Fetal Heart Failure

High-output states
  Primary fetal anemias
  Acute fetal–maternal or fetal–fetal   transfusion
  Arterio-venous malformations
    Vein of Galen aneurysm
    Sacrococcygeal teratoma
    Hepatic AVM
    Chorioangioma
  Agenesis of the ductus venosus
  Acardiac twins
Altered ventricular filling
  Intrathoracic pathology
    Cystic adenomatous malformations
    Diaphragmatic hernia
    Pericardial teratoma
    Bilateral pleural effusions
    Ectopia cordis
Altered ventricular afterload
  Severe placental insufficiency

(43,45). Onset at less than 32 weeks, an incessant nature
(>50% of the time) and the presence of structural heart
pathology such as Ebstein's anomaly of the tricuspid valve
and fetal cardiac rhabdomyomas, are the factors that are most
associated with the development of heart failure (46). While
higher ventricular rate, at least for atrial flutter (46) has been
suggested as a risk factor for heart failure, mechanism of the
supraventricular tachyarrhythmia has not (45,46). In fetal
supraventricular tachycardia, while central venous pressures
are increased, assessment of systemic venous flow is not so
useful there is usually a to and fro inferior vena cava and
hepatic venous flow pattern observed in affected fetuses with
and without hydrops fetalis. Umbilical venous flow, however,
should not be affected unless there is a critical elevation in
central venous pressure (Fig. 8).

Less is understood about ventricular tachyarrhythmias
as they are rarely encountered before birth. Ventricular ectopy

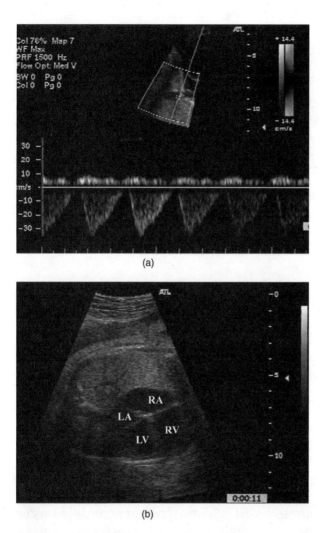

(a)

(b)

Figure 8 The 28-week fetus with supraventricular tachycardia demonstrated shown in Fig. 1 with bilateral pleural effusions, ascites, and skin and placental edema, also had (a) umbilical venous pulsations confirming the presence of significantly elevated central venous pressures and absent diastolic flow in the umbilical artery. Two weeks after initiation of maternal sotalol and digoxin therapy with conversion of the fetal rhythm to sinus, (b) the effusions and skin edema had completely resolved although there was still cardiomegaly, and (c) the umbilical venous flow had normalized. (*Continued next page*)

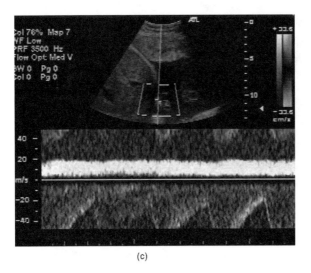

(c)

Figure 8 (*Continued*)

and tachycardia in utero have been observed in the presence of primary myocardial disease or tumors, which may contribute or be the primary cause of heart failure (12). It has also been observed in cases of postnatally confirmed long-QT syndrome (47) and idiopathic ventricular tachycardia (48).

Fetal atrioventricular block may also be associated with heart failure. This is particularly true for fetuses with coexisting structural heart disease, and most often in left atrial isomerism in which ventricular rates can be extremely low (49). A fetus with single ventricle physiology may be particularly compromised if a slower rate demands a larger stroke volume that the single ventricle, already generating the equivalent of a combined ventricular output, cannot accommodate. Most fetuses with isolated atrioventricular block associated with maternal autoantibodies tolerate the slower rates by increasing the stroke volume. The hearts are invariably dilated reflecting changes in preload, but the systolic function if anything is hyperdynamic and the diastolic function typically normal (50). The coexistence of more diffuse myocardial pathology usually associated with endocardial fibroelastosis which occurs in up to 14% of prenatally presenting cases, however, is associated with fetal hydrops and overall a worse prognosis (51,52). In this condition, the heart is unable to increase the stroke volume to sustain a normal biventricular output as a result of altered systolic and diastolic function (12).

Primary myocardial disease has been associated with development of fetal heart failure and is an important cause of mortality among affected fetuses (12). Primary cardiomyopathies include those with intrinsic etiologies such as single gene and mitochondrial disorders. There may also be extrinsic etiologies that lead to myocardial disease including maternal–fetal infection with development of myocarditis, maternal conditions including autoimmune disease and diabetes, and twin–twin transfusion syndrome. Significant atrioventricular valve regurgitation is present in the majority of fetuses with primary myocardial disease and may further compromise the fetus. One of the more unique pathologies associated with the development of ventricular dysfunction is twin–twin transfusion syndrome which occurs typically in monochorionic, diamniotic twins. In this disease, the recipient fetus develops biventricular hypertrophy with signs of abnormal left and right ventricular filling early in the course of the disease and systolic dysfunction occurring only late (12,53). The cardiovascular pathology is a form of hypertrophic cardiomyopathy that can lead to severe heart failure which accounts for much of the morbidity and mortality associated with this condition both for the recipient as well as the donor twin (54,55) (Fig. 9). Investigations into its etiology suggest a critical role for vasoactive peptides and growth factors (e.g., endothelin I and angiotension II) that might be expressed by the placenta in response to these abnormal vascular connections (56–59). Much like the hypertrophic cardiomyopathy observed in the infant of a diabetic mother, following delivery of the recipient twin, the biventricular hypertrophy and dysfunction resolves within the first few months of life.

Finally, many extracardiac conditions can also compromise myocardial function. Such conditions may lead to an increased workload as occurs in high-output states associated with anemia, arterio-venous malformations (Fig. 10), agenesis

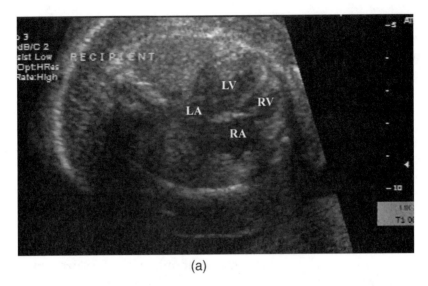

(a)

Figure 9 These images were obtained in the recipient of a pregnancy complicated by twin–twin transfusion syndrome. At 23 weeks, there was evidence of significant heart failure associated with (a) biventricular hypertrophy with diastolic and systolic dysfunction. There was severe skin edema (seen around the fetal chest wall) and ascites (not shown) as well as (b) significant A wave reversal in the ductus venosus and (c) umbilical venous pulsations. (d) Within 2 weeks of laser therapy, there was a significant reduction in the skin edema concomitant with normalization of the ductus venosus and umbilical venous flow patterns. Mildly increased A wave reversal in the inferior vena cava persisted, however, for an additional 2–3 weeks suggesting some degree of elevated central venous pressures, albeit less than observed prior to intervention. The twins were subsequently delivered at 35 weeks of gestation.

of the ductus venosus and acardiac twining (60–66). There are other lesions that result in inadequate ventricular filling as a result of compression including congenital cystic adenomatous malformation, pericardial teratoma, and large bilateral pleural effusions (63,67–69). Finally, an increase in afterload as occurs with severe placental insufficiency may also compromise myocardial function and output (22), although usually this is associated with acute demise rather than evolving fetal heart failure.

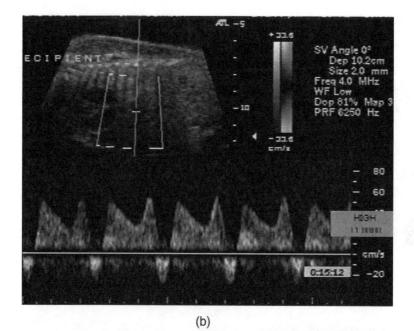

(b)

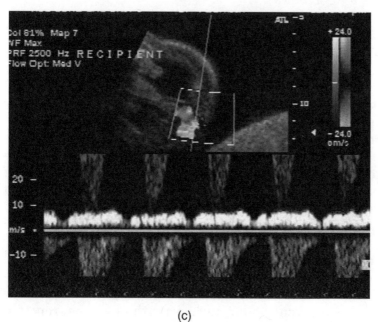

(c)

Figure 9 (*Continued next page*)

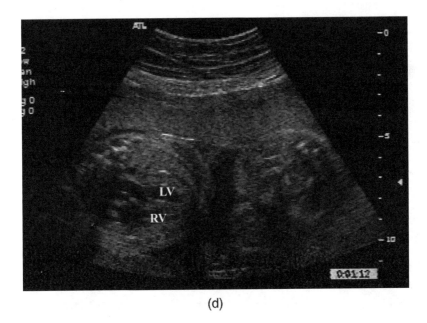

(d)

Figure 9 (*Continued*)

TREATMENT STRATEGIES AND OUTCOME

Strategies for prenatal and perinatal intervention in fetal heart failure are determined largely by the specific etiology of the myocardial dysfunction (Fig. 11). The overall goal of the intervention is to improve cardiovascular function, prolong the pregnancy to as close to term as possible, and improve associated perinatal mortality and fetal, neonatal, and maternal morbidity. Most critical to the management of any affected pregnancy is a multidisciplinary approach with excellent communication between and collaboration of the obstetrical, pediatric, and surgical subspecialists.

Improved outcome as a result of changes in perinatal management has best been demonstrated for fetal arrhythmias. Prior to the advent of maternal/transplacental therapy for fetal supraventricular tachyarrhythmias, the reported mortality associated with supraventricular tachycardia and hydrops fetalis was as high as 50%. With successful treatment, which is possible in at least 80% of affected pregnancies with fetal hydrops (41), however, the mortality associated with fetal supraventricular tachycardia and heart failure has decreased to less than 10% (43). Improvements in outcome have also been observed in autoimmune-associated fetal heart block. Retrospective investigations suggest that the routine use of corticosteroids in this condition results in less severe disease and a reduction in heart failure (70,71). Use of β sympathomimetics, in increasing the fetal ventricular heart rate and potentially improving myocardial function, may also reduce the incidence of heart failure and sudden fetal death in fetal atrioventricular block (70,72,73).

Treatment of myocardial dysfunction through maternal or transumbilical pharmacological therapy in many different conditions has been attempted in isolated cases. Digoxin has been administered both transplacentally and intraumbilically in an effort to improve fetal ventricular function in cases of atrioventricular block, structural heart defects, twin–twin transfusion syndrome, and high-output conditions. The results have been variable (74–79). Use of diuretics administered intraumbilically to grossly hydropic fetuses has also been reported with some success (74,75,80). Finally, in the setting of fetal myocardial disease of unclear etiology, particularly where an inflammatory process is suspected (e.g., infectious myocarditis or immune-mediated cardiomyopathy), intraumbilical and transplacental corticosteroids with or without gammaglobulin have been administered and/or considered as a potential treatment option (12,52).

In certain circumstances, when observed at a viable gestational age, fetal heart failure may be best managed by early delivery. This is only true if the hemodynamic issues can be alleviated by delivery, as occurs in the context of an abnormal fetal shunt (constriction of the ductus arteriosus, foramen ovale restriction, agenesis of the ductus venosus) and twin–twin transfusion syndrome, or can be improved through postnatal medical and/or surgical intervention. Certain structural heart defects may be best managed with early delivery if medical (or surgical) intervention would improve their hemodynamic condition. Critical pulmonary or aortic

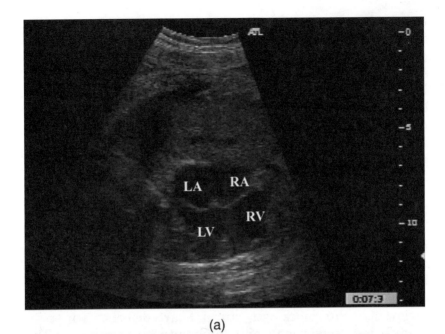

(a)

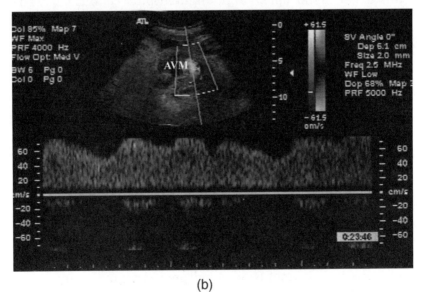

(b)

Figure 10 (*Caption on facing page*)

stenosis associated worsening atrioventricular valve regurgitation and evolving hydrops may best be treated with early delivery followed by emergent balloon valvuloplasty. Even fetuses with Ebstein's anomaly of the tricuspid valve and evolving heart failure may fair better being removed from the fetal circulation if there is evidence of worsening left ventricular diastolic function. After delivery, medical intervention aimed at alleviating right ventricular outflow tract obstruction and lowering the pulmonary artery pressure, including early ductus arteriosus ligation when necessary, may improve survival of this condition (81), which has a reported 45% incidence of fetal demise in the early third trimester (32). Evolving hydrops where there is either structural heart disease with atrioventricular block or autoimmune-mediated atrioventricular block may warrant an early delivery with pacemaker implantation. However, as the hemodynamic issues may not be fully resolved with increasing the ventricular rate alone, improved survival for these conditions is not assured. Early delivery should only be seriously considered at a truly viable gestational age and in the setting where one is certain that the hemodynamic condition can be improved. Otherwise, following delivery progressive hydrops with demise is inevitable. As well, in any affected pregnancy that is within a viable age of delivery where early delivery is likely, maternal corticosteroids should be considered to accelerate fetal lung maturation. Late in the third trimester, delivery with planned immediate ECMO

Figure 10 (*Facing page*) These images demonstrate the findings in a high-output state associated with a large hepatic arteriovenous malformation at 39 weeks of gestation. (a) There was cardiomegaly without obvious structural heart disease, and high flow velocities through both ventricular inflow and outflow tracts consistent with increased preload and ventricular stroke volumes. This prompted a search for an arterio-venous malformation. (b) Flow through the hepatic arterio-venous malformation was continuous and of high velocity as shown. LA—left atrium; LV—left ventricle; RA—right atrium; RV—right ventricle.

(a)

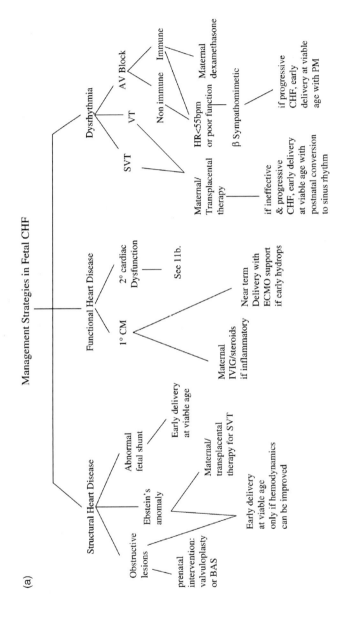

Management Strategies in Fetal CHF

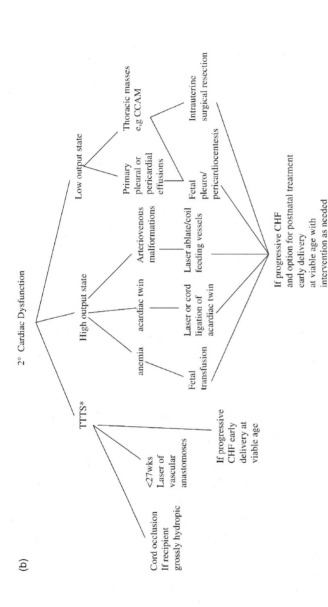

Figure 11 This diagram demonstrates several potential management algorithms given the presence of (a) primary or (b) secondary cardiovascular pathology associated with heart failure. AV—atrioventricular; BAS—balloon atrial septostomy; CCAM—congenital cystic adenomatous malformation; CHF—congestive heart failure; ECMO—extracorporeal membrane oxygenator; IVIG—intravenous gammaglobulin; PM—pacemaker; SVT—supraventricular tachycardia; TTTS—twin-twin transfusion syndrome. *It is not entirely clear whether the cardiomyopathy that evolves in the recipient fetus is primary or secondary, or both.

assistance bridging to transplant might be considered for certain uncorrectable conditions such as fetal cardiomyopathies and structural heart lesions without options for correction or palliation associated with evolving (early) hydrops.

Finally, invasive prenatal intervention has evolved dramatically over the past decade. While for many years fetal blood transfusion through cordocentesis has improved the perinatal outcome associated with fetal anemia, invasive strategies have only recently been applied for other pathologies associated with hemodynamic compromise in utero. Open and minimal access techniques for the treatment of sacrococcygeal teratoma are now feasible and effective (82,83). Antenatal resection of lung masses and placement of thoracoamniotic shunts for massive pleural effusions and pericardial effusions associated with hydrops have been effective in reversing the hydrops (84–86). Ligation or laser ablation of the umbilical cord of the acardiac twin can reverse the negative cardiovascular impact on the "pump" twin (87,88). Finally selective laser ablation of placental vascular anastomosis in twin–twin transfusion can reverse the profound cardiovascular pathology in the recipient twin with rapid improvement in systolic function and gradual recovery of diastolic function (89,90). Interventional strategies to relieve ventricular outflow tract obstruction, while in its infancy, may ultimately lead to improved survival and reduced morbidity for selected fetuses (92,93). Such strategies are aimed at preventing or reducing the evolution of secondary pathology including progressive ipsilateral ventricular and great artery hypoplasia. Clearly, if the primary lesion can be ameliorated in a timely fashion, and the normal or near normal hemodynamic condition restored, hydrops may resolve. The most appropriate gestational age for intervention for fetal outflow tract obstruction and the best timing in the course of the disease has yet to be fully determined.

When there is no prenatal or postnatal treatment option that would improve the hemodynamic situation for the fetus, progressive heart failure and intrauterine demise is likely. The family should be prepared for the loss of their baby providing the necessary supportive services. Serial assessment may or may not be warranted depending upon the need of the pregnant woman and her family. If the diagnosis is made early in pregnancy, termination of pregnancy should be offered as a reasonable option.

Despite improvements in the perinatal management of affected pregnancies, structural heart disease and cardiomyopathies associated with hydrops fetalis continue to have a poor prognosis with an 86% and 59% perinatal mortality, respectively, based on a recent assessment of 98 cases of cardiac pathology associated with fetal heart failure (29). This is an area that requires further attention if we are to make an important impact in the outcome of prenatally diagnosed cardiovascular disorders. Further investigation into the pathogenesis of fetal heart failure through the use of animal models, biochemical analysis of affected human pregnancies, and assessment of cardiovascular changes on a cellular and molecular level may lead to novel strategies to treat affected pregnancies.

REFERENCES

1. Rudolph AM. Distribution and regulation of blood flow in the fetal and neonatal lamb. Circ Res 1985; 57:811–821.
2. Kenny JF, Plappert T, Doubilet P, Saltzman DH, Cartier M, Zollars L, Leatherman GF. St John Sutton MG Changes in intracardiac blood flow velocities and right and left ventricular stroke volumes with gestational age in the normal human fetus: a prospective Doppler echocardiographic study. Circulation 1986; 74:1208–1216.
3. Fishman NH, Hof RB, Rudolph, et al. Models of congenital heart disease in fetal lambs. Circulation 1978; 58:354–364.
4. Rudolph AM, Heyman MA. Cardiac out in the fetal lamb: the effects of spontaneous and induced changes of heart rate on right and left ventricular output. Am J Obstetr Gynecol 1976; 124:183–192.
5. Reuss ML, Rudolph AM, Dae MW. Phasic blood flow patterns in the superior and inferior venae cavae of fetal sheep. Am J Obstetr Gynecol 1983; 143:70–78.
6. Kanzaki T, Chiba Y. Evaluation of the preload condition of the fetus by inferior vena caval blood flow pattern. Fetal Diagn Ther 1990; 5: 168–174.
7. Johnson P, Sharland G, Allan LD, Tynan MJ, Maxwell DJ. Umbilical venous pressure in non-immune hydrops fetalis: correlation with cardiac size. Am J Obstetr Gynecol 1992; 167:1309–1313.

8. Brace RA. Effects of outflow pressure on fetal lymph flow. Am J Obstetr Gynecol 1989; 160:494–497.

9. Brace RA, Valenzuela GJ. Effects of outflow pressure and vascular volume loading on thoracic duct lymph flow in adult sheep. Am J Physiol 1990; 258:R240–R244.

10. Rudolph AM. The Fetal Circulation and Postnatal Adaptation. Congenital Disease of the Heart: Clinical–Physiological Considerations. Chapter 1. Armonk, NY: Futura Publishing Co., 2001:38–43.

11. Jaeggi ET, Fouron J-C, Hornberger LK, Proulx F, Iberhaensli-Weiss I, Fermont L. Agenesis of the ductus venosus associated with extrahepatic umbilical vein drainage: clinical presentation, echocardiographic features and fetal outcome. Am J Obstetr Gynecol 2002; 187: 1031–1037.

12. Fontes-Pedra SRF, Smallhorn J, Ryan G, Chitayat D, Morghani H, Khan R, Hornberger LK. Fetal cardiomyopathies: etiologies, hemodynamic findings and clinical outcome. Circulation 2002; 106:585–591.

13. Turkel SB. Conditions associated with nonimmune hydrops fetalis. Clin Perinatol 1982; 9(3):613–625.

14. Allan LD, Crawford DC, Sheridan R, Chapman MG. Aetiology of non-immune hydrops: the value of echocardiography. Br J Obstetr Gynaecol 1986; 93:223–225.

15. Machin GA. Hydrops revisited: literature review of 1414 cases published in the 1980s. Am J Med Genet 1989; 34:366–390.

16. Jauniaux E. Diagnosis and management of early non-immune hydrops fetalis. Prenatal Diagn 1997; 17:1261–1268.

17. Respondek M, Respondek A, Huhta JC, Wilczynski J. 2D echocardiographic assessment of the fetal heart size in the 2nd and 3rd trimester of uncomplicated pregnancy. Eur J Obstetr Gynaecol Reprod Biol 1992; 44:185–188.

18. Allan L. The normal fetal heart. Allan L, Hornberger L, Sharland G, eds. Textbook of Fetal Cardiology. Chapter 5. London, UK: Greenwich Medical Media, 2000:95–97.

19. Reed KL, Meijboom EJ, Sahn DJ, Scagnelli SA, Valdes-Cruz LM, Shenker L. Cardiac Doppler flow velocities in human fetuses. Circulation 1986; 73:41–46.

20. Reed KL, Sahn DJ, Scagnelli S, Anderson CF, Shenker L. Doppler echocardiographic studies of diastolic function in the human fetal heart: changes during gestation. J Am Coll Cardiol 1986; 8:391–395.

21. Carcellar-Blanchard AM, Fouron JC. Determinants of Doppler velocity profile through the mitral valve of the human fetus. Br Heart J 1993; 70:457–460.

22. Reed KL, Appleton CP, Anderson CF, Shenker L, Sahn DJ. Doppler of vena cava flows in human fetuses. Circulation 1990; 81:498–505.

23. Okamura K, Murotsuki J, Kobayashi M, et al. Umbilical venous pressure and Doppler flow pattern of inferior vena cava in the fetus. Fetal Diagn Ther 1990; 5:168–174.

24. Huisman TWA, Stewart PA, Wladimiroff JW. Flow velocity waveforms in the fetal inferior vena cava during the second half of normal pregnancy. Ultrasound Med Biol 1991; 17:679–682.
25. Gudmundsson S, Huhta JC, Wood DC, Tulzer G, Cohen AW, Weiner S. Venous Doppler ultrasonography in the fetus with non-immune hydrops. Am J Obstetr Gynecol 1991; 164:33–37.
26. Hecher K, Campbell S, Doyle P, Harrington K, Nicolaides K. Assessment of fetal compromise by Doppler ultrasound investigation of the fetal circulation. Circulation 1995; 918:129–138.
27. Tulzer G, Gudmundsson S, Wood DC, Cohen AW, Weiner S, Huhta JC. Doppler in non-immune hydrops fetalis. Ultrasound Obstetr Gynecol 1994; 4:279–283.
28. Kleinman CS, Connerstein RL, DeVore GR, Jaffe CC, Lynch KC, Berkowitz RL, Talner NS, Hobbins JC. Fetal Echocardiography for evaluation of in utero congestive heart failure: a technique for study of nonimmune fetal hydrops. N Engl J Med 1982; 306:568–575.
29. Tsang W, van der Velde Mary, Windrim R, Smallhorn JF, Hornberger LK. Hydrops fetalis: primary cardiovascular etiologies and clinical outcome in 98 affected pregnancies. American College of Cardiology Scientific Session, Atlanta, GA. J Am Coll Cardiol 2002; 39(suppl A): 415A.
30. Hornberger LK, Sander SP, Rein AJJT, Spevak JP, Parness IA, Colan SD. Left heart obstructive lesions and left ventricular growth in the midtrimester fetus. A longitudinal study. Circulation 1995; 92: 1531–1538.
31. Hornberger LK, Need L, Benacerraf BR. Hornberger LK, Need L, Benacerraf BR. Development of significant left and right ventricular hypolasia in the second and third trimester fetus. J Ultrasound Med 1996; 15:655–659.
32. Hornberger LK, Sahn DJ, Kleinman CS, Copel JA, Reed KL. Tricuspid valve disease with significant tricuspid insufficiency in the fetus: Diagnosis and outcome. J Am Coll Cardiol 1991; 17(1):167–173.
33. Sharland G, Chita SK, Allan LD. Tricuspid valve dysplasia or displacement in intrauterine life. J Am Coll Cardiol 1991; 17:944–949.
34. Inamura N, Taketazu M, Smallhorn JF, Hornberger LK. Left ventricular myocardial performance in the fetus with severe tricuspid valve disease and tricuspid insufficiency. J Am Coll Cardiol 2002; 39:414A.
35. Pavlova M, Fouron JC, Drblik PD, van Doesburg NH, Bigras JL, Smallhorn J, Harder J, Robertson M. Factors affecting the prognosis of Ebstein's anomaly during fetal life. Am Heart J 1998; 135: 1081–1085.
36. Silverman NH, Kleinman CS, Rudolph AM, Copel JA, Weinstein AM, Enderlein MA, Golbus M. Fetal atrioventricular valve insufficiency associated with nonimmune hydrops: a two-dimensional echocardiographic and pulsed Doppler ultrasound study. Circulation 1985; 72(4):825–832.

37. Iskaros J, Jauniaux E, Rodeck C. Outcome of nonimmune hydrops fetalis diagnosed during the first half of pregnancy. Obstetr Gynecol 1997; 90(3):321–325.

38. Landrum BG, Johnson DE, Ferrara B, Boros SJ, Thompson TR. Hydrops fetalis and chromosomal trisomies. Am J Obstetr Gynecol 1986; 154:1114–1115.

39. Saller DN, Canick JA, Schwartz S, Blitzer MG, Moerman P, Vandenberghe K, Devlieger H, Van Hole C, Fryns JP, Lauweryns JM. Congenital pulmonary lymphangiectasis with chylothorax: a heterogeneous lymphatic vessel abnormality. Am J Med Genet 1993; 47(1):54–58.

40. Kleinman CS. Prenatal diagnosis and management of intrauterine arrhythmias. Fetal Ther 1986; 1:92–95.

41. Van Engelen AD, Weijtens O, Brenner JI, et al. Management, outcome and follow-up of fetal tachycardia. J Am Coll Cardiol 1994; 24: 1371–1375.

42. Jaeggi E, Fouron JC, Drblik SP. Fetal atrial flutter: diagnosis, clinical features, treatment, and outcome. J Pediatr 1998; 132:335–339.

43. Simpson JM, Sharland GK. Fetal tachycardias: management and outcome of 127 consecutive cases. Heart 1998; 79:576–581.

44. Jaeggi E, Fouron JC, Fournier A, van Doesburg NH, Drblik SP, Proulx F. Ventriculo-atrial time interval measured on M-mode echocardiography: a determining element in the diagnosis, treatment and prognosis of fetal supraventricular tachycardia. Heart 1998; 79:582–587.

45. Krapp M, Kohl T, Simpson JM, Sharland GK, Katalinic A, Gembruch U. Review of diagnosis, treatment, and outcome of fetal atrial flutter compared with supraventricular tachycardia. Heart 2003; 89:913–917.

46. Naheed ZJ, Strasburger JF, Deal BJ, Benson DW Jr, Gidding SS. Fetal tachycardia: mechanisms and predictors of hydrops fetalis. J Am Coll Cardiol 1996; 27:1736–1740.

47. Chang IK, Shyu MK, Lee CN, Kau ML, Ko YH, Chow SN, Hsieh FJ. Prenatal diagnosis and treatment of fetal long QT syndrome: a case report. Prenat Diagn 2002; 22(13):1209–1212.

48. Lopez LM, Cha SC, Scanavacca MI, Tuma-Cali VM, Zugaib M. Fetal idiopathic ventricular tachycardia with nonimmune hydrops: benign course. Pediatr Cardiol 1996; 17:192–193.

49. Schmidt KG, Ulmer HE, Silverman NH, Kleinman CS, Copel JA. Perinatal outcome of fetal complete atrioventricular block: a multicenter experience. J Am Coll Cardiol 1991; 17:1360–1366.

50. Koyanagi T, Hara K, Satoh S, Yoshizato T, Nakano H. Relationship between heart rate and rhythm, and cardiac performance assessed in the human fetus in utero. Int J Cardiol 1990; 28(2):163–171.

51. Jaeggi ET, Hamilton RM, Silverman ED, Zamora SA, Hornberger LK. Outcome of children with fetal, neonatal or childhood diagnosis of isolated congenital atrioventricular block. A single institution's experience of 30 years. J Am Coll Cardiol 2002; 39:130–137.

52. Nield LE, Silverman ED, Taylor GP, Smallhorn JF, Mullen JB, Silverman NH, Finley JP, Law YM, Human DG, Seaward PG, Hamilton RM, Hornberger LK. Maternal anti-Ro and anti-La antibody associated endocardial fibroelastosis. Circulation 2002; 105:843–848.

53. Barrea C, Ryan G, McCrindle BW, Smallhorn JF, Hornberger LK. Prenatal cardiovascular manifestations in the recipient twin of pregnancies complicated by twin-to-twin transfusion syndrome and the impact of therapeutic amnio reduction. Circulation 2001; 104:II–517.

54. Dickinson JE, Evans SF. Obstetric and perinatal outcomes from the Australian and New Zealand twin–twin transfusion syndrome registry. Am J Obstetr Gynecol 2000; 182:706–712.

55. Mari G, Detti L, Oz U, Abuhamad AZ. Long-term outcome in twin–twin transfusion syndrome treated with serial aggressive amnioreduction. Am J Obstetr Gynecol 2000; 183:211–217.

56. Bajoria R, Sullivan M, Fisk NM. Endothelin concentrations in monochorionic twins with severe twin–twin transfusion syndrome. Human Reprod 1999; 14:1614–1618.

57. Bajoria R, Ward S, Chatterjee R. Natriuretic peptides in the pathogenesis of cardiac dysfunction in the recipient fetus of twin–twin transfusion syndrome. Am J Obstetr Gynecol 2002; 186:121–127.

58. Porepa L, Barrea C, Singhroy S, Hornberger LK. Cellular insights into the role of Endothelin-1 in the cardiovascular pathology of twin–twin transfusion syndrome. J Am Coll Cardiol 2002; 39(suppl 5):415A.

59. Mahieu-Caputo D, Muller F, Joly D, Gubler MC, Lebidois J, Fermont L, et al. Pathogenesis of twin–twin transfusion syndrome: the renin–angiotensin system hypothesis. Fetal Diagn Ther 2001; 16:241–24.

60. Rodriguez MM, Chaves F, Romaguera RL, Ferrer PL, de la Guardia C, Bruce JH. Value of autopsy in nonimmune hydrops fetalis: series of 51 stillborn fetuses. Pediatr Dev Pathol 2002; 5(4):365–374.

61. Henrich W, Fuchs I, Buhrer C, van Landeghem FK, Albig M, Stoever B, Dudenhausen JW. Isolated cardiomegaly in the second trimester as an early sign of fetal hydrops due to intracranial arteriovenous malformation. J Clin Ultrasound 2003; 31(8):445–449.

62. Tonkin IL, Setzer ES, Ermocilla R. Placental chorioangioma: a rare cause of congestive heart failure and hydrops fetalis in the newborn. AJR Am J Roentgenol 1980; 134(1):181–183.

63. Walton JM, Rubin SZ, Soucy P, Benzie R, Ash K, Nimrod C. Fetal tumors associated with hydrops: the role of the pediatric surgeon. J Pediatr Surg 1993; 28(9):1151–1153.

64. Silverman NH, Schmidt KG. Ventricular volume overload in the human fetus: observations from fetal echocardiography. J Am Soc Echocardiogr 1990; 3(1):20–29.

65. Osborn P, Gross TL, Shah JJ, Ma L. Prenatal diagnosis of fetal heart failure in twin reversed arterial perfusion syndrome. Prenatal Diagn 2000; 20(8):615–617.

66. Brassard M, Fouron JC, Leduc L, Grignon A, Proulx F. Prognostic markers in twin pregnancies with an acardiac fetus. Obstetr Gynecol 1999; 94(3):409–414.

67. Mahle WT, Rychik J, Tian ZY, Cohen MS, Howell LJ, Crombleholme TM, Flake AW, Adzick NSE. Echocardiographic evaluation of the fetus with congenital cystic adenomatoid malformation. Ultrasound Obstetr Gynecol 2000; 16:620–624.

68. Riskin-Mashiah S, Moise KJ, Wilkins I, Ayres NA, Fraser CD. In utero diagnosis of intrapericardial teratoma: a case for in utero open fetal surgery. Prenatal Diagn 1998; 18(12):1328–1330.

69. Weber AM, Philipson EH. Fetal pleural effusion: a review and meta-analysis for prognostic indicators. Obstetr Gynecol 1992; 79(2): 281–286.

70. Jaeggi, ET, Fouron J-C, Smallhorn J, Proulx F, Hornberger LK. Prenatally diagnosed complete atrioventricular block with and without structural heart disease in the 1990s—management and impact on outcome. J Am Coll Cardiol 2003; 41:482A.

71. Saleeb S, Copel J, Friedman D, Buyon JP. Comparison of treatment with fluorinated glucocorticoids to the natural history of autoantibody associated congenital heart block. Arth Rheum 1999; 42:2335–2345.

72. Groves AMM, Allan LD, Rosenthal E. Therapeutic trial of sympathomimetics in three cases of complete heart block in the fetus. Circulation 1995; 92:3394–3396.

73. Räsänen J. The effects of ritodrine infusion on fetal myocardial function and fetal hemodynamics. Acta Obstetr Gynecol Scand 1990; 69:487–492.

74. Harris JP, Alexson CG, Manning JA, Thompson HO. Medical therapy for the hydropic fetus with congenital complete atrioventricular block. Am J Perinatol 1993; 10:217–219.

75. Zosmer N, Bajoria R, Weiner E, Rigby M, Vaughan J, Fisk NM. Clinical and echographic features of in utero cardiac dysfunction in the recipient twin in twin–twin transfusion syndrome. Br Heart J 1994; 72:74–79.

76. Anandakumar C, Biswas A, Chew SS, Chia D, Wong YC, Rantam SS. Direct fetal therapy for hydrops secondary to congenital atrioventricular heart block. Obstetr Gynecol 1996; 87: 835–837.

77. Chavkin Y, Kupfersztain C, Ergaz Z, Guedj P, Finkel AR, Stark M. Successful outcome of idiopathic nonimmune hydrops treated by maternal digoxin. Gynecol Obstetr Invest 1996; 42:137–139.

78. Koike T, Minakami H, Shiraishi H, Ogawa S, Matsubara S, Honma Y, Sato I. Digitalization of the mother in treating hydrops fetalis in monochorionic twin with Ebstein's anomaly. Case report. J Perinat Med 1997; 25:295–297.

79. Hsieh YY, Lee CC, Chang CC, Tsai HD, Yeh LS, Tsai CH. Successful prenatal digoxin therapy for Ebstein's anomaly with hydrops fetalis. A case report. J Reprod Med 1998; 43(8):710–712.

80. Harlass FE, Duff P, Brady K, Read J. Hydrops fetalis and premature closure of the ductus arteriosus: a review. Obstetr Gynecol Surv 1989; 44:541–543.
81. Wald R, Adatia I, Van Arsdell G, Hornberger LK. J Am Coll Cardiol 2004.
82. Hinrose S, Farmer DL. Fetal surgery for sacrococcygeal teratoma. Clin Perinatol 2003; 30:493–506.
83. Paek BW, Jennings RW, Harrison MR, Filly RA, Tacy TA, Farmer DI, Albanese CT. Radiofrequency ablation of human fetal sacrococcygeal teratoma. Am J Obstetr Gynecol 2001; 184:503–507.
84. Adzick NS, Kitano Y. Fetal surgery for lung lesions, congenital diaphragmatic hernia, and sacrococcygeal teratoma. Semin Pediatr Surg 2003; 12:154–167.
85. Morrow RJ, Macphail S, Johnson JA, Ryan G, Farine D, Knox Ritchie JW. Midtrimester thoracoamniotic shunting for the treatment of fetal hydrops. Semin Pediatr Surg 2003; 12(3):182–189.
86. Wilson RD, Johnson MP. Prenatal ultrasound guided percutaneous shunts for obstructive uropathy and thoracic disease. Ultrasound Obstetr Gynecol 2003; 22(5):484–488.
87. Gallot D, Laurichesse H, Lemery D. Selective feticide in monochorionic twin pregnancies by ultrasound-guided umbilical cord occlusion. Ultrasound Obstetr Gynecol 2003; 22(4):409–419.
88. Tan TY, Sepulveda W. Acardiac twin: a systematic review of minimally invasive treatment modalities. Ultrasound Obstetr Gynecol 2003; 22(4):409–419.
89. Quintero RA. Twin–twin transfusion syndrome. Clin Perinatol 2003; 30:591–600.
90. Alkazaleh F, Barrea C, Hornberger LK, Seaward G, Greg R. Outcome and acute changes of the cardiovascular manifestations in the recipient twin after laser therapy for severe twin-to-twin transfusion syndrome (TTTS). J Soc Gynecol Invest 2002; 9:70A.
91. Kohl T, Sharland G, Allan LD, Gembruch U, Chaoui R, Lopes LM, Zielinsky P, Huhta J, Silverman NH. World experience of percutaneous ultrasound-guided balloon valvuloplasty in human fetuses with severe aortic valve obstruction. Am J Cardiol 2000; 85(10):1230–1233.
92. Tworetzky W, Marshall AC. Balloon valvuloplasty for congenital heart disease in the fetus. Clin Perinatol 2003; 30(3):541–550.

7

Heart Failure in the Neonate

DANA CONNOLLY, MARCELO AUSLENDER,
and MICHAEL ARTMAN
Department of Pediatrics, New York University
School of Medicine, New York, New York, U.S.A.

INTRODUCTION

This chapter focuses on the heart failure syndrome in
neonates, recognizing that compared to the plethora of data
in adults, far less information is available regarding heart
failure in newborn infants. The roles of physiologic and
neurohormonal compensatory mechanisms in heart failure
have been studied largely in chronic compensated states in
adult patients and mature animal models. Clearly, the etiologies of heart failure in neonates differ from the etiologies of
heart failure in other age groups. Furthermore, it is likely
that normal developmental changes during the neonatal
period will impact upon the nature and magnitude of the
compensatory physiological responses and the responses to

therapy. Lastly, there are marked differences in the psychosocial aspects of chronic disease and the impact of heart failure on growth, development, and quality of life.

PATHOPHYSIOLOGY

It is important to consider neonatal heart failure as a syndrome that encompasses a variety of disorders of the cardiovascular system. Heart failure develops as a consequence of compensatory physiological and neurohormonal mechanisms that become overwhelmed or exhausted in response to inadequate systemic blood flow (1–7). The signs and symptoms of heart failure result from these compensatory responses and may change with changes in acuity of the disease process. The following definitions can be used as a practical basis for considering heart failure in neonates.

Acute Heart Failure Syndrome

Acute (or decompensated) heart failure can be defined as a state in which compensatory physiological and neurohormonal mechanisms are completely overwhelmed and inadequate, resulting in cardiogenic shock (2,3). Additional myocardial injury, increased metabolic demands, or changes in loading conditions may trigger decompensation from a stable compensated state. Sodium and water retention results from activation of the renin–angiotensin–aldosterone system (RAAS), resulting in a congested circulatory state. Pulmonary congestion is an important feature of heart failure in newborns. In contrast to adults, peripheral edema is uncommon and neonates accumulate excessive fluid in the liver. Neonates with acute heart failure exhibit restlessness, irritability, tachypnea, tachycardia, diminished peripheral perfusion, and decreased urine output. As decompensation progresses, these signs become worse and without therapeutic intervention, may be followed by hypotension, respiratory failure, and circulatory collapse.

Chronic Heart Failure Syndrome

The chronic heart failure syndrome occurs when compensatory hemodynamic and neurohormonal responses are sufficient to maintain near normal cardiovascular homeostasis. Therefore, these patients may exhibit little evidence of a congested circulatory state. However, sustained activation of the sympathetic nervous system (SNS) and RAAS ultimately contribute to progressive (and often silent) deterioration of myocardial function. Chronic heart failure is a common manifestation of many types of structural and acquired cardiac defects in neonates resulting from the abnormal distribution of blood flow or abnormal myocardial function.

Neonates represent a unique population in terms of cardiopulmonary function, clinical presentation, and approaches to management. It is important to have a firm understanding of these developmental differences in order to understand the pathophysiology of heart failure in neonates and age-appropriate approaches to therapy.

Maturation of Cardiac Function: Molecular and Cellular Aspects

The developing heart undergoes a series of complex morphological and functional changes that begin at the earliest stages of embryonic development. After morphogenesis is complete, functional maturation continues into the postnatal period. Age-related changes occur in the pattern of cardiac responses to virtually every pharmacological or physiological intervention that has been tested in each of the mammalian species studies to date. Numerous reports have been published describing the functional responses elicited by many different pharmacological agents in various species, age groups, and experimental models. Consequently, a more thorough understanding of the developmental aspects of regulation of contractility has been obtained over the past few years. However, in many instances, a complete mechanistic explanation for the observed changes in cardiac responses is lacking. In particular, there is relatively little known about fundamental mechanisms of excitation–contraction (EC) coupling and regulation of contractile function in the newborn human heart. Several recent reviews provide additional information regarding developmental changes in cardiac structure, ultrastructure, metabolism, mechanics, electrophysiology, morphogenesis, and responses to pathophysiological states (8–12).

Excitation–Contraction Coupling

Depolarization of the sarcolemmal membrane ultimately results in a rise in intracellular cytosolic calcium, binding of calcium to the contractile protein complex in the myofibrils, and cell shortening (contraction). Relaxation is achieved by a fall in intracellular cytosolic calcium and dissociation of calcium from the contractile proteins. These processes must be tightly regulated in order to maintain calcium homeostasis and control of contraction and relaxation. During the past several years, it has become clear that many of the pathways involved in these processes undergo developmental regulation. Thus, there are significant age-related differences in the fundamental mechanisms of cardiac contraction, relaxation, and regulation of contractile function.

In mature mammalian ventricular myocardium, it has been well established that the rise in intracellular calcium that triggers contraction is mediated by the release of calcium from sarcoplasmic reticulum (SR) stores (13,14). The opening of specific SR calcium release channels (ryanodine receptors) is triggered by an influx of calcium across the sarcolemma through L-type calcium channels in a process known as calcium-induced calcium release (CICR). This model depends upon the close physical relationship between L-type calcium channels in the sarcolemmal membrane, concentrated predominately in the transverse-tubules (T-tubules), and ryanodine receptors in the SR (15,16). Localized, nonpropagating SR calcium release events (either evoked or spontaneously occurring) have been commonly termed "calcium sparks." It is now commonly believed that contraction in mature cardiac myocytes takes place as a result of the graded summation of "calcium sparks" that increase intracellular calcium homogeneously throughout the cell. Relaxation occurs because of the reuptake of cytosolic calcium into the SR through SR calcium pumps and to a much lesser extent, calcium extrusion from the cell via sodium–calcium exchange and sarcolemmal calcium pumps.

A large body of literature indicates that in contrast to the adult heart, immature myocytes depend much less on SR calcium release for the initiation of contraction. The profound differences between contraction and relaxation processes in the developing and mature heart (8–10) are probably related to fundamental developmental differences in the spatial arrangement and expression of key cellular components involved in producing the mature EC coupling phenotype. The concept that the SR plays a lesser role in EC coupling in the developing heart is supported by results from experiments employing ultrastructural, pharmacological, biochemical, electrophysiological, and molecular biological approaches (for a review, see Ref. 17).

The major structural components of EC coupling in mature ventricular myocardium are (i) sarcolemmal L-type calcium channels (mostly clustered in the T-tubules), (ii) the diadic junction of T-tubules with the junctional SR, and (iii) calcium release channels in the junctional SR (ryanodinereceptors). T-tubules do not appear until approximately 10–14 days after birth in rabbits (18,19), suggesting that a lack of diadic junctional coupling may be a key factor in the inadequate coupling of calcium influx pathways with SR calcium release in the neonatal heart. Thus, although the SR at birth in the rabbit is capable of releasing substantial amounts of calcium in response to pharmacological stimulation (e.g., rapid application of a high concentration of caffeine to open SR calcium release channels), the relative paucity of T-tubules, sarcolemmal L-type calcium channels, and SR calcium release channels appears to functionally isolate the SR from participating in EC coupling under physiological conditions. Furthermore, morphological considerations in immature myocytes support the feasibility of transsarcolemmal calcium influx serving as a direct source of activator calcium. Despite a lack of T-tubules, fetal and newborn myocytes are relatively small and have a much higher cell surface area-to-volume ratio than adult myocytes (20). A high surface area-to-volume ratio and the subsarcolemmal position of myofibrils in fetal and newborn myocytes (21,22) could support direct transsarcolemmal calcium delivery to (and from) the contractile proteins.

There is general agreement that the main functional role of the sarcolemmal sodium–calcium exchanger (NCX) in mature cardiac cells is to extrude calcium during relaxation (13,14). However, NCX can function bidirectionally and bring calcium into the cell during depolarization. It has been shown that NCX activity in sarcolemmal vesicles, sarcolemmal NCX protein content, and steady-state mRNA levels were highest in late fetal and early newborn rabbits and declined postnatally to adult levels by two to three weeks of age (23,24). Subsequent immunohistochemical studies in intact myocytes confirmed that NCX protein expression is high at birth in rabbits and that the exchanger is homogeneously distributed over the cell surface (19,25). During the first few weeks after birth, NCX is down-regulated and the sarco(endo)plasmic reticulum calcium-ATPase (SERCA2) is up-regulated (26,27), consistent with a postnatal transition from the sarcolemma to the SR as the predominant source of activator calcium. In addition, NCX current density is high at birth and declines during the first 3 weeks after birth in rabbit ventricular myocytes (20,28). The time course of the down-regulation of NCX and up-regulation of SERCA2 coincides with that of the postnatal acquisition of T-tubules. Experiments performed under conditions wherein the other major calcium transport pathways are blocked demonstrate that NCX alone is sufficient for normal contraction and relaxation in neonatal rabbit ventricular myocytes. Thus, it has been proposed that NCX is the predominant route for sarcolemmal calcium entry and efflux in the immature heart.

Regulation of Contractile Function in the Neonatal Heart

If these concepts described above are correct, then graded control of contraction amplitude is predicted to be achieved in immature myocytes predominantly by factors that modulate NCX activity. NCX activity may be influenced by several factors (e.g., ATP, pH, PIP_2, PKC, redox state) (29–31), but the extent and duration of membrane depolarization and the transsarcolemmal gradients of sodium and calcium are the primary determinants of NCX activity. Therefore, control of contractile function in the immature heart is likely to be substantially different from the mechanisms operative in the fully mature heart.

In the fully mature heart, β-adrenergic receptor agonists produce positive inotropic and lusitropic effects mediated by activation of protein kinase A and phosphorylation of key proteins involved in CICR and SR reuptake (e.g., L-type calcium channels, ryanodine receptors, phospholamban) (13,14). However, these molecular targets are thought to play a minimal role in normal contraction and relaxation in the immature rabbit heart. Despite this apparent lack of targets, newborn rabbit myocardium responds to β-adrenergic receptor agonists with increases in the force of contraction and the rate of relaxation (10,32,33). The recent report of modest stimulation of sodium–calcium exchange current by the β-adrenergic signaling pathway in mature cardiac myocytes (34) leads to the speculation that this mechanism might be of central importance in the newborn heart, which is highly dependent on sodium–calcium exchange. This hypothesis remains to be tested and again, relatively little information is available regarding these concepts in human newborns.

A family of phosphodiesterase (PDE) enzymes mediates hydrolysis of cAMP. As cAMP increases within the myocyte, PKA is activated. This activation is terminated primarily by hydrolysis of cAMP with a return to basal cAMP levels and basal PKA activity. Phosphodiesterases are expressed in various cytosolic or membrane compartments within the myocyte.

The isoform that has commanded most of the interest as an inotropic target is PDE3 because it is localized predominately to the SR and plays a major role in regulating the phosphorylation state of phospholamban. It is this isoform that is the target of selective PDE inhibitors, such as amrinone and milrinone. However, PDE isoforms undergo developmental changes in expression and activity. In most mammalian species that have been studied, PDE3 activity is either absent or markedly diminished at birth (35). Consequently, PDE3 inhibitors have relatively little effect on the inotropic or lusitropic state in immature mammalian myocardium (10,32,33). It therefore seems likely that the beneficial hemodynamic effects of milrinone observed in neonates are largely due to reduction in afterload and systemic and pulmonary vasodilation. However, the developmental expression of PDE isoforms in the human heart has not been studied.

In summary, our present understanding of the regulation of contractile function in the immature human heart is based on extrapolation from animal studies. Whether or not these concepts are valid and operational in the human preterm newborn, neonate and young infant remain to be defined. Furthermore, the response of the neonatal heart in the setting of the heart failure syndrome has not been characterized, even in animal models. There is increasing evidence that fundamental molecular and cellular processes involved in contraction and relaxation are deranged in myocytes isolated from adult humans with heart failure (36). Much additional research is needed to define these mechanisms and responses in the failing neonatal heart.

Neonatal Pulmonary Function

Neonates differ from older children and adults with regard to alveolar stability and oxygenation. Functional residual capacity (FRC), or the volume of gas present in the lungs at the end of a normal expiration, is derived from the inward recoil of the lung balanced by the outward recoil of the chest wall. In neonates, the chest wall generates little outward recoil making the relaxation volume of the thorax smaller than that of the adult. Closing capacity (the point at which small conducting airways begin to collapse) exceeds FRC, making neonatal lungs susceptible to atelectasis. Furthermore, anesthesia, deep sedation, and failure to thrive often lead to muscle weakness that can compromise alveolar stability and pulmonary compliance. Reduced outward recoil of the chest can also limit the amplitude of the pleural pressure variation during breathing, resulting in an increased cardiovascular tolerance of many neonates to high levels of positive airway pressure.

ETIOLOGIES OF NEONATAL HEART FAILURE

Heart failure in newborns and young infants can be due to a variety of different causes, including congenital cardiovascular structural malformations, heart muscle dysfunction, rhythm disturbances, and metabolic or hematologic disorders (37). Heart failure present at birth is rare and is generally attributed to those conditions that can produce heart failure and hydrops fetalis in utero. However, there are a few structural abnormalities that can present with heart failure at the time of birth. In formulating a diagnostic approach and differential diagnosis for the neonate with signs of heart failure, it is helpful to consider the age at which the onset of heart failure was first noted. Age at onset can provide important clues to the etiology and helps to narrow the differential diagnosis and focus the diagnostic approach. Table 1 lists the various causes of heart failure in the first two months, categorized according to the age of the infant when heart failure began.

As mentioned previously, heart failure that is present at birth is generally due to heart muscle dysfunction caused by birth asphyxia with myocardial ischemia, neonatal sepsis, hypoglycemia, or severe anemia or polycythemia (Table 1). Overall, fetal/neonatal arrhythmias (either sustained tachycardia or bradycardia) are much less common causes of heart failure at birth. Least common are the rare congenital cardiovascular structural defects that may present with heart failure at birth (Ebstein's anomaly with severe tricuspid

Table 1   Etiology of Neonatal Heart Failure by Age

Age	Etiology
Birth	1. Neonatal heart muscle dysfunction Asphyxia; transient myocardial ischemia Sepsis and/or myocarditis Hypoglycemia Hypocalcemia 2. Neonatal hematological abnormalities Anemia or hyperviscosity syndrome 3. Neonatal heart rate abnormalities SVT or congenital complete AV block 4. Structural abnormalities Tricuspid regurgitation Pulmonary regurgitation Systemic arteriovenous fistula
1 week	1. Structural abnormalities Critical aortic stenosis Coarctation or interrupted aortic arch Hypoplastic left-heart syndrome TAPVC (with obstruction) PDA (preterm infants) Ductal-dependent lesions with a large PDA 2. Heart muscle dysfunction or arrhythmias 3. Renal abnormalities Renal failure or systemic hypertension 4. Endocrine disorders Hyperthyroidism or adrenal insufficiency
2 weeks–2 months	1. Shunt defects Septal defects (ASD, VSD, AVSD) Aortopulmonary shunt (PDA, AP window, truncus) 2. Single ventricle 3. Obstructive lesions (see above) 4. Myocardial dysfunction Cardiomyopathy Anomalous origin of the left coronary artery Metabolic diseases 5. Pulmonary disease

regurgitation, absent pulmonary valve syndrome, and large systemic arteriovenous malformations).

Onset of heart failure in the first week of life (Table 1) is most likely to be due to a structural defect involving the left heart [critical aortic stenosis, severe coarctation or interrupted aortic arch, hypoplastic left-heart syndrome (HLHS)]. Less common are other forms of congenital structural defects and heart muscle dysfunction. Renal disorders that cause profound renal failure or neonatal systemic hypertension may present in the first week of life with signs of heart failure. Similarly, certain endocrine abnormalities may cause heart failure in neonates during the first week or two after birth.

Previously well newborns that develop heart failure in the first two to eight weeks of life are most likely to have some type of structural defect that results in a left-to-right shunt (Table 1). These infants are generally asymptomatic until the pulmonary vascular resistance (PVR) falls postnatally and the magnitude of the shunt becomes sufficiently large to cause signs and symptoms of heart failure due to maldistribution of blood flow (pulmonary overcirculation with or without inadequate systemic blood flow). Other forms of congenital cardiovascular malformations can present in the first two weeks to two months of life, including complex defects such as various forms of single ventricle, obstructive lesions that are not critical at birth but gradually produce symptoms, heart muscle dysfunction, and rarely, heart failure due to severe pulmonary problems.

Clinical Manifestations of Neonatal Heart Failure

Recognized signs and symptoms of heart failure in neonates generally include respiratory signs such as tachypnea, dyspnea with feeding, slow feeding, poor weight gain, diaphoresis, hepatomegaly, cool extremities, and poor peripheral perfusion. The signs and symptoms and heart failure severity depend largely on etiology, severity and age at onset (Table 1). Early signs of heart failure can be subtle and variable in the timing of presentation. For example, neonates with ductal-dependent lesions will most likely present with acute decompensation several days after birth when the ductus arteriosus constricts or closes completely. However, ductal-dependent left-heart obstructive lesions can present in the first few hours after birth. In contrast, neonates with significant left-to-right shunt lesions will develop progressive heart failure due to the steady decline in pulmonary vascular resistance over the first few weeks and months of life.

General Approaches to Management Based on Physiological Considerations

Although it is common to consider heart failure in the neonate with a large left-to-right shunt and/or compromised systemic circulation, neonates with structural defects resulting in decreased pulmonary circulation, right-to-left shunt or parallel circulation physiology (e.g., transposition complex) may also develop heart failure. It is important to consider that the presence of a large patent ductus arteriosus in the setting of dependency on the ductus for either pulmonary blood flow (Q_p) or systemic blood flow (Q_s) transforms the physiologic scenario into one of left-to-right shunt physiology. The same holds true for neonates with parallel circulation lesions such as d-transposition of the great arteries. Thus, pulmonary overcirculation, heart failure, and shock can occur even in "cyanotic" lesions. These concepts are illustrated in Fig. 1.

Neonates that experience cardiovascular collapse in the first week or two of life may respond well enough to treatments so as to allow withdrawal of ventilatory and parenteral pharmacological support. The infant then transitions from an acutely decompensated state (shock) to chronic compensation (chronic heart failure). During the shock phase, preservation and recovery of end-organ function is the goal. Maintenance of appropriate cardiac output and maximization of oxygen delivery using mechanical ventilation, parenteral inotropic drugs, and, when needed, prostaglandin E_1 (PGE_1) may be necessary during this period. Metabolic acidosis and major organ dysfunction often will resolve with aggressive management. The patient can then be gradually transitioned

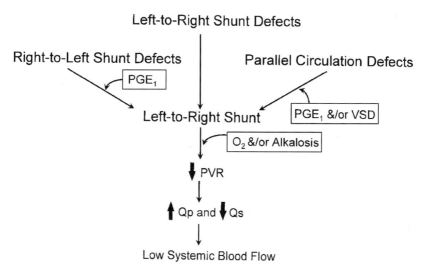

Figure 1 Physiological considerations in neonates with congenital cardiovascular malformations. Heart failure can occur in neonates with a variety of congenital cardiovascular malformations. Neonates with structural defects that initially result in predominately right-to-left shunting can be converted into a left-to-right shunting physiological condition when the ductus arteriosus is dilated (either naturally or as a consequence of administration of PGE_1). Similarly, infants with transposition complex (parallel circulation defects) and a large VSD or large PDA will exhibit physiological manifestations of a left-to-right shunt with excessive pulmonary blood flow and inadequate systemic flow. In either of these two conditions, or in the setting of structural defects that produce a left-to-right shunt, hyperoxygenation, and hyperventilation can reduce pulmonary vascular resistance (PVR), resulting in increased pulmonary flow and reduced systemic blood flow.

from parenteral to oral therapy with attention to maximizing nutrition. Failure to favorably progress along this path generally results to decompensation and may indicate the need for surgical intervention in the form of repair or palliation.

Classifying congenital heart defects as cyanotic vs. acyanotic often leaves many physiologic characteristics ill-defined and may lead to fundamental errors in clinical and presurgical management of the neonate with heart failure

(2,3). In order to more accurately describe the physiologic conditions and better understand the clinical manifestations that predominate for a given congenital cardiovascular malformation, it is helpful to consider the following five general circulatory models: series circulation, left-to-right shunt circulation, right-to-left shunt circulation, parallel circulation, venous obstruction, and ventricular dysfunction. In addition, each of these models may be modified by the presence of outflow obstruction, atrioventricular or semilunar valve regurgitation, and/or cardiac muscle dysfunction.

Series Circulation

Series circulation is the normal circulatory pattern and is characterized by the absence of mixing between deoxygenated and oxygenated blood. If heart failure occurs in this setting, it is generally due to either structural malformations that cause obstruction to blood flow or to heart muscle dysfunction. In these patients, hypoxemia is the result of ventilation/perfusion (V/Q) mismatch leading to end-organ hypoxia. Acidosis results from low cardiac output. Primary cardiac dysfunction may be present in both normal and abnormal cardiac anatomy. Treatment is directed at improving pulmonary status using diuresis, supplemental oxygen, and positive pressure ventilation. Cardiac pump dysfunction can be improved with manipulation of loading conditions and inotropic support (3,37).

Left-to-Right Shunt Circulation

Left-to-right shunt circulation is characterized by the presence of a certain volume of oxygenated blood that recirculates between the lungs and the heart, never making it through the peripheral systemic circulation. The volume of blood shunted away from the general circulation is determined by the anatomic size of the communication between the circulations, the interaction of the systemic and pulmonary vascular resistances (SVR, PVR, respectively) as well as by the presence and degree of outflow tract obstruction. Decreased PVR due to hyperoxygenation, hyperventilation, chemical alkalosis, and/or systemic vasoconstriction results in an increased left-to-right shunt at the expense of the systemic circulation. This also results in a greater degree of pulmonary overcirculation, worsening of the heart failure syndrome, and in some cases cardiogenic shock. While this scenario is common in the patient with HLHS, in which case the entire ventricular output is directed into the pulmonary system, aspects of this condition can occur in other less complex forms of left-to-right shunt lesions (Fig. 1). Treatment is directed at obtaining adequate levels of oxygenation that are usually lower than normal, as well as maintaining adequate cardiac pump function.

Right-to-Left Shunt Circulation

Right-to-left shunt circulation is characterized by the presence of deoxygenated blood that recirculates between the body and the heart without passing through the pulmonary circulation. The volume of blood shunted away from the pulmonary circulation is determined by anatomic size of the communication between the circulations, the interaction of the SVR and PVR, the degree of mechanical obstruction to the pulmonary circulation, and the presence, absence, and status of the pulmonary arteries. Neonates with right-to-left shunt lesions have traditionally been classified as cyanotic. However, it is possible for patients with this circulatory arrangement to display little or no cyanosis. For example, a neonate with right-to-left shunt physiology and unobstructed flow to the lungs (certain forms of tricuspid atresia, for example) will fail a hyperoxia test, but as the PVR decreases, symptoms of pulmonary overcirculation and left-to-right shunt circulatory model will predominate and clinical cyanosis may not be evident.

Any maneuver to increase Q_p, such as administration of PGE_1 would be appropriate for the patient with right-to-left shunt circulation and hypoxemia. However, if Q_p is excessive, this may promote pulmonary overcirculation, heart failure, and possibly cardiogenic shock (Fig. 1). Treatment of the neonate with right-to-left shunt physiology is based on the degree of oxygenation and pulmonary blood flow. When severe hypoxemia and low Q_p is present, PGE_1 therapy must be initiated. It should be recognized that this will change the circulatory condition to that of left-to-right shunt physiology and that normal levels of oxygenation can only be achieved at the expense of the systemic circulation. When the level of Q_p is adequate to maintain systemic oxygenation (e.g., lower than normal arterial saturation but with adequate oxygen delivery and no acidosis), stabilization occurs. Relief of congestion and treatment of heart failure is needed when Q_p is elevated. In neonates with single ventricle physiology with high pulmonary flow and near systemic pulmonary artery pressure, the pulmonary artery circuit must be protected. Pulmonary artery banding or separation of the pulmonary artery from the single ventricle and placement of an aorto-pulmonary shunt may be necessary to treat heart failure in these situations.

Parallel Circulation

Parallel circulation occurs when blood recirculates through the pulmonary circuit, never providing oxygenated blood to the body, and another pool circulates through the body, never providing deoxygenated blood to the lungs. Obviously, this situation is not compatible with life unless there is some volume of pulmonary venous blood that enters the systemic circulation. Congenital heart defects that produce parallel circulation include transposition of the great arteries, double outlet right ventricle with malposition of the great arteries, and some forms of single ventricle. In such cases, profound hypoxemia develops as the ductus arteriosus and foramen ovale begin to close in postnatal life. Neonates with this circulatory configuration require the presence of a systemic–pulmonary connection to allow bidirectional shunting for survival. Due to the physiologically normal elevated PVR at birth, patency of the ductus arteriosus or presence of a VSD allows bidirectional shunting and oxygenation. However, during the days and weeks following birth as the PVR drops and Q_p increases at the expense of Q_s (left-to-right shunt physiology; Fig. 1). The patient paradoxically develops clinical signs of pulmonary overcirculation and yet oxygenation remains the same or even drops. For these reasons, therapeutic hyperoxia and hyperventilation have no role in this circulatory scenario. In fact, administration of oxygen may actually worsen the clinical status of the patient and precipitate decompensation or even shock with very little gain in oxygenation.

Shunts across atrial septal defects or a patent foramen ovale meet the bidirectional criterion needed for adequate oxygenated–deoxygenated blood exchange. Factors such as atrial wall compliance (left atrium < right atrium), timing of ventricular activation (right before left), and right ventricular afterload greater than left ventricular afterload contribute to bidirectional shunting and thereby provide palliation for neonates with parallel circulation.

Venous Obstruction

In neonates with total anomalous pulmonary venous connection (TAPVC) or single ventricle physiology due to tricuspid and/or pulmonary atresia, cardiac output and oxygenation depend on right-to-left shunting at the atrial level. Compromised pulmonary or systemic venous return due to extracardiac or intracardiac obstruction reduces systemic cardiac output. The RAAS and SNS are then activated, promoting fluid retention with pulmonary and/or systemic venous congestion. Under these circumstances, the neonate is dependent on adequate preload to ensure some degree of right-to-left shunting at the atrial level in order to maintain Q_s and systemic oxygenation. Therefore, diuresis may be induced to improve symptoms secondary to congestion, with particular attention to preload. In this regard, central venous pressure monitoring can be extremely helpful in guiding fluid management in the acute phase. Administration of intotropic agents with a significant chronotropic effect may not be helpful due to the shortening of diastolic filling time, which may further compromise cardiac output in this setting. If immediate surgical repair is not possible, atrial balloon septostomy may be necessary to facilitate adequate right-to-left shunting in order to maintain adequate cardiac output and oxygenation.

Ventricular Dysfunction

Systolic ventricular dysfunction in neonates can be caused by a variety of etiologies, including bacterial and viral sepsis and a number of metabolic disorders. Isolated diastolic ventricular dysfunction characterized by decreased ventricular compliance can also occur in neonates, but is unusual and generally occurs as a consequence of severe hypertrophy due to pressure overload. Heart failure is often the presenting manifestation of anomalous origin of the left coronary artery from the pulmonary artery. In this condition, heart failure is due to severe ischemic cardiomyopathy. Treatment of heart failure due to ventricular function includes manipulation of loading conditions [diuretics and angiotensin converting enzyme (ACE) inhibitors] and inotropic support.

GENERAL GUIDELINES FOR MEDICAL THERAPY

The treatment objectives for a neonate with heart failure may be somewhat different than those for older children. Often, heart failure in infants with structural heart disease is managed for a relatively short period of time until surgical or catheter-based intervention is undertaken. For example, an infant with left ventricular failure as a result of severe aortic stenosis will be treated medically until stabilized and then referred for definitive therapy. However, heart failure may persist in some of these infants because of pre-existing myocardial dysfunction or incomplete relief of structural abnormalities (e.g., residual aortic stenosis and aortic insufficiency after aortic valvuloplasty).

Chronic Heart Failure Syndrome

During the past decade, treatment of adult patients with compensated congestive heart failure has been directed at modifying or interrupting the excessive neurohormonal activity (4–6). Treatment objectives in adults include reduction of morbidity and hospitalization, increased long-term survival, and improved quality of life (enhanced exercise capacity and reduction in symptoms). Drugs such as ACE inhibitors, angiotensin receptor blockers, aldosterone antagonists, and β-adrenergic receptor blockers have all emerged as important agents in the treatment of adult patients with heart failure (5,6). Whether or not and to what extent these processes play a role in newborns with heart failure remain to be determined. However, based upon studies in adults and animal experiments, it is reasonable to predict that similar mechanisms are operative in human neonates with heart failure, although there may be both qualitative and quantitative age-related differences. A great deal of additional research is needed to characterize the neurohormonal responses to heart failure and to heart failure therapy in preterm and term infants. The major classes of drugs used to treat chronic heart failure in neonates include diuretics, positive inotropic agents, vasodilators, and neurohormonal modulators.

Diuretics

Diuretics produce symptomatic improvement in neonates with pulmonary congestion. Three classes of diuretics are commonly used for the treatment of congestion related to heart failure in neonates (38). Loop diuretics, mainly furosemide, are potent drugs that retain their effectiveness even at very low glomerular filtration rates. The neonatal response to these loop diuretics is reduced because of immaturity of renal secretory mechanisms. Thiazide diuretics (e.g., hydrochlorothiazide, chlorothiazide) are diuretics that act in the distal tubules. They are less potent than loop diuretics and are more affected by low cardiac output and thus low glomerular filtration rate. Potassium sparing diuretics (e.g., spironolactone) also act in the distal tubules. Spironolactone has recently been shown to diminish myocardial fibrosis by blocking aldosterone receptors in heart tissue. Potassium sparing diuretics should be used with caution in infants being treated concomitantly with an ACE inhibitor because of the potential for hyperkalemia.

Diuretic therapy in neonates is commonly initiated with a loop diuretic. However, in resistant cases, a thiazide diuretic is added to the use of a loop diuretic agent. This combination impairs postdiuretic sodium retention and blocks the adaptive processes that develop during chronic loop diuretic therapy. When a thiazide is combined with a loop diuretic, the thiazide should be given approximately 30–60 min before the loop diuretic to permit transport in the downstream segment to be blocked fully before it is flooded with solute from the thick ascending limb. This strategy will optimize the natriuretic response.

Positive Inotropic Agents

For the longer-term management of impaired contractility in neonates, the most commonly used drug is digoxin. Although digoxin is often thought of as a positive inotropic agent in infants, the effect on contractility is minimal. Furthermore, digoxin may improve symptoms even in the absence of a measurable change in cardiac contractile function. For these reasons, it has been proposed that the major beneficial effects of digoxin therapy in chronic heart failure are attributable largely to neurohormonal modulation.

Vasodilators

Vasodilator therapy with ACE inhibitors has emerged as a mainstay of heart failure treatment in adult patients. More recently, vasodilator treatment has assumed an important role in the management of chronic heart failure in newborn and young infants. Vasodilators are used in the treatment of heart failure in neonates with, impaired ventricular function, atrioventricular or semilunar valve regurgitation, and left-to-right shunts (39).

In situations of depressed cardiac contractile function, the administration of a vasodilator may reduce impedance to ejection and improve cardiac output. In a neonate with a large left-to-right shunt, the magnitude of the shunt is dependent on the relative ratio of systemic to pulmonary vascular resistance. Cardiac contractile function is generally normal or only mildly depressed. An arteriolar dilator may improve systemic output by decreasing systemic vascular resistance, thereby increasing left ventricular output into the aorta and diminishing the magnitude of left-to-right shunt. However, it is important to note that systemic vascular resistance is low in the normal newborn and in newborns with large left-to-right shunts who have warm and well-perfused extremities. The benefit of vasodilators in these infants may be questionable. Moreover, the reduction in left-to-right shunt volume depends upon the reactivity of the pulmonary vascular bed as well. If the pulmonary vascular resistance is normal or only mildly elevated (which is commonly the case), then a reduction in systemic vascular resistance by arteriolar dilatation results in increased systemic output and reduction of left-to-right shunt. However, if the pulmonary vascular resistance is elevated and also decreases in response to drug therapy (a less common scenario), there may not be any overall change in the magnitude of the left-to-right shunt.

ACE inhibitors have emerged as the drug class of choice for vasodilator therapy of chronic heart failure in neonates (39,40). Presently, it is not known whether ACE inhibitor therapy will have the same long-term beneficial effects in infants as has been shown in adults. Furthermore, safety, efficacy, impact of maturational changes in the RAAS on drug responses and pharmacokinetics of various drugs in this class remain to be defined in human newborns.

Neurohormonal Modulation

As described above, the heart failure syndrome is characterized by generalized and organ-specific increases in sympathetic efferent discharge, activation of the RAAS, and activation of other mediators of myocardial remodeling. The current treatment of chronic heart failure is directed at "resetting" this neurohormonal imbalance. Drugs currently used for this purpose in adults include digoxin, ACE inhibitors,

β-adrenergic receptor blockers, aldosterone antagonists, and angiotensin receptor blockers.

Many of these drugs have not been studied in neonates with heart failure. Even old drugs such as digoxin have not been studied in appropriately designed prospective clinical trials of heart failure in infants and children. Although the neurohormonal responses to digoxin have not been defined in infants, the beneficial effects of digoxin in infants with heart failure due to a left-to-right shunt and apparently normal cardiac contractility suggest that neurohormonal modulation by digoxin may play a role in this population, as well. Similarly, no prospective randomized controlled trials of ACE inhibitor therapy for heart failure have been conducted in infants. However, published reports of infants and children with left-to-right shunts or dilated cardiomyopathy describe beneficial hemodynamic and clinical responses to ACE inhibitors (mainly captopril or enalapril) (37,39,40).

Clinical studies have confirmed increased SNS activity in infants with heart failure due to both congenital defects and acquired causes. At present, there is relatively little information available regarding the use of β-adrenergic blockers for the treatment of heart failure in newborns (41). Additional studies will be necessary to define the role of β-adrenergic blocker therapy in this patient population.

Spironolactone, an aldosterone receptor antagonist, decreases ventricular fibrosis that occurs as part of cardiac remodeling in heart failure in adult patients. However, these responses to heart failure and to therapeutic interventions have not been formally studied in infants and children. Although spironolactone has been used routinely as a potassium sparing diuretic in infants with heart failure, it is not known whether these additional beneficial effects occur in this population.

Angiotensin receptor blockers are a newer class of drugs (e.g., losartan and candesartan) that have been tested in adult patients with heart failure. Theoretically, these drugs may provide incremental benefits over ACE inhibitors, but these drugs have not been studied in neonates with heart failure.

In summary, despite an enlarging body of evidence in adult patients related to the favorable effects of drugs targeted at the neurohormonal derangements observed in heart failure, little or no information is available to support the use of these drugs in infants. Extrapolating from adult studies can be misleading and inappropriate due to important developmental differences in receptor–effector systems and circulatory physiology. However, it is important to recognize that neurohormonal activation and its pharmacological modulation may be important in the chronic heart failure syndrome in newborn and young infants. Infants with refractory heart failure and failure to thrive despite intensive medical management should undergo surgical repair or palliation (if a surgical approach is possible) without further delay.

Nutritional Therapy

Nutritional therapy is perhaps one of the most important (and often overlooked) aspects of the management of neonates with chronic heart failure (37,42,43). Acute and chronic malnutrition is common in infants with congenital and acquired heart disease and may be related to the complexity of the medical condition (80% of infants with complex single ventricle exhibit chronic malnutrition). When caring for a neonate with significant structural heart disease, caretakers may focus on the acute medical and surgical aspects of the condition and not give the nutritional aspects of neonatal heart failure care sufficient priority. Early attention to nutritional needs may ultimately have important positive influences on overall growth, well being, and long-term outcome. Failure to establish adequate growth in an infant awaiting surgical repair or palliation should be considered a failure of medical therapy, and constitutes an indication for surgical intervention.

In general, the most common cause for failure to thrive in infants with heart failure is a combination of decreased caloric intake and increased energy expenditure. Infants with heart failure simply do not feed well. Newborn and young infants with heart failure tire easily and may be unable to nipple effectively. Fatigue may also result from chronic hypoxia and diminished energy reserves. In addition, pronounced tachypnea may interfere with feeding in young infants, as they are unable to coordinate sucking, swallowing, and breathing. The increased work of breathing causes increased intra-abdominal pressure, which may explain the higher frequency of vomiting in these infants, another cause of decreased caloric intake. Discoordination of sucking and swallowing, delayed gastric emptying, vomiting, and increased total energy expenditure all contribute to growth failure in neonates with heart disease. Although resting energy expenditure may be normal or only slightly elevated, total energy expenditure is significantly increased in infants with heart failure due to increased energy requirements associated with the work of breathing and feeding.

Calorie and protein requirements of neonates with heart failure are greater than those of normal infants. Infants with heart failure may require 120–160 kcal/kg/day to maintain appropriate weight gain (approximately 30 g/day in term neonates). Standard infant formulas and breast milk contain 20 kcal/ounce. Infants with significant heart failure may not be able to tolerate the fluid load necessary to provide sufficient calories. In this setting, formula (or breast milk) with a higher caloric density should be employed. Fluid requirements must be individualized and may change, depending on the course of the disease and changes in diuretic therapy. In general, sodium restriction is not recommended for neonates with heart failure since provision of less than 2 mEq/kg/day may result in hyponatremia and growth impairment.

The caloric density of standard infant formula or breast milk may be increased to 24–30 kcal/ounce using either of two general methods (formula greater than 30 kcal/ounce can be used, but this often produces an osmotic diarrhea). One method is to prepare concentrated or powdered formula with less water. This has the advantage of being relatively simple, but carries the disadvantage of high solute (and sodium) load. In a similar fashion, breast milk can be supplemented with powdered formula. Generally, infants will tolerate formula or breast milk concentrated to

24–27 kcal/ounce. If the caloric density required exceeds 27 kcal/ounce, then the concentration method should not be used to further increase caloric density. Instead, the alternative method of adding supplements to the concentrated formula or breast milk should be employed. Corn oil, glucose polymers, and/or lipids may be added in measured amounts to increase the caloric density of standard infant formulas. Several commercial breast milk fortifiers are available that have been developed for preterm infants. Caloric density should not be increased abruptly as that is likely to produce emesis and/or diarrhea. Instead, caloric density should be increased by 2–3 kcal/ounce every 24 hr as tolerated (defined as minimal emesis and no diarrhea). Thus, it will take about 3–5 days to incrementally advance an infant from 20 to 30 kcal/ounce.

Increasing the caloric content of infant formula or breast milk may increase the respiratory quotient if all of the added calories are in the form of a glucose polymer. Infants with chronic heart failure are prone to contraction alkalosis (secondary to diuretic therapy), which, if combined with an increased carbohydrate load, may lead to either inadequate ventilation or to even greater caloric expenditure from excessive use of respiratory muscles.

Comprehensive nutritional therapy includes not only provision of sufficient calories and nutrients, but also involves attention to specific feeding problems and educational efforts to ensure the family's ability to provide specialized care at home. It is often helpful to enlist the assistance of nutritionists and social workers for infants with especially difficult or demanding nutritional needs. In addition, occupational and physical therapists with special expertise in infant oral-motor feeding techniques may provide invaluable advice and practical assistance.

If a neonate is failing to thrive despite attention to feeding issues and increased caloric density, it may be necessary to intensify nutritional support by providing nasogastric or orogastric feeds. The most effective method of improving nutritional status is by 24-hr continuous enteral feeding. If the neonate is home, it is easier for the family if the feeding is for a total of 18–20 hr per day to allow time for bathing, formula preparation, and travel. A potential disadvantage to strict tube feeding and avoidance of all oral feeding is that this approach may contribute to poor oral-motor function and delay progression of adequate oral intake. It is therefore recommended that tube feeding be combined with strategies to maintain oral-motor feeding skills.

Education and Counseling

The concept of family-centered care is based on the principle that a neonate with heart failure is a member of a family unit and that the illness will impact upon all members of the family. Thus, it is important to involve siblings and other close family members in education and counseling efforts. Family members must be knowledgeable and engaged in the care of the infant with heart failure. As much as is practical and possible, the family and primary care-givers at home should be engaged in decision-making, as well. This helps create a sense of empowerment and minimizes the stress that results from a sense of a lack of control. Another important factor in lessening parental anxiety is information. It is important to provide specific information about the infant's condition, status, progress, care plans, medical therapy, and prognosis. Specific information should be provided with regard to each medication and how to administer medicines at home. In addition to teaching about the infant's particular medical condition and needs, education regarding routine well baby care should not be neglected. Teaching normal well baby and primary care needs are also essential to facilitate the transition to home and to help parents see their neonate as a person, and to not just focus on heart failure. Open-ended sessions with time for parent's questions are helpful in dispelling common myths and reducing stress and anxiety within the home. Most neonatal nurseries offer formal training in basic infant cardiopulmonary resuscitation to parents. This should be incorporated into the predischarge teaching for parents of neonates with heart failure.

APPENDIX A

Dosage Guidelines for Selected Cardiovascular Drugs in Neonates

Drug	Dose
Diuretics	
Bumetanide	0.01–0.05 mg/kg/dose IV or PO (daily or every other day; maximum 0.1 mg/kg/day)
Chlorothiazide	20–40 mg/kg/day PO divided into two daily doses
	1–4 mg/kg/dose IV every 6–12 hr
Ethacrynic acid	0.5–1.0 mg/kg IV; every 12–24 hr
Furosemide	1–2 mg/kg IV or PO every 4–12 hr
	Continuous infusion: 0.01– 0.05 mg/kg/hr
Hydrochlorothiazide	2–3 mg/kg/day PO in two divided doses
Mannitol	0.5–1 g/kg IV. After urine flow is established, lower doses (0.25– 0.5 g/kg) are recommended. Repeat every 6 hr as clinically indicated. Use with caution in newborns due to hyperosmolarity.
Metolazone	0.2–0.4 mg/kg PO once daily
Spironolactone	1–3.5 mg/kg/day PO. Caution in combination with ACE inhibitors (may produce hyperkalemia).
Inotropic agents and vasopressors	
Amrinone	Loading dose: 1–3 mg/kg IV over 30 min
	Continuous infusion: 5–10 µg/kg/min
	Loading dose may promote hypotension
Digoxin	Total digitalizing dose: Preterm infant 10 µg/kg PO Term infant 10–20 µg/kg PO

(Continued)

Drug	Dose
	Maintenance dose:
	5–10 µg/kg/day PO
	Reduce dose in renal dysfunction.
	IV dose is 75–80% of oral dose.
Dobutamine	2–20 µg/kg/min continuous infusion IV
Dopamine	2–20 µg/kg/min continuous infusion IV
Epinephrine	Acute: 0.1 ml/kg of 1:10,000 solution (0.01 mg/kg)
	Continuous IV infusion: 0.1–1 µg/kg/min
Isoproterenol	0.05–1 µg/kg/min continuous infusion IV
Milrinone	Loading dose: 0.1 mg/kg IV over 15–30 min
	Continuous infusion: 0.5–0.75 µg/kg/min
	Loading dose may promote hypotension
Norepinephrine	0.05–1 µg/kg/min continuous infusion IV
Phenylephrine	0.5–5 µg/kg/min continuous infusion IV
Vasodilators and antihypertensives	
Atenolol	0.5–2 mg/kg/day PO
Captopril	0.1–0.5 mg/kg/dose PO every 8 hr
	Maximum neonatal dose: 3 mg/kg/24 hr
Enalapril	0.1–0.4 mg/kg/day PO
Enalaprilat	5–10 µg/kg/dose IV q8–24 hr
Esmolol	Loading dose: 500 µg/kg IV over 2–4 min; initial maintenance: 50–200 µg/kg/min
	May increase in 50–100 µg/kg/min increments up to maximum of 1000 µg/kg/min. Mean effective dose ~500 µg/kg/min
Hydralazine	0.1–0.5 mg/kg/dose IV

Drug	Dose
	0.25–0.75 mg/kg/dose PO
	For chronic therapy, administer every 6–8 hr PO or every 4–6 hr IV
Nifedipine	0.1–0.5 mg/kg PO every 8 hr
	May depress cardiac contractility in neonates
Nitric oxide	1–40 ppm via inhalation
Nitroglycerin	0.5–3 μg/kg/min IV
Nitroprusside	0.5–3.0 μg/kg/min IV
Phentolamine	0.05–0.1 mg/kg/dose IV
	2.5–15 μg/kg/min continuous infusion IV
	Treatment of extravasation (due to dopamine, dobutamine, norepinephrine, epinephrine, or phenylephrine); dilute 5–10 mg in 10 ml normal saline and infiltrate area subcutaneously. Do not exceed 0.1–0.2 mg/kg or 5 mg total.
Propranolol	0.5–1 mg/kg/day PO (divided three or four times daily)
Prostaglandin E_1	Initial dose 0.05 μg/kg/min
	May increase to 0.1–0.15 μg/kg/min
	Lower doses (as low as 0.01 μg/kg/min) may be effective and tapering to lowest effective dose is recommended. May cause apnea and/or hypotension.

REFERENCES

1. Packer M. Pathophysiology of chronic heart failure. Lancet 1992; 340:88–92.
2. Auslender M, Artman M. Overview of the management of pediatric heart failure. Prog Pediatr Cardiol 2000; 11:231–241.
3. Balaguru D, Artman M, Auslender M. Management of heart failure in children. Curr Prob Pediatr 2000; 30:5–30.

4. Bolger AP, Sharma R, Li W, Leenarts M, Kalra PR, Kemp M, Coats AJS, Anker SD, Gatzoulis MA. Neurohormonal activation and the chronic heart failure syndrome in adults with congenital heart disease. Circulation 2002; 106:92–99.

5. Mehra MR, Uber PA, Francis GS. Heart failure therapy at the crossroads: are there limits to the neurohormonal model? J Am Coll Cardiol 2003; 41:1606–1610.

6. Konstam MA. Improving clinical outcomes with drug treatment in heart failure: what have trials taught? Am J Cardiol 2003; 91:9D–14D.

7. Bolger AP, Coats AJ, Gatzoulis MA. Congenital heart disease: the original heart failure syndrome. Eur Heart J 2003; 24:970–976.

8. Anderson PA. The heart and development. Semin Perinatol 1996; 20:482–509.

9. Teitel DF. Physiologic development of the cardiovascular system in the fetus. In: Polin RA, Fox WW, eds. Fetal and Neonatal Physiology. Philadelphia: W.B. Saunders Co. 1998.

10. Artman M. Developmental Changes in Myocardial Inotropic Responsiveness. Austin, TX: R.G. Landes Company, 1994.

11. Riva E, Hearse DJ. The Developing Myocardium. Mt. Kisco, New York: Futura Publishing, 1991.

12. Harvey RP, Rosenthal N. Heart Development. San Diego: Academic Press, 1999.

13. Bers DM. Excitation–Contraction Coupling and Cardiac Contractile Force. 2nd ed. Dordrecht, The Netherlands: Kluwer Academic Publishers, 2001.

14. Bers DM. Cardiac excitation–contraction coupling. Nature 2002; 415:198–205.

15. Sun X, Protasi F, Takahashi M, Takeshima H, Ferguson DG, Franzini-Armstrong C. Molecular architecture of membranes involved in excitation–contraction coupling of cardiac muscle. J Cell Biol 1995; 129:659–671.

16. Carl SL, Felix K, Caswell AH, Brandt NR, Ball WJ Jr, Vaghy PL, Meissner G, Ferguson DG. Immunolocalization of sarcolemmal dihydropyridine receptor and sarcoplasmic reticular triadin and ryanodine receptor in rabbit ventricle and atrium. J Cell Biol 1995; 129:672–682.

17. Artman M, Henry G, Coetzee WA. Cellular basis for age-related differences in cardiac excitation–contraction coupling. Prog Pediatr Cardiol 2000; 11:185–194.

18. Page E, Buecker JL. Development of dyadic junctional complexes between sarcoplasmic reticulum and plasmalemma in rabbit left ventricular myocardial cells. Circ Res 1981; 48:519–522.

19. Haddock PS, Coetzee WA, Cho E, Porter L, Katoh H, Bers DM, Jafri MS, Artman M. Subcellular $[Ca^{2+}]_i$ gradients during excitation–contraction coupling in newborn rabbit ventricular myocytes. Circ Res 1999; 85:415–427.

20. Haddock PS, Coetzee WA, Artman M. Na^+/Ca^{2+} exchange current and contractions measured under Cl^--free conditions in developing rabbit hearts. Am J Physiol 1997; 273:H837–H846.

21. Nassar R, Reedy MC, Anderson PA. Developmental changes in the ultrastructure and sarcomere shortening of the isolated rabbit ventricular myocyte. Circ Res 1987; 61:465–483.

22. Kim H, Kim D, Lee I, Rah B, Sawa Y, Schaper J. Human fetal heart development after mid-term: morphometry and ultrastructural study. J Mol Cell Cardiol 1992; 24:949–965.

23. Artman M. Sarcolemmal $Na^+–Ca^{2+}$ exchange activity and exchanger immunoreactivity in developing rabbit hearts. Am J Physiol 1992; 263:H1506–H1513.

24. Boerth SR, Zimmer DB, Artman M. Steady-state mRNA levels of the sarcolemmal $Na^+–Ca^{2+}$ exchanger peak near birth in developing rabbit and rat hearts. Circ Res 1994; 74:354–359.

25. Chen F, Mottino G, Klitzner TS, Philipson KD, Frank JS. Distribution of the Na^+/Ca^{2+} exchange protein in developing rabbit myocytes. Am J Physiol 1995; 268:C1126–C1132.

26. Vetter R, Studer R, Reinecke H, Kolár F, Ostádalová I, Drexler H. Reciprocal changes in the postnatal expression of the sarcolemmal $Na^+–Ca^{2+}$-exchanger and SERCA2 in rat heart. J Mol Cell Cardiol 1995; 27:1689–1701.

27. Boerth SR, Artman M. Thyroid hormone regulates $Na^+–Ca^{2+}$ exchanger expression during postnatal maturation and in adult rabbit ventricular myocardium. Cardiovasc Res 1996; 31(suppl S):E145–E152.

28. Artman M, Ichikawa H, Avkiran M, Coetzee WA. Na^+/Ca^{2+} exchange current density in cardiac myocytes from rabbits and guinea pigs during postnatal development. Am J Physiol 1995; 268:H1714–H1722.

29. Hryshko LV, Philipson KD. Sodium–calcium exchange: recent advances. Basic Res Cardiol 1997; 92(suppl 1):45–51.

30. Matsuda T, Takuma K, Baba A. $Na^+–Ca^{2+}$ exchanger: physiology and pharmacology. Jpn J Pharmacol 1997; 74:1–20.

31. Hilgemann DW, Ball R. Regulation of cardiac Na^+, Ca^{2+} exchange and K_{ATP} potassium channels by PIP_2. Science 1996; 273:956–959.

32. Artman M, Kithas PA, Wike JS, Strada SJ. Inotropic responses change during postnatal maturation in rabbit. Am J Physiol 1988; 255:H335–H342.

33. Artman M. Developmental changes in myocardial contractile responses to inotropic agents. Cardiovasc Res 1992; 26:3–13.

34. Perchenet L, Hinde AK, Patel CKR, Hancox JC, Levi AJ. Stimulation of Na/Ca exchange by the β-adrenergic/protein kinase A pathway in guinea-pig ventricular myocytes at 37°C. Pflugers-Arch Eur J Physiol 2000; 439:822–828.

35. Kithas PA, Artman M, Thompson WJ, Strada SJ. Subcellular distribution of high-affinity type IV cyclic AMP phosphodiesterase activity in

rabbit ventricular myocardium: relations to postnatal maturation. J Mol Cell Cardiol 1989; 21:507–517.

36. Piacentino V, Weber CR, Chen X, Weisser-Thomas J, Margulies KB, Bers DM, Houser SR. Cellular basis of abnormal calcium transients of failing human ventricular myocytes. Circ Res 2003; 92:651–658.

37. Artman M, Mahony L, Teitel DF. Neonatal Cardiology. New York: The McGraw-Hill Companies, 2002.

38. Lowrie L. Diuretic therapy of heart failure in infants and children. Prog Pediatr Cardiol 2000; 12:45–55.

39. Balaguru D, Auslender M. Vasodilators in the treatment of pediatric heart failure. Prog Pediatr Cardiol 2000; 12:81–90.

40. Grenier MA, Fioravanti J, Truesdell SC, Mendelsohn AM, Vermillion RP, Lipshultz SE. Angiotensin-converting enzyme inhibitor therapy for ventricular dysfunction in infants, children and adolescents: a review. Prog Pediatr Cardiol 2000; 12:91–111.

41. Shaddy RE. Beta-adrenergic blockers in the treatment of pediatric heart failure. Prog Pediatr Cardiol 2000; 12:113–118.

42. Leitch CA. Growth, nutrition and energy expenditure in pediatric heart failure. Prog Pediatr Cardiol 2000; 11:195–202.

43. Abad-Sinden A, Sutphen JL. Growth and nutrition. In: Allen HD, Gutgesell HP, Clark EB, Driscoll DJ, eds. Moss and Adams' Heart Disease in Infants, Children and Adolescents 6th ed. Philadelphia: Lippincott Williams & Wilkins, 2001:325–332.

8

Metabolic Causes of Pediatric Heart Failure

BRIAN D. HANNA

Department of Pediatrics, Division of Cardiology, Children's Hospital of Philadelphia, University of Pennsylvania School of Medicine, Philadelphia, Pennsylvania, U.S.A.

INTRODUCTION

This discussion of inherited metabolic causes of pediatric cardiac failure will encompass processes affecting energy production, and the storage diseases that affect cardiac systolic and/or diastolic function. Several diseases have a component of cardiac hypertrophy without cardiac failure in the presentation (Table 1). Only those with clear cardiac pathology are included. Metabolic derangements can cause arrhythmogenesis either associated with, or as a result of, cardiac failure, and these will be noted. Genetic abnormalities of contractile

241

Table 1 Syndromes and Diseases that are Associated with
Radiographic Cardiomegaly and/or Ventricular Hypertrophy
on Echocardiography

Contractile protein	Storage disorders	Mitochondrial diseases
Mutation	Hurler, Hurler–Scheie,	Carnitine deficiencies[a]
Familial HCM	Scheie (MPS I)[a]	OXPHOS complex
Beta-myosin	Hunter (MPS II)[a]	I–V defects[a]
heavy chain	Maroteaux–Lamy	MELAS[a]
Troponin T	(MPS VI)[a]	MERRF[a]
Alpha-tropomyosin	Sly (MPS VII)[a]	Fatty acid
Desmin accumulation	I-cell disease (ML II)[a]	beta-oxidation
syndromes	Alpha-mannosidosis[a]	defects[a]
Associated syndromes	Fucosidosis[a]	Friedreich ataxia[a]
Noonan	Sialidosis type II[a]	
LEOPARD	Multiple sulfatase	
Beckwith-Wiedemann	deficiency	
Infant of a diabetic	Fabry disease[a]	
mother	Gangliosidoses[a]	
Cardio-facial-cutaneous	Glycogen storage	
syndrome	type II, III, IV[a]	
Costello syndrome	Cardiac phosphorylase b	
	kinase deficiency[a]	

HCM: hypertrophic cardiomyopathy; MPS: mucopolysaccharidosis; ML, muco-
lipidosis.
[a]Entities with abnormal metabolism and cardiac symptomatology that are discussed
in the text.

force generation and transmission, now thought to be the
basis of many types of idiopathic hypertrophic and dilated
cardiomyopathy, fall out of the scope of this discussion of
altered myocardial metabolism. Recent reviews of the point
mutations and deletions that affect the cytoskeletal and sarcomere structure and function in inherited hypertrophic and
dilated cardiomyopathies are available (1–5). An exhaustive
database of these gene defects is available on the web site
http://www.angis.org.au.

Normal myocardial energy production involves the mitochondrial pathways of pyruvate oxidation, the Krebs cycle,
beta-oxidation of fatty acids, and the inner mitochondrial
membrane oxidative phosphorylation (OXPHOS) complexes
(electron transport chain complexes I–IV, ATP synthase com-

plex V, and the adenosine nucleotide translocator). After the early postnatal change from fetal myocardial utilization of glucose and lactate, the vast majority of myocardial ATP is produced by beta-oxidative phosphorylation of fatty acids. The translocation of fatty acids through the myocyte into mitochondria involves several important transporters [fatty acid translocase, carnitine acyltransferase (CAT), carnitine and carnitine palmitoyl transferases (CPTs)]. In addition, mitochondrial RNA transport of specific amino acids is crucial to mitochondrial structure and function. Derangements in many of these processes have now been identified with ramifications to cardiac function and will be discussed in relation to the affected process in the section on Mitochondrial Cardiomyopathies.

Storage diseases with cardiac ramifications are the result of specific enzymatic dysfunction and involve lysosomes and the cytosol. The cardiac abnormalities can be the result of either the accumulation of nondegraded substrates in macrophages and myocytes engorged with lysosomes, the metabolic effect of deficient enzyme function or coronary vasculopathy. These diseases will be discussed in relationship to the stored product.

CLINICAL PRESENTATION

Although specific clinical presentations do occur with some metabolic cardiomyopathies, most historical and physical findings are nonspecific and related to the physiology of decreased systolic function, reduced lisotropy (decreased relaxation), and/or arrhythmogenesis. Especially, in the case of ventricular dilation and dysfunction, there is little that differentiates myocarditis from a genetic cardiomyopathy. It should be recognized that the cardiac decompensation that leads to the first clinical presentation is frequently precipitated by an intercurrent illness. This continues to be important into adulthood. In the Pediatric Heart Failure Program of our institution, several symptomatic children have significant family histories of adult-onset heart failure requiring prolonged treatment or cardiac transplantation; all of these adult patients carried a "firm" diagnosis of myocarditis as the etiology of the heart failure and none had been diagnosed as having a genetic etiology for their disease.

The age at presentation with heart failure can assist in narrowing the differential diagnosis. Most storage diseases, caused by enzyme deficiencies, will present early in life but later presentation does occur within each subgroup when there is more residual enzyme activity. Furthermore, the physical features that are disease specific often are not clear in infancy but become more so with age. Reevaluation of nondiagnosed patients at frequent intervals is helpful. Defects that significantly affect energy production, e.g., glycogen storage diseases, will manifest during times of stress: fasting, gastrointestinal illnesses, extreme exercise, etc. However, true biochemical crises are most common with mitochondrial diseases.

Historical evidence should be sought for other organ involvement: (1) skeletal muscle: myotonia (decreased muscle relaxation), myopathy (weakness either congenital or after infancy); (2) brain: seizures, ataxia (loss of motor control), encephalopathy, delay or regression in neurodevelopment, failure to thrive (FTT); (3) biochemical crises: syncope, seizures, episodic vomiting, symptoms with fasting, lethargy; (4) GI: pseudo-obstruction; and (5) prolonged cardiac dysfunction: syncope, palpitations, activity intolerance, FTT. In the event that the patient presents in cardiac failure, few of the above features will pinpoint a diagnosis but the timing to the presentation is important. Most of these findings predate significant cardiac dysfunction and therefore can direct biochemical and genetic testing. In addition to these historical features of the proband, a thorough family history is crucial and best carried out by metabolic genetics consultants.

The relevant physical findings, outside of the cardiac examination, are often subtle, nonspecific, and related to other organ involvement. Unfortunately, prolonged cardiac dysfunction is often overlooked until a significant decompensation is triggered. An example is skeletal muscle wasting and weakness, where the myopathy can be due to disuse, or myotonic as in Becker muscular dystrophy. Hypotonia and weakness are most consistently associated with mitochondrial disorders and in infancy are causes of respiratory failure. On the other hand, recurrent respiratory infections, FTT, coarse features, short stature with multiple skeletal changes, and corneal clouding are hallmarks of the mucopolysaccharidoses and glycoproteinoses and predate the cardiac symptomatology. Hepatomegaly, out of proportion to the cardiac failure, is a prominent feature of the lipidoses and most patients with glycogen storage diseases.

Patients with cardiomyopathy and associated dysmorphism syndromes, e.g., Noonan syndrome, are not commonly symptomatic at presentation. At present, none are known to have etiologies within the scope of this chapter; however, dysmorphism may be seen with some of the metabolic diseases discussed here. There is an excellent review by Schwartz et al. (6) with an exhaustive listing of these syndromes, as well as online Mendelian inheritance in man (OMIM) (TM) (7).

INVESTIGATIONS

It is important to recognize that the complexity in the differential diagnosis of pediatric cardiac failure requires the assistance of several key consulting services: cardiology, metabolic genetics, neurology, and ophthalmology. Most patients come to the attention of these consultants with basic testing completed, including chest x-ray and basic blood tests (CBC, electrolytes, BUN, creatinine). In addition, EEG, brain imaging (MRI and/or MRS chemical assays via magnetic resonance spectroscopy), relevant skeletal survey, and an expert, comprehensive ophthalmologic examination are important.

Standard EKG and echocardiography examinations are indicated in all patients with suspected metabolic cardiac involvement. In most metabolic cardiomyopathies, the EKG shows increased precordial voltages; this occurs maximally in Pompe disease (glycogen storage disease type II). The PR interval is abnormal in most, but not all of the metabolic diseases: either short but without pre-excitation or too long with first degree AV block. Nonspecific ST-T wave abnormalities are common. Evidence for myocardial infarction is a late finding in several of the lysosomal disorders presenting with ventricular dysfunction. The echocardiographic findings are disease specific; however, most storage diseases show an element of ventricular hypertrophy and atrial enlargement. Most lysosomal disorders affect valve structure and function long before ventricular dysfunction is noted, whereas this is not seen in the glycogen storage diseases or mitochondrial disorders.

Unfortunately, the biochemical investigations are complex and time consuming to perform. Most require the services of specialized laboratories. Knowledgeable metabolic genetics consultants should direct specific testing. Table 2 lists the

Table 2 Blood, Urine, and Cerebral Spinal Fluid Testing that Help Differentiate the Metabolic Causes of Heart Failure: Test Immediately on Presentation

---

Blood
    Blood gas and electrolytes with attention to pH and anion gap
    Glucose
    Ketones
    Lactate[a]
    Pyruvate[a]
    Ammonia
    Hepatic enzymes
    Creatine phosphokinase: total and isoenzymes
    Acyl-carnitine quantification (before starting carnitine)
    Carnitine: total and free (before starting carnitine)
    Quantitative amino acids[a] (before starting intravenous amino acids)
Urine
    Ketones
    Carnitine
    Quantitative organic acids
Cerebral spinal fluid (if presentation includes encephalopathy)
    Glucose
    Lactate
    Pyruvate
    Total protein
    Quantitative amino acids
    Cell count

---

[a]Optimally obtain 1–1.5 hr after a meal.

Table 3 Specialized Testing for Metabolic Causes of Heart Failure: As Directed by the Results from the Testing in Table 2

Blood: White cells (sampled before transfusion)
  Mitochondrial DNA analysis for mutations and deletions
  Lysosomal enzyme analysis
  DNA banking
Urine
  Acyl-glycine derivatives
Tissue biopsies
  Skeletal muscle[a]
  Cardiac muscle[a]
  Skin for fibroblast culture
  Liver[a]
Consultations
  Neurology
  Ophthalmology
  Metabolic genetics

---

[a]Must be examined fresh; however, if this is not possible, freeze immediately in liquid nitrogen and store at −70 F. Post-mortem specimens must be obtained and processed within 20 min.

blood, urine, and cerebral spinal fluid testing that help differentiate the different metabolic causes of heart failure. Table 3 lists more specialized testing that is recommended, based on the clinical features and the test results from Table 2. Early catheterization and myocardial biopsy carry significant risk and should be deferred. The risk for death of the procedure is highest in infants < 6 months old and patients requiring mechanical ventilation and/or significant inotropic support. Often a period of stabilization can decrease the risk. Furthermore, the utility of skeletal muscle biopsy has proven to be greater: more tissue is available for histologic, histochemical, enzyme, and DNA studies. Even if there is no overt skeletal muscle dysfunction, the genetic defect is present. Notable exceptions include an adult-onset form of Fabry disease, phosphorylase kinase deficiency that is limited to the heart and maternally inherited mitochondrial cardiomyopathies, where because of heteroplasmy, these defects may not be adequately expressed in skeletal muscle.

The pathologic investigation for cardiac and/or skeletal muscle should include the following: (1) four samples are preserved in formalin for light microscopy for evaluation of inflammation, fibrosis, myofiber disarray and size, ragged red fibers (RRF), viral inclusions, and vacuolization. Special stains and processing are necessary to determine the characteristics of storage material in vacuoles, e.g., lipid, abnormal forms of glycogen, etc; (2) one sample for electron microscopy to look for mitochondrial structural abnormalities, mitochondrial number and location, storage material, abnormal lysosomes, etc; (3) one sample is sent for viral PCR to exclude at least entero-, parvo- and adeno-viruses; and (4) immediately on biopsy, two samples should be examined for mitochondrial enzyme analysis. If this is not possible, the muscle samples should be flash frozen in liquid nitrogen and saved for future enzyme and mitochondrial DNA analysis as directed by the metabolic geneticist.

INITIAL TREATMENT

For the most part, treatment is symptomatic, according to the specific cardiac dysfunction: acidosis, low output, congestion, reduced lisotropy, and arrhythmia. Specific treatment for the metabolic derangements is limited and discussed with the specific disease. However, in general patients should not be enterally fed but given intravenous 5% glucose to rapidly counter catabolic states and move energy production away from lipid and glycogen. Higher glucose concentrations are not recommended in case the failure is due to pyruvate dehydrogenase deficiency. Continuous insulin infusions have also been advocated, especially if the acidosis persists or if there is severe hyperglycemia. The use of intravenous or oral L-carnitine (50–300 mg/kg/day) on presentation of the cardiac failure seems well supported (8). Endogenously provided L-carnitine may improve mitochondrial energy metabolism by esterifying accumulated acyl-CoA metabolites, whether or not there is a defect in carnitine metabolic pathways. Furthermore, it is safe and well tolerated. Oral carnitine should start at 50 mg/kg/day with gradual increases to prevent diarrhea.

MITOCHONDRIAL CARDIOMYOPATHIES

Mitochondria are crucial to normal myocyte function. Almost 40% of the myocyte volume is made up of these energy-producing organelles. The structure includes an outer membrane and an inner membrane that is folded into cristae. Fifteen percent of all cellular proteins reside within the mitochondria, 65% within the matrix [fatty acid beta-oxidation, pyruvate dehydrogenase, and Krebs tricarboxylic acid (TCA) cycle], 25% associated with the inner membrane (electron transport chain respiratory complexes I–V), and 10% associated with the outer membrane (carnitine translocation system and the apoptosis-associated mitochondrial permeability transition pore). Each mitochondrion contains circular DNA with genes that encode two ribosomal RNAs, 22 transfer RNAs, and 13 proteins that form part of OXPHOS complexes I, III, IV, and V. All other proteins involved in mitochondrial transcription, translation, and enzymatic functions are encoded by the chromosomes in the nucleus and require protein transport into the mitochondria.

Histologic abnormalities of mitochondria include abnormally large or swollen mitochondria with distended cristae, inclusion bodies, abnormal number, aggregation, or location. By light microscopy and staining with Gomori dye, "RRF" which are abnormal mitochondrial aggregations can be seen in defects of mitochondrial protein synthesis (9). Enzyme immunoassays can assess specific enzyme activity.

Mitochondrial DNA is maternally inherited and has a high rate of spontaneous mutation, most likely associated with the high concentration of oxygen free radicals, the result of mitochondrial respiration, and the low rate of mitochondrial DNA repair (10). The number of mutations and the severity of symptoms increase with age (11). Therefore, mitochondria within any cell or organ can have several different DNA and protein structures. Furthermore, the amount of enzyme dysfunction can vary among mitochondria, among cells, and among organs: this is the etiology of the heteroplasmy (or mosaicism) in maternally inherited mitochondrial diseases. Genes from both the nucleus and mitochondrion encode proteins for mitochondrial complexes I, III, IV and V: therefore, a single clinical phenotype can have varied inheritance patterns.

Mitochondrial abnormalities associated with heart failure fall into five areas: (a) defects within the respiratory electron transport chain; (b) oxidative phosphorylation (OXPHOS complexes); (c) defects in mitochondrial beta-oxidation of fatty acids; (d) abnormality in the apoptosis-associated mitochondrial permeability transition pore; and (e) abnormalities in mitochondrial structure and/or location associated with abnormal energy utilization. A current listing of mitochondrial DNA mutations and deletions can be found at http://www.mitomap.org. Only defects that are associated with cardiac failure, at presentation or as a significant component of the clinical course, are discussed here.

Respiratory Transport Chain Defects (Autosomal Recessive Inheritance)

Electron transfer flavoprotein (ETF) (either subunit a or b) and ETF dehydrogenase catalyze the electron transport between acyl-CoA dehydrogenases and the respiratory transport chain resulting in multiple acyl-CoA dehydrogenase deficiencies (MADD or glutaric aciduria type II). This presents with cardiomyopathy (histology: cardiac fatty infiltration without RRF) without encephalopathy, metabolic acidosis, nonketotic hypoglycemia, and accumulation of the corresponding urinary organic acids that cannot be metabolized. Three characteristic clinical patterns occur: lethal neonatal presentation either with or without dysmorphism and polycystic kidneys, and late onset with a variable course (12). No linkage between the three affected proteins and the phenotype has been found. Treatment of the neonatal disease may be possible with carnitine, insulin, and low-fat, low-protein diet (13); however, the ultimate outcome is poor.

OXPHOS Defects

OXPHOS complexes I–V catalyze the transfer of electrons to ATP. Defects of these complexes occur because of mutations in either nuclear or mitochondrial DNA. The clinical hallmarks of these defects include nonspecific signs and symptoms of both energy deficiency and lactic acidosis affecting multiple organ systems. Patients can present with biochemical crises. A current classification of these diseases utilizes the mutation in the encoding DNA: Class I: disorders of the nuclear OXPHOS genes; Class II: point mutations in mitochondrial DNA; and Class III: deletions in mitochondrial DNA (14). However, it should be noted that these are not distinct or specific clinical manifestations. Variable presentations within a kindred can encompass several syndromes.

Class I Mutations: Disorders of the Nuclear
OXPHOS Genes (Autosomal Recessive
Inheritance)

Lethal infantile mitochondrial syndrome (15,16) may be caused by several different enzyme defects that lead to the same phenotype: NADH dehydrogenase (complex I), ubiquinol-cytochrome *c* reductase (complex III), and cytochrome *c* oxidase (complex IV). This presents over the first several weeks of life with progressive feeding difficulties, FTT, hypotonia, lethargy, lactic acidosis and cardiomyopathy (histology: cardiac and skeletal lipid and glycogen without RRF but with abnormal mitochondria), skeletal muscle, liver and kidney involvement without encephalopathy. In addition to the expected autosomal recessive inheritance, maternal inheritance can be seen because genes for some subunits exist on mitochondrial DNA. Current medical treatment does not change the clinical course of progressive lactic acidosis and death at <1 year. However, milder forms exist with reduced complex IV activity but the survival potential is unknown.

Leigh "disease" (sub acute necrotizing encephalomyelopathy) (16) is caused by defects in several different proteins that lead to the same phenotype: ATPase 6 (complex V); mitochondrial lysine transfer RNA; cytochrome *c* oxidase (complex IV); and subunits of pyruvate dehydrogenase complex (autosomal and X-linked inheritance). This is a rapidly progressive disease of early childhood with stress related crises with seizures, ataxia, weakness, and cardiac failure from hypertrophic cardiomyopathy (histology: normal to hypertrophic myocytes with distended mitochondria and abnormal cristae). High blood and cerebral spinal fluid levels of lactate and pyruvate with metabolic acidosis and hypoglycemia can occur during crises; elevated lactate is seen on magnetic resonance spectroscopy.

Hypertrophic cardiomyopathy with late cardiac failure has been reported in patients with propionic aciduria (17). This association is not currently a known component of the phenotype; however, as many as half the patients may be affected (P. Kaplan, personal communication, 2004). The pathogenesis of the cardiac failure is not known and it is not clear whether this is an epiphenomenon. Point mutations in the A or B subunits of the biotin-requiring propionyl-CoA carboxylase are associated with defects in the metabolism of valine, isoleucine, methionine, threonine, and fatty acids with odd numbered chain lengths. Infants present with hypotonia, lethargy, vomiting, and/or respiratory distress but not with signs or symptoms of cardiac failure. There is hyperketotic acidosis, hyperammonemia, and low total and free serum carnitine levels.

Class II Mutations: Mitochondrial DNA Point Mutations (Maternal Inheritance)

Mitochondrial encephalomyopathy, lactic acidosis, and stroke-like episodes (MELAS) are associated with a point mutation in the leucine transfer RNA in 85% of cases (18). The common presentation is between 3 and 11 years of age with headaches, seizures, vomiting and in 85% loss of consciousness associated with lactic acidosis. Weakness, renal insufficiency, and cardiomyopathy (hypertrophic or dilated) are progressive (histology: RRF). Familial involvement can occur, in fact since the presentation is quite variable, a child can present before the mother. Treatment is symptomatic and avoidance of the situations associated with the crises. The related disease, myoclonic epilepsy and RRF (MERRF), is associated with a mutation in the lysine transfer RNA, and rarely has a cardiac involvement that is milder than MELAS.

Oncocytic cardiomyopathy (infantile xanthomatous cardiomyopathy) is a rare disease of infancy with dysrhythmia, cardiac arrest, and hepatic steatosis and acute renal tubular necrosis. Histology of the affected organs shows foamy cytoplasm caused by the massive numbers of abnormal mitochondria. This disease may be caused by a defect in cytochrome *b*, a subunit of complex III that is encoded on mitochondrial DNA; however, only one patient has had extensive testing (19).

Mitochondrial cardiomyopathy, associated with cardiac failure, has been reported with more than 20 substitution mutations in transfer RNA (16). Mutations of transfer RNAs for leucine, isoleucine, and lysine seem to be more commonly associated with cardiac failure compared to those for glycine, alanine, and arginine. All have reduced OXPHOS activity and histologic findings of cardiac hypertrophy (histology: abnormal mitochondria and cristae). Cardiac failure, arrhythmias, pre-excitation, and AV node disease have been reported. Elevated lactate and heteroplasmy in organs are common.

Class III: Mitochondrial DNA Deletion

Kearns–Sayre syndrome and chronic progressive external ophthalmoplegia are usually caused by mitochondrial deletions (common 5 kb deletion) with sporadic inheritance; however, Mendelian inheritance rarely can occur. The deletion involves genes encoding subunits of complexes I, IV, and V. Significant heteroplasmy has been seen (20). The syndrome can be defined as a presentation, before age 20 years, of chronic progressive external ophthalmoplegia associated with retinitis pigmentosa, mitochondrial myopathy with RRF, cardiac conduction defect, cerebellar ataxia, and cerebral spinal fluid protein >100 mg/dl; however, the manifestations are variable and can include renal tubular acidosis and diabetes. The cardiac conduction defects are progressive and require close monitoring and early pacemaker placement. The cardiac failure is a late manifestation of the dilated and hypertrophied heart.

Pearson syndrome is also caused by mitochondrial DNA deletions. It is an infantile disease characterized by sideroblastic anemia, lactic acidosis, and reduced exocrine pancreatic function. Rare cases of worsening cardiac function have been reported (21); however, this is not a usual feature of the syndrome and may represent a different deletion or a case of cardiac failure unrelated to the metabolic disorder. Late survivors have been known to demonstrate the arrhythmias seen in Kearns–Sayre syndrome, so close clinical followup is indicated.

Smaller mitochondrial deletions associated with cardiomyopathy but not ophthalmoplegia have been found in patients with cardiomyopathy and myopathy, usually with OXPHOS activity defects and RRF (9). The prevalence of these deletions that cause cardiac failure is probably underestimated by current technology. It addition to deletions, newer data suggest that rearrangements of mitochondrial DNA also occur and can be associated with this clinical presentation.

Fatty Acid Oxidation Defects

Beta-oxidation of long-chain fatty acids is the primary pathway for cardiac ATP production. The short- and medium-chain fatty acids are able to pass directly through the outer and inner mitochondrial membranes without specific transport processes. However, the long-chain fatty acids undergo several membrane-bound transport steps requiring carnitine metabolism: (1) transport of carnitine into the cell by carnitine transporter; outer membrane conjugation to carnitine requiring carnitine palmitoyl transferase I (CPT I); (2) by carnitine–acyl-carnitine translocase mediated transport to the inner membrane of long-chain fatty acids acyl-carnitine in exchange for free carnitine; (3) cleavage of the carnitine from the long-chain fatty acid acyl-CoA mediated by carnitine palmitoyl transferase II (CPT II). Once within the mitochondrial matrix, fatty acid acyl-CoA chains undergo beta-oxidation by four enzymes that are moderately specific for the fatty acid chain length: very-long-chain, long-chain, medium-chain, and short-chain. First, a chain-length-specific dehydrogenase converts acyl-CoA to enoyl-CoA. The enoyl-CoA is catabolized by acyl-CoA hydrase, hydroxyacyl-CoA dehydrogenase, and acyl-CoA ketothiolase into acetyl-CoA and a fatty acid acyl-

CoA that is two carbons shorter. The latter three enzymes function separately for the shorter chain fatty acids, but a trifunctional protein complex metabolizes the long-chain fatty acids. The electrons generated from beta-oxidation are captured by ETF and ETF dehydrogenase.

Defects in many of these fatty acid oxidation enzymes have been associated with cardiac failure (22). The inheritance patterns are autosomal recessive. The age at presentation is predominantly determined by the effect on beta-oxidation by the residual enzyme activity, or by the effect of enzyme deficiency on "down stream" events. The presentations are similar with biochemical crises precipitated by fasting, cold stress, strenuous physical activity, or infections. In infancy, this often becomes evident when nighttime feeding is stopped. Cardiomyopathy, hepatomegaly, muscle weakness, coma and/or seizures with apnea, mimicking sudden death, and SIDS, are common presentations. Biochemical findings during crises include severe hypoketotic hypoglycemia with low serum insulin, and frequently hyperammonemia and elevated creatine phosphokinase. Plasma carnitine levels are lesion specific but frequently are low with high urine carnitine and dicarboxylic aciduria. The dicarboxylic acids are elevated because fatty acids that are not metabolized by the deficient enzyme will be metabolized down the omega oxidative pathway. Analysis of these dicarboxylic acids may localize the chain-length-specific defects. Plasma acylcarnitines often are elevated for similar reasons. Pathologic findings in muscle and myocardium show fat vacuolization, usually with normal mitochondria. Myocardial biopsy is not necessary as the defects are expressed in skeletal muscle and skin fibroblasts.

Carnitine Transport Defects: These Defects Affect the Oxidation Only of Long-Chain Fatty Acids

Carnitine transporter deficiency is the only primary defect in carnitine metabolism. Both myopathic and more generalized systemic forms are known. Presentation occurs either in infancy when it is rapidly lethal or later childhood with rapidly progressive cardiac failure. The defect is diagnosed with absent carnitine uptake in cultured fibroblasts, and the muscle biopsy shows abnormal mitochondria and fatty vacuolization. High dose oral carnitine can be life-sustaining treatment (23).

Translocase deficiency presents in infancy after a prolonged fast with hypoketotic hyopglycemic seizures and coma, frequently with characteristic ventricular arrhythmias, atrioventricular node block, and at times left bundle branch block. Rapid deterioration to death is the most common outcome; however, an infant treated with frequent high carbohydrate, low-fat meals, and carnitine, has been reported to be well at 2 years of age. This child and several others with mild phenotypes were shown to have enzyme activities in the range of 6% (24).

Carnitine palmitoyl transferase deficiencies result from an abnormality in either of the two forms of the enzyme. One enzyme is associated with the outer mitochondrial membrane (transferase I: CPT I) and one is associated with the inner membrane (transferase II: CPT II). Different genes encode these enzymes. CPT I deficiency has a presentation similar to Reye syndrome and has not been associated with cardiac failure or cardiomyopathy. Deficiency of CPT II leads to accumulation of arrhythmogenic long-chain acyl-carnitines. Severe reduction in CPT II enzyme activity and block of beta-oxidation of long-chain fatty acids results in the lethal infantile form affecting liver, muscle, and heart; less reduction of enzyme activity without a block in beta-oxidation manifests in a mild adult-onset muscular form with stress associated rhabdomyolysis and myoglobinuria (25).

Dehydrogenases: A Specific Enzyme Processes Each Chain Length Class of Fatty Acid

The presentation includes hepatocellular and cardiac failure (hypertrophic cardiomyopathy) and myopathy. Low total plasma carnitine, dicarboxylic aciduria, and marked fatty infiltration of most tissues are seen.

Very-long-chain acyl-CoA dehydrogenase deficiency (VLCAD) most often presents in infancy with severe hepatocellular disease and cardiac failure; however, milder enzyme deficiency manifests later in adolescence and adulthood with activity-related muscle pain, rhabdomyolysis, and myoglobinuria associated with the cardiac and hepatic failure. Renal failure can be the result of the myoglobinuria. This deficiency is differentiated from long-chain acyl-CoA dehydrogenase deficiency (LCAD), as the enzyme is associated with the inner mitochondrial membrane not the matrix. This is the only dehydrogenase deficiency that may respond to treatment: avoidance of fasting and treatment with low-fat diets supplemented with medium-chain triglycerides and carnitine (26).

Long-chain acyl-CoA dehydrogenase deficiency is a neonatal disease where the C8–C18 fatty acids cannot undergo beta-oxidation. Although specific diets reduce the frequency and severity of the biochemical crises, the cardio-respiratory failure is progressive and eventually lethal.

Medium-chain acyl-CoA dehydrogenase deficiency (MCAD) has been described with hypertrophic changes of the heart from accumulation of fatty acids, but the arrhythmias seen in the longer chain defects do not develop. Cardiac failure occurs only when total plasma carnitine levels are extremely low enough to decrease beta-oxidation. The more usual manifestation resembles Reye syndrome: hypoketotic hypoglycemia, hyperammonemia, and hepatic failure.

Short-chain acyl-CoA dehydrogenase deficiency (SCAD) presents predominantly with FTT, myopathy, and neurological symptoms rather than with cardiac failure. However, fatty acid accumulation in the myocardium does give the appearance of hypertrophy in some affected individuals.

Trifunctional protein deficiency (LCHAD) is caused by abnormalities in either the alpha or beta subunit. This protein is involved in the degradation of only long-chain fatty acids. The presentation includes cardiac failure associated with a hypertrophied and dilated heart, Reye syndrome-like symptoms, myopathy with high serum CK, and myoglobinuria during biochemical crises. Characteristically, there is 3-hydroxydicarboxylic aciduria. There is a loose correlation between genotype and phenotype: cardiac failure is present only in the most severe neonatal presentation and the severity of presentation seems to be related to the reduction in ketothiolase activity (27). Previous reports of a separate long-chain hydroxyacyl-CoA dehydrogenase deficiency, with a picture of severe cardiac failure, preceded the characterization of the trifunctional protein and most likely do not represent a separate disease. Neither cardiomyopathy nor cardiac failure has been associated with a deficiency of the separate proteins that perform these functions for medium- and short-chain fatty acids.

Mitochondrial Apoptosis

Mitochondrial DNA encodes for the antiapoptosis protein DCL-2, the mitochondrial permeability transition pore, and the spatially related, adenosine nucleotide translocator. DCL-2 prevents apoptosis by reducing the pore permeability. The pore opens and releases the proapoptosis enzyme cytochrome c during the stress of anoxia, ischemia, excess concentrations of reactive oxygen species, and plasma membrane binding of TNF-alpha (17). Clinically significant dilated cardiomyopathy has been associated with alteration of the mitochondrial permeability transition pore function by doxorubicin (28) and viral alteration of adenosine nucleotide translocator function (29).

A recent report links this mitochondrial role in apoptosis to cardiac failure (30). A mouse model that demonstrates an age-related increase in mitochondrial DNA point mutations was examined. The resulting dilated cardiomyopathy was associated with release of cytochrome c from the mitochondria, interstitial fibrosis, and apoptosis, without a change in mitochondrial structure or respiratory function. DCL-2 levels were consistently high. Although the authors did not make a conclusion as to how increased mitochondrial DNA point mutations caused the biochemical and physiologic changes in these mice, the fact that apoptosis is controlled by an interaction between DCL-2 and the mitochondrial permeability transition pore, both encoded by mitochondrial DNA, suggests that these mutations could affect the structure and function of this interaction.

Sengers syndrome may be a disease related to abnormalities of the mitochondrial permeability transition pore and the adenine nucleotide translocator, in that it is characterized by reduced adenine nucleotide translocator activity (31) and involvement of increased oxygen free radicals (32). It presents in an autosomal recessive inheritance pattern with congenital cataracts, muscular hypotonia from a mitochondrial myopathy, a hypertrophic cardiomyopathy, and stress related lactic acidosis. Premature death, often in infancy, is related to cardiac failure. The histology is one of abnormal mitochondria, and abnormal storage of lipid and normal glycogen.

Abnormalities Associated with Mitochondrial Structure or Location

When the biochemical results do not confirm a diagnosis compatible with a defect in mitochondrial energy production, several defects in the contractile protein complex have been characterized and are associated with cardiac failure (1). However, ultrastructurally abnormal mitochondria occur in a high percentage of myocardial biopsies even without known pathogenic mitochondrial DNA mutations (33). Decreased beta-oxidation has been reported in some of these cases suggesting that reduced mitochondrial energy production is also involved in the cardiac failure seen with structural gene mutations. Furthermore, these same structural proteins determine the intracellular location and movement of mitochondria. This has been confirmed to affect overall mitochondrial respiratory function in a desmin defect (34). These two factors, mitochondrial structure and location, may play a role in the phenotypic variability of known myocardial structural and myofilament defects, especially during periods of metabolic stress.

Other Unclassified Defects

Two additional diseases, associated with abnormal mitochondrial function and cardiomyopathy, cannot be easily classified: Friedreich ataxia and Barth syndrome. The first is associated with an abnormality of the mitochondrial iron transport protein, frataxin and the second is associated with an abnormality in the acyltransferase-like proteins, tafazzins, associated with phospholipid synthesis.

Friedreich Ataxia

Friedreich ataxia has autosomal recessive inheritance caused by homozygous GAA expansion in the FRDA gene. The size of the GAA expansion may be directly related to disease severity, including the significance of the concentric hypertrophic cardiomyopathy. Rarely, patients with familial ataxia have one of the several allelic variants without GAA expansions. FRDA encodes a mitochondrial protein that controls intramitochondrial iron. Several respiratory chain complexes with iron-sulfur containing subunits are damaged by the resulting iron overload (35).

Presentation occurs in the second decade with spinocerebellar degeneration and selective loss of large myelinated fibers in the dorsal root, cerebellum, and medulla. Hypoactive knee and ankle reflexes, progressive cerebellar dysfunction, and preadolescent onset are the hallmarks of the clinical diagnosis. In approximately 10% of patients with familial ataxia, retained reflexes, later onset, and less cardiac dysfunction have been found. Cardiac involvement is an important aspect of the disease (36). The EKG changes (repolarization abnormalities, ventricular hypertrophy, and various levels of conduction block) are present in 100% of patients with the GAA expansion, but less frequently in the rare patient without the genetic marker. Echocardiographic LVH has been reported in 22–75% of patients. Cardiac failure occurs late in life in over 70% of patients. There is no definitive treatment; however, because the mitochondrial defect is associated with reactive oxygen species, idebenone (a free radical scavenger) was evaluated in a small number of patients and may protect the heart from iron overload injury (37).

Barth Syndrome (38) (X-Linked Cardio-Skeletal
Myopathy with Neutropenia and Abnormal
Mitochondria or 3-Methylglutaconic Aciduria,
Type II)

Barth syndrome is inherited as an X-linked trait. The genetic defect is in the tafazzin gene (G4.5), mapped to Xq28 and highly expressed in both myocardium and muscle, which encodes an unusual protein class, tafazzins. Their intracellular role has not been defined but they may be a new family of acyltransferases involved in phospholipid synthesis. This could explain the low cardiolipin levels in affected individuals (39).

The disease manifests in neonates or infants with dilated cardiomyopathy, severe growth retardation, cyclical neutropenia, and persistently elevated urinary levels of 3-methylglutaconic acid. Low cardiolipin levels are frequently present. Abnormal mitochondria are found in granulocyte precursors, skeletal muscle, myocardium, liver, kidney, and fibroblasts. Left ventricular noncompaction occurs frequently. The cardiomyopathy may be severe to require transplantation, although in some individuals it stabilizes in adolescence. Furthermore, with the adolescent growth spurt, some individuals will reach their mid-parental height. Treatment with carnitine has been reported to worsen the cardiomyopathy.

STORAGE DISEASES ASSOCIATED WITH CARDIAC FAILURE

Mucopolysaccharidoses

The mucopolysaccharidoses make up the largest class of lysosomal storage diseases. Most are due to autosomal recessive inherited enzyme deficiencies, the exception being type II: Hunter disease which has X-linked recessive inheritance. There is deficient catabolism of one or more of the glycosaminoglycans (GAGs), heparan sulfate, dermatan sulfate, and keratan sulfate. The lysosomes become engorged with nondegraded GAGs that interfere with normal cell function. The phenotype depends on the specific enzyme deficiency, the severity of the deficiency, and the tissues where the enzyme is expressed. The specific defects are listed in Table 4 with the affected enzyme and the cardiovascular involvement. To more or lesser extent all affected individuals have short stature, characteristic coarse faces, dysostosis multiplex skeletal changes, and, except Hunter syndrome, corneal clouding. These abnormalities develop with age and therefore are not usually apparent in infancy, making early diagnosis difficult.

Table 4 Enzyme Deficiencies and Cardiac Phenotypes of the Mucopolysaccharidoses with Prominent Cardiovascular Presentations

Disease	Enzyme deficiency and inheritance pattern	Biochemical and clinical phenotype
Type I: Hurler; Hurler–Scheie; Scheie	Alpha-L-iduronidase deficiency: compound heterozygosity exists with a severe and a mild form	Accumulation of heparan and dermatan sulfates in tissues and urine Aortic and mitral regurgitation; aortic and coronary intima thickening to the point of severe stenosis causing hypertension, infarction and failure Hurler is the most severe; Scheie is the mildest without CNS involvement
Type II: Hunter	Iduronate sulfatase deficiency: a form with deletions and frame shift mutations is more severe than missense mutations	Accumulation of excess chondroitin sulfate B in tissues and urine No corneal clouding, otherwise phenotypically similar to Hurler
Type III: Sanfilippo—four subtypes	A: Heparan *N*-sulfatase B: Alpha *N*-acety glucosaminidase C: Acetyl-CoA: alpha glucosaminide acetyl transferase	Accumulation of heparan sulfate Mild cardiovascular involvement, e.g., mild mitra regurgitation

Type IV: Morquio—two subtypes	D: *N*-acetylglucosamine 6-sulfatase A: Galactosamine 6-sulfate sulfatase B: Beta-galactosidase	Accumulation of keratan sulfate Mainly skeleta involvement with normal facies and CNS Prominent coronary intima sclerosis and possible infarction
Type VI: Maroteaux–Lamy	Aryl-sulfatase B	Accumulation of dermatan sulfate Infant presentation: dilated cardiomyopathy and endocardiofibrosis Late presentation: mild valvar regurgitation
Type VII: Sly	Beta-glucuronidase	Accumulation of dermatan and Keratan sulfates Arterial intima hypertrophy and aortic valvar regurgitation

The progressive CNS deterioration is most severe in Hurler (type I), Hunter (type II), and Sanfilippo (type III) syndromes. In Morquio (type IV) and Maroteaux–Lamy (type VI) intelligence is preserved. Growth initially may be normal but growth velocity decreases after a few years in most affected children. Odontoid process hypoplasia is prevalent and can be clinically important. Respiratory system abnormalities including infections, sleep apnea, and severe tracheal hypoplasia are common causes of morbidity.

The most common cause of death in mucopolysaccharidoses is cardio-respiratory failure. The cardiac involvement is usually limited to the cardiac valves and chordal apparatus. Aortic and mitral regurgitation and mitral stenosis are common. As noted in Table 4, there are individuals with progressive intimal thickening that leads to stenosis of the coronary arteries and the aorta itself. Myocardial infarction and severe hypertension lead to life threatening cardiac failure. Although left ventricular hypertrophy is seen by echocardiography and histologically the myocardium has storage disease cells with hypertrophy and clear cytoplasm, primary systolic and/or diastolic dysfunction is limited to infants with type VI, Maroteaux–Lamy disease. On EKG, most of these diseases have short PR intervals, the etiology is still under debate.

Treatment of the mucopolysaccharidoses is imperfect. Bone marrow transplantation has been used in Hurler (40) and Hunter (41) syndromes. Transplantation in Hurler syndrome has slowed or halted the CNS deterioration in most patients, with the best outcomes in patients who were engrafted before the age of 24 months. Hepatosplenomegaly and airway narrowing improve but the bony involvement is not altered. For Hunter syndrome, nonsignificant improvement in the skeletal involvement, and continued regression of the CNS has been seen post-transplantation. Intravenous recombinant alpha-iduronidase enzyme replacement in a study of 10 patients with mild Hurler, Hurler–Sheie, and Sheie syndromes showed improvement in somatic involvement (42). Skeletal involvement was unchanged and, since the enzyme cannot pass the blood–brain barrier, neurologic benefits do not occur. Additional benefit may occur prebone marrow or stem-cell transplantation; its value after transplantation has not been tested.

Additional Lysosomal Storage Diseases with Cardiac Presentations

Few of the other lysosomal storage diseases have significant cardiac disease or the potential for cardiac failure. It can be assumed that the connective tissue of all organs, including the heart, will be affected in all of these diseases because of the importance of GAG in the extracellular matrix. There is a larger pool of GAG in cardiac valve tissue compared with the myocardium. Lysosomal diseases that do not develop more than a short PR interval, mild ventricular hypertrophy and/or mild aortic and mitral regurgitation are not included in this discussion. The remaining lysosomal storage diseases with cardiac presentations are presented in Table 5 .

The glycogen storage diseases that have significant cardiac disease include type II, type IIb, type III, type IV, and cardiac phosphorylase kinase b deficiency (Table 6). In all of these diseases, the cardiac abnormality is global ventricular hypertrophy from accumulation of glycogen or glycogen analogues. EKGs universally show biventricular hypertrophy with T-wave abnormalities. Typical phenotypes occur for each disease, but several patients have been reported with milder forms of each disease, and biochemical evidence for decreased but not absent, enzyme activity. The diagnosis can be made from white cell, fibroblast, or skeletal muscle assays in all except the cardiac phosphorylase kinase deficiency that requires cardiac biopsy for diagnosis.

No current treatment modality has successfully altered the progressive course of any of these diseases; however, there are results from a phase I/II clinical trial of enzyme replacement for type II in three infants (43). The cardiac hypertrophy and skeletal muscle disease seemed to progressively regress over the year-long study. A late onset adult form of type II has been treated with high protein diets, but no dietary changes alter the lethal infant form (44). Type IV classically

Table 5 Additional Lysosomal Storage Diseases with Cardiovascular Compromise

Disease	Enzyme deficiency and inheritance pattern	Biochemical and clinical phenotype
I-cell disease (mucolipidosis II)	N-acetyl-glucosamine-1-phosphotransferase Autosomal recessive No mannose-6-phosphate receptor, resulting in a lack of post-translational modification of acid hydrolases so that they are not incorporated into the lysosome but secreted into plasma Increased levels of acid hydrolases in plasma Lysosomal accumulation of GAG substrates of these enzymes	Hurler-like phenotype Neonatal CHF from LVH and aortic and mitral valve stenosis Arterial stenoses present A milder form exists as pseudo-Hurler polydystrophy with minimal cardiac involvement (ML III) Histologic: I-cells (fibroblasts with inclusions)
Sialidosis, type II	Neuraminidase Autosomal recessive Lysosomal accumulation of sialyl-hexasaccharide	Coarse faces, dysostosis multiplex, and cherry-red macular spots Infant presentation Neonatal hydrops fetalis Ventricular hypertrophy Varying severity of mitral regurgitation
Gaucher disease, type I (nonneuropathic form)	Acid beta-glucosidase Autosomal recessive Lysosomal accumulation of glucocerebroside	Painless splenomegaly, hypersplenism, bone lesions, growth retardation Restrictive cardiac disease due to Gaucher cell infiltration of the myocardium, or more likely, hemorrhagicand constrictive pericarditis and valvar disease (46)

Fabry disease	Alpha-galactosidase A X-linked affecting males and some females Accumulation of neutral glycosphingolipids Female heterozygotes tend to have a milder form A cardiac variant of Fabry (without coronary disease or ventricular hypertrophy) presents late, fourth decade, with total loss of the enzyme isolated to the heart and is diagnosed only by cardiac biopsy (47)	Liver transplantation has been shown to improve all aspects of the disease (45) Recombinant enzyme replacement has also been effective Presentation in first decade with acroparesthesias, angiokeratomata, corneal opacities, renal failure End stage congestive heart failure from asymmetric ventricular hypertrophy, ischemic disease from coronary narrowing and/or dilation from severe aortic or mitral regurgitation Recombinant enzyme replacement may be an effective treatment
Gangliosidoses G_{M1} type I	Type I G_{M1}: beta-galactosidase	Neurologic deterioration with developmental retardation, followed by paralysis, dementia and blindness before 3 years old
G_{M2}: Tay-Sachs and Sandhoff	G_{M2}: hexosaminidase (A in Tay-Sachs; A and B in Sandhoff) Autosomal recessive Lysosomal accumulation of gangliosides: "zebra bodies"	Cardiac involvement seen in cases with early infant presentations: LV dilation and failure with thickened aortic and mitral valves. Coronary occlusion with intimal lipid-laden fibroblasts may be the cause of the failure.

CHF, congestive heart failure; LVH, left ventricular hypertrophy; LV, left ventricle.

Table 6 Glycogen Storage Diseases with Cardiac Symptomatology

Disease	Enzyme deficiency and inheritance pattern	Biochemical and clinical phenotype
Type II: Pompe	Alpha-1,4-glucosidase Autosomal recessive Lysosomal and cytoplasmic deposits of normal glycogen	HCM, short PR interval, neonatal muscle weakness Large tongue, minimal liver enlargement except with CHF The cardio-respiratory failure is lethal Recombinant enzyme therapy trials are ongoing
Type IIB: Danon	Lysosome-associated membrane protein-2 X-linked recessive Normal alpha-1,4-glucosidase activity Intracytoplasmic vacuoles containing autophagic material and glycogen	HCM, myopathy, ± mental retardation Cardiomyopathy can predominate with late CHF, death or transplantation (48)
Type III: Cori or Forbes	Debrancher enzyme (amylo-1,6-glucosidase activity and oligo-1,4-1,4-glucanotransferase activity) Autosomal recessive Cytoplasmic deposits of limit dextrans	Childhood presentation with FTT, fasting hypoglycemia, HSM, seizures, HCM CHF is a late finding Type IIIa involves liver and muscle Type IIIb involves only liver
Type IV: Andersen	Glycogen branching enzyme (amylo(1,4 to 1,6) transglucosidase) Autosomal recessive Cytoplasmic deposits of amylopectin-like polysaccharides	Presents in the first 18 months of life with failure to thrive, HSM, and liver cirrhosis HCM, neurologic syndromes and myopathy can be observed Variability in presentation and age is common
Deficient cardiac phosphorylase kinase	Isoforms of phosphorylase kinase are different in muscle, liver, and heart Probably X-linked recessive Cytoplasmic deposits of granular glycogen	Neonatal hypoglycemia, FTT, HCM with early CHF Rapidly progressive CHF leads to early death

HCM, hypertrophic cardiomyopathy; CHF, congestive heart failure; FTT, failure to thrive; HSM, hepatosplenomegaly.

progresses to hepatic failure with worsening cardiac failure, but liver transplantation in a limited number of patients has been associated with regression of the cardiac hypertrophy, possibly on the basis of lymphocyte chimerism (45).

ACKNOWLEDGMENT

The assistance of Dr. Paige Kaplan is gratefully acknowledged.

REFERENCES

1. Fatkin D, Graham RM. Molecular mechanisms of inherited cardiomyopathies. Physiol Rev 2002; 82:945–980.
2. Franz WM, Muller OJ, Katus HA. Cardiomyopathies: from genetics to the prospect of treatment. Lancet 2001; 358:1627–1637.
3. Seidman JG, Seidman C. The genetic basis for cardiomyopathy: from mutation identification to mechanistic paradigms. Cell 2001; 104:557–567.
4. Towbin JA, Bowles NE. The failing heart. Nature 2002; 415:227–233.
5. Watkins H. Genetic clues to disease pathways in hypertrophic and dilated cardiomyopathies. Circulation 2003; 107:1344–1346.
6. Schwartz ML, Cox GF, Lin AE, Korson MS, Perez-Atayde A, Lacro RV, Lipshultz SE. Clinical approach to genetic cardiomyopathy in children. Circ 1996; 94:2021–2038.
7. McKusick-Nathans Institute for Genetic Medicine, Johns Hopkins University (Baltimore, MD) and National Center for Biotechnology Information, National Library of Medicine (Bethesda, MD), 2000. World Wide Web URL: http://www.ncbi.nlm.nih.gov/omim/.
8. Winter SC, Buist NRM. Cardiomyopathy in childhood, mitochondrial dysfunction, and the role of L-carnitine. Am Heart J 2000; 139: S63–S69.
9. Marvin-Garcia J, Goldenthal MJ. Mitochondrial Cardiomyopathy: molecular and biochemical analysis. Pediatr Cardiol 1997; 18: 251–260.
10. Rozwodowska M, Drewa G, Zbytniewski Z, Wozniak A, Krzyzynska-Malinowska E, Maciak R. Mitochondrial diseases. Med Sci Monit 2000; 6:817–822.
11. Graff C, Clayton DA, Larsson NG. Mitochondrial medicine—recent advances. J Int Med 1999; 246:11–23.
12. Frerman FE, Goodman SI. Defects of electron transfer flavoprotein and electron transfer flavoprotein-ubiquinone oxidoreductase: glutaric aciduria type II. In: Scriver CR, Beaudet AJ, Sly WS, Valle D, eds. The

Metabolic and Molecular Basis of Inherited Disease. NY: McGraw-Hill, 2001:2357–2365.

13. Moody PD. Glutaric aciduria type II: treatment with riboflavin, carnitine and insulin. Eur J Pediatr 1984; 143:92–95.

14. Shoffner JM, Wallace DC. Oxidative phosphorylation diseases: disorders of two genomes. Adv Hum Genet 1990; 19:267–275.

15. Shoffner JM, Wallace DC. Oxidative phosphorylation diseases. In: Scriver CR, Beaudet AL, Sly WS, Valle D, eds. The Metabolic and Molecular Basis of Inherited Disease. NY: McGraw-Hill, 1995: 1535–1609.

16. Marvin-Garcia J, Goldenthal MJ. Understanding the impact of mitochondrial defects in cardiovascular disease: a review. J Card Fail 2002; 8:347–361.

17. Massoud AF, Leonard JV. Cardiomyopathy in propionic acidemia. Eur J Pediatr 1993; 152:441–445.

18. Goto Y, Nonaka I, Horai S. A mutation in the tRNA (Leu[UUR]) gene associated with the MELAS subgroup of mitochondrial encephalomyopathies. Nature 1990; 348:651–653.

19. Andreu AL, Checcarelli N, Iwata S, Shanske S, DiMauro S. A missense mutation in the mitochondrial cytochrome b gene in a revisited case with histiocytoid cardiomyopathy. Pediat Res 2000; 48:311–314.

20. Moraes CT, DiMauro S, Zeviani M, Lombes A, Shanske S, Miranda AF, Nakase H, Bonilla E, Werneck LC, Servidei S, Nonaka I, Koga Y, Spiro AJ, Brownell AKW, Schmidt B, Schotland DL, Zupanc M, DeVivo DC, Schon EA, Rowland LP. Mitochondrial DNA deletions in progressive external ophthalmoplegia and Kearns-Sayre syndrome. N Engl J Med 1989; 320:1293–1299.

21. Krauch G, Wilichowski E, Schmidt KG, Mayatepek E. Pearson marrow-pancreas syndrome with worsening cardiac function caused by pleiotropic rearrangement of mitochondrial DNA. Am J Med Genet 2002; 110:57–61.

22. Kelly DP, Strauss AW. Mechanisms of disease. N Engl J Med 1994; 330:913–919.

23. Lamhonwah A-M, Olpin SE, Pollitt RJ, Vianey-Saban C, Divry P, Guffon N, Besley GTN, Onizuka R, De Meirleir LJ, Cvitanovic-Sojat L, Baric I, Dionisi-Vici C, Fumic K, Maradin M, Tein I. Novel OCTN2 mutations: no genotype-phenotype correlations: early carnitine therapy prevents cardiomyopathy. Am J Med Genet 2002; 111:271–284.

24. Olpin SE, Bonham JR, Downing M, Manning NJ, Pollitt RJ, Sharrard MJ, Tanner NS. Carnitine-acyl carnitine translocase deficiency—a mild phenotype. J Inherit Metab Dis 1997; 20:714–715.

25. Bonnefont J-P, Taroni F, Cavadini P, Cepanec C, Brivet M, Saudubray J-M, Leroux J-P, Demaugre F. Molecular analysis of carnitine palmitoyl transferase II deficiency with hepatocardiomuscular expression. Am J Hum Genet 1996; 58:971–978.

26. Cox KB, Souri M, Aoyama T, Rockenmacher S, Varogli L, Rohr F, Hashimoto T, Korson MS. Reversal of severe hypertrophic cardiomyopathy and excellent neurophysiologic outcome in very-long-chain acylcoenzyme A dehydroge nase deficiency. J Pediat 1998; 133:247–253.

27. Spiekerkoetter U, Sun B, Khuchua Z, Bennett BJ, Strauss AW. Molecular and phenotypic heterogeneity in mitochondrial trifunctional protein deficiency due to beta-subunit mutations. Hum Mutat 2003; 21:598–607.

28. Wang GW, Klein JB, Kang YJ. Metallothionein inhibits doxorubicininduced mitochondrial cytochrome c release and caspase-3 activation in cardiomyocytes. J Pharmacol Exp Ther 2001; 298:461–468.

29. Schulze K, Schultheiss HP. The role of the ADP/ATP carrier in the pathogenesis of viral heart disease. Eur Heart J 1995; 16(suppl O):64–67.

30. Zhang D, Mott JL, Farrar P, Ryerse JS, Change S-W, Stevens M, Denniger G, Zassenhaus HP. Mitochondrial DNA mutations activate the mitochondrial apoptotic pathway and cause dilated cardiomyopathy. Cardiovasc Res 2003; 57:147–157.

31. Jordens EZ, Palmieri L, Huizing M, van den Heuvel LP, Sengers RCA, Dorner A, Ruitenbeek W, Trijbels FJ, Valsson J, Sigfusson G, Palmieri F, Smeitink JAM. Adenine nucleotide translocator 1 deficiency associated with Senger's syndrome. Ann Neurol 2002; 52:95–99.

32. Luo X, Pitkanen S, Kassovska-Bratinova S, Robinson BH, Lehotay DC. Excessive formation of hydroxyl radicals and aldehydic lipid peroxidation products in cultured skin fibroblasts from patients with complex I deficiency. J Clin Invest 1997; 99:2877–2882.

33. Turner LF, Kaddoura S, Harrington D, Cooper JM, Poole-Wilson PA, Schapira AH. Mitochondrial DNA in idiopathic cardiomyopathy. Eur Heart J 1998; 19:1725–1729.

34. Milner DJ, Mavroidis M, Weisleder N, Capetanaki Y. Desmin cytoskeleton linked to muscle mitochondrial distribution and respiratory function. J Cell Biol 2000; 150:1283–1298.

35. Rotig A, de Lonlay P, Chretien D, Foury F, Koenig M, Sidi D, Munnich A, Rustin P. Aconitase and mitochondrial iron-sulfur protein deficiency in Friedreich ataxia. Nat Genet 1997; 17:215–217.

36. Albano LMJ, Nishioka SAD, Moyses RL, Wagenfuhr J, Bertola D, Sugayama SMM, Kim CA. Friedreich's ataxia. Cardiac evaluation of 25 patients with clinical diagnosis and literature review. Arg Bras Cardiol 2002; 78:444–451.

37. Rustin P, von Kleist-Retzow J-C, Chantrel-Groussard K, Sidi D, Munnich A, Rotig A. Effect of idebenone on cardiomyopathy in Friedreich's ataxia: a preliminary study. Lancet 1999; 354:477–479.

38. Barth PG, Scholte HR, Berden JA, Van der Klei-Van Moorsel JM, Luyt-Houwen IE, Van't Veer-Korthof ET, Van der Harten JJ, Sobotka-Plojhar MA. An X-linked mitochondrial disease affecting

cardiac muscle, skeletal muscle and neutrophil leucocytes. J Neurol
Sci 1983; 62:327–355.

39. Neuwald AF. Barth syndrome may be due to an acyltransferase
deficiency. Curr Biol 1997; 7:R465-R466.

40. Peters C, Shapiro EG, Anderson J, Henslee-Downey J, Klemperer MR,
Cowan MJ, Saunders EF, deAlarcon PA, Twist C, Nachman JB, Hale
GA, Harris RE, Rozans MK, Kurtzberg J, Grayson GH, Williams TE,
Lenarsky C, Wagner JE, Krivit W. Hurler syndrome. II. Outcome of
HLA-genotypically identical sibling and HLA-haploidentical related
donor bone marrow transplantation in fifty-four children. Blood
1998; 91:2601–2608.

41. Vellodi A, Young E, Cooper A, Lidchi V, Winchester B, Wraith JE.
Long-term follow-up following bone marrow transplantation for
Hunter disease. J Inherit Metab Dis 1999; 22:638–648.

42. Kakkis ED, Muenzer J, Tiller GE, Waber L, Belmont J, Passage M,
Izykowski B, Phillips J, Doroshow R, Walot I, Hoft R, Neufeld EF.
Enzyme-replacement therapy in mucopolysaccharidosis I. N Engl J
Med 2001; 344:182–188.

43. Amalfitano A, Bengur AR, Morse RP, Majure JM, Case LE, Veerling
DL, Mackey J, Kishnani P, Smith W, McVie-Wylie A, Sullivan JA,
Hoganson GE, Phillips JA III, Schaefer GB, Charrow J, Ware RE,
Bossen EH, Chen Y-T. Recombinant human acid alpha-glucosidase
enzyme therapy for infantile glycogen storage disease type II: results
of a phase I/II clinical trial. Genet Med 2001; 3:132–138.

44. Margolis ML, Hill AR. Acid maltase deficiency in an adult: evidence
for improvement in respiratory function with high-protein dietary
therapy. Am Rev Respir Dis 1986; 134:328–331.

45. Starzl TE, Demetris AJ, Trucco M, Ricordi C, Ildstad S, Terasaki PI,
Murase N, Kendall RS, Kocova M, Rudert WA, Zeevi A, Van Thiel
D. Chimerism after liver transplantation for type IV glycogen storage
disease and type 1 Gaucher's disease. N Engl J Med 1993; 328:
745–749.

46. Chabas A, Cormand B, Grinberg D, Burguera JM, Balcells S, Merino
JL, Mate I, Sobrino JA, Gonzalez-Duarte R, Vilageliu L. Unusual
expression of Gaucher's disease: cardiovascular calcifications in three
sibs homozygous for the D409H mutation. J Med Genet 1995; 32:
740–742.

47. Ogawa K, Sugamata K, Funamoto N, Abe T, Sato T, Nagashima K,
Ohkawa S. Restricted accumulation of globotriaosylceramide in the
hearts of atypical cases of Fabry's disease. Hum Path 1990;
21:1067–1073.

48. Dworzak F, Casazza F, Mora CM, De Maria R, Gronda E, Baroldi G,
Rimoldi M, Morandi L, Cornelio F. Lysosomal glycogen storage with
normal acid maltase: a familial study with successful heart transplant.
Neuromuscul Disord 1994; 4:243–247.

9

Cardiomyopathy and Myocarditis

**J.A. TOWBIN, MATTEO VATTA, and
N.E. BOWLES**
Department of Pediatrics (Cardiology),
Baylor College of Medicine,
Houston, Texas, U.S.A.

OVERVIEW

Cardiomyopathies in children are major causes of morbidity and mortality and over the past 20 years, limited improvements in outcome have been reported. However, on the basis of improvements in the understanding of several of the major forms of cardiomyopathy in adults, as well as the treatment of these disorders, a variety of concepts have been tested (or are currently being tested) in childhood forms of these disorders. In addition, various forms of cardiomyopathy commonly present early in childhood, and these disorders are being described in detail by pediatric cardiologists.

The major classifications of the forms of cardiomyopathies include: (1) dilated cardiomyopathy, which includes approximately 55% of all cardiomyopathies, (2) hypertrophic cardiomyopathy, which accounts for approximately 35% of all cardiomyopathies (3) restrictive cardiomyopathy, an uncommon form accounting for < 5% of cases, and (4) arrhythmogenic right ventricular cardiomyopathy an uncommon form of disease as well, particularly during childhood. An unclassified form of cardiomyopathy, left ventricular noncompaction, is considered to be quite rare but recent evidence suggests that this disorder is actually relatively common but only rarely diagnosed.

These classified and unclassified disorders are generally considered diseases primarily affecting systolic function (dilated cardiomyopathy affecting the left ventricle, arrhythmogenic right ventricular cardiomyopathy affecting the right ventricle), diastolic function (hypertrophic cardiomyopathy and restrictive cardiomyopathy), or both (left ventricular noncompaction). Based on these functional considerations, therapies have been devised which focus on affecting systole or diastole directly or indirectly.

Over the past decade, advances in molecular genetics and mouse modeling efforts have occurred and have resulted in modifications of our understanding of these disorders as well as the therapies designed to treat these disorders. In this chapter, the clinical description, therapies, molecular basis, and functional abnormalities of these disorders will be discussed. The goal of this chapter is to acquaint the reader with these disorders and a variety of new considerations regarding form and function of the heart and the potential new diagnostic and therapeutic horizons of the future for these potentially devastating diseases.

INTRODUCTION

The cardiomyopathies are heart muscle disorders associated with significant morbidity and mortality. These disorders are classified by the World Health Organization (WHO) into four forms (1): (1) dilated cardiomyopathy (DCM), (2) hypertrophic cardiomyopathy (HCM), (3) restrictive cardiomyopathy (RCM), and (4) arrhythmogenic right ventricular cardiomyopathy (ARVC). Recently, another cardiomyopathy, left ventricular noncompaction (LVNC), has gained attention although it does not meet criteria for a separate classification currently.

The most common cardiomyopathy is DCM, accounting for approximately 55% of cases (1). Hypertrophic cardiomyopathy is second most common, approximately 35%, with the remaining forms accounting for approximately 5% or less in each case (1). The importance of these disorders lies in the fact that they are responsible for a high proportion of cases of congestive heart failure and sudden death, as well as the need for transplantation. The mortality rate in the United States due to cardiomyopathy is greater than 10,000 deaths per annum, with DCM being the major contributor to this death rate (2). The total cost of health care in the United States focused on cardiomyopathies is in the billions of dollars and only limited success has been achieved (3). In order to achieve improved care and outcomes in children and adults, understanding of the causes of these disorders has been sought in earnest over the past decade.

Physiologically, HCM and RCM are primarily diastolic disorders, while DCM and ARVC are primarily systolic disorders (1). Left ventricular noncompaction is a combination overlap disorder with evidence of both systolic and diastolic dysfunction (4). The molecular basis of HCM has been well studied since the early 1990s and to date, 11 genes have been identified as disease. Interestingly, nearly all of these genes encode proteins comprising the sarcomere including β-myosin heavy chain, α-tropomyosin, cardiac troponin T, cardiac troponin I, myosin binding protein-C, myosin essential light chain, myosin regulatory light chain, actin, muscle LIM protein, and titin (5). Hence, the disease is now considered a disease of the sarcomere (6). One recently identified gene appears to question whether the sarcomere is the only region of the heart causing HCM when altered. This gene, called AMP-kinase (AMPK), is important in metabolic regulation, participating in energy utilization and appears to be similar to a glycogen storage disease (7).

Dilated cardiomyopathy has become a popular target of research over the past 7–8 years, with multiple genes identified during that time period. These genes appear to encode two major subgroups of proteins, cytoskeletal, and sarcomeric proteins (6). The cytoskeletal proteins identified to date include dystrophin, desmin, lamin A/C, δ-sarcoglycan, metavinculin, muscle LIM protein, and α-actinin. In the case of sarcomere-encoding genes, the same genes identified for HCM appear to be culprits in select patients. A new gene, cypher/ZASP, a Z-line protein, has been identified recently as well (8). In addition, two genes with uncertain mechanisms (including phospholamban and G4.5/Tafazzin) are also reported. Another form of DCM, the acquired disorder viral myocarditis, has the same clinical features as DCM including heart failure, arrhythmias, and conduction block (9). The most common causes of myocarditis are viral, including the enteroviruses (coxsackie viruses and echovirus), adenoviruses, and parvovirus B19, amongst other cardiotropic viruses (10). Evidence currently exists that suggests that viral myocarditis and DCM (genetic) have similar mechanisms of disease based on the proteins targeted.

Restrictive cardiomyopathy, ARVC, and LVNC are the "new kids on the block" scientifically but progress is being made in unraveling the underlying mechanisms of these disorders. Once the cardiomyopathies are understood at the molecular and cellular level, targeted therapies can be developed in addition to current strategies, with the hope for improved outcomes. In this chapter, we will review the clinical and scientific characteristics of these disorders and describe potential novel therapeutic approaches for future consideration.

In order to understand the mechanisms responsible for the development of the clinical phenotype, an understanding of normal cardiac structure is necessary.

NORMAL CARDIAC STRUCTURE

Cardiac muscle fibers are comprised of separate cellular units (myocytes) connected in series (11). In contrast to skeletal muscle fibers, cardiac fibers do not assemble in parallel arrays but bifurcate and recombine to form a complex three-dimensional network. Cardiac myocytes are joined at each end to adjacent myocytes at the intercalated disc, the specialized area of interdigitating cell membrane (Fig. 1). The intercalated disc contains gap junctions (containing connexins), and mechanical junctions, comprised of adherens junctions (containing N-cadherin, catenins, and vinculin) and desmosomes (containing desmin, desmoplakin, desmocollin, desmoglein). Cardiac myocytes are surrounded by a thin membrane

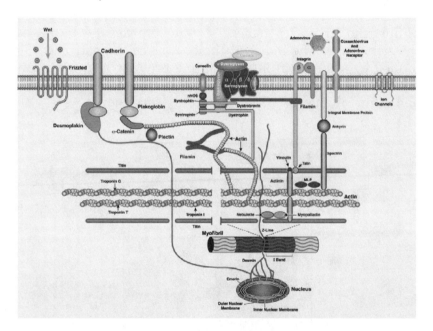

Figure 1 Cardiac myocyte cytoarchitecture. Schematic of the interactions between dystrophin and the dystrophin-associated proteins in the sarcolemma and intracellular cytoplasm (dystroglycans, sarcoglycans, syntrophins, dystrobrevin, sarcospan) at the C-terminal end of the dystrophin. The integral membrane proteins interact with the extracellular matrix via α-dystroglycan-laminin $\alpha2$ connections. The N-terminus of dystrophin binds actin and connects dystrophin with the sarcomere intracellularly, the sarcolemma and extracellular matrix. N = amino terminus; C = carboxy terminus; MLP = muscle LIM protein.

(sarcolemma) and the interior of each myocyte contains bundles of longitudinally arranged myofibrils. The myofibrils are formed by repeating sarcomeres, the basic contractile units of cardiac muscle comprised of interdigitating thin (actin) and thick (myosin) filaments (Fig. 1) that give the muscle its characteristic striated appearance (12,13). The thick filaments are composed primarily of myosin but additionally contain myosin binding proteins C, H, and X. The thin filaments are composed of cardiac actin, α-tropomyosin (α-TM), and troponins T, I, and C (cTnT, cTnI, cTnC). In addition, myofibrils contain a third filament formed by the giant filamentous protein, titin, which extends from the Z-disc to the M-line and acts as a molecular template for the layout of the sarcomere. The Z-disc at the borders of the sarcomere is formed by a lattice of interdigitating proteins that maintain myofilament organization by cross-linking antiparallel titin and thin filaments from adjacent sarcomeres (Fig. 2).

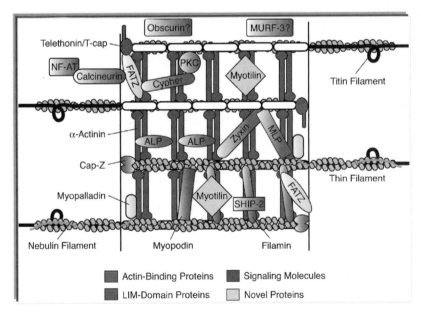

Figure 2 Z-disc architecture. The Z-disc of the sarcomere is comprised of multiple interacting proteins that anchor the sarcomere. (Reported with permission from Ref. 13)

Other proteins in the Z-disc include α-actinin, nebulette, telethonin/T-cap, capZ, MLP, myopalladin, myotilin, Cypher/ZASP, filamin, and FATZ (12–15).

Finally, the extrasarcomeric cytoskeleton, a complex network of proteins linking the sarcomere with the sarcolemma and the extracellular matrix (ECM), provides structural support for subcellular structures and transmits mechanical and chemical signals within and between cells. The extrasarcomeric cytoskeleton has intermyofibrillar and subsarcolemmal components, with the intermyofibrillar cytoskeleton composed of intermediate filaments (IFs), microfilaments, and microtubules (14–19). Desmin IFs form a three-dimensional scaffold throughout the extra-sarcomeric cytoskeleton with desmin filaments surrounding the Z-disc, allowing for longitudinal connections to adjacent Z-discs and lateral connections to subsarcolemmal costameres (18,19). Microfilaments composed of nonsarcomeric actin (mainly γ-actin) also form complex networks linking the sarcomere (via α-actinin) to various components of the costameres. Costameres are subsarcolemmal domains located in a periodic, grid-like pattern, flanking the Z-discs and overlying the I bands, along the cytoplasmic side of the sarcolemma. These costameres are sites of interconnection between various cytoskeletal networks linking sarcomere and sarcolemma and are thought to function as anchor sites for stabilization of the sarcolemma and for integration of pathways involved in mechanical force transduction. Costameres contain three principal components: the focal adhesion-type complex, the spectrin-based complex, and the dystrophin/dystrophin-associated protein complex (DAPC) (20,21). The focal adhesion-type complex, comprised of cytoplasmic proteins (i.e., vinculin, talin, tensin, paxillin, zyxin), connect with cytoskeletal actin filaments and with the transmembrane proteins α-, β-dystroglycan, α-, β-, γ-, δ-sarcoglycans, dystrobrevin, and syntrophin (16,17). Several actin-associated proteins are located at sites of attachment of cytoskeletal actin filaments with costameric complexes, including α-actinin and the muscle LIM protein, MLP. The C-terminus of dystrophin binds β-dystroglycan (Fig. 1), which in turn interacts with α-dystroglycan to link to the ECM (via α-2-laminin). The

N-terminus of dystrophin interacts with actin. Also notable, voltage gated sodium channels colocalize with dystrophin, β-spectrin, ankyrin, and syntrophins, while potassium channels interact with the sarcomeric Z-disc and intercalated discs (22–24). Since arrhythmias and conduction system diseases are common in children and adults with DCM, this could play an important role. Hence, disruption of the links from the sarcolemma to ECM at the dystrophin C-terminus and those to the sarcomere and nucleus via N-terminal dystrophin interactions could lead to a "domino effect" disruption of systolic function and development of arrhythmias.

Z-DISC ORGANIZATION

The precise organization of Z-discs, the borders of individual sarcomeres in vertebrate striated muscle, defines a supramolecular assembly of eukaryotic cell structure (Fig. 2). Z-discs contain the barbed ends of actin thin filaments, the N-terminal ends of titin filaments, the C-terminal ends of nebulette/nebulin in cardiac and skeletal muscle, respectively, as well as a variety of other regulatory and structural proteins. In addition to being a boundary between successive sarcomeres, Z-discs are responsible for transmitting tension generated by individual sarcomeres along the length of the myofibril, allowing for efficient contractile activity (i.e., the primary conduits of the force generated by contraction) (12–15). Z-disc associated proteins also appear to be crucial for early stages of myofibril assembly since I-Z-I structures (i.e., Z-disc precursors) form the earliest identifiable protein assemblies observed during muscle differentiation (12,25–27). Detailed ultrastructural and biochemical investigations of the Z-disc and its various components have yielded valuable information concerning its structural architecture. The width of the Z-disc can vary from $\sim$30 nm in fish skeletal muscle to $>1\,\mu$m in patients with Nemaline myopathy (15,28,29). The thin filaments from adjacent sarcomeres fully overlap within the Z-disc and are cross-linked by the direct interaction of actin filaments and the actin filament barbed end-capping protein,

CapZ, with α-actinin (30,31). Titin filaments from adjacent sarcomeres also fully overlap in the Z-lines and are cross-linked by α-actinin (14). In vitro studies have identified two distinct α-actinin-binding sites within titin's N-terminal, 80 kD, Z-disc integral segment. These binding sites may link together titin and α-actinin filaments both inside the Z-disc and its periphery (32–37). A direct interaction between the Z-disc peripheral region of nebulin /nebulette and the intermediate filament protein desmin has been identified and it is believed that this link contributes to the lateral connections between adjacent Z-discs (38). Another protein, myopalladin interacts with nebulette and α-actinin, as well as with tinin and the thin filaments, forming intra-Z-disc meshworks. Myopalladin complex and α-actinin appear to form a linking system, tethering the barbed ends of actin–titin filaments, the N-terminal ends of titin filaments, and the C-terminal ends of nebulin/nebulette within the Z-disc and provide the anchor to stabilize these structures against stress and other forces.

Another important interaction within the Z-disc occurs between titin and telethonin (T-cap), an interaction critical for sarcomeric function (32). Telethonin has recently been shown to interact with α-actinin as well as muscle LIM protein (MLP), another Z-disc protein (39). This complex (T-cap/MLP/α-actinin/titin) appears to stabilize Z-disc function via mechanical stretch sensing. Loss of the MLP/T-cap/titin-dependent mechanical stress sensor pathway (due to MLP mutations) is thought to result in destabilization of the anchoring of the Z-disc to the proximal end of the T-cap/titin titin complex, which leads to conformational alteration of the intrinsic titin molecular spring elements (9). In turn, this loss of elasticity results in the primary defect in the endogenous cardiac muscle stretch sensor machinery. The over-stretching of individual myocytes leads to activation of cell death pathways, at a time when stretch-regulated survival cues are diminished due to defective stretch sensing, leading to myocyte cell death and progression of heart failure (40).

Disruption of cardiac cytoarchitecture by genetic mutations or acquired abnormalities leads to clinical cardiomyopathic disorders. These disorders will be discussed.

DISORDERS OF VENTRICULAR SYSTOLIC DYSFUNCTION

Dilated Cardiomyopathy

Clinical Aspects

Congestive heart failure (CHF) due to myocardial dysfunction is a serious malady which is a major cause of morbidity and mortality in children and adults (41). In these conditions, ventricular arrhythmias commonly occur and, in many instances, result in sudden death. These disorders are the most common diseases leading to cardiac transplantation, with an associated cost of billions of dollars annually in the United States (3). Dilated cardiomyopathy is the most common cause of CHF (41,42) and although the overall incidence varies, it is believed that DCM occurs in at least 40 per 100,000 population (43–45). The prevalence and incidence of DCM appear to be increasing (45). Depending on the diagnostic criteria used, the annual incidence varies between 5 and 8 cases per 100,000 population (42,44–48); the true incidence is probably underestimated by these figures, since many asymptomatic cases go unrecognized. Nearly five million Americans have heart failure currently with an increasing incidence with age (41). Individuals older than 65 years, the incidence approaches 10 per 1000 population, and accounts for more than 20% of all hospital admissions in this age group (41). In the pediatric population, newborns and infants have the highest rates of disease, with an annual incidence of 4.58 per 100,000 children (range 5.98–10.72 per 100,000) (42,49,50). Symptomatic heart failure at all ages continues to confer a poor prognosis with one year mortality rates still reported to be 45% (41,44).

Clinical Features

Idiopathic DCM (IDCM) is characterized by increased ventricular size (i.e., left ventricular or biventricular dilation) and reduced ventricular contractility (Fig. 3) in the absence of coronary artery disease, valvular abnormalities, or pericardial disease (1). Mitral regurgitation is common, as is ventricular

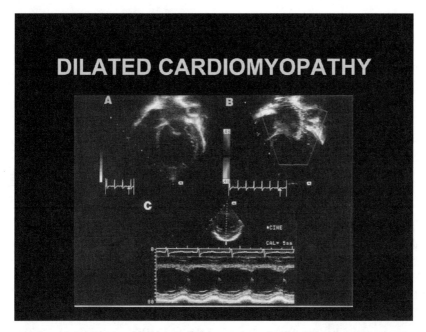

Figure 3   Echocardiography in dilated cardiomyopathy: (A) apical four chamber view demonstrating dilated left ventricle; (B) similar view showing mitral regurgitation; (C) M-mode showing poor systolic function.

arrhythmias, particularly ventricular tachycardia (VT), *torsade de pointes* (TdP), and ventricular fibrillation (VF). Clinical features include the signs and symptoms of CHF, which include breathlessness, fatigue, orthopnea, diaphoresis, chest pain, palpitations, exercise intolerance, and syncope (51). On physical exam, tachypnea, tachycardia, diaphoresis, an S3 or summation of S3 and S4 gallop, and hepatomagly are common with or without peripheral edema or ascites. Supportive data include radiographic evidence of cardiomegaly (with or without pulmonary edema), and reduced cardiac contractility with (or without) ventricular dilation on echocardiography (41,45). In adults, it is more frequently seen in men (2.5:1) and in African-Americans (2.5:1), but the causes of these differences are not well understood (6). In childhood, this appears to be different, with the male-to-female ratio being

60% males, 40% females (42). The clinical course of DCM, almost regardless of etiology, may be progressive, with approximately 50% of individuals reported to die within five years of diagnosis without transplantation (41). The cause of death is evenly divided between sudden death and pump failure. Longer survival has been accomplished more recently with improved medical therapies (i.e., ACE inhibitors, β-blockers) and interventions (i.e., implantable defibrillators, ventricular assist devices).

Clinical Evaluation

The usual evaluation includes chest radiography, electrocardiography, echocardiography, and Holter monitoring. Exercise testing and cardiac catheterization, with or without endomyocardial biopsy, may also be performed. Blood and urine testing, particularly in young children, is mandatory in order to define an underlying etiology.

Chest radiography: Chest x-rays typically identify cardiomegaly and pulmonary edema with increased pulmonary vascular markings and Kerley B lines. In patients with a dilated left atrium, tracheal narrowing and atelectasis may occur. In some cases, pleural effusions are notable.

Electrocardiography: Sinus tachycardia is most common. In patients with a dilated left atrium, left atrial enlargement may occur. Ventricular arrhythmias and, on occasion, preexcitation may be identified, as well as bundle-branch block or atrioventricular block.

Echocardiography: Classic features include a dilated left ventricle with poor ventricular function. Doppler and color Doppler interrogation may demonstrate atrioventricular valve regurgitation (particularly mitral regurgitation, Fig. 3). A pericardial effusion may also be seen along with atrial dilation.

Holter monitoring: The purpose of 24 hr electrocardiographic monitoring is to identify episodes of ventricular arrhythmias or bradycardia/atrioventricular block.

Cardiac catheterization: This is not typically used as a diagnostic modality except to obtain endomyocardial biopsies to evaluate for possible myocarditis or, rarely, for mitochondrial abnormalities. Hemodynamic evaluation may identify elevated left ventricular end diastolic pressure and pulmonary wedge pressures; in some cases, pulmonary vascular resistance may be elevated substantially. If endomyocardial biopsies are obtained, polymerase chain reaction analysis for viral genome should be considered.

Metabolic studies: In children, the underlying etiology of DCM may include mitochondrial or metabolic derangement. For this reason, urine analysis for lactate, amino acids, and organic acid elevations may be useful and in some cases, such as Barth syndrome, may help to narrow the differential diagnosis. In Barth syndrome, for instance, elevated 3-methylglutaconic acid in a male with neutropenia would be diagnostic. Blood studies, including complete blood count, acylcarnitine profile (for fatty acid oxidation defects), pyruvate dehydrogenase complex, electrolyte profile, creatine kinase (with isoform analysis if elevated), plasma amino acids, and blood for genetic testing are all reasonable to obtain. Elevation of creatine kinase muscle isoform (CK-MM) is useful to identify associated skeletal myopathy and may lead to identification of dystrophin (or other) mutations. Viral serologies may or may not be helpful. In some patients, particularly young children, skeletal muscle biopsy for microscopy, electron microscopy, and electron transport chain biochemistry can be useful and, if abnormal, should suggest the need for blood studies to evaluate for mitochondrial DNA mutations.

ARRHYTHMIAS AND CONDUCTION SYSTEM DISEASE IN DILATED CARDIOMYOPATHY

The rate of sudden cardiac death in individuals with heart failure has been reported by Stevenson and Stevenson (52) to be six to nine times that seen in the general population. The basis of this sudden demise is thought to occur due to ventricular tachyarrhythmias or severe bradyarrhythmias in children. The cause of these rhythm disturbances is currently unknown but it has been speculated that myocardial

irritability due to remodeling and fibrosis is a common incit-
ing event. In addition, the myocardial conduction system is
likely to be vulnerable to the same pathologic processes affecting the myocytes and interstitial elements, resulting in
altered conduction. Furthermore, patients with dilated cardiomyopathy develop atrial stretching resulting from elevated
end-diastolic ventricular pressure due to poor systolic function and from mitral regurgitation, with electrical instability
ensuing. In adults, this leads to atrial fibrillation (53), a decidedly uncommon event in children. However, abnormal myocardial conduction may also lead to ventricular conduction
delays and bundle-branch block, leading in some patients to
worsening mechanical coupling, ventricular activation and
contraction, ventricular dyssynchony, abnormal diastolic
function and significant hemodynamic consequences which
could trigger ventricular arrhythmias (54). These arrhythmias increase the risk of sudden death dramatically and
currently are treated with internal defibrillators (ICDs)
and/or antiarrhythmic drugs. In adults, left bundle-branch
block is a significant predictor of sudden death and a common
finding in adults with heart failure (55); however, this does
not appear to be the case in children.

HEART FAILURE WITH PRESERVED SYSTOLIC
FUNCTION

The usual teaching regarding heart failure specifies the need
for either systolic dysfunction (pump failure) or volume overload. However, another form of heart failure has become
increasingly common in adults (20–50% of heart failure
patients) and is beginning to crop up in a small number of
children with heart failure. In this patient cohort, the usual
systolic function indices (shortening fraction, ejection fraction) is preserved. Despite these patients having normal contractility, diastole (relaxation) is impaired and cardiac output
is therefore limited by the abnormal filling characteristics of
the ventricles, particularly during exercise. For a given ventricular volume, ventricular pressures are elevated, leading

to pulmonary congestion, dyspnea, and edema. These symptoms are identical to patients with pump failure (56–59). This disorder is unusual in childhood, most commonly being seen in elderly, usually female individuals with obesity, hypertension, and diabetes. Mortality is similar to typical CHF.

SYNDROME OF HEART FAILURE

Traditionally, the syndrome of heart failure has been viewed as a constellation of clinical findings resulting from inadequate systolic function ("pump function"). However, over the past decade, this view has been altered by a variety of clinical and basic data including the continued poor outcomes of patients despite therapies designed to improve systolic function (60). In addition, information regarding inflammatory mediators, apoptosis, structure–function studies, and genetics has resulted in a concept that the syndrome of heart failure occurs due to a complex interaction of structural, functional, and biologic disturbances of the heart.

The current concepts regarding the syndrome of heart failure integrate a series of models of heart failure, including the hemodynamic model, neurohormonal model, structural model, and autocrine–paracrine model of heart failure (41,51). In the hemodynamic model, alterations in load on the failing ventricle are central to the hypothesis and rely heavily on pump dysfunction as the key contributor. Based on this model, therapies were developed which focused on inotropic agents and vasodilators, with the goal of improving contractility. In distinction to this model, the neurohormonal model (see also Chapter 4) focused on the importance of the renin–angiotensin–aldosterone system (RAAS) and the sympathetic nervous system as central to the development of heart failure and resulted in attempts to pharmacologically antagonize the effect of circulating norepinephrine and angiotensin II. The autocrine–paracrine model was developed due to the findings that norepinephrine, angiotensin II, and other vasoactive substances such as brain natriuretic peptide (BNP) are also synthesized within the myocardium, therefore acting in an autocrine and paracrine manner in addition to their actions in the circulation. Finally, the structural model focuses on the necessity of proper interactions between the sarcomere and sarcolemma via cytoskeletal and other proteins. These, as well as models relying on inflammatory mediators and apoptosis, have all been used to explain the features of heart failure; it is likely that all play a role in the clinical disorder.

Despite the probable complexity of interactions resulting in heart failure, a major abnormality at the center of the disorder and its reversal is the process of remodeling. Improved outcomes appear to be linked to the ability to reverse this process ("reverse-remodeling"). Remodeling of the left ventricle is a process in which ventricular size, shape, and function is altered due to mechanical, genetic, and neurohormonal factors that lead to hypertrophy, myocyte loss, and interstitial fibrosis (61). In dilated cardiomyopathy, the process of progressive ventricular dilation and changes of the shape of the ventricle to a more spherical shape, associated with changes in ventricular function and/or hypertrophy, occur without known initiating disturbance except in patients with myocardial infarction. Due to this remodeling event, mitral regurgitation may develop as the geometric relation between the mitral valve apparatus, mitral ring and papillary muscles are altered. The presence of mitral regurgitation results in increasing volume overload on an already compromised ventricle, further contributing to remodeling, symptoms, disease progression, and left atrial dilation.

CLINICAL GENETICS OF DILATED CARDIOMYOPATHY

Dilated cardiomyopathy was initially believed to be inherited in a small percentage of cases (48,62,63) until Michels et al. (64) showed that approximately 20% of probands had family members with echocardiographic evidence of DCM when family screening was performed. More recently, inherited, familial DCM (FDCM) has been shown to occur in over 30%

of cases (65–67). In the remaining cases, a large percentage is acquired, with viral myocarditis playing a significant role (68–71).

As noted, over 30% of patients with DCM have a familial form of disease (48,62–67). Autosomal dominant inheritance is the predominant pattern of transmission, with X-linked, autosomal recessive, and mitochondrial inheritance less common (48,62–67,72). Mitochondrial inheritance is seen most commonly in childhood forms of FDCM, while X-linked and autosomal recessive forms are probably evenly mixed between childhood and adult forms of disease.

MOLECULAR GENETICS OF DILATED CARDIOMYOPATHY

Over the past decade, progress has been made in the understanding of the genetic etiology of FDCM (Table 1). Initial progress was made studying families with X-linked forms of DCM, with the autosomal dominant forms of DCM beginning

Table 1 Dilated Cardiomyopathy (DCM) Genetics

CHR Locus	Gene	Protein
Xp21.2	DYS	Dystrophin
Xq28	G4.5	Tafazzin
1q21	LMNA	Lamin A/C
1q32	TNNT2	Cardiac Troponin T
1q42–43	ACTN	a-Actinin
2q31	TTN	Titin
2q35	DES	Desmin
5q33	SGCD	δ-Sarcoglycan
6q22.1	PLN	Phospholamban
10q22.3–23.2	ZASP/cypher	ZASP
10q22–q23	VCL	Metavinculin
11p11	MYBPC3	Myosin binding protein C
11p15.1	MLP	Muscle LIM protein
14q12	MYH7	β-Myosin heavy chain
15q14	ACTC	Cardiac actin
15q22	TPM1	α-Tropomyosin

to unravel over the past few years. In the case of X-linked forms of DCM, two disorders have been well characterized, X-linked cardiomyopathy (XLCM) which presents in adolescence and young adults, and Barth syndrome, which is most frequently identified in infancy (70–72).

X-LINKED CARDIOMYOPATHIES

X-Linked Dilated Cardiomyopathy (XLCM)

First described in 1987 by Berko and Swift (73) as DCM occurring in males in the teen years and early 20s with rapid progression from CHF to death due to VT/VF or transplantation, these patients are distinguished by elevated serum creatine kinase muscle isoforms (CK-MM). Female carriers tend to develop mild to moderate DCM in the fifth decade and the disease is slowly progressive. Towbin et al. (74) were the first to identify the disease-causing gene and characterize the functional defect. In this report, the dystrophin gene was shown to be responsible for the clinical abnormalities and protein analysis by immunoblotting demonstrated severe reduction or absence of dystrophin protein in the heart of these patients. These findings were later confirmed by Muntoni et al. (75) when a mutation in the muscle promoter and exon 1 of dystrophin was identified in another family with XLCM. Subsequently, multiple mutations have been identified in dystrophin in patients with XLCM (76–81).

Dystrophin is a cytoskeletal protein which provides structural support to the myocyte by creating a lattice-like network to the sarcolemma (82). In addition, dystrophin plays a major role in linking the sarcomeric contractile apparatus to the sarcolemma and extracellar matrix (83–86). Furthermore, dystrophin is involved in cell signaling, particularly through its interactions with nitric oxide synthase (87). The dystrophin gene is responsible for Duchenne and Becker muscular dystrophy (DMD/BMD) when mutated as well (88). These skeletal myopathies present early in life (DMD is diagnosed before age 12 years, while BMD is seen in teenage males older than 16 years of age) and the vast majority of patients develop DCM before the 25th birthday. In most patients, CK-MM is elevated similar to that seen in XLCM; in addition, manifesting female carriers develop disease late in life, similar to XLCM. Furthermore, immuno-histochemical analysis demonstrates reduced levels (or absence) of dystrophin, similar to that seen in the hearts of patients with XLCM.

Murine models of dystrophin deficiency demonstrate abnormalities of muscle physiology based on membrane structural support abnormalities. In addition to the dysfunction of dystrophin, mutations in dystrophin secondarily affect proteins which interact with dystrophin. At the amino-terminus (N-terminus), dystrophin binds to the sarcomeric protein actin, a member of the thin filament of the contractile apparatus. At the carboxy-terminus (C-terminus), dystrophin interacts with α-dystroglycan, a dystrophin-associated membrane-bound protein which is involved in the function of the dystrophin-associated protein complex (DAPC), which includes β-dystroglycan, the sarcoglycan subcomplex (α, β, γ, δ, and ε sarcoglycan), syntrophins, and dystrobrevins (Fig. 1). In turn, this complex interacts with α2-laminin and the extracellular matrix (89). Like dystrophin, mutations in these genes lead to muscular dystrophies with or without cardiomyopathy, supporting the contention that this group of proteins is important to the normal function of the myocytes of the heart and skeletal muscles (85,89–91). In both cases, mechanical stress (92) appears to play a significant role in the age-onset dependent dysfunction of these muscles. The information gained from the studies on XLCM, DMD, and BMD led us to hypothesize that DCM is a disease of the cytoskeleton/sarcolemma which affects the sarcomere (93). We also have suggested that dystrophin mutations play a role in idiopathic DCM in males. Recently, we showed that 3/22 boys with DCM studied for dystrophin mutations using a rapid DNA mutation screening method had mutations and all had elevated CK-MM as well (94). In addition, eight families with DCM and possible X-linked inheritance were also screened and in 3/8 families, dystrophin mutations were noted. Again, CK-MM was elevated in all subjects carrying mutations (81).

BARTH SYNDROME

Initially described as X-linked cardioskeletal myopathy with abnormal mitochondria and neutropenia by Neustein et al. (95) and Barth et al. (96), this disorder typically presents in male infants as CHF associated with neutropenia (cyclic) and 3-methylglutaconic aciduria (97). Mitochondrial dysfunction is noted on EM and electron transport chain biochemical analysis. Recently, abnormalities in cardiolipin have been noted (98–100). Echocardiographically these infants typically have left ventricular dysfunction with left ventricular dilation, endocardial fibroelastosis, or a dilated hypertrophic left ventricle. In some cases, these infants succumb due to CHF/sudden death VT/VF, or sepsis due to leukocyte dysfunction. The majority of these children survive infancy and do well clinically, although DCM usually persists. In some cases, cardiac transplantation has been performed. Histopathologic evaluation typically demonstrates the features of DCM, although endocardial fibroelastosis may be prominent and the mitochondria are abnormal in shape and abundance.

The genetic basis of Barth syndrome was first described by Bione et al. (101) who cloned the disease-causing gene, G4.5. This gene encodes a novel protein called tafazzin, whose function is not currently known. It has been speculated, however, that the gene product is an acyltransferase based on the cardiolipin abnormalities (102). Mutations in G4.5 result in a wide clinical spectrum, which includes apparent classic DCM, hypertrophic DCM, endocardial fibroelastosis (EFE), or left ventricular noncompaction (LVNC) (103–107). In the latter case, the left ventricular noncompaction is characterized by deep trabeculations giving the appearance of a "spongiform" myocardium (Fig. 4) (4,108). The mechanisms responsible for this clinical heterogeneity are not currently known. More detail will be provided regarding LVNC in the section on this disorder.

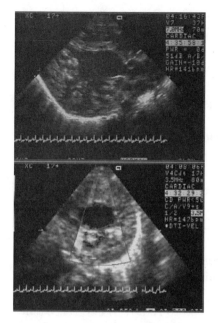

LV NONCOMPACTION

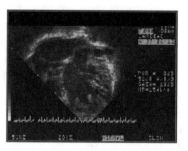

Figure 4 Left ventricular noncompaction. Echocardiogram with Doppler tissue imaging. Note the highly trabeculated left ventricle with deep recesses in the free wall creating the appearance of holes in the myocardium in left ventricular noncompaction or "spongy myocardium" (top left). The trabeculations are well seen by color, with blood noted in some of the trabeculations. In the apical four chamber view (right panel), the hypertrophic, trabeculated, dilated left ventricule is well seen. RA, RV = right atrium, right ventricle; LA, LV = left atrium, left ventricle.

AUTOSOMAL DOMINANT DILATED CARDIOMYOPATHY

The most common form of inherited DCM is the autosomal dominant form of disease (6). These patients present as classic "pure" DCM or DCM associated with conduction system disease (CDDC). In the latter case, patients usually present in the third decade of life with mild conduction system disease which can progress to complete heart block over decades. Dilate cardiomyopathy usually presents late in the course but is out-of-proportion to the degree of conduction system disease (109). The echocardiographic and histologic findings in both subgroups are classic for DCM, although the conduction system may be fibrotic in patients with CDDC. In both groups of DCM patients, VT, VF, and TdP occur and may result in sudden death.

Genetic heterogeneity exists for autosomal dominant DCM with 15 loci mapped for pure DCM and five loci for CDDC (6). In the case of pure DCM, 10 genes have been identified to date, including three by our group (δ-sarcoglycan, α-actinin-2, ZASP), (8,110,111), as well as actin (112), desmin (113), troponin T (114), β-myosin heavy chain (114); titin, (115) metavinculin (116), myosin binding protein C (117), α-tropomyosin (118), muscle LIM protein (MLP) (8,39), and phospholamban (119) (Table 1).

The majority of genes identified to date encode either cytoskeletal or sarcomeric proteins. In the case of cytoskeletal proteins (desmin, δ-sarcoglycan, metavinculin, MLP), defects of force transmission are considered to result in the DCM phenotype, while defects of force generation have been speculated to cause sarcomeric protein-induced DCM (114,120).

Cardiac actin is a sarcomeric protein that is a member of the sarcomeric thin filament interacting with tropomyosin and the troponin complex. As previously noted, actin plays a significant role in linking the sarcomere to the sarcolemma via its binding to the N-terminus of dystrophin. Interestingly, the mutations in actin which resulted in DCM as described by Olson et al. (112) appear to be directly involved in the binding of dystrophin while mutations in the sarcomeric end of actin result in hypertrophic cardiomyopathy (121). The DCM-causing mutations are believed to result in DCM by causing force transmission abnormalities. Further, actin interacts in the sarcomere with TnT and β-MHc, two other genes resulting in either DCM or HCM depending on the position of the mutation (114,122,123). In the case of TnT and β-MHC, force generation abnormalities have been speculated as the responsible mechanism.

Desmin is a cytoskeletal protein that forms intermediate filaments specific for muscle (18). This muscle-specific 53 kDa subunit of class III intermediate filaments forms connections between the nuclear and plasma membranes of cardiac, skeletal, and smooth muscle. Desmin is found at the Z lines and intercalated disk of muscle and its role in muscle function appears to involve attachment or stabilization of the sarcomere. Mutations in this gene appear to cause abnormalities of force and signal transmission similar to that believed to occur with actin mutations (113).

Another DCM-causing gene, δ-sarcoglycan is a member of the sarcoglycan subcomplex of the DAPC (89,110). This gene encodes for a protein involved in stabilization of the myocyte sarcolemma as well as signal transduction. Mutations identified in familial and sporadic cases resulted in reduction of the protein within the myocardium. In the absence of δ-sarcoglycan, the remaining sarcoglycans (δ, β, γ, Σ) cannot assemble properly in the endoplasmic reticulum. Mouse models of δ-sarcoglycan deficiency demonstrate dilated, hypertrophic cardiomyopathy, sarcolemmal fragility, and disrupted vasculin smooth muscle which leads to vascular spasm, including coronary spasm (124,125). In addition, mutations in this gene lead to the phenotype of the cardiomyopathic Syrian hamster (126–128). Other human mutations in δ-sarcoglycan cause a form of autosomal recessive limb girdle muscular dystrophy (LGMD2F) which rarely is associated with heart disease (129,130).

The final cytoskeletal protein-encoding gene, metavinculin, encodes vinculin and its splice variant metavinculin. Vinculin is ubiquitously expressed and metavinculin is coexpressed with vinculin in heart, skeletal and smooth muscle, with this protein complex localized to subsarcolemmal costameres in the heart where they localized to subsarcolemmal costameres in the heart where they interact with α-actinin, talin, and γ-actin to form a microfilamentous network linking cytoskeleton and sarcolemma. In addition, these proteins are present in adherens junctions in intercalated disks and participate in cell–cell adhesion. Mutations in metavinculin has been shown to disrupt the intercalated disks and alter actin filament cross-linking (116,131).

As previously noted, mutations in the sarcomere may produce hypertrophic cardiomyopathy or dilated cardiomyopathy.

In the latter case, abnormalities in force generation or transmission are thought to contribute to the development of this phenotype. In addition to mutations in the thin filament protein actin, mutations in the thick filament protein-encoding gene β-myosin heavy chain have been shown to cause DCM with associated sudden death in at least one infant, as well as DCM in older children and adults (114,117). Mutations in this gene are thought to perturb the actin–myosin interaction and force generation or alter cross-bridge movement during contraction. Mutations in cardiac troponin T, a thin filament protein, have been speculated to disrupt calcium-sensitive troponin C binding (114). Mutations in phospholamban (119) have also been identified which further support calcium handling as a potentially important mechanism in the development of DCM. Interestingly, Haghighi et al. (132) identified homozygous mutations causing dilated cardiomyopathy and heart failure, while heterozygoes had cardiac hypertrophy. Recessive mutation in troponin I, which is thought to impair the interaction with troponin T, α-tropomyosin mutations have also been identified and were predicted to alter the surface charge of the protein leading to impaired interaction with actin (133).

A recent area of interest for evaluation at the molecular level is the Z-disc (36). Knoll et al. (39) identified mutations in muscle LIM protein (MLP) and demonstrated that this results in defects in the interaction with telethonin (39). Using mouse models, they also demonstrated that MLP acts as a stretch sensor and that mutant MLP causes defects in this activity. More recently, Mohapatra et al. (111) demonstrated mutations in MLP in families and sporadic cases and identified abnormalities in the T-tubule system and Z-disc architecture by electron microscopy, which correlates with the histopathology seen in MLP-knockout mice (134). This was further supported by the finding of reduced expression of MLP in chronic human heart failure (135,136). In addition, mutations in α-actinin-2, which is involved in cross-linking actin filaments and shares a common actin binding domain with dystrophin, were also identified in familial DCM which disrupts its binding to MLP (134). Finally, Vatta et al. (8) identified mutations in the Z-band alternatively spliced PDZ-motif protein ZASP, the human homolog of the mouse cypher gene which when disrupted leads to DCM (137). Multiple mutations in this gene were identified in families and sporadic cases of DCM and with LV noncompaction. This protein, which interacts with α-actinin-2, disrupts the actin cytoskeleton when mutated. Another gene, titin, which encodes the giant sarcomeric cytoskeletal protein titin that contributes to the maintenance of the sarcomere organization and myofibrillar elasticity, interacts with these proteins at the Z-disc/I band transition zone (37). Mutations have been identified in familial DCM as well (115).

As seen in pure autosomal dominant DCM, genetic heterogeneity also exists for CDDC. To date, CDDC genes have been mapped to chromosomes 1p1–1q1 (138), 2q14–21 (139), 3p25–22 (140), and 6q23 (141). The only gene thus far identified was initially reported by Fatkin et al. (142) and Brodsky et al. (143) to be lamin A/C on chromosome 1q21 which encodes a nuclear envelope intermediate filament protein (138).

LAMIN A/C

The lamins are located in the nuclear lamina at the nucleoplasmic side of the inner nuclear membrane, and lamin A and C are expressed in heart and skeletal muscle (144). Mutations in this gene were initially reported to cause the autosomal dominant form of Emery–Dreifuss muscular dystrophy (145,146), which has skeletal myopathy associated with DCM and conduction system disease. It has also been found to cause a form of autosomal dominant limb girdle muscular dystrophy (LGMD1B), which is also associated with conduction system disease (147). Multiple mutations have been identified in patients with DCM and conduction system disease which, in some cases, had mildly elevated CK. This gene defect appears to be relatively common in patients with CDDC (142,143,148,149). The mechanisms responsible for the development of DCM and conduction system abnormalities are currently unknown.

MUSCLE IS MUSCLE: CARDIOMYOPATHY AND
SKELETAL MYOPATHY GENES OVERLAP

Interestingly, nearly all of the genes identified for inherited DCM are also known to cause skeletal myopathy in humans and/or mouse models. In the case of dystrophin, mutations cause Duchenne and Becker muscular dystrophy (82–89) while δ-sarcoglycan mutations cause limb girdle muscular dystrophy (LGMD2F) (85,86,89,91,129,130). Lamin A/C has been shown to cause autosomal dominant Emery–Dreifuss muscular dystrophy (EDMD) (145,146) and LGMD1B (147) while actin mutations are associated with nemaline myopathy (150). Desmin, G4.5, α-dystrobrevin, Cypher/ZASP, MLP, α-actinin-2, titin, β-sarcoglycan mutations also have associated skeletal myopathy (151–158) suggesting that cardiac and skeletal muscle function is interrelated and that possibly the skeletal muscle fatigue seen in patients with DCM with and without CHF may be due to primary skeletal muscle disease and not only related to the cardiac dysfunction. It also suggests that the function of these muscles has a "final common pathway" and that cardiologists and neurologists should consider evaluation of both sets of muscles (159).

Further support for this concept comes from studies of animal models. Mutations in δ-sarcoglycan in hamsters result in cardiomyopathy (126–128) while mutations in all sarcoglycan subcomplex genes in mice cause skeletal and cardiac muscle disease (85–87,91,124,125,155,156). Mutations in other DAPC genes as well as dystrophin in murine models also consistently demonstrate abnormalities of skeletal and cardiac muscle function (85,86,91). Arber et al. (134) also produced a mouse deficient in muscle LIM protein (MLP), a structural protein that links the actin cytoskeleton to the contractile apparatus. The resultant mice develop severe DCM, CHF, and disruption of cardiac myocyte cytoskeletal architecture. Murine mutations in titin (157), cypher (137), α-dystrobrevin (154), desmin (18), and other all demonstrate cardiac and skeletal muscle disease. Finally, Badorff et al. (160) have shown that the DCM that develops after viral myocarditis has a mechanism similar to the inherited forms. Using coxsackievirus B3 (CVB3) infection of mice, the authors showed that the CVB3 genome encodes for a protease (enteroviral protease 2A) which cleaves dystrophin at the third hinge region of dystrophin, resulting in force transmission abnormalities and DCM. In addition, Xiong et al. (161) showed that abnormal dystrophin increases susceptibility to viral infection and resultant myocarditis. Interestingly, a similar dystrophin mutation which affects the first hinge region of dystrophin in patients with XLCM was previously reported by our laboratory (77), demonstrating a consistent mechanism of DCM development, abnormalities of the cytoskeleton/sarcolemma and sarcomere. In addition, we have shown that N-terminal dystrophin is reduced or absent in hearts of patients with all forms of DCM (ischemic, acquired, genetic, idiopathic) and that reduction of mechanical stress by use of left ventricular assist devices (LVADS) results in reverse remodeling of dystrophin and of the heart itself (162,163).

Therapy of Dilated Cardiomyopathy

The therapy for DCM has changed over the past decade from focusing on improving systolic function to improving cardiac efficiency (164). In the past, inotropic therapy was a mainstay of therapy (165) while today this is less popular (166). We tend to avoid inotropic medications as much as possible, using combinations of medication aimed at avoiding arrhythmias. Low dose (renal dose) dopamine in addition to milrinone and diuretics has been useful. More recently, neseritide, a BNP synthetic has been useful in improving urine output and cardiac function. In children requiring intubation and mechanical ventilation, calcium infusion with or without vasopressin has worked well in selected patients. In some centers, dobutamine and epinephrine remain mainstays.

In patients in whom these therapies are ineffective, mechanical assist device therapies using left ventricular assist (LVAD) device or ECMO have been life-saving (167). We have hypothesized that LVAD treatment reduces mechanical stress on the myocardium, enabling reverse remodeling via dystrophin (162). We have previously shown that the

N-terminus of dystrophin is lost in DCM and, after weeks of LVAD treatment, reversal occurs, resulting in relinkage of the sarcolemma and sarcomere at the actin binding domain of dystrophin (162). More recently, we demonstrated similar findings in the right ventricle as well and showed biventricular reversal using either pulsatile or continuous flow-type LVADs (163). In patients well enough to be treated as outpatients, angiotensin-converting enzyme (ACE) inhibitors and β-blockers have been shown to be efficacious (168–170). The use of diuretics may also be useful (170–173). The certainty of efficacy of digoxin has come into question and controversy also exists regarding the use of "vitamins" such as coenzyme Q10, carnitine, thiamine, riboflavin, and others. In the latter case, these medications are usually reserved for patients with mitochondrial or metabolic-based disease.

Other novel approaches currently under investigation include biventricular pacing (also known as resynchronization therapy). In those with atrioventricular block, a pacemaker is also appropriate while patients with VT currently are considered for internal defibrillators (173).

MYOCARDITIS

Definition

Myocarditis is a process characterized by inflammatory infiltrate of the myocardium with necrosis and/or degeneration of adjacent myocytes not typical of the ischemic damage associated with coronary artery disease. This definition does not account for the underlying etiology (174).

Etiology

Most cases of myocarditis in the United States and western Europe result from viral infections (10,175,176). The most common viral causes include adenovirus (particularly serotype 2 and 5) (10,177,178) and enterovirus (coxsackieviruses A and B, echovirus, poliovirus), particularly coxsackievirus B (178–181) (Table 2). However, a wide variety of other viral causes of myocarditis (10,178,182) in children and adults have

Table 2 Viral PCR Analysis of Myocarditis and Dilated Cardiomyopathy (DCM): Detection of Viruses by PCR in Myocardial Samples

Diagnosis	Number of samples	Number of PCR+samples	PCR amplimer (Number)
Myocarditis	624	239 (38%)	Adenovirus 142 (23%) Enterovirus 85 (14%) CMV 18 (3%) Parvovirus 6 (<1%) Influenza A 5 (<1%) HSV 5 (<1%) EBV 3 (<1%) RSV 1 (<1%)
DCM	149	30 (20%)	Adenovirus 18 (12%) Enterovirus 12 (8%)
Controls	215	3 (1.4%)	Enterovirus 1 (<1%) CMV 2 (<1%)

been described, including influenza (183,184), cytomegalovirus (CMV) (185,186), herpes simplex virus (HSV) (187), parvovirus (188), hepatitis C (HCV) (189), rubella (190), varicella (191,192), mumps (193,194), Epstein–Barr Virus (EBV) (195), human immunodeficiency virus (HIV) (196–198), and respiratory syncytial virus (RSV) (199), amongst others. Other nonviral etiologies include other infectious agents such as Rickettsiae, bacteria, protozoa, and other parasites, fungi, and yeast (Table 3) (174); various drugs including antimicrobial medications (174); hypersensitivity, autoimmune or collagen-vascular diseases such as systemic lupus erythematosus, mixed connective tissue disease, rheumatic fever, rheumatoid arthritis, and scleroderma; toxic reactions to infectious agents (e.g., diphtheria); or other disorders such as Kawasaki disease and sarcoidosis (Table 3). In most cases, however, "idiopathic" myocarditis is encountered (174).

Epidemiology

Myocarditis is a disorder that is underdiagnosed (174), but the incidence of the usual lymphocytic form of myocarditis

Table 3   Causes of Myocarditis

Viral
- Coxsackievirus A
- Coxsackievirus B
- Echoviruses
- Rubella virus
- Measles virus
- Parvovirus
- Adenovirus
- Polio viruses
- Vaccinia virus
- Mumps virus
- Herpes Simplex virus
- Epstein–Barr virus
- Cytomegalovirus
- Rhinoviruses
- Hepatitis viruses
- Arboviruses
- Influenza viruses
- Varicella virus

Rickettsial
- *Rickettsia Ricketsi*
- Rickettsia Tsutsugamushi

Bacterial
- Meningococcus
- Klebsiella
- Leptospira
- Diphtheria
- Salmonella
- Clostridia
- Tuberculosis
- Brucella
- *Legionella Pneumophila*
- Streptococcus

Protozoal
- *Trypanosoma Cruzi*
- Toxoplasmosis
- Amebiasis

Other Parasites
- Toxocara canis
- Schistosomiasis
- Heterophyiasis
- Cysticercosis
- Echinococcus
- Visceral larva migrans

Fungi and Yeasts
- Actinomycosis
- Coccidioidomycosis
- Echinococcus
- Histoplasmosis
- Candida

Toxic
- Scorpion
- Diphtheria

Drugs
- Sulfonamides
- Phenylbutazone
- Cyclophosphamide
- Neomercazole
- Acetazolamide
- Amphotericin B
- Indomethacin
- Tetracycline
- Isoniazid
- Methyldopa
- Phenytoin
- Penicillin

Hypersensitivity/autoimmune
- Rheumatoid arthritis
- Rheumatic fever
- Ulcerative colitis
- Systemic lupus erythematosus

Other
- Sarcoidosis
- Scleroderma
- Idiopathic
- Cornstarch

has been reported to be from 4% to 5% (as obtained from reports of young men dying of trauma) (200) to as high as 16–21% (as found in autopsy series of children dying suddenly) (179,201–203). In adults with unexplained DCM, the reported incidence varies between 3% and 63% (204), although the large multicenter Myocarditis Treatment Trial (205), which was strictly based on the "Dallas criteria" (206), reported a 9% incidence.

Usually sporadic, viral myocarditis can also occur as an epidemic. Epidemics usually are seen in newborns, most commonly in association with coxsackievirus B (CVB). Intrauterine myocarditis has also been seen during epidemics as well as sporadically (207,208). Postnatal spread of coxsackievirus is via the fecal/oral or airborne route (174,209). The World Health Organization (WHO) reports that this ubiquitous family of viruses results in cardiovascular sequelae in less than 1% of infections, although this increases to 4% when CVB is considered (210). Other important viral causes, such as adenovirus and Influenza A, are transmitted through the air (209,211,212). Although the disease can occur equally throughout the year, the exact etiology is probably season-dependent [in other words, certain viral causes are seasonal (i.e., coxsackievirus) while others are year-round (i.e., adenovirus)].

Clinical Manifestations

Differences in presentation are seen depending on the age of the child (i.e., newborn/infant vs. child or adolescent), making the diagnosis challenging (179,209). Adults and adolescents present with similar findings. In general, myocarditis should be considered in all children and adults with new-onset congestive heart failure (CHF) in whom no other etiology is found (176). In many cases, an antecedent, nonspecific flu-like illness or episode of gastroenteritis may precede the symptoms of CHF.

Newborns and Infants

Newborns or infants typically present with fever, irritability or listlessness, periodic episodes of pallor (which may precede the sudden onset of cardiorespiratory symptoms including tachypnea or respiratory distress), and diaphoresis. Poor appetite or vomiting can also be seen frequently. Sudden death may occur in this subgroup of children (179,212). On physical examination, pallor and mild cyanosis are commonly noted. The skin is usually cool and mottled (and sometimes clammy), consistent with poor perfusion due to decreased cardiac output. Respirations are usually rapid and labored; grunting may be prominent but rales are uncommon (in fact, if rales are auscultated, strongly consider pneumonia with or without sepsis as the diagnosis). The cardiovascular exam is consistent with congestive heart failure and includes resting tachycardia and a gallop rhythm, muffled heart sounds, and frequently an apical systolic murmur due to mitral regurgitation. In some of these young children, particularly newborns, a tricuspid regurgitation murmur may also be identified. The pulses are usually thready and hepatomegaly is usually obvious. Depending on the underlying etiology, splenomegaly may also be prominent, but this is very uncommon when myocarditis is the cause of heart failure. Arrhythmias (supraventricular or ventricular tachycardia) or atrioventricular block (AVB) may also occur (209).

It is important to keep in mind that the younger the child, the more likely that intrauterine myocarditis occurred and that the findings may be more associated with chronic disease than otherwise expected in acute disease (213,214).

Children, Adolescents, and Adults

Older children, adolescents, and adults commonly report a recent history of viral disease, generally 10–14 days prior to presentation. Initial symptoms include lethargy, low grade fever, and pallor; the child usually has decreased appetite and may complain of abdominal pain. Diaphoresis, palpitations, rashes, exercise intolerance, and general malaise are common signs and symptoms. Later in the course of illness, respiratory symptoms become predominant; syncope or sudden death may occur due to cardiac collapse. Physical exam findings are consistent with congestive heart failure. Unlike newborns, jugular venous distention and pulmonary rales may be found, and resting tachycardia may be prominent. Arrhythmias, including atrial fibrillation, supraventricular tachycardia or ventricular tachycardia, as well as AVB, may occur (215–217).

Diagnostic Tests

The diagnosis of myocarditis is often difficult to establish but should be suspected in any infant or child who presents with unexplained congestive heart failure or ventricular tachycardia. Appropriate diagnostic studies include:

Chest x-ray: Cardiomegaly with prominent pulmonary vascular markings suggestive of pulmonary edema, possibly consistent with congestive heart failure, is notable. Comparisons over time may demonstrate significant improvement or normalization of the chest X-ray within a few months of presentation, suggesting a transient disease state (most typically myocarditis).

Electrocardiogram: Sinus tachycardia with low-voltage QRS complexes (less than 5 mm total amplitude in all limb leads) with or without low-voltage or inverted T waves are classically described. A pattern of myocardial infarction with wide Q waves (>35 msec) and S-T segment changes may also be seen. Ventricular tachycardia, supraventricular tachycardia, atrial fibrillation, or atrioventricular block occur in some children.

Echocardiogram: A dilated and dysfunctional left ventricle consistent with DCM (i.e., left ventricular end-diastolic and end-systolic dimensions are increased, shortening and ejection fractions are decreased) is seen on two-dimensional and M-mode echocardiography (Fig. 3). Segmental wall motion abnormalities are relatively common, but global hypokinesis is predominant. Pericardial effusion frequently occurs. Doppler and color-Doppler commonly demonstrate mitral regurgitation (Fig. 3). Dilation of other chambers may also be seen. Cardiac output calculations may also be obtained and are typically reduced. Coronary artery or structural abnormalities which could result in these features should be excluded.

Endomyocardial biopsy: A cardiac catherization and endomyocardial biopsy (Fig. 5) may be performed to obtain cardiac output and intracardiac pressure measurements. Low cardiac output is commonly seen along with elevated end-diastolic ventricular pressures. Endomyocardial biopsy (EMB) (218,219), usually obtained from the right ventricle, is used to directly evaluate the myocardium for evidence of inflammation histologically (Fig. 6). Usually five tissue specimens are obtained for analysis (as outlined by the "Dallas criteria") (206) since the inflammatory infiltrate is usually patchy and scattered in the ventricular myocardium. Evidence of significant mononuclear cell infiltrate is diagnostic of myocarditis, although this does not delineate etiology (220). Unfortunately the results of EMB are commonly nondiagnostic, with the incidence of "biopsy-proven" myocarditis in patients presenting with new-onset CHF and DCM

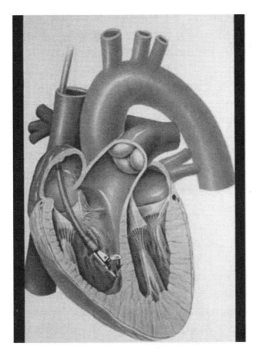

Figure 5   Endomyocardial biopsy technique.

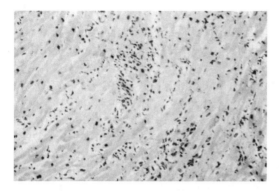

Figure 6 Histologic findings in myocarditis. Note the diffuse inflammatory infiltrate, myocyte necrosis, and edema.

ranging from 3% to 63% of cases (221–223). This lack of sensitivity has been clearly shown by Hauck et al. (224), Chow et al. (225), Lie et al. (226), and others; in fact, using the usual number of specimens (i.e., five biopsy specimens) outlined by the "Dallas criteria," only approximately 50% of all true cases of myocarditis will be identified. In order to identify 80% of cases, 17 or more specimens must be obtained. Since there is risk associated with EMB, particularly in young children or those with severe ventricular dilatation, many centers have abandoned this procedure.

The **"Dallas criteria":** In order to minimize the discrepancy or disagreement in diagnosis (227,228), this standardized histopathologic definition and classification scheme was devised (206). This defines myocarditis as "a process characterized by an inflammatory infiltrate of the myocardium with necrosis and/or degeneration of adjacent myocytes not typical of ischemic damage" due to coronary artery or other disease. At the time of initial biopsy, a specimen may be classified either as *active myocarditis-borderline myocarditis-* or *no myocarditis,* depending on whether an inflammatory infiltrate occurs in association with myocyte degeneration or necrosis (*active*) or too spase of an infiltrate or no myocyte degeneration occurs (*borderline*). Repeat EMB may be appropriate in cases where strong suspicion of myocarditis exists clinically (229); on repeat EMB, histology may be classified as *ongoing myocarditis* (similar or worse findings compared to the initial biopsy), *resolving myocarditis* (inflammatory infiltrate is diminished), or *resolved myocarditis* (cellular infiltrate or myocyte necrosis no longer present).

Viral studies: The diagnostic gold standard of the viral etiology is positive viral culture from the myocardium; this is rare, however. Viral cultures of peripheral specimens, such as blood, stool, or urine are commonly performed but are unreliable at identifying the causative infection. Other studies used to delineate the viral etiology include serologic studies in which a fourfold rise in antibody titer is required (209). Antibody studies commonly performed include type-specific neutralizing, hemagglutination inhibiting, or complement-fixing antibody studies. However, these studies are nonspecific, since prior infection with the causative virus is commonplace. Molecular analysis using in situ hybridization has been used to identify coxsackievirus B sequences in myocardial samples (230–232), but this method never gained popularity. Currently, polymerase chain reaction (PCR) (177–179) has been used to rapidly and specifically amplify viral sequences from cardiac tissue samples (see Molecular Aspects section).

Molecular diagnostics: In 1986, the first molecular diagnostic approach was reported by Bowles et al. (230) in which in situ hybridization was performed on myocardial tissue using probes for coxsackievirus. Subsequently other reports noted the utility of this method in identifying coxsackievirus RNA within cardiac tissue specimens (231,232). However, the difficulty of using this technique in the hospital-based setting reduced the interest in pursuing this technique. In 1990, Jin et al. (233) first reported the use of PCR in identification of viral genome within the myocardium. This amplification process allows for specific portions of the viral genome of interest to be identified on an agarose gel after electrophoresis and is quite sensitive and specific (Fig. 7). During the past decade, a large number of investigators have demonstrated the ability to identify enteroviral genome by PCR (234–237) and, in fact, 20–50% of cases are reportedly identified as enterovirus PCR-positive in these studies. Polymerase chain reaction

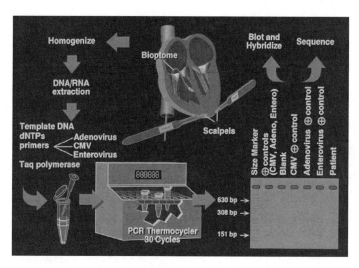

Figure 7 Polymerase chain reaction (PCR) approach to viral genome identification in myocarditis.

has also been used to screen for other viral genomes within cardiac tissue specimens and, using this method, Towbin and colleagues have showed adenovirus to be at least as common as enterovirus in heart tissue specimens of patients with myocarditis or DCM (177,179,237). This was confirmed by other laboratories as well (238–240). In addition, other viral genomes have been identified using PCR, including cytomegalovirus, parvovirus, respiratory syncytial virus, Epstein–Barr virus, Herpes simplex virus, and influenza A virus (179,188,241). Further, this method has been used to identify mumps virus (Fig. 8) as the responsible agent in endocardial fibroelastosis (EFE) (241), a previously important cause of heart failure in children which has disappeared over the past 20 years (193,194,213).

PCR analysis usually does not identify viral genome in peripheral blood of patients with myocarditis; however, Akhtar et al. (242) demonstrated the ability of this method to identify viral genome in tracheal aspirates of intubated children with myocarditis, potentially reducing the need for EMB.

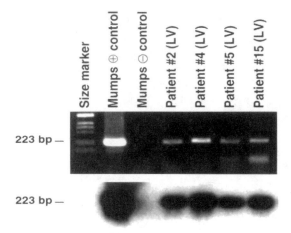

223 bp —

223 bp —

Figure 8 Viral PCR demonstrating mumps viral genome in endocardial fibroelastosis.

The Role of Cytokines in Myocarditis and DCM

Over the last few years, there has been considerable interest in the role of cytokines in the pathogenesis of myocarditis and DCM. Animal studies have suggested that a relationship may exist between subclinical viral infection and later development of DCM. This process is presumed to occur by an autoimmune-like mechanism triggered by the initial viral insult (243–245). Several murine models have been studied which suggest that cytokine-mediated modulation of the immune response to viral infection may lead to induction of chronic autoimmune myocarditis (246–249). Among their many immunomodulatory activities, cytokines contribute to regulation of antibody production and maintenance of "self-tolerance." Certain susceptible murine strains, when infected with CVB3, are known to develop myocyte necrosis and an acute inflammatory response consisting mainly of neutrophils and macrophages within the heart. After the initial viral infection, resolution of inflammation eventually occurs. In other strains, however, a second autoimmune phase of myocarditis appears later with findings of diffuse mononuclear cell infiltrates within the heart. These mononuclear cells are a significant source of the cytokine interleukin-1 (IL-1) and tumor necrosis factor-α (TNF-α), and work by Henke et al. (250) demonstrated that release of large amounts of TNF-α and IL-1β by human monocytes exposed to CVB3 occurs. Both of these cytokines are known to participate in leukocyte activation which may be beneficial in promoting a specific lymphocyte response to viral infection. However, these cytokines may also promote cardiac fibroblast activity and therefore it has been speculated that local secretion of cytokines in the myocardium perpetuates the inflammatory process, which secondarily leads to the fibrosis associated with DCM and resultant deterioration of cardiac function. Studies by Gulick et al. (251) initially implicated IL-1 and TNF-α as potential inhibitors of cardiac myocyte β-adrenergic responsiveness, and further studies have shown IL-1 and TNF-α to be the macrophage factors mediating this effect. In particular, TNF-α has been studied in some detail, resulting in reports of elevated TNF-α levels in the serum of patients with chronic heart disease (252), including a subset of patients with myocarditis or DCM (253). TNF-α is able to potentiate the immune response and induce apoptosis in cells, both of which appear to hold special importance in the pathogenesis of myocarditis. Other inflammatory mediators, including interleukin-1 (IL-1) and granulocyte colony-stimulating factor (GCSF), are also elevated in myocarditis patients (253) and have received attention as well. Other studies have suggested that inflammatory cytokines may actually cause a direct negative inotropic response (254).

The Role of Cell Adhesion Molecules in Myocarditis and DCM

Molecules now known to play a major role in many processes of inflammation, the distinct classes of cell adhesion molecules (CAMs), may also play a role in the pathogenesis of myocarditis. One molecule which is well known to play a major role in cell–cell adhesion, particularly leukocyte adherence and transendothelial migration, is intercellular adhesion molecule-1 (ICAM-1). ICAM-1 is a member of the immunoglobulin supergene family of CAMs and is a single chain glycoprotein of 80–115 kd with an extracellular domain made up of five immunoglobulin-like repeats (255,256). ICAM-1 is predominantly expressed on endothelial cells, but also on fibroblasts, epithelial cells, mucosal cells, lymphocytes, monocytes, and cardiac myocytes after inflammatory injury. Expression of ICAM-1 on endothelial cells is known to be upregulated by cytokines such as IL-1 and TNF-α. A well-established binding ligand of ICAM-1 is lymphocyte function-associated antigen-1 (LFA-1), is a molecule which is part of the β-2 integrin family and consists of a 180 kd α subunit (CD11a) and a 95 kd β subunit (CD18). LFA-1 is expressed on virtually all leukocytes, including monocytes. The adhesive interaction between LFA-1 and ICAM-1 is known to mediate adhesion-dependent helper T cell, cytotoxic T cell, and NK cell functions. Antibody to LFA-1 has been used for therapy in animal models of myocarditis with resultant blockade of the inflammatory response.

Apoptosis

Apoptosis, or programmed cell death, has an important role in embryogenesis, tissue homeostasis, and regulation of immunologic responses, among normal physiologic processes, and is associated with the growth and regression of tumors (257). Cells undergoing apoptosis exhibit characteristic morphologic and biochemical features, including chromatin aggregation, nuclear and cytoplasmic aggregation, and formation of apoptotic bodies resulting from the partition of the cytoplasm and nucleus into membrane bound-vesicles. These apoptotic bodies are rapidly phagocytosed by adjacent macrophages or epithelial cells, without resulting in an inflammatory response. Apoptotic cells are detectable by terminal transferase labeling [terminal deoxynucleotide transferase-mediated biotin-deoxyuridine triphosphate nick end labeling (TUNEL)] in myocardial tissue samples from patients with DCM. It has been shown that up to 0.1% of cells stained positive by this technique.

A number of viruses have been implicated in the induction of apoptosis, including human immunodeficiency virus (HIV), Epstein–Barr virus (EBV), and adenovirus. Apoptotic cells have been detected in myocardial sections from patients with adenovirus-associated myocarditis and DCM, the areas of staining are usually focal, and a number of positively staining areas may be detected within each section. Within such areas, up to 1% of cells may stain positive, including myocytes, infiltrating inflammatory cells, and endothelial cells. In the tissue sections from control patients, either unstained or sporadic (one or two per section) stained cells may be detected. These data suggest a relationship between infection of the myocardium by adenovirus and the onset of apoptosis, which could result in pathologic processes associated with myocarditis and DCM (258). Further, a number of inflammatory cells may be seen to be undergoing apoptosis. Although this could reflect the natural defense mechanism of the host against the virus, it also raises the possibility of virus-induced apoptosis as a mechanism of immune system avoidance. Strand et al. (259) reported that in tumors, infiltrating immune cells are destroyed by the induction of apoptosis through the expression of Fas ligand on the tumor cell that binds Fas on the lymphocyte.

Long-Term Sequelae

In those cases in which resolution of cardiac dysfunction does not occur, chronic DCM results (177,179). It has been unclear what the underlying etiology of this long-term sequelae could be, but viral persistence and autoimmunity have been widely speculated. Recently, Badorff et al. (260) demonstrated that enteroviral protease 2A directly cleaves the cytoskeletal protein dystrophin, resulting in dysfunction of this protein (Fig. 9). Since mutations in dystrophin are known to cause an inherited form of DCM (261), as well as the DCM associated with the neuromuscular diseases Duchenne and Becker muscular dystrophy, it is likely that this is to a large extent responsible for the chronic DCM seen in enteroviral myocarditis. Other viruses, such as adenoviruses, also have enzymes which cleave membrane structural proteins or result in activation or inactivation of transcription factors, cytokines or adhesion molecules to cause chronic DCM. Therefore, it appears as if a complex interaction between the viral genome

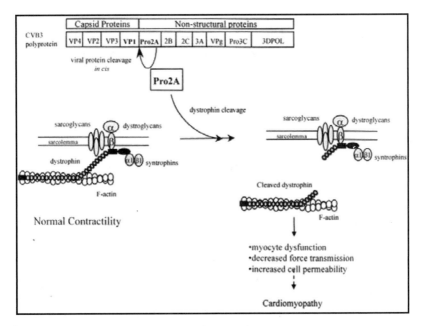

Figure 9 Coxsackievirus B3 protease 2A cleaves dystrophin, resulting in dilated cardiomyopathy in viral myocarditis.

and the heart occurs and results in the long-term outcome of affected patients.

There are some reports which suggest myocarditis could be inherited (262,263). Support for this includes the frequent finding of myocardial lymphocytic infiltrate in patients with familial and sporadic DCM, as well as the few reports of families in which two or more individuals have been diagnosed with myocarditis on EMB. The recent finding of a common receptor for the four most common viral causes of myocarditis (coxsackievirus B3 and B4 and adenovirus 2 and 5), the human Coxsackie and Adenovirus Receptor (HCAR) (Fig. 1) (264,265) which if mutated could result in responsible host differences leading to myocarditis, is intriguing and requires study.

Treatment

Care of a patient presenting with a clinical picture and history strongly suggestive of myocarditis depends on the severity of myocardial involvement. Many patients will present with a relatively mild disease, with minimal or no respiratory compromise and only mild signs of congestive heart failure. These patients require close monitoring to assess whether the disease will progress to worsening heart failure and the need for intensive medical care. Experimental animal studies suggest that bed rest may prevent an increase in intra-myocardial viral replication in the acute stage; thus, it appears prudent to place patients under this restriction at the time of diagnosis. Normal arterial blood oxygen levels should be maintained for any patient with compromised hemodynamics resulting in hypoxemia. Although no specific therapy aimed at reversing myocardial injury is currently widely recommended, maintenance of cardiac output at levels that supply adequate tissue perfusion and prevent metabolic disturbances is essential. In cases of congestive heart failure, the same general approaches to supportive care as described for heart failure associated with dilated cardiomyopathy are relevant.

The use of immunosuppressive agents in suspected or proven viral myocarditis is controversial (266–271). Some animal studies have suggested an exacerbation of virus-induced cytotoxicity in the presence of immunosuppressive drugs, possibly due to interference with interferon production (267). In 1995, Camargo et al. (270) described 68 children with DCM, including 43 with active myocarditis diagnosed by endomyocardial biopsy. These children were divided into four treatment groups including standard therapy (Group I), prednisone plus standard therapy (Group II), azathioprine (Group III) plus prednisone plus standard therapy, and cyclosporine (Group IV) plus prednisone and conventional therapy. The authors noted the best results with prednisone plus either azathioprine or cyclosporine therapy. Support for this was shown by Wojnicz et al. (271) who also showed improvement in echocardiographic criteria, NYHA class but no difference in outcome vs. control patients in an older group of patients with DCM. Other studies have shown no improvement, however.

Another potential therapeutic option is the use of intravenous gamma-globulin in children with myocarditis. This study is based on the early results of Drucker et al. (272) who investigated the use of this agent in 21 of 46 children with myocarditis. Patients who received this drug had better left ventricular function at follow-up. In addition, survival tended to be higher at 1 year though the data did not reach statistical significance because of the small number of patients in the study. Whether this proves to be beneficial or whether these early results mirror the early published experience with corticosteroids remains to be seen.

Left ventricular assist devices (LVAD) and aortic balloon pumps have been used to support the cardiovascular system in some cases, while extracorporeal membrane oxygenator (ECMO) therapy has been used in others. When necessary, the devices may be life-saving and should be considered an option in children large enough to allow placement of the device successfully. In some circumstances, transplantation becomes necessary. The prognosis of acute myocarditis in newborns, infants and children, however, remains poor (179).

ARRHYTHMOGENIC RIGHT VENTRICULAR DYSPLASIA/CARDIOMYOPATHY (ARVD/ARVC)

ARVD/ARVC is a primary disorder of the right ventricle characterized by myocyte loss, fibrofatty infiltration of the right ventricular wall, with associated dilation and systolic dysfunction of the right ventricle, although the left ventricle may be affected as well (Fig. 10) (273–275). Ventricular arrhythmias commonly occur (usually left bundle-branch morphology VT and VF) and sudden death, particularly in athletes, is an important and tragic outcome in many patients (275).

Clinical Presentation

Arrhythmogenic right ventricular dysplasia/cardiomyopathy typically presents in young adult men, with 80% or more diagnosed before 40 years of age. It is uncommon in childhood and is rare in prepubertal individuals. The clinical phenotype is quite variable, including arrhythmic or heart failure

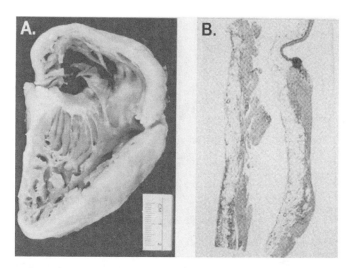

Figure 10 Features of arrhythmogenic right ventricular cardiomyopathy: (A) gross specimen with thin right ventricular wall with fatty infiltrate; (B) histology with fibrofatty infiltration of the right ventricular myocardium.

symptoms. A common presentation is syncope with occasional individuals presenting with sudden death. In the United States, ARVD/ARVC accounts for 5% of sudden cardiac deaths in subjects less than 65 years of age and is responsible for at least 3–5% of deaths associated with physical activity in athletes and younger persons. In the Veneto region of Italy, the disorder is the most common cause of sudden death in patients less than 35 years of age, particularly athletes, usually due to ventricular tachyarrhythmias. In addition, patients with ARVD/ARVC may develop isolated right heart failure or biventricular failure, typically presenting in the fourth or fifth decade of life.

Clinical Evaluation

This is a difficult diagnosis to make and for this reason, an expert consensus group proposed diagnostic criteria (276). The diagnosis requires clinical, electrocardiographic, histopathologic, and imaging abnormalities (Table 4).

Table 4 Arrhythmogenic Right Ventricular Dysplasia Consensus Diagnostic Criteria

Major criteria	Minor criteria
1. Global and/or regional dysfunction and structural alterations	
Severe dilatation and reduction of right ventricular ejection with no (or only mild) LV impairment	Mild global right ventricular dilation and/or ejection fraction reduction with normal left ventricle.
Localized right ventricular aneursym (akinetic or dyskinetic areas diastolic buldging)	Mild segmental dilation of the right ventricle
Severe segmental dilation of the right ventricle	Regional right ventricular hypokinesia
2. Tissue characterization of wall	
Fibrofatty replacement of myocardium on endomyocardial biopsy, autopsy, or explant	
3. Repolarization abnormalities	Inverted T waves in right precordial leads (V_1 and V_2)people aged > 12 years, in absence of right bundle-branch block
4. Depolarization/conduction abnormalities	
Epsilon waves or localized prolongation (> 110 msec) of the QRS complex in right precordial leads ($V_1 - V_2$)	Late potentials (SAECG)
5. Arrhythmias	Left bundle-branch block type ventricular tachycardia (sustained and nonsustained) by ECG, Holter, or exercise testing
	Family history of premature sudden death (< 35 years) due to suspected right ventricular dysplasia
6. Family history	
Familial disease confirmed at necropsy or surgery	Familial history (clinical diagnosis based on present criteria)

LV: left ventricle; SAECG: signal-averaged ECG.

Electrocardiography: The diagnosis is most definitive when epsilon waves, postexcitation electrical potentials of small amplitude occurring at the end of the QRS complex and the beginning of the ST segment, are seen as these are highly specific for this disorder (273–275,277). However, epsilon waves, reflecting delayed right ventricular activation, are only seen in approximately one-third of cases. Other usual features include right bundle-branch block with extensive QRS precordial dispersion, inverted T waves in the right precordial leads (V2, V3) in the absence of right bundle-branch block, and ST-segment elevation in the right precordial leads similar to that seen in Brugada syndrome (277). Left bundle-branch block-type VT seen on electrocardiogram, Holter monitor or stress test is also suggestive of this diagnosis. Supportive data include late action potentials on signal-averaged ECG, the equivalent of epsilon waves on the surface ECG.

Histopathology

The diagnosis of ARVD/ARVC is dependent on tissue diagnosis when available. Right ventricular biopsy diagnosis may be difficult as the most frequently involved region is the posterior tricuspid area (275–277), with the apex and infundibulum also affected (the "triangle of dysplasia"); the interventricular septum is usually not affected. The disease process primarily affects the epicardium and mid-myocardial layers with endocardial sparing. Tabib et al. (278) recently demonstrated fatty infiltration in 75%, and with associated lymphocytic infiltrate in 5% of cases. Cardiac hypertrophy was noted in 15% of cases and, in most cases, the bundle of HIS was abnormal.

Imaging

Echocardiography commonly overlooks the diagnosis unless a severely hypokinetic, dilated RV is seen. In some cases, localized aneurysms are seen. In addition, left ventricular disease can be seen in some patients. Cardiac magnetic resonance imaging has been touted as the imaging modality of choice but inconsistencies exist. Cardiac MRI can identify the morphologic abnormalities of the RV better than echocardiography, noting RV dilation, aneurysms and fatty infiltrate, as well as the poor RV function. However, intraobserver variability has limited the technique (279). Finally, angiography has been reported by many to be the modality of choice, identifying the diagnostic abnormalities in a high percentage of cases.

Therapy of ARVD/ARVC

Current management of ARVD/ARVC has shifted in recent years to consideration of implantable defibrillators due to the high risk of arrhythmia-induced syncope and sudden death (280). Pharmacologic therapy has included Sotolol, Verapamil, and Amiodarone most commonly. In addition, radiofrequency ablation has been reported with variable success. It is possible that understanding of the disease at the cellular and molecular level will enable improved therapies to be developed.

Genetics of ARVD/ARVC

The prevalence of ARVD/ARVC in the general population is reportedly 1 in 5000, with 30–50% of cases being inherited (275). A significant percentage of patients with ARVD/ARVC ARVC have autosomal dominant transmission of disease (285). In one subgroup of patients with ARVD/ARVC associated with wooly hair, palmoplantar keratosis and autosomal recessive inheritance, known as Naxos disease because of its identification in individuals from Naxos, Greece, the disorder is complex (282). In another subpopulation, a similar complex phenotype associated with DCM has been identified and called Carvajal Syndrome (283).

ARVD/ARVC is another genetically heterogeneous disorder with genetic loci identified for pure ARVD/ARVC [chromosomes 14q24 (284), 1q42 (285), 14q12–22 (296), 2q35 (286), 10p12–14 (288), 3p23 (289) (Table 5). In addition, one locus for Naxos disease (chromosome 17q21) (290) and another for Carvajal Syndrome (chromosome 6p24) have been

Table 5 Genetic Basis of Arrhythmogenic Right Ventricular Cardiomyopathy

Locus name	Inheritance	Map position	Gene
ARVD1	AD	14q23	?
ARVD2	AD	1q42–q43	RYR2
ARVD3	AD	14q12	?
ARVD4	AD	2q32	?
ARVD5	AD	3p23	?
ARVD6	AD	10p12	?
ARVD7	AD	10q22	?
ARVD8	AD	6p24	DESMOPLAKIN
Naxos	AR	17q21	PLAKOGLOBIN
Naxos-like	AR	6p24	DESMOPLAKIN

identified (291). A gene for Naxos disease has been identified, with mutations in plakoglobin, an intermediate filament, desmosomal protein, reported (290). Another desmosomal protein, desmoplakin, has also been identified in patients with Carvajal Syndrome (291) (Table 5). For the autosomal dominant form of disease, only two genes have been identified. Tiso et al. (292) reported mutations in the ryanodine receptor (RyR2), which encodes a protein integral to calcium channel function, as the cause of chromosome 1q42-linked ARVD2, suggesting ARVD to be a primary rhythm disorder (Table 5). Interestingly, RyR2 was subsequently shown to cause catecholamine-sensitive VT (bi-directional VT), further supporting this concept (293). Corrado et al. (277) has shown that ST-segment elevation in V_1–V_3 commonly occurs in ARVD, similar to the ECG abnormalities in Brugada syndrome, another primary electrical disorder (294,295). The second gene, desmoplakin, suggests that the desmosome/gap junctions are important "final common pathways." Rampazzo et al. (296) have also identified mutations in desmoplakin in pure ARVD/ARVC.

Nongenetic causes have also been identified. Bowles et al. (297) demonstrated enteroviral and adenoviral genome within the heart of patients with this disorder, supporting the claims of Grumbach et al. (298).

DISEASES OF VENTRICULAR DIASTOLIC FUNCTION

Hypertrophic Cardiomyopathy

Hypertrophic cardiomyopathy is a complex cardiac disease with unique pathophysiological characteristics and a great diversity of morphologic, functional, and clinical features (299,300). Although hypertrophic cardiomyopathy has been regarded largely as a relatively uncommon cardiac disease, the prevalence of echcocardiographically defined hypertrophic cardiomyopathy in a large cohort of apparently healthy young adults selected from a community-based general population was reported to be as high as 0.2% (301). The disorder is considered to occur due to diastolic dysfunction, a disease of relaxation of the ventricular myocardium. Systolic function is preserved or hypercontractile and left ventricular outflow tract obstruction may occur.

Clinical Aspects of Hypertrophic Cardiomyopathy

Hypertrophic cardiomyopathy is a primary myocardial disorder with an autosomal dominant pattern of inheritance that is characterized by hypertrophy of the left (± right) ventricle with histological features of myocyte hypertrophy, myofibrillar disarray, and interstitial fibrosis (300). Hypertrophic cardiomyopathy is one of the most common inherited cardiac disorders, with a prevalence in young adults of 1 in 500 (302). Various names have been given to this disorder including hypertrophic obstructive cardiomyopathy (HOCM) and diopathic subaortic stenosis (IHSS). These names reflect "textbook" features of asymmetric septal hypertrophy and left ventricular outflow tract obstruction. This description of the disease is based primarily on patients with severe symptoms seen in tertiary hospital referral centers. Epidemiological studies now suggest that a wide spectrum of clinical manifestations of varying severity and prognosis is present in community populations. The first clinical description of HCM was reported in 1869 (303) in France, and was recognized to be a genetic disorder in the late 1950s. Since then, numerous clinical and pathological studies of HCM have been performed. During the last 15 years, molecular genetic studies have given important insights into the pathogenesis of HCM and have provided a new perspective for the diagnosis and management of patients with this disorder (304).

Diagnosis of HCM

Affected individuals with HCM exhibit significant variability in their clinical presentation. They may be asymptomatic or present with symptoms ranging from palpitations and dizziness to syncope and sudden death. The age of onset of symptoms varies with some children presenting at birth or during childhood, with others presenting late in life, such as the fifth or sixth decade. Most commonly, patients present in the first two decades of life (305). The physical examination in subjects with HCM may or may not be fruitful. Due to the ventricular relaxation disorder, the ventricular stiffness may result in an S4 gallop. In patients with left ventricular outflow tract obstruction, an outflow murmur may be heard. Otherwise, the examination is typically normal unless a restrictive component or heart failure exists, in which case jugular venous distention, hepatomegaly (and other signs of heart failure) may be in evidence.

The diagnosis of HCM relies on echocardiography, Holter monitoring, and exercise testing; histopathology may also be useful. In addition, in small children, metabolic studies may be useful in determining the etiology of disease (305).

Echocardiography: The primary modality for the diagnosis of HCM is transthoracic echocardiography. The hallmark diagnostic feature of HCM is asymmetric hypertrophy of the interventricular septum, with or without systolic anterior motion of the mitral valve and hypercontractile systolic function as seen by M-mode (Fig. 11). Doppler and color Doppler interrogation identifies outflow tract obstruction when it occurs. It is now recognized that the obstructive form of HCM occurs in <25% of affected individuals. Studies of kindreds with HCM have shown that the distribution and severity of left ventricular hypertrophy may vary considerably,

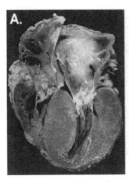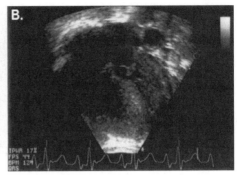

Figure 11 Hypertrophic cardiomyopathy. Anatomic (A) and echo-cardiographic features (B) of hypertrophic cardiomyopathy with thickened interventricular septum and left ventricular posterior wall.

that asymmetric hypertrophy is no longer an essential requirement for the diagnosis of this disorder, and that even within the same family, the features may differ. The diagnosis of HCM generally requires exclusion of secondary causes of hypertrophy, such as hypertension or aortic stenosis; however, in some individuals, particularly in older age groups, these conditions may coexist. The differentiation of HCM from physiological left ventricular hypertrophy may be difficult, particularly in competitive athletes. The extent of left ventricular hypertrophy also may vary between different mutant genes. For example, individuals with β-MHC gene mutations usually develop moderate or severe hypertrophy with a high disease penetrance, whereas those with cardiac troponin T gene mutations reportedly have only mild or clinically undetectable hypertrophy (306,307). Unusual forms of hypertrophy have been reported, localized to the left ventricular apex (cardiac troponin I mutations) (308) or midcavity (cardiac actin and MLC gene mutations) (309,310). The extent of left ventricular hypertrophy may also vary between members of a single family with the same gene mutation, as previously noted. These observations may be explained by a modifying role of additional genetic and environmental factors, such as blood pressure, exercise, diet, and body mass.

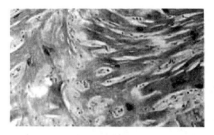 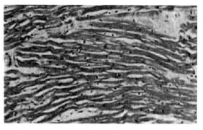

Figure 12   Histologic features of hypertrophic cardiomyopathy including myocyte hypertrophy and myofibril disarray.

Electrocardiography: The ECG may be normal in HCM or have associated left ventricular hypertrophy or biventricular hypertrophy. Giant QRS complexes are common in patients with Pompe disease or LV noncompaction (4). Pre-excitation may also be noted in patients with HCM (305,311,312). Ventricular, atrial or supraventricular arrhythmias may be seen onsurface ECG as well. Patients with restrictive physiology may demonstrate atrial enlargement. Holter monitoring may demonstrate arrhythmias as well.

Exercise testing: Risk stratification has been reported with the use of exercise testing, with blunting or reduction of blood pressure and or blunting of heart rate response to exercise being associated with increased risk (313). In particular, blood pressure reduction by more than 15 mmHg or failure to increase blood pressure more than 25 mmHg is associated with increased risk. Other associated risk factors include syncope, nonsustained VT, severe LVH on echocardiography (>3 cm in adults), and family history of premature death (314).

Histopathology: The classic features of HCM include myocyte hypertrophy, myofiber disarray, and patchy fibrosis (302) (Fig. 12). In some patients, mitochondrial proliferation or morphologic abnormalities with or without inclusion material, glycogen stores, vacuolization, or desmin deposits may be seen (305).

Metabolic studies: Similar to DCM, metabolic and mitochondrial abnormalities may be causative and therefore, the same blood, urine and muscle studies should be obtained. In addition, fibroblasts for α-1, 4-glycosidase (acid maltase) deficiency to diagnose Pompe disease should be considered (305).

Natural History of HCM

The natural history of HCM is variable; some individuals remain asymptomatic throughout life, and others may develop progressive symptoms with or without heart failure or experience sudden death. Longitudinal echocardiographic studies have documented left ventricular remodeling with age. Progressive increases to left ventricular wall thickness have been reported in individuals during adolescence and early adult life. In some individuals, left ventricular wall thickness may increase in later life (315). Age-related reductions in left ventricular wall thickness, associated with myocyte loss and fibrosis, have also been described in individuals with long-standing disease ("burnt out" HCM). Ten to twenty percent of individuals with HCM may develop dilated cardiomyopathy. Ten to sixteen percent of affected adult individuals develop atrial fibrillation, and this risk of atrial fibrillation is increased in those with left atrial enlargement.

Hypertrophic cardiomyopahy is a frequent cause of sudden death, particularly in young individuals and competitive athletes (316). Estimates of the prevalence of sudden death vary according to the population studied, ranging from $<1\%$ in the general community to 3–6% in tertiary care hospital referral centers. Various mechanisms for sudden death have been proposed, including ventricular bradyarrhythmias due to sinus node and atrioventricular conduction abnormalities and tachyarrhythmias triggered by re-entrant depolarization pathways related to myofibrillar disarray and fibrosis, abnormal Ca^{2+} homeostasis, myocardial ischemia, left ventricular diastolic dysfunction, or left ventricular outflow tract obstruction. Various risk stratification algorithms based on clinical parameters have been proposed to identify individuals with an increased propensity for sudden death. Given the complexity of mechanisms that may precipitate sudden death, it is not surprising that no single risk factor has been identified. Conflicting results have been found for the positive predictive value of young age at diagnosis, history of syncope, severity of symptoms, left ventricular wall thickness, left ventricular outflow tract gradient, left atrial size, atrial fibrillation, exercise response of blood pressure and heart rate. Genotype has also been suggested to predict outcome. The mechanisms whereby HCM gene mutations influence prognosis are unknown. Although some HCM mutations that alter the charge of the encoded amino acid have been associated with a poor outcome, other mutations that alter charge have a good prognosis (317,318). Genetic studies and animal model studies including electrophysiological studies in mouse models may provide important insights into the differential propensity for sudden death between different HCM gene mutations.

Genetics of Familial Hypertrophic Cardiomyopathy

The first gene for familial hypertrophic cardiomyopathy (FHC) was mapped to chromosome 14q11.2–q12 using genome-wide linkage analysis in a large Canadian family (319). Soon afterwards, FHC locus heterogeneity was reported (320) and subsequently confirmed by the mapping of the second FHC locus to chromosome 1q3 and of the third locus to chromosome 15q2 (321,322). Carrier et al. (323) mapped the fourth FHC locus to chromosome 11p11.2. Multiple other loci were subsequently reported, including loci on chromosomes 7q3 (324), 3p21.2– 3p21.3 (325), 12q23–q24.3 (325), 19p13.2–q13.2 (326), and 15q14 (327) (Fig. 13). Several other families are not linked to any known FHC loci, indicating the existence of additional FHC-causing genes (Table 6).

Gene Identification in Familial Hypertrophic Cardiomyopathy

All the disease-causing genes identified to date code for proteins that are part of the sarcomere, which is a complex structure with an exact stoichiometry and multiple sites of protein–protein interactions (5,6,304). These include three myofilament proteins: the β-myosin heavy chain (β-MyHC), the ventricular myosin essential light chain 1 (MLC-1s/v)

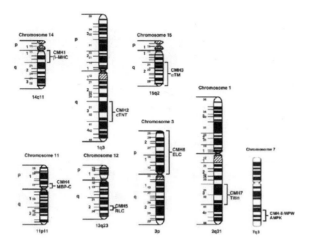

Figure 13 Genetic location of hypertrophic cardiomyopathy-causing genes.

and the ventricular myosin regulatory light chain 2 (MLC-2s/v); four thin filament proteins: cardiac actin, cardiac troponin T (cTnT), cardiac troponin I (cTnI), and α-tropomyosin (α-TM); and one myosin-binding protein, the cardiac myosin binding protein C (cMyBP-C) (Table 6). Each of these proteins is encoded by multigene families which exhibit tissue specific, developmental, and physiologically regulated patterns of

Table 6 Hypertrophic Cardiomyopathy Genetics

CHR locus	Gene	Protein
1q32	TNNT2	Cardiac troponin T
2q31	TTN	Titin
3p21.2	MLC-1	Myosin essential light chain
7q31	PRGKγ	AMP kinase
11p11	MYBPC3	Myosin binding protein C
11p15.1	MLP	Muscle LIM protein
12q2.3	MLC-2	Myosin regulatory light chain
14q12	MYH7	β-Myosin heavy chain
15q14	ACTC	Cardiac actin
15q22	TPM1	α-Tropomyosin
19p13.2	TNNI3	Cardiac troponin I

expression (328). The giant protein titin and its interactive Z-disc protein, muscle LIM protein (MLP) have also been identified (329). In addition, the gene located on chromosome 7q3 associated with HCM and Wolff–Parkinson–White (WPW) syndrome was identified as AMP Kinase (AMPK), which has been suggested to play a role in energy metabolism and cause infiltration of a glycogen-like substance similar to that seen in Pompe disease (7,311,312).

Thick Filament Proteins

Myosin Subunits

Myosin is the molecular motor that transduces energy from the hydrolysis of ATP into directed movement and that, by doing so, drives sarcomere shortening and muscle contraction. Cardiac myosin consists of two heavy chains (MyHC) and two pairs of light chains (MLC), referred to as essential (or alkali) light chains (MLC-1) and regulatory (or phosphorylatable) light chains (MLC-2), respectively (328). The myosin molecule is highly asymmetric, consisting of two globular heads joined to a long rod-like tail. The light chains are arranged in tandem in the head–tail junction. Their function is not fully understood. Neither myosin light chain type is required for the adenosine triphosphatase (ATPase) activity of the myosin head, but they probably modulate it in the presence of actin and contribute power stroke. Mutations have been found in the heavy chains and in the two types of ventricular light chains.

Concerning the heavy chains, the β isoform (β-MyHC) is the major isoform of the human ventricle and of slow-twitch skeletal fibers. It is encoded by *MYH7*. This gene appears to be the most commonly mutated HCM gene and hot spots for mutations have been identified (5,304). The majority of mutations are missense mutations located either in the head or in the head–rod junction of the molecule. Based on their structural location in the myosin head, the majority of mutations are likely to disrupt both mechanical and catalytic components of actin–myosin interactin, resulting in reduced force generation. Sarcomere assembly is also likely to be disrupted.

Mutations in the light meromyosin domain have also been identified and Blair et al. (330) speculated that HCM develops in this case due to abnormalities of myosin filament assembly or interactions with thick filament binding proteins.

The myosin light chain isoforms are expressed in the ventricular myocardium and in the slow-twitch muscles and are the so-called ventricular myosin regulatory light chains (MLC-2 s/v) encoded by *MYL2*, and the ventricular myosin essential light chain (MLC-1 s/v) encoded by *MYL3*. The myosin light chains are thought to influence the mechanical efficiency of cross-bridge cycling and speed of contraction. It is believed that these proteins regulate power output via a calcium-dependent mechanism and disruption leads to the HCM phenotype.

Myosin-Binding Protein C (MyBP-C)

MyBP-C is part of the thick filaments of the sarcomere, being located at the level of the transverse stripes, 43 nm apart, seen by electron microscopy in the sarcomere A band. Its function is uncertain, but, for over a decade, evidence has existed to indicate both structural and regulatory roles. Partial extraction of cMyBP-C from rat skinned cardiac myocytes and rabbit skeletal muscle fibers alters Ca^{2+}-sensitive tension (331), and it has shown that phosphorylation of cMyBP-C alters myosin cross-bridges in native thick filaments, suggesting that cMyBP-C can modify force production in activated cardiac muscles. The cardiac isoform is encoded by the *MYBPC3* gene.

Thin Filament Proteins

The thin filament contains actin, the troponin complex, and tropomyosin. The troponin complex and tropomyosin constitute the Ca^{2+}-sensitive switch that regulates the contraction of cardiac muscle fibers. Mutations have been found in α-TM and in two of the subunits of the troponin complex: cTnI, the inhibitory subunit, and cTnT, the tropomyosin-binding subunit.

α-TM is encoded by *TPM1*. The cardiac isoform is expressed both in the ventricular myocardium and in fast twitch skeletal muscles (332). It shares the overall structure of other tropomyosins that are rod-like proteins that possess a simple dimeric α-coiled-coil structure of other tropomyosins that are rod-like proteins that possess a simple dimeric α-coiled-coil structure in parallel orientation along their entire length (332). It is believed that some mutations in this gene could alter tropomyosin binding to actin

cTnT is encoded by *TNNT2*. In human cardiac muscle, multiple isoforms of cTnT have been described which are expressed in the fetal, adult, and diseased heart, and which result from alternative splicing of the single gene *TNNT2* (333,334). The precise physiological relevance of these isoforms is currently poorly understood. Mutations in this gene are predicted to influence the inhibitory regulatory effect of the tropomyosin–troponin complex.

cTnl is encoded by *TNNl3*. The cTnl isoform is expressed only in cardiac muscles (335). Cooperative binding of cTnl to actin–tropomyosin is a unique property of the cardiac variant, it is thought that mutations disrupt the calcium-sensitive switch mediated by this protein, resulting in increased calcium sensitivity and reduced maximum tension.

α-Cardiac actin (ACTC) mutations also cause of FHC. Mogensen et al. (327) identified mutations in a family with heterogeneous phenotypes, ranging from asymptomatic with mild hypertrophy to pronounced septal hypertrophy and left ventricular outflow tract obstruction. Mutations in titin and MLP have also been identified suggesting the Z-disc to be important in the development of HCM although the mechanism is uncertain.

Genotype–Phenotype Relations in Familial
Hypertrophic Cardiomyopathy

The pattern and extent of left ventricular hypertrophy in patients with HCM vary greatly even in first-degree relatives and a high incidence of sudden death is reported in selected families. An important issue therefore is to determine whether the genotype heterogeneity observed in HCM accounts for the phenotypic diversity of the disease. However, the results must be seen as preliminary, because the available data relate to only a few hundred individuals, and it is obvious that although a given phenotype may be apparent in a small family, examining large or multiple families with the same mutation is required before drawing unambiguous conclusions. Several concepts have been published for mutations in the *MYH7-TNNT2-* and *MYBPC3* genes. For *MYH7*, the prognosis for patients with different mutations has been shown to vary. For example, the R403Q mutation was felt to be associated with markedly reduced survival (336), whereas some others, such as V606M, appeared more benign. The disease caused by *TNNT2* mutations was reportedly associated with a 20% incidence of nonpenetrance, a relatively mild and sometimes subclnical hypertrophy, but a high incidence of sudden death which occurred even in the absence of significant clinical left ventricular hypertrophy (337,338). Mutations in *MYBPC3*, on the other hand, have been characterized by specific clinical features with a mild phenotype in young subjects, a delayed age at the onset of symptoms and a favorable prognosis before the age of 40 (339–342). However, despite these assertions, the notion of mutation-specific clinical outcomes was challenged by Van Diest and colleagues who demonstrated that "benign" mutations were uncommon (5/253) and that the mutations studied all had severe clinical disease (343).

Genetic studies have also revealed the presence of clinically healthy individuals carrying the mutant allele, which is associated in first-degree relatives with a typical phenotype of the disease. Several mechanisms could account for the large variability of the phenotypic expression of the mutations: the role of environmental differences and acquired traits (e.g., differences in lifestyle, risk factors, and exercise) and finally the existence of modifier genes and/or polymorphisms that could modulate the phenotypic expression of the disease. Significant results have been obtained thus far regarding the influence of the angiotensin I converting enzyme insertion/deletion (ACE I/D) polymorphism. Association studies showed that, compared to a control population, the D allele is more common in patients with hypertrophic cardiomyopathy and in patients with a high incidence of sudden cardiac death (344,345). It was also shown that the association between the D allele and hypertrophy was seen in the case of *MYH7* R403 codon mutations, but not with *MYBPC3* mutation carriers (346), raising the concept of multiple genetic modifiers in HCM.

THERAPY IN HYPERTROPHIC CARDIOMYOPATHY

The mainstay of therapy in children with HCM has been pharmacologic approaches. The two major medication classes used include beta-blockers and calcium-channel blockers (347–349). In small children, we have used propranolol as our drug of choice due to ease of access, liquid formulation, and low side-effect profile. Therapy in these children is monitored by heart rate response, with the goal being approximately 80–100 beats per minute. Therapy typically ranges in dosage from 2 to 5 mg/kg/day divided three times daily. Verapamil has been popular in some institutions and reportedly results in good outcomes. In older children, we typically treat with atenolol. In children with excessive hypertrophy and severe outflow tract obstruction, we occasionally consider use of combination therapy (beta-blocker plus calcium-channel blocker) although this is not without risk. However, the risk:benefit ratio must be determined for each patient.

When standard pharmacologic therapy fails, there are limited options, although the size of the child plays a role. In small children, myomectomy is the only proven option (350). Again, this is not without risk. In older patients, pacing protocols have been used but are controversial (351–353). In adults, alcohol septal ablation has been utilized but this has not yet been championed in children due to the uncertainties associated with creating an infarct in a young individual regarding long-term outcome (354–356).

In patients with syncope, ventricular arrhythmias, or other presumed high risk, ICD implantation should be considered (357). In some patients, pacing is necessary as well.

Finally, in children with metabolic or mitochondrial dysfunction underlying the HCM, metabolic therapies have been successful on occasion. Similar to the therapy in DCM caused by these deficiencies, carnitine, coenzyme Q10, riboflavin, and thiamine may be considered (305).

RESTRICTIVE CARDIOMYOPATHY

Restrictive cardiomyopathy is a relatively rare form of cardiomyopathy, affecting only approximately 5% of individuals with heart muscle disease (358). However, the disorder appears to have the worst outcome of all forms of cardiomyopathy (especially in children), with sudden death occurring within 2–5 years of diagnosis in over half the cases (359). In some instances, ventricular tachycardia has been shown as the etiology of demise. In the remaining patients, congestive heart failure with or without pulmonary hypertension is notable.

Clinical Features

Restrictive cardiomyopathy most commonly presents with syncope or sudden death in children (359–363). Rarely does this disorder present in the first two years of life, with the majority of children identified before puberty. Later-onset patients tend to present with signs and symptoms of CHF, particularly dyspnea, orthopnea, and abdominal pain. Chest pain and palpitations may also be prominent features. On physical examination, these children have a quiet precordium, regular rhythm, and nondisplaced apical impulse associated with a gallop rhythm, usually an S4. If a murmur exists, it is usually due to AV valve regurgitation. The liver tends to be significantly enlarged and tender without splenomegaly. The lungs are usually clear to auscultation and peripheral edema is rare.

Clinical Evaluation

The usual evaluation includes chest radiography, electrocardiography, echocardiography, and Holter monitoring. Exercise testing and cardiac catheterization may also be performed.

Chest radiography: Chest x-rays commonly demonstrate mild cardiomegaly and, in children with CHF, increased pulmonary vascular markings, and Kerley B lines. Due to the enlarged atria, pulmonary atelectasis is common.

Electrocardiography: The ECG has classic features including biatrial enlargement. Usually the QRS complexes, QT interval, and T wave morphology are normal but atrial and ventricular arrhythmias may be noted along with ST-segment abnormalities.

Echocardiography: Restrictive cardiomyopathy is characterized by atrial dilation bilaterally with normal sized ventricles (Fig. 14). Systolic function is usually preserved but diastolic dysfunction is usually evident with abnormal mitral inflow patterns. Atrioventricular valve regurgitation is common and evidence of elevated right heart pressures is typical. Cardiac hypertrophy, including asymmetric septal hypertrophy, occurs in some patients. Whether this is true RCM or HCM with restrictive physiology remains a conundrum.

Holter monitoring: In some children, 24 hr Holter monitors will demonstrate atrial or ventricular tachyarrhythmias. In addition, ST-segment abnormalities may occur, particularly at higher heart rates.

Cardiac catheterization: Elevated atrial and ventricular end diastolic pressures are typical and worsen with volume challenge. A so-called "square root sign" is confirmatory of

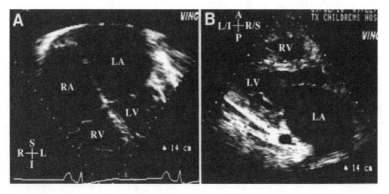

Figure 14 Echocardiographic features of restrictive cardiomyopathy, including biatrial enlargement with normal ventricular size and thickness. (A) apical four-chamber view; (B) parasternal long axis view.

restrictive physiology. Pulmonary hypertension may be identified and AV valve regurgitation is commonly seen on angiography. Coronary angiography and contractile function are also normal. In some patients, endomyocardial biopsy may be performed. Myocyte hypertrophy and fibrosis may occur, but, unlike adults, infiltrative processes (such as amyloid and sarcoid) are not seen.

Exercise testing: Although a normal exercise test may be seen, this test may be dangerous in some due to propensity for ST-segment changes, particularly at higher heart rates, which may lead to serious ventricular arrhythmias. Reduced exercise capacity and abnormal oxygen consumption are also common.

Genetics of RCM

When RCM is inherited, autosomal dominant inheritance is most common although autosomal recessive transmission has been reported (364). However, inherited disease appears to occur in ≤10% of cases. Two genes have been identified in autosomal dominant RCM thus far, troponin I (365) and desmin (366). In the cases with troponin I mutations, interventricular septal hypertrophy consistent with HCM with restrictive physiology was seen in several individuals while others had normal septal and wall thicknesses (365). The patients with desmin mutations had pure RCM. Normal skeletal muscle function was clinically found in subjects with these gene defects. Clearly other genes exist which cause this disorder, but these remain elusive. In some cases, RCM coexists with skeletal myopathy and/or conduction system disease (152,153). In these cases, mutations in desmin have been described (152,153). Mouse models of desmin knockouts are confirmatory (367–369). In elderly patients with RCM, mutations in the prealbumin gene, tranthyretin, have been described (370,371).

Therapy and Outcome of RCM

Children with RCM are possibly the highest risk-population in pediatrics for sudden cardiac death. Therapy tends to be unsuccessful. Based on treatment results in patients with HCM, the other disorder associated with predominant diastolic dysfunction, β-blocker therapy or calcium-channel blocking agents were initially thought to be the treatment of choice. However, these agents have had little impact on outcome and, in some children, have added to the symptomatology. For instance, the use of β-blockers has caused hypoglycemia with associated seizures and syncope in several children. No other pharmacologic agents have been useful in children without CHF; therapy of CHF in this subgroup is efficacious, however. The use of antiarrhythmic agents and implantable cardioverter defibrillators (ICDs) may protect some children at-risk for arrhythmogenic sudden death. Unfortunately, most of these approaches have not reduced mortality and, in our institution, children are listed for transplantation at the time of diagnosis with extremely good outcomes occurring. In those waiting for transplantation in whom evidence of heart rate-related ischemia is noted, intravenous esmolol infusion has been useful.

OVERLAP DISORDERS

Left Ventricular Noncompaction

This disorder has been considered to be a rare disease and has been identified by a variety of names including spongy myocardium, fetal myocardium, and noncompaction of the left ventricular myocardium (372–374). The abnormality is believed to represent an arrest in the normal process of myocardial compaction, the final stage of myocardial morphogenesis, resulting in persistence of multiple prominent ventricular trabeculations and deep intertrabecular recesses. This cardiomyopathy is somewhat difficult to diagnose unless the physician has a high level of suspicion during echocardiographic evaluation. In fact, on careful review of echocardiograms and other clinical data, it appears that left ventricular noncompaction is relatively common in children and is also seen in adults (4).

Two forms of left ventricular noncompaction occur: (1) isolated noncompaction and (2) noncompaction associated with congenital heart disease such as septal defects (ventricular and/or atrial septal defect), pulmonic stenosis, hypoplastic left heart syndrome, amongst others. In the isolated form and the form associated with congenital heart disease, metabolic derangements may be notable (372–374).

Clinical Features

Left ventricular noncompaction most commonly presents in infancy with signs and symptoms of heart failure but some patients are identified during later childhood, adolescence, or adulthood. Pignatelli et al. (4) recently reported the findings on 36 children identified over a five-year period, with the median age at presentation being 90 days (range 1 day to 17 years). In this study, 40% of the children presented with low cardiac output or congestive heart failure and only one child (3%) presented with syncope. The most common presenting symptom other than heart failure was asymptomatic electrocardiographic or radiographic abnormalities, with 42% being asymptomatic. In addition, 14% of children had associated dysmorphic features while 19% of affected children had first-degree relatives with cardiomyopathy. The children with dysmorphic features were diagnosed with DiGeorge syndrome in one child and one child had congenital adrenal hyperplasia.

Clinical Evaluation

The usual evaluation includes an electrocardiogram, chest radiograph, and echocardiogram, as well as Holter monitoring, blood and urinary studies, and skeletal muscle biopsy. These studies, in addition to the clinical evaluation and a high degree of suspicion, should lead to a higher likelihood of correct diagnosis.

Chest radiography: Chest x-rays commonly demonstrate cardiomegaly (20%) or signs of heart failure such as increased pulmonary vascular markings (40%).

Metabolic testing: Blood and urine studies, as well as muscle biopsy with biochemical analysis, are important diagnostic tests in patients with left ventricular noncompaction. Due to the association of LV noncompaction with Barth syndrome, mitochondrial or other metabolic syndromes, abnormalities may be notable with all such studies. These may include cyclic neutropenia (Barth syndrome), lactic acidosis (Barth syndrome, mitochondrial or metabolic disorders), 3-methylglutaconic aciduria (Barth syndrome, mitochondrial disease), carnitine or fatty acid oxidation defects; skeletal muscle biopsies are commonly abnormal, demonstrating evidence of mitochondrial proliferation and morphology abnormalities (with or without inclusions). Electron transport chain biochemistry may also be abnormal with deficiencies identified in complexes I–IV of the respiratory chain in association with elevated citrate synthase and succinate dehydrogenase. Cytochrome C deficiencies have also been reported.

Electrocardiography: A high prevalence of ECG abnormalities, thought to be as high as 75% or more, are noted. The most prominent features seen are marked biventricular hypertrophy with extreme QTS voltage (Fig. 15) similar to that seen in Pompe disease (~30%), T-wave inversion (20%), pre-excitation (15–20%), and premature atrial and ventricular contractions (~10%). On rare occasions, children present with supraventricular or ventricular tachycardia.

Echocardiography: Two-dimensional echocardiography demonstrates the classic features of noncompaction including noncompaction morphology of deep trabeculations and inter-trabecular recesses, ventricular hypertrophy (especially apical hypertrophy) with or without dilation (Fig. 4). In nearly

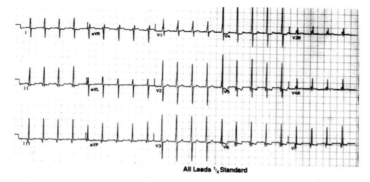

All Leads ¼ Standard

Figure 15 Electrocardiogram in left ventricular noncompaction. Giant QRS complex voltages are noted (1/4 standard).

90% of patients, systolic dysfunction is noted at presentation. Most commonly, the left ventricle alone is affected (80%) while biventricular noncompaction occurs in approximately 20% of children. Congenital heart disease occurs in 10–20% of children and should be specifically evaluated. Doppler interrogation identifies abnormal mitral inflow velocities consistent with restrictive physiology (decreased E/A ratio) in approximately half of the cases. Interestingly, several children demonstrate with increased hypertrophy and systolic function normalizes (or becomes hypercontractile) before reverting to the initial phenotype. In rare instances, thrombi (particularly in the inter-trabecular apical recesses) are noted.

Genetics

When LV noncompaction is inherited, it can be transmitted as an X-linked, mitochondrial, autosomal recessive or autosomal dominant trait. In approximately 20–30% of cases, familial inheritance has been identified. The X-linked form usually is associated with isolated noncompaction and a mutation in the G4.5 (tafazzin) gene located on chromosome Xq28 (375). This gene has also been identified in patients with Barth syndrome.

In autosomal dominant inherited cases, mutations in the Z-line protein encoding ZASP, located on chromosome 10q22, have been identified in isolated noncompaction (8), while mutations in the gene encoding α-dystrobrevin, a cytoskeletal protein located on chromosome, have been identified in patients with noncompaction associated with congenital heart disease (106). No genes have been identified thus far for autosomal recessive-inherited noncompaction while mutations in mitochondrial DNA have been seen in patients with noncompaction (372–374).

Therapy and Outcome

The specific therapy depends on the clinical and echocardiographic findings. In patients with systolic dysfunction and heart failure, anticongestive therapy identical to those used in patients with dilated cardiomyopathy is appropriate. In particular, angiotensin-converting enzyme inhibitors such as captopril and enalapril, as well as β-adrenergic blocking agents such as metoprolol or carvedilol, are useful. Diuretics may also be needed. However, in those patients exhibiting findings more consistent with a hypertrophic cardiomyopathy or diastolic dysfunction physiologic phenotype, β-blocker therapy alone with propranolol or atenolol is more appropriate. In patients with either of these forms of noncompaction with associated mitochondrial or metabolic dysfunction some investigators add a "vitamin cocktail" to the cardiac therapy with coenzyme Q10, carnitine, riboflavin, and thiamine commonly used alone or in combination.

In patients having associated congenital heart disease, appropriate therapeutic approaches may include simple pharmacologic therapy with diuretics for volume overload associated with left to right shunts, more complex pharmacologic therapy for patients with restrictive physiology and pulmonary hypertension, or invasive therapy with catheter intervention or surgical repairs, depending on the lesions. Intimate understanding of the cardiac function abnormalities, evidence of thrombi (which should be treated with anticoagulation), and the metabolic status of the patient must be attended to by the interventional cardiologist, cardiac anesthesiologist, and surgeon in approaching these patients invasively. In addition, cardiac rhythm disturbances need to be identified and therapies such as pacemakers, implantable defibrillators, and intracardiac ablations considered.

The clinical outcome of patients with noncompaction has been reported to be poor with death occurring due to heart failure or sudden death presumably arrhythmia-related or stroke-related due to embolization of left ventricular thrombi (108,375). However, Pignatelli et al. (4) demonstrated a five-year survival rate of 86%; when transplanted patients were added, the five-year survival free of death or transplantation was 75%.

FINAL COMMON PATHWAY HYPOTHESIS

Clearly, familial hypertrophic cardiomyopathy of adults is a disease of the sarcomere (5,6). Similarly, patients with other cardiac disorders, such as familial dilated cardiomyopathy (FDCM) and familial ventricular arrhythmias (i.e., long QT syndromes and Brugada syndrome), have been shown to have mutations in genes encoding a consistent family of proteins (6,295). In familial ventricular arrhythmias, ion channel gene mutations (i.e., ion channelopathy) have been found in all cases thus far reported. In FDCM, cytoskeletal protein-encoding genes and sarcomeric proteins have been speculated to be causative (i.e., cytoskeletal/sarcomyopathy) [6,45,93]. Hence, the final common pathways of these disorders include ion channels and cytoskeletal proteins, similar to the sarcomyopathy in HCM. Intermediate disorders, such as ARVD/ARVC ARVC appear to connect the primary electrical and primary muscle disorders mechanistically. Although it is not yet certain what the underlying pathways and targets are for RCM, hints have been forthcoming. Desmin and other intermediate filament proteins appear to be at play in RCM as has been shown in animal models. The sarcomere is an additional target. In addition, it appears that cascade pathways are involved directly in some cases (i.e., mitochondrial abnormalities in HCM, DCM) while secondary influences are likely to result in the wide clinical spectrum seen in patients with similar mutations. In HCM, mitochondrial and metabolic influences are probably important (Fig. 16). Additionally, molecular interactions with such molecules as calcineurin, sex hormones, growth factors, amongst others, are probably involved in development of clinical signs, symptoms, and age of presentation. In the future, these factors are expected to be uncovered, allowing for development of new therapeutic strategies.

RELEVANCE OF THE FINAL COMMON PATHWAY HYPOTHESIS

The relevance of the hypothesis is its ability to classify disease entities on a molecular and mechanistic basis. This reclassification of disorders on the basis of molecular abnormalities

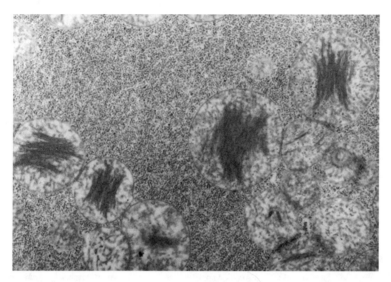

Figure 16 Skeletal muscle biopsy histology demonstrating abnormal sizes, numbers, and inclusions of mitochondria, as well as increased lipid and glycogen.

such as "dystrophinopathies," "ion channelopathies," "sarcomyopathies," or "cytoskeletopathies" could lead to more focused approaches to gene discovery and future therapeutic interventions. For instance, on the basis of the understanding of the molecular aspects of long QT syndrome, we considered the possibility that all ventricular arrhythmias are the result of ion channel abnormalities. On the basis of the hypothesis, we studied the possibility that the cardiac sodium channel gene (*SCN5A*) was mutated in patients with the idiopathic ventricular fibrillation disorder called Brugada syndrome, identifying mutations in three separate, unrelated families (376). Use of this hypothesis for disorders such as inherited DCM has enabled our group to more narrowly focus efforts at gene identification. Once the genes for all of these disorders are known, and the mechanisms causing the clinical phenotype and natural history are known, improved pharmacologic therapies based on the actual disease mechanism can be produced and utilized.

REFERENCES

1. Report of the 1995 World Health Organization/International Society and Federation of Cardiology Task Force on the Definition and Classification of Cardiomyopathies. Circulation 1996; 93:841–842.

2. Abelman WH, Lorrell BH. The challenge of cardiomyopathy. J Am Coll Cardiol 1989; 13:1219.

3. O'Connell JB, Bristow MR. Economic impact of heart failure in the United States: Time for a different approach. J Heart Lung Transplant 1994; 13:S107–S112.

4. Pignatelli RH, McMahon CJ, Dreyer WJ, et al. Clinical characterization of left ventricular noncompaction in children. A relatively common form of cardiomyopathy. Circulation 2003; 108:2672–2678.

5. Seidman JG, Seidman C. The genetic basis for cardiomyopathy from mutation identification to mechanistic paradigms. Cell 2001; 108:557–567.

6. Towbin JA, Bowles NE. The failing heart. Nature 2002; 415:227–233.

7. Arad M, Benson DW, Perez-Atayde AR, et al. Constitutively active AMP kinase mutations cause glycogen storage disease mimicking hypertrophic cardiomyopathy. J Clin Invest 2002; 109:357–362.

8. Vatta M, Mohapatra B, Jimenez S, et al. Mutations in cypher/ZASP in patients with dilated cardiomyopathy and left ventricular noncompaction. J Am Coll Cardiol 2003; 42:2014–2027.

9. Towbin JA (MC Chapter) In: Towbin JA. Myocarditis. In: Finberg L, Kleinman R, eds. Saunders Manual of Pediatric Practice. 2nd ed. , Philadelphia: Saunders Co. Publishers, 2002:660–663.

10. Bowles NE, Bowles NE, Ni J, et al. Detection of viruses in myocardial tissues by polymerase chain reaction: evidence of adenovirus as a common cause of myocarditis in children and adults. J Am Coll Cardiol 2003; 42:466–472.

11. Schwartz SM, Duffy JY, Pearl JM, Nelson DP. Cellular and molecular aspects of myocardial dysfunction. 2001; 29:S214–S219.

12. Gregorio CC, Antin PB. To the heart of myofibril assembly. Trends Cell Biol 2000; 10:355–362.

13. Squire JM. Architecture and function in the muscle sarcomere. Curr Opin Struct Biol 1997; 7:247–257.

14. Clark KA, McElhinny AS, Beckerle MC, Gregorio CC. Striated muscle cytoarchitecture: An intricate web of form and function. Annu Rev Cell Dev Biol 2002; 18:637–706.

15. Vigoreaux JO. The muscle Z band: lessons in stress management. J Muscle Res Cell Motil 1994; 15:237–255.

16. Barth AL, Nathke IS, Nelson WJ. Cadherins, catenins and APC protein; interplay between cytoskeletal complexes and signaling pathways. Curr Opin Cell Biol 1997; 9:683–690.

17. Burridge K, Chrzanowska-Wodnicka M. Focal adhesions, contractility, and signaling. Annu Rev Cell Dev Biol 1996; 12:463–518.
18. Capetanaki Y. Desmin cytoskeleton: a potential regulator of muscle mitochondrial behaviour and function. Trends Cardiovasc Med 2002; 12:339–348.
19. Stewart M. Intermediate filament structure and assembly. Curr Opin Cell Biol 1993; 5:3–11.
20. Sharp WW, Simpson DG, Borg TK, Samarel AM, Terracio L. Mechanical forces regulate focal adhesion and costamere assembly in cardiac myocytes. Am J Physiol 1997; 273:H546–H556.
21. Straub V, Campbell KP. Muscular dystrophies and the dystrophin - glycoprotein complex. Curr Opin Neurol 1997; 10:168–175.
22. Furukawa T, Ono Y, Tsuchiya H, et al. Specific interaction of the potassium channel beta-subunit iph with the sarcomeric protein T-cap suggests a T-tuble-myofibril linking system. 2001; 313:775–784.
23. Kucera JP, Rohr S, Rudy Y. Localization of sodium channels in intercalated disks modulates cardiac conduction. Circ Res 2002; 91:1176–1182.
24. Ribaux P, Bleicher F, Couble ML, et al. Voltage-gated sodium channel (SkM1) content in dystrophin-deficient muscle. Pflugers Arch 2001; 441:746–755.
25. Ehler E, Rothen BM, Hammerle SP, Komiyama M, Perriard JC. Myofibrillogenesis in the developing chicken heart: assembly of Z-disk, M-line and the thick filaments. J Cell Sci 1999; 112(Pt 10): 1529–1539.
26. Epstein HF, Fischman DA. Molecular analysis of protein assembly in muscle development. Science 1991; 251:1039–1044.
27. Holtzer H, Hijikata T, Lin ZX, et al. Independent assembly of 1.6 microns long bipolar MHC filaments and I-Z-I bodies. Cell Struct Funct 1997; 22:83–93.
28. Franzini-Armstrong C. The structure of a simple Z line. J Cell Biol 1973; 58:630–642.
29. Rowe RW. The ultrastructure of Z disks from white, intermediate, and red fibers of mammalian striated muscles. J Cell Biol 1973; 57: 261–277.
30. Goll DE, Dayton WR, Singh I, Robson RM. Studies of the alpha-actinin/actin interaction in the Z-disk by using calpain. J Biol Chem 1991; 266:8501–8510.
31. Papa I, Astier C, Kwiatek O, et al. Alpha-actinin-CapZ, an anchoring complex for thin filaments in Z-line. J Muscle Res Cell Motil 1999; 20:187–197.
32. Gregorio CC, Trombitas K, Centner T, et al. The NH2 terminus of titin spans the Z-disc: lts interaction with a novel 19-kD ligand (T-cap) is required for sarcomeric integrity. J Cell Biol 1998; 143:1013–1027.

33. Ohtsuka H, Yajima H, Maruyama K, Kimura S. Binding of the N-terminal 63 kDa portion of connectin/titin to alpha-actinin as revealed by the yeast two-hybrid system. FEBS Lett 1997; 401:65–67.

34. Sorimachi H, Freiburg A, Kolmerer B, et al. Tissue-specific expression and alpha-actinin binding properties of the Z-disc titin: implications for the nature of vertebrate Z-discs. J Mol Biol 1997; 270:688–695.

35. Young P, Ferguson C, Banuelos S, Gautel M. Molecular structure of the sarcomeric Z-disk: two types of titin interactions lead to an asymmetrical sorting of alpha-actinin. EMBO J 1998; 17:1614–1624.

36. Pyle WG, Solaro RJ. At the crossroads of myocardial signaling: the role of Z-discs in intracellular signaling and cardiac function. Circ Res 2004; 94:296–305.

37. Granzier H, Labeit S. The grant protein titin: a major player in myocardial mechanics, signaling, and disease. Circ Res 2004; 94:284–295.

38. Bang ML, Mudry RE, McElhinny AS. Myopalladin, a novel 145-kilodalton sarcomeric protein with multiple roles in Z-disc and I-band protein assemblies. J Cell Biol 2001; 153:413–427.

39. Knoll R, Hoshijima M, Hoffman HM, et al. The cardiac mechanical stretch sensor machinery involves a Z disc complex that is defective in a subset of human dilated cardiomyopathy. Cell 2002; 11:943–955.

40. Chien KR. Stress pathways and heart failure. Cell 1999; 98:555–558.

41. Jessup M, Brozena S. Heart failure. N Engl J Med 2003; 348:2007–2018.

42. Lipshultz SE, Sleeper LA, Towbin JA, et al. The incidence of pediatric cardiomyopathy in two regions of the United States. N Engl J Med 2003; 348:1647–1655.

43. Konstam MA. Progress in heart failure management? Lessons from the real world. Circulation 2000; 102:1076–1078.

44. Khand A, Gemmel I, Clark AL, Cleland JG. Is the prognosis of heart failure improving? J Am Coll Cardiol 2000; 36:2284–2286.

45. Towbin JA. Familial dilated cardiomyopathy. In: Berul CI, Towbin JA, eds. The Molecular and Clinical Genetics of Cardiac Electrophysiological Disease. Chapter 13. Kluwer Academic Publishers, 2000:195–218.

46. Wynn J, Braunwald E. The cardiomyopathies and myocarditis. In: Braunwald E, ed. Heart Disease: A Textbook of Cardiovascular Medicine. W.B: Saunders, 1987.

47. Coughlin SS, Szklo M, Baughman K, Pearson TA. The epidemiology of idiopathic dilated cardiomyoypathy in a biracial community. Am J Epidemiol 1990; 131:48–56.

48. Michels VV, Driscoll DJ, Miller FA Jr. Familial aggregation of idiopathic dilated cardiomyopathy. Am J Cardiol 1985; 55:1232–1233.

49. Arola A, Touminen J, Ruuskanen O, Jokinen E. Idiopathic dilated cardiomyopathy in children: prognostic indicators and outcome. Pediatrics 1998; 101:369–376.

50. Nugent AW, Danbeney PEF, Chondros P, et al. The epidemiology of childhood cardiomyopathy in Australia. N Engl J Med 2003; 348:1639–1646.

51. Francis GS, Wilson-Tang WH. Pathophysiology of congestive heart failure. Rev Cardiovasc Med 2003; 4(supp 2):S14–S20.

52. Stevenson WG, Stevenson LW. Prevention of sudden death in heart failure. J Cardiovasc Electrophysiol 2001; 12:112–114.

53. Benjamin EJ, Wolf PA, D'Agostino RB, Silbershatz H, Kannel WB, Levy D. Impact of atrial fibrillation on the risk of death: the Framingham Heart Study. Circulation 1998; 78:946–952.

54. Aaronson KD, Schwartz JS, Chen TM, Wong KL, Goin JE, Mancini DM. Development and prospective evaluation of a clinical index to predict survival in ambulatory patients referred for cardiac transplant evaluation. Circulation 1997; 95:2660–2667.

55. Gerber TC, Nishimura RA, Holmes DR Jr, et al. Left ventricular and biventricular pacing in congestive heart failure. Mayo Clin Proc 2001; 76:803–812.

56. Banergee P, Banergee T, Khand A, Clark AL, Cleland JG. Diastolic heart failure: neglected or misdiagnosed? J AM Coll Cardiol 2001; 39:138–141.

57. Vasan RS, Levy D. Defining diastolic heart failure: A call for standardized diagnostic criteria. Circulation 2000; 101: 2118–2121.

58. Zile MR, Brutsaert DL. New concepts in diastolic dysfunction and diastolic heart failure. II. Causal mechanisms and treatment. Circulation 2002; 105:1503–1508.

59. Senni M, Redfield MM. Heart failure with preserved systolic function: a different natural history? J Am Coll Cardiol 2001; 38:1277–1282.

60. Hunt SA, Baker DW, Chin MH, et al. ACC/AHA guidelines for the evaluation and management of chronic heart failure in the adult: Executive summary: a Report of the American College of Cardiology/American Heart Association Task Force on Practice Guidelines. J Am Coll Cardiol 2001; 38:2101–2103.

61. Sutton MGSJ, Sharpe N. Left ventricular remodeling after myocardial infarction: pathophysiology and therapy. Circulation 2000; 101:2981–2988.

62. Valentine HA, Hunt SA, Fowler MB, Billingham ME, Schroeder JS. Frequency of familial nature of dilated cardiomyopathy and usefulness of cardiac transplantation in this subset. Am J Cardiol 1989; 63:959–963.

63. Mestroni L, Miani D, DiLenarda A, et al. Clinical and pathologic study of familial dilated cardiomyopathy. Am J Cardiol 1990; 65:1449–1453.

64. Michels VV, Moll PP, Miller FA, et al. The frequency of familial dilated cardiomyopathy in a series of patients with idiopathic dilated cardiomyopathy. N Engl J Med 1992; 326:77–82.

65. Keeling PJ, McKenna WJ. Clinical genetics of dilated cardiomyopathy. Herz 1994; 19:91–96.

66. Baig MK, Goldman JH, Caforio ALP, et al. Familial dilated cardiomyopathy: cardiac abnormalities are common in asymptomatic relatives and may represent early disease. J Am Coll Cardiol 1998; 31: 195–201.

67. Grunig E, Tasman JA, Kucherer H, et al. Frequency and phenotypes of familial dilated cardiomyopathy. J Am Coll Cardiol 1998; 31:186–194.

68. Bowles NE, Towbin JA. Molecular aspects of myocarditis. Curr Infect Dis Rep 2000; 2:134–140.

69. Kasper EK, Agema WR, Hutchins GM, et al. The causes of dilated cardiomyopathy: a clinicopathologic review of 673 consecutive patients. J Am Coll Cardiol 1994; 23:586–590.

70. Towbin JA. Pediatric myocardial disease. Pediatr Clin North Am 1999; 46:289–312.

71. Towbin JA, Bowles KR, Bowles NE. Etiologies cardiomyopathy and heart failure. Nat Med 1999; 5:266–267.

72. Towbin JA. Molecular genetic aspects of cardiomyopathy. Biochem Med Metab Biol 1993; 49:285–320.

73. Berko BA, Swift M. X-linked dilated cardiomyopathy. N Engl J Med 1987; 316:1186–1191.

74. Towbin JA, Hejtmancik JF, Brink P, et al. X-linked dilated cardiomyopathy (XLCM): molecular genetic evidence of linkage to the Duchenne muscular dystrophy gene at the Xp21 locus. Circulation 1993; 87:1854–1865.

75. Muntoni F, Cau M, Ganau A, et al. Brief report: deletion of the dystrophin muscle-specific promoter region associated with X-linked dilated cardiomyopathy. N Engl J Med 1993; 329:921–925.

76. Milasin J, Muntoni F, Severini CM, et al. A point mutation in the 5′ splice site of the dystrophin gene first intron responsible for X-linked dilated cardiomyopathy. Hum Mol Genet 1996; 5:73–79.

77. Ortiz-Lopez R, Li H, Su J, Goytia V, Towbin JA. Evidence for a dystrophin missense mutation as a cause of X-linked dilated cardiomyopathy. Circulation 1997; 95:2434–2440.

78. Ferlini A, Galie N, Merlini L, et al. A novel Alu-like element rearranged in the dystrophin gene causes a splicing mutation in a family with X-linked dilated cardiomyopathy. Am J Hum Genet 1998; 63:436–460.

79. Yoshida K, Nakamura A, Yazak M, et al. Insertional mutation by transposable element, L1, in the DMD gene results in X-linked dilated cardiomyopathy. Hum Molec Med 1998; 7:1129–1132.

80. Franz W-M, Muller M, Muller AJ, et al. Association of nonsense mutation of dystrophin gene with disruption of sarcoglycan complex in X-linked dilated cardiomyopathy. Lancet 2000; 355:1781–1785.

81. Feng J, Yan J, Buzin CH, Sommer SS, Towbin JA. Comprehensive mutation scanning of the dystrophin gene in patients with nonsyndromic X-linked dilated cardiomyopathy. J Am Coll Cardiol 2002; 40:1120–1124.

82. Hoffman EP, Brown RH, Kunkel LM. Dystrophin: The protein product of the Duchenne muscular dystrophy locus. Cell 1987; 51:919–928.

83. Meng H, Leddy JJ, Frank J, Holland P, Tuana BS. The association of cardiac dystrophin with myofibrils/z-discs regions in cardiac muscle suggests a novel role in the contractile apparatus. J Biol Chem 1996; 271:12364–12371.

84. Kaprielian RR, Stevenson S, Rothery SM, Cullen MJ, Severs NJ. Distinct patterns of dystrophin organization in myocyte sarcolemma and transverse tubules of normal and diseased human myocardium. Circulation 2000; 101:2586–2594.

85. Campbell KP. Three muscular dystrophies: loss of cytoskeleton-extracellular matrix linkage. Cell 1995; 80:675–679.

86. Cox GF, Kunkel LM. Dystrophies and heart disease. Curr Opin Cardiol 1997; 12:329–343.

87. Chang WJ, Iannaccone ST, Lau KS, et al. Neuronal nitric oxide synthase and dystrophin-deficient muscular dystrophy. Proc Natl Acad Sci USA 1996; 93:9142–9147.

88. Koenig M, Hoffman EP, Bertelson CJ, et al. Complete cloning of the Duchenne muscular dystrophy (DMD) cDNA and preliminary genomic organization of the DMD gene in normal and affected individuals. Cell 1987; 50:509–517.

89. Emery AE. The muscular dystrophies. Lancet 2002; 359:687–695.

90. Klietsch R, Ervasti JM, Arnold W, Campbell KP, Jorgensen AO. Dystrophin-glycoprotein complex and laminin colocalize to the sarcolemma and transverse tubules of cardiac muscle. Circ Res 1993; 72:349–360.

91. Ozawa E, Yoshida M, Suzuki A, Mizuno Y, Hagiwara Y, Noguchi S. Dystrophin-associated proteins in muscular dystrophy. Hum Mol Genet 1995; 4:1711–1716.

92. Petrof BJ, Shrager JB, Stedman HH, Kelly AM, Sweeny HL. Dystrophin protects the sarcolemma from stresses developed during muscle contraction. Proc Natl Acad Sci USA 1993; 90:3710–3714.

93. Towbin JA. The role of cytoskeletal proteins in cardiomyopathies. Curr Opin Cell Biol 1998; 10:131–139.

94. Feng J, Yan J, Buzin CH, Towbin JA, Sommer SS. Mutations in the dystrophin gene are associated with sporadic dilated cardiomyopathy. Molec Genet Metab 2002; 77:119–126.

95. Neustein HD, Lurie PR, Dahms B, Takahashi M. An X-linked recessive cardiomyopathy with abnormal mitochondria. Pediatrics 1979; 64:24–29.

96. Barth PG, Scholte HR, Berden JA, et al. An X-linked mitochondrial disease affecting cardiac muscle, skeletal muscle and neutrophil leucocytes. J Neurol Sci 1983; 62: 327–355.

97. Kelley RI, Cheatham JP, Clark BJ, et al. X-linked dilated cardiomyopathy with neutropenia, growth retardation, and 3-methylglutaconic aciduria. J Pediatr 1991; 119:738–747.

98. Schlame M, Towbin JA, Heerdt PM, Jehle R, DiMauro S, Blanck TJJ. Deficiency of tetralinoleoyl-cardiolipin in Barth syndrome. Ann Neurol 2002; 51:634–637.

99. Vreken P, Valianpour F, Nijtmans LG, et al. Defective remodeling of cardiolipin and phosphatidyl-glycerol in Barth syndrome. Biochem Biophys Res Commun 2000; 279:378–382.

100. Schlame M, Kelley R, Feigenbaum A, et al. Phospholipid abnormalities in children with Barth syndrome. J Am Coll Cardiol 2003; 42:1994–1999.

101. Bione S, D'Adamo P, Maestrini E, Gedeon AK, Bolhuis PA, Toniolo D. A novel X-linked gene, G4.5, is responsible for Barth syndrome. Nat Genet 1996; 12:385–389.

102. Neuwald AF. Barth syndrome may be due to an acyltransferase deficiency. Curr Biol 1997; 7:R465–R466.

103. D'Adamo P, Fassone L, Gedeon A, et al. The X-linked gene G4.5 is responsible for different infantile dilated cardiomyopathies. Am J Hum Genet 1997; 61:862–867.

104. Johnston J, Kelley RI, Feigenbaum A, et al. Mutation characterization and genotype-phenotype correlation in Barth syndrome. Am J Hum Genet 1997; 61:1053–1058.

105. Bleyl SB, Mumford BR, Thompson V, et al. Neonatal, lethal noncompaction of the left ventricular myocardium is allelic with Barth syndrome. Am J Hum Genet 1997; 61:868–872.

106. Ichida F, Tsubata S, Bowles KR, et al. Novel gene mutations in patients with left ventricular noncompaction or Barth syndrome. Circulation 2001; 103:1256–1263.

107. Chen R, Tsuji T, Ichida F, et al. Mutation analysis of the G4.5 gene in patients with isolated left ventricular noncompaction. Mol Genet Metab 2002; 77:319–325.

108. Chin TK, Perloff JK, Williams RG, Jue K, Mohrmann R. Isolated noncompaction of left ventricular myocardium. A study of eight cases. Circulation 1990; 82:507–513.

109. Graber HL, Unverferth DV, Baker PB, Ryan JM, Baba N, Wooley CF. Evolution of hereditary cardiac conduction and muscle disorder:

a study involving a family with 6 generations affected. Circulation 1986; 74:21–35.

110. Tsubata S, Bowles KR, Vatta M, et al. Mutations in the human delta-sarcoglycan gene in familial and sporadic dilated cardiomyopathy. J Clin Invest 2000; 106:655–662.

111. Mohapatra B, Jimenez S, Lin JH, et al. Mutations in the muscle LIM protein and α-actinen-2 genes in dilated cardiomyopathy and endocardial fibroelastosis. Mol Genet Metab 2003; 80:207–215.

112. Olson TM, Michels VV, Thibodeau SN, Tai YS, Keating MT. Actin mutations in dilated cardiomyopathy, a heritable form of heart failure. Science 1998; 280:750–752.

113. Li D, Tapscott T, Gonzalez O, et al. Desmin mutations responsible for idiopathic dilated cardiomyopathy. Circulation 1999; 100:461–464.

114. Kamisago M, Sharma SD, DePalma SR, et al. Mutations in sarcomere protein genes as a cause of dilated cardiomyopathy. N Engl J Med 2000; 343:1688–1696.

115. Gerul B, Gramlich M, Atherton J, et al. Mutations of TTN encoding the giant muscle filament titin, cause familial dilated cardiomyopathy. Nat Genet 2002; 30:201–204.

116. Olson TM, Illenberger S, Kishimoto NY, Huttelmaier S, Keating MT, Jockusch BM. Metavinculin mutations alter actin interaction in dilated cardiomyopathy. Circulation 2002; 105:431–437.

117. Regitz-Zagrosek V, Daehmlow S, Knueppel T, et al. Novel mutations in the myosin heavy chain and myosin binding protein C gene are associated with dilated cardiomyopathy. Circulation 2001; 104(supp II):II–572.

118. Olson TM, Kishimoto NY, Whitby FG, Michels VV. Mutations that alter the surface charge of alpha-tropomyosin are associated with dilated cardiomyopathy. J Mol Cell Cardiol 2001; 33:723–732.

119. Schmitt JP, Kamisago M, Asahi M, et al. Dilated cardiomyopathy and heart failure caused by a mutation in phospholamban. Science 2003; 299:1410–1413.

120. Fatkin D, Graham RM. Molecular mechanisms of inherited cardiomyopathies. Physiol Ref 2002; 82:945–980.

121. Mogensen J, Klausen IC, Pedersen AK, et al. α-Cardiac actin is a novel disease gene in familial hypertrophic cardiomyopathy. J Clin Invest 1999; 103:R39–R43.

122. Thierfelder L, Watkins H, MacRae C, et al. α-tropomyosin and cardiac troponin T mutations cause familial hypertrophic cardiomyopathy: a disease of the sarcomere. Cell 1994; 77:701–712.

123. Geisterfer-Lowrance AA, Kass S, Tanigawa E, et al. A molecular basis for familial hypertrophic cardiomyopathy: a β-cardiac myosin heavy chain gene missense mutation. Cell 1990; 62:999–1006.

124. Coral-Vazquez R, Cohn RD, Moore SA, et al. Disruption of the sarcoglycan-sarcospan complex in vascular smooth muscle: A novel

mechanism for cardiomyopathy and muscular dystrophy. Cell 1999; 98:465–474.

125. Wheeler MT, Allikian MJ, Heydemann A, Hadhazy M, Zarnegar S, McNally EM. Smooth muscle cell-extrinsic vascular spasms arise from cardiomyocyte degeneration in sarcoglycan-deficient cardiomyopathy. J Clin Invest 2004; 113:668–675.

126. Nigro V, Okazaki Y, Belsito A, et al. Identification of the Syrian hamster cardiomyopathy gene. Hum Mol Genet 1997; 6:601–607.

127. Sakamoto A, Ono K, Abe M, et al. Both hypertrophic and dilated cardiomyopathies are caused by mutation of the same gene, delta-sarcoglycan, in hamster: an animal model of disrupted dystrophin-associated glycoprotein complex. Proc Natl Acad Sci USA 1997; 94:13873–13878.

128. Sakamoto A, Abe M, Masaki T. Delineation of genomic deletion in cardiomyopathic hamster. FEBS Lett 1999; 447:124–128.

129. Jung D, Duclos F, Apostal B, et al. Characterization of delta-sarcoglycan, a novel component of the oligomeric sarcoglycan complex involved in limb–girdle muscular dystrophy. J Biol Chem 1996; 271:32321–32329.

130. Nigro V, de Sa Moreira E, Piluso G, et al. Autosomal recessive limb–girdle muscular dystrophy, LGMD2F, is caused by a mutation in the delta-sarcoglycan gene. Nat Genet 1996; 14:195–198.

131. Maeda M, Holder E, Lowes B, Valent S, Bies RD. Dilated cardiomyopathy associated with deficiency of the cytoskeletal protein metavinculin. Circulation 1997; 95:17–20.

132. Haghighi K, Kolokathis F, Pater L, et al. Human phospholamban null results in lethal diliated cardiomyopathy revealing a critical difference between mouse and human. J Clin Invest 2003; 111:869–876.

133. Murphy RT, Mogensen J, Shaw A, et al. Novel mutation in cardiac troponin I in recessive idiopathic dilated cardiomyopathy. Lancet 2004; 363:371–372.

134. Arber S, Hunter JJ, Ross J Jr, et al. MLP-deficient mice exhibit a disruption of cardiac cytoarchitectural organization, dilated cardiomyopathy, and heart failure. Cell 1997; 88:393–403.

135. Zolk O, Caroni P, Bohm M. Decreased expression of the cardiac LIM domain protein MLP in chronic human heart failure. Circulation 2000; 101:2674–2677.

136. Katz AM. Cytoskeletal abnormalities in the failing heart. Out on a LIM? Circulation 2000; 101:2672–2673.

137. Zhou Q, Chu PH, Huang C, et al. Ablation of ipher, a PDZ-LIM domain Z-line protein, cause a severe form of congenital myopathy. J Cell Biol 2001; 155:605–612.

138. Kass S, MacRae C, Graber HL, et al. A gene defect that causes conduction system disease and dilated cardiomyopathy maps to chromosome 1p1–1q1. Nat Genet 1994; 7:546–551.

139. Jung M, Poepping I, Perrot A, et al. Investigation of a Family with autosomal dominant dilated cardiomyopathy defines a novel locus on chromosome 2q14–q22. Am J Hum Genet 1999; 65:1068–1077.

140. Olson TM, Keating MT. Mapping a cardiomyopathy locus to chromosome 3p22–p25. J Clin Invest 1996; 97:528–532.

141. Messina DN, Speer MC, Pericak-Vance MA, McNally EM. Linkage of familial dilated cardiomyopathy with conduction defect and muscular dystrophy to chromosome 6q23. Am J Hum Genet 1997; 61:909–917.

142. Fatkin D, MacRae C, Sasaki T, et al. Missense mutations in the rod domain of the lamin A/C gene as causes of dilated cardiomyopathy and conduction-system disease. N Engl J Med 1999; 34: 1715–1724.

143. Brodsky GL, Muntoni F, Miocic S, Sinagra G, Sewry C, Mestroni L. Lamin A./C gene mutation associated with dilated cardiomyopathy with variable skeletal muscle involvement. Circulation 2000; 101:473–476.

144. Stuurman N, Heins S, Aebi U. Nuclear iamins: their structure, assembly and interactions. J Struct Biol 1998; 122:42–66.

145. Bonne G, DiBarletta MR, Varnous S, et al. Mutations in the gene encoding lamin A/C cause autosomal dominant Emery–Dreifuss muscular dystrophy. Nat Genet 1999; 21:285–288.

146. Di Barletta R, Ricci E, Galluzzi G, et al. Different mutations in the LMNA gene cause autosomal dominant and autosomal recessive Emery–Dreifuss muscular dystrophy. Am J Hum Genet 2000; 66:1407–1412.

147. Muchir A, Bonne G, van der Kooi AJ, et al. Identification of mutations in the gene encoding lamin A/C in autosomal dominant limb girdle muscular dystrophy with atrioventricular conduction disturbance (LGMD1B). Hum Mol Genet 2000; 9:1453–1459.

148. Arbustini E, Pilotto A, Repetto A, et al. Autosomal dominant dilated cardiomyopathy with atrioventricular block: a lamin A/C defect related disease. J Am Coll Cardiol 2002; 39:981–990.

149. Taylor MR, Fain PR, Sinagra G, et al. Natural history of dilated cardiomyopathy due to lamin A/C gene mutations. J Am Coll Cardiol 2003; 41:771–780.

150. Novak KJ, Wattanasikichaigood D, Goebel HH, et al. Mutations in the skeletal muscle alpha-actin gene in patients with actin myopathy and nemaline myopathy. Nat Genet 1999; 23:208–212.

151. Barresi R, Di Blasi C, Negri T, et al. Disruption of heart sarcoglycan complex and severe cardiomyopathy caused by beta sarcoglycan mutations. J Med Genet 2000; 37:102–107.

152. Goldfarb LG, Park K-Y, Cervenakova L, et al. Missense mutations in desmin associated with familial cardiac and skeletal myopathy. Nat Genet 1998; 19:402–403.

153. Dalakas MC, Park K-Y, Semino-Mora C, Lee HS, Sivakumar K, Goldfarb LG. Desmin myopathy a skeletal myopathy with cardiomyopathy

caused by mutations in the desmin gene. N Engl J Med 2000; 342: 770–780.

154. Grady RM, Grange RW, Lau KS, Maimone MM, Nichol MC, Stull JT, Sanes JR. Role for α-dystrobrevin in the pathogenesis of dystrophin-dependent muscular dystrophies. Nat Cell Biol 1999; 1:215–220.

155. Araishi K, Sasaoka T, Imamura M, et al. Loss of the sarcoglycan complex and sarcospan leads to muscular dystrophy in beta-sarcoglycan-deficient mice. Hum Mol Genet 1999; 8:1589–1598.

156. Hack AA, Cordier L, Shoturma DI, Lam MY, Sweeney HL, McNally EM. Gamma-sarcoglycan deficiency leads to muscle membrane defects and apoptosis independent of dystrophin. J Cell Biol 1999; 142:1279–1287.

157. Garvey SM, Rajan C, Lerner AP, Frankel WN, Cox GA. The muscular dystrophy with myositis (mdm) mouse mutation disrupts a skeletal muscle-specific domain of titin. Genomics 2002; 79:146–149.

158. Hackman P, Vihola A, Haravuori H, et al. Tibial muscular dystrophy is a titinopathy caused by mutations in TTN, the gene encoding the grant skeletal muscle protein titin. Am J Hum Genet 2002; 71:492–500.

159. Bowles NE, Bowles KR, Towbin JA. The "Final Common Pathway" hypothesis and inherited cardiovascular disease: the role of cytoskeletal proteins in dilated cardiomyopathy. Herz 2000; 25:168–175.

160. Badorff C, Lee GH, Lamphear BJ, et al. Enteroviral protease 2A cleaves dystrophin's evidence of cytoskeletal disruption in an acquired cardiomyopathy. Nat Med 1999; 5:320–326.

161. Xiong D, Lee GH, Badorff C, et al. Dystrophin deficiency markedly increases enterovirus-induced cardiomyopathy: a genetic predisposition to viral heart disease. Nat Med 2002; 8:872–877.

162. Vatta M, Stetson SJ, Perez-Verdra A, et al. Molecular remodeling of dystrophin in patients with end-stage cardiomyopathies and reversal for patients on assist device therapy. Lancet 2000; 359:936–941.

163. Vatta M, Stetson SJ, Jimenez S, et al. Molecular normalization of dystrophin in the failing left and right ventricle of patients treated with either pulsatile or continuous flow-type ventricular assist devices. J Am Coll Cardiol 2004; 43:811–817.

164. Heart Failure Society of American (HFSA) Practice Guidelines. HFSA guildelines for management of patients with heart failure caused by left ventricular systolic dysfunction—pharmacological approaches. J Card Fail 1999; 5:357–382.

165. Gaffney TE, Braunwals EB. Importance of the adrenergic nervous system in the support of circulatory function in patients with congestive heart failure. Am J Med 1963; 34:320–324.

166. Kaye DM, Lefkovits J, Jennings GL, et al. Adverse consequences of high sympathetic nervous activity in the failing human heart. J Am Coll Cardiol 1995; 26:1257–1263.

167. Reinlib L, Abraham W. Recovery from heart failure with circulatory assist: a working group of the National Heart, Lung, and Blood Institute. J Card Fail 2003; 9:459–463.
168. Braunwald E. Expanding indications for beta-blockers in heart failure. N Engl J Med 2001; 344:1711–1712.
169. Poole-Wilson PA, Swedberg K, Cleland JFG, et al. Comparison of carvedilol and metoprolol on clinical outcomes in patients with chronic heart failure in the Carvedilol Q2 Metoprolol European Trial (COMET): randomized controlled trial. Lancet 2003; 362:7–13.
170. Konstam MA, Rousseau MF, Kroneberg MW, et al. Effects of the angiotensin converting enzyme inhibitor enalapril on the long-term progression of left ventricular dysfunction in patients with heart failure. Circulation 1992; 86:431–438.
171. Channer KS, McLean KA, Lawson-Matthew P, Richardson M. Combination diuretic treatment in severe heart failure: randomized controlled trial. Br Heart J 1994; 71:146–150.
172. Pitt B, Zannad F, Remme WJ, et al. The effect of spironolactone on morbidity and mortality in patients with severe heart failure. N Engl J Med 1999; 341:709–717.
173. Lejemtel TH, Sonnenblick EH, Frishman WH. Diagnosis and management of heart failure. In: Fuster V, Alexander RW, O'Rourke RA, eds. Hurst's The Heart. 10th eds. Chapter 21. Philadelphia: McGraw-Hill, 2001:687–724.
174. Wynn J, Braunwald E. The cardiomyopathies and myocarditides. In: Braunwald E, ed. Heart Disease: A Textbook of Cardiovascular Medicine. WB Saunders, 1997:1404–1463.
175. Berkovich S, Rodriguez-Torres R, Lin JS. Virologic studies in children with acute myocarditis. Am J Dis Child 1968; 115:207–221.
176. Dec GW, Palacios IF, Fallon JT, et al. Active myocarditis in the spectrum of acute dilated cardiomyopathies: clinical features, histologic correlates, and clinical outcome. N Engl J Med 1985; 312:885–890.
177. Martin AB, Webber S, Fricker FJ, et al. Acute myocarditis: rapid diagnosis by PCR in children. Circulation 1994; 90:330–333.
178. Bowles NE, Towbin JA. Molecular aspects of myocarditis. Curr Opin Cardiol 1998; 13:179–184.
179. Woodruff JF. Viral myocarditis: a review. Am J Pathol 1980; 101:427–484.
180. Rosenberg HS, McNamara DG. Acute myocarditis in infancy and childhood. Prog Cardiovasc Dis 1964; 7:179–197.
181. Hirschman ZS, Hammer SG. Coxsackie virus myopericarditis: a microbiological and clinical review. Am J Cardiol 1974; 34:224–232.
182. Perez, Pulido S. Acute and subacute myocarditis. Cardiovasc Rev Rep 1984; 5:912–926.
183. Karjalainen J, Nieminen MS, Heikkila J. Influenza A1 myocarditis in conscripts. Acta Med Scand 1980; 20:27–30.

184. Proby CM, Hackett S, Gupta S, Cox TM. Acute myopericarditis in influenza A infection. QJ Med 1986; 60:887–892.

185. Tiula E, Leinikki P. Fatal cytomegalovirus infection in a prevously healthy boy with myocarditis and consumption coagulopathy as a presenting sign. Scand J Infect Dis 1972; 4:57–60.

186. Schonian U, Crombach M, Maser S, Maisch B. Cytomegalovirus associated heart muscle disease. Eur Heart J 1995; 16(suppl 0):46–49.

187. Lowry PJ, Thompson RA, Littler WA. Humoral immunity in cardiomyopathy. Br Heart J 1983; 50:390–394.

188. Schowengerdt KO, Ni J, Denfield SW, et al. Parvovirus B19 infection as a cause of myocarditis and cardiac allograft rejection: diagnosis using the polymerase chain reaction (PCR). Circulation 1997; 96:3549–3554.

189. Okabe M, Fukuda K, Arakawa K, Kikuchi M. Chronic variant myocarditis associated with hepatitis C virus infection. Circulation 1997; 96:22–24.

190. Ainger LE, Lawyer NG, Fitch CW. Neonatal rubella myocarditis. Br Heart J 1966; 28:691–697.

191. Osama SM, Krishnamurti S, Gupta DN. Incidence of myocarditis in varicella. Ind Heart J 1979; 31:315–320.

192. Lorber A, Zonis A, Maisuls E, et al. The scale of myocardial involvement in varicella myocarditis. Int J Cardiol 1988; 20:257–262.

193. Chaudary S, Jaski BE. Fulminant mumps myocarditis. Ann Intern Med 1989; 110:569–570.

194. Noren GR, Adams P Jr, Anderson RC. Positive skin reactivity to mumps virus antigen in endocardial fibroelastosis. J Pediatr 1963; 62:604–606.

195. Frishman W, Kraus ME, Zabkar J, et al. Infectious mononucleosis and fatal myocarditis. Chest 1977; 72:535–538.

196. Lipshultz SE, Easley KA, Orav EJ. Left ventricular structure and function in children infected with human immunodeficiency virus. Circulation 1998; 97:1246–1256.

197. Herskowitz A, Wu T-C, Willoughby SB, et al. Myocarditis and cardiotropic viral infection associated with severe left ventricular dysfunction in late-stage infection with human immunodeficiency virus. J Am Coll Cardiol 1994; 24:1025–1032.

198. Barbaro G, Di Lorenzo G, Grisorio B, Barbarini G, for the Gruppo Italiano per Lo Studio Cardiologico dei Pazienti Affeti da AIDS. Incidence of dilated cardiomyopathy and detection of HIV in myocardial cells of HIV-positive patients. N Engl J Med 1998; 339:1093–1099.

199. Puchkov GF, Minkovich BM. A case of respiratory syncytial infection in a child by interstitial myocarditis with lethal outcome. Arkh Patol 1972; 34:70–73.

200. Stevens PJ, Underwood Ground KE. Occurrence and significance of myocarditis in trauma. Aerospace Med 1970; 41:770–780.

201. Noren GR, Staley NA, Bandt CM, Kaplan EL. Occurrence of myocarditis in sudden death in children. J Forensic Sci 1977; 22:188–196.
202. Molander N. Sudden natural death in later childhood and adolescence. Arch Dis Child 1982; 57:572–576.
203. Neuspiel DR, Kuller LH. Sudden and unexpected natural death in childhood and adolescence. J Am Med Assoc 1985; 254:1321–1325.
204. Zee-Cheng CS, Tsai CC, Palmer DC, et al. High incidence of myocarditis by endomyocardial biopsy in patients with idiopathic congestive cardiomyopathy. J Am Coll Cardiol 1984; 3:63–70.
205. Mason JW, O'Connell JB, Herskowitz A, et al. A clinical trial of immunosuppressive therapy for myocarditis. N Engl J Med 1995; 333:269–275.
206. Aretz HT, Billingham ME, Edwards WD, et al. Myocarditis: a histopathologic definition and classification. Am J Cardiovasc Pathol 1987; 1:3–14.
207. Towbin JA, Griffin LD, Martin AB, et al. Intrauterine adenoviral myocarditis presenting as non-immune hydrops fetalis: diagnosis by polymerase chain reaction. Pediatr Infect Dis J 1993; 13:144–150.
208. Van den Veyver IB, Ni J, Bowles N, et al. Detection of intrauterine viral infection using the polymerase chain reaction (PCR). Molec Genet Metab 1998; 63:85–95.
209. Friedman RA, Schowengerdt KO, Towbin JA. Myocarditis. In: Bricker JT, Garson A Jr, Fisher DJ, Neish SR, eds. The Science Practice of Pediatric Cardiology. Chapter 79. 2nd ed. Williams & Wilkins Publishers, 1998:1777–1794.
210. Grist NR, Reid D. General pathogenicity and epidemiology. In: Bendinelli M, Friedman H, eds. Coxsackieviruses: A General Update. New York: Plenum Press, 1962:241–252.
211. Sterner G. Adenovirus infections in childhood: an epidemiological and clinical survey among Swedish children. Acta Paediat 1962; 142:1–30.
212. Shimizu C, Rambaud C, Cheron G, et al. Molecular identification of viruses in sudden infant death associatied with myocarditis and pericarditis. Pedatr Infec Dis J 1995; 14:584–588.
213. Hutchins GM, Vie SA. The progression of interstitial myocarditis to idiopathic endocardial fibroelastosis. Am J Pathol 1972; 66:483–496.
214. Gardner AJS, Short D. Four faces of acute myopericarditis. Br Heart J 1973; 35:433–442.
215. Kimby AG, Sodermark T, Volpe U, Zetterquist S. Stokes–Adams attacks requiring pacemaker treatment in three patients with acute nonspecific myocarditis. Acta Med Scand 1980; 207:177–181.
216. Karjalainen J, Viitasalo M, Kala R, Heikkila J. 24-hour electrocardiographic recordings in mild acute infectious myocarditis. Ann Clin Res 1984; 16:34–39.
217. Vignola PA, Aonuma K, Swaye PS, et al. Lymphocytic myocarditis presenting as unexplained ventricular arrhythmias: diagnosis with

endomyocardial biopsy and response to immunosuppression. J Am Coll Cardiol 1984; 4:812–819.

218. Konno S, Sakakibara S. Endomyocardial biopsy. Chest 1963; 44:345–350.

219. Lurie PR, Fujita M, Neustein HB. Transvascular endomyocardial biopsy in infants and small children: description of a new technique. Am J Cardiol 1978; 42:453–457.

220. Please give details.

221. Grogan M, Redfield MM, Bailey KR, et al. Long-term outcome of patients with biopsy-proven myocarditis: comparison with idiopathic dilated cardiomyopathy. J Am Coll Cardiol 1995; 26:80–84.

222. Mason JW. Distinct forms of myocarditis. Circulation 1991; 83:1110–1111.

223. French WJ, Criley JM. Caution in the diagnosis and treatment of myocarditis. Am J Cardiol 1984; 54:445–446.

224. Hauck AJ, Kearney DL, Edwards WD. Evaluation of postmortem endomyocardial biopsy specimens from 38 patients with lymphocytic myocarditis: implication for role of sampling error. Mayo Clin Proc 1989; 64:1235–1245.

225. Chow LH, Radio SJ, Sears TD, McManus BM. Insensitivity of right ventricular biopsy in the diagnosis of myocarditis. J Am Coll Cardiol 1989; 14:915–920.

226. Lie JT. Myocarditis and endomyocardial biopsy in unexplained heart failure: a diagnosis in search of a disease [editorial]. Ann Intern Med 1988; 109:525–528.

227. Shanes JG, Ghali J, Billingham ME, et al. Inter-observer variability in the pathologic interpretation of endomyocardial biopsy results. Circulation 1987; 75:401–405.

228. Tazalaar HD, Billingham ME. Myocardial lymphocytes: fact, fancy or myocarditis? Am J Cardiovase Pathol 1986; 1:47–50.

229. Dec GW, Fallon JT, Southern JF, Palacios I. "Borderline" myocarditis: An indication for repeat endomyocardial biopsy. J Am Coll Cardiol 1990:283–289.

230. Bowles NE, Richardson PJ, Olsen EGJ, Archard LC. Detection of Coxsackie-B virus specific RNA sequences in myocardial biopsy samples from patients with myocarditis and dilated cardiomyopathy. Lancet 1986; 1:1120–1123.

231. Bowles NE, Rose ML, Taylor P. End-stage dilated cardiomyopathy: persistence of enterovirus RNA in myocardium at cardiac transplantation and lack of immune response. Circulation 1989; 80:1128–1136.

232. Archard LC, Bowles NE, Olsen EGJ, Ricardson PJ. Detection of persistent coxsackie B virus in dilated cardiomyopathy and myocarditis. Eur Heart J 1987; 8:437–440.

233. Jin O, Sole M, Butany J. Detection of enterovirus RNA in myocardial biopsies from patients with myocarditis and cardiomyopathy using

gene amplification by polymerase chain reaction. Circulation 1990; 82:8–16.

234. Hilton DA, Variend S, Pringle JH. Demonstration of coxsackie virus RNA in formalin-fixed tissue sections from childhool myocarditis by in situ hybridization and the polymerase chain reaction. J Pathol 1993; 170:45–51.

235. Archard LC, Khan MA, Soteriou BA, et al. Characterization of coxsackie B virus RNA in myocardium from patients with dilated cardiomyopathy by nucleotide sequencing of reverse transcription-nested polymerase chain reaction products. Hum Pathol 1998; 29:578–584.

236. Kyu BS, Matsumori A, Sato Y. Cardiac persistence of enteroviral RNA detected by polymerase chain reaction in a murine model of dilated cardiomyopathy. Circulation 1992; 86:522–530.

237. Griffin LD, Kearney D, Ni J, et al. Analysis of formalin-fixed and frozen myocardial autopsy samples for viral genome in childhood myocarditis and dilated cardiomyopathy with endocardial fibroelastosis using polymerase chain reaction (PCR). Cardiovasc Pathol 1995; 4:3–11.

238. Pauschinger M, Bowles NE, Fuentes-Garcia FJ, et al. Detection of adenoviral genome in the myocardium of adult patients with idiopathic left ventricular dysfunction. Circulation 1999; 99:1348–1354.

239. Lozinski GM, Davis GC, Krous HF, Billman GF, Shimizu H, Burns JC et al. Adenovirus myocarditis: retrospective, diagnosis by gene amplification from formalin-fixed, paraffin-embedded tissues. Hum Pathol 1994; 25:831–834.

240. Calabrese F, Rigo E, Milanesi O, et al. Molecular diagnosis of myocarditis and dilated cardiomyopathy in children: clinicopathologic features and prognostic implications. Diagn Mol Pathol 2002; 11:212–221.

241. Ni J, Bowles NE, Kim Y-H, et al. Viral infection of the myocardium in endocardial fibroelastosis: molecular evidence for the role of mumps virus as an etiological agent. Circulation 1997; 95:133–139.

242. Akhtar N, Ni J, Langston C, et al. PCR diagnosis of viral pneumonitis from fixed-lung tissue in children. Biochem Mol Med 1996; 58:66–76.

243. Kubota T, McTiernan CF, Frye CS, et al. Cardiospecific overexpression of tumor necrosis factor-alpha causes lethal myocarditis. J Card Fail 1997; 3:117–124.

244. Neumann DA, Lane JR, Allen GS, et al. Viral myocarditis leading to cardiomyopathy: do cytokines contribute to pathogenesis? Clin Immunol Immunopath 1993; 68:181–191.

245. Lane JR, Neumann DA, Lafond-Walker A, et al. Role of IL-I and tumor necrosis factor in coxsackie virus-induced autoimmune myocarditis. J Immunol 1993; 151:1682–1690.

246. Lane JR, Neumann DA, Lafond-Walker A, et al. Interleukin 1 or tumor necrosis factor can promote coxsackie B3-induced myocarditis in resistant B10.A mice. J Exp Med 1992; 175:1123–1129.

247. Smith SC, Allen PM. Neutralization of endogenous tumor necrosis factor ameliorates the severity of myosin-induced myocarditis. Circ Res 1992; 70:856–863.

248. Kroemer G, Martinez AC. Cytokines and autoimmune disease. Clin Immunol Immunopathol 1991; 61:275–295.

249. Huber SA. Autoimmunity in myocarditis: rlevance of animal models. Clin Immuol Immunopathol 1997; 83:93–102.

250. Henke A, Nain M, Stelzner A, et al. Induction of cytokine release from human monocytes by coxsackievirus infection. Eur Heart J 1991; 12(suppl D):134–136.

251. Gulick T, Chung MK, Pieper SJ, et al. Interleukin-1 and tumor necrosis factor inhibit cardiac myocyte β-adrenergic responsiveness. Proc Natl Acad Sci USA 1989; 86:6753–6757.

252. Torre-Amione G, Kapadia S, Lee J, et al. Tumor necrosis factor-alpha and tumor necrosis factor receptors in the failing human heart. Circulation 1996; 93:704–711.

253. Matsumori A, Yamada T, Suzuki H, et al. Increased circulating cytokines in patients with myocarditis and cardiomyopathy. Br Heart J 1994; 72:561–566.

254. Bowles NE, Vallejo J. Viral causes of cardiac inflammation. Curr Opin Cardiol 2003; 18:182–188.

255. Springer TA. Adhesion receptors of the immune system. Nature 1990; 346:425–434.

256. Seko Y, Matsuda H, Kato K, et al. Expression of intercellular adhesion molecule-1 in murine hearts with acute myocarditis caused by coxsackievirus B3. J Clin Invest 1993; 91:1327–1336.

257. Cohen JJ. Apoptosis. Immunol Today 1993; 14:126–130.

258. White E. Regulation of apoptosis by the transforming genes of the DNA tumor virus adenovirus. Proc Soc Exp Biol Med 1993; 204:30–39.

259. Strand S, Hofmann WJ, Hug H, et al. Lymphocyte apoptosis induced by CD95 (APO-1/Fas) ligand-expressing tumor cells—a mechanism of immune evasion? Nat Med 1996; 2:1361–1366.

260. Badorff C, Lee G-H, Lamphear BJ, et al. Enteroviral protease 2A cleaves dystrophin: evidence of cytoskeletal disruption in an acquired cardiomyopathy. Nat Med 1999; 5:320–326.

261. Towbin JA, Hejtmancik JF, Brink P et al. X-linked dilated cardiomyopathy (XLCM): molecular genetic evidence of linkage to the Duchenne muscular dystrophy gene at the Xp21 locus. Circulation 1993; 87:1854–1865.

262. Shapiro LM, Rozkovec A, Cambridge G, et al. Myocarditis in siblings leading to chronic heart failure. Eur Heart J 1983; 4:742–746.

263. O'Connell JB, Fowles RE, Robinson JA, et al. Clinical and pathologic findings of myocarditis in two families with dilated cardiomyopathy. Am Heart J 1984; 167:127–135.

264. Bergelson JM, Cunningham JA, Drouguett G, et al. Isolation of a common receptor for coxsackie B viruses and adenoviruses 2 and 5. Science 1997; 275:1320–1323.

265. Tomko RP, Xu R, Philipson L. HCAR and MCAR: the human and mouse cellular receptors for subgroup C adenoviruses and group B coxsackieviruses. Proc Natl Acad Sci USA 1997; 94:3352–3356.

266. Kleinert S, Weintraub RG, Wilkinson JL, Chow CW. Myocarditis in children with dilated cardiomyopathy: incidence and outcome after duel therapy immunosuppression. J Heart Lung Transplant 1997; 16:1248–1254.

267. Weller AH, Hall M, Huber SA. Polyclonal immunoglobulin therapy protects against cardiac damage in experimental coxsackievirus-induced myocarditis. Eur Heart J 1992; 13:115–119.

268. Chan KY, Iwahara M, Benson LN, et al. Immunosuppressive therapy in the management of acute myocarditis in children: a clinical trial. J Am Coll Cardiol 1991; 17:458–460.

269. Parillo JE, Cunnion RE, Epstein SE, et al. A prospective, randomized, controlled trial of prednisone for dilated cardiomyopathy. N Engl J Med 1989; 321:1061–1068.

270. Camargo PR, Snitcowsky R, da Luz PL, Mazzieri R, Higuchi ML, Rati M, Stolf N, Ebaid M, Pileggi F. Favorable effects of immunosuppressive therapy in children with dilated cardiomyopathy and active myocarditis. Pediatr Cardiol 1995; 16:61–68.

271. 'Wojnicz R, Nowalany-Kozielska E, Wojciechowska C, Glanowska G, Eilczewski P, Niklewski T, Zembala M, Polonski L, Rozek MM, Wodniecki J. Randomized, placebo-controlled study for immunosuppressive treatment of inflammatory dilated cardiomyopathy: two-year follow-up results. Circulation 2001; 104:4–6.

272. Drucker NA, Colan SD, Lewis AB, et al. α-globulin treatment of acute myocarditis on the pediatric population. Circulation 1994; 89:52–257.

273. Marcus FI, Fontaine G, Guiraudon G, et al. Right ventricular dysplasia. A report of 24 adult cases. Circulation 1982; 65:384–398.

274. Corrado D, Basso C, Thiene G, et al. Spectrum of clinicopathologic manifestations of arrhythmogenic right ventricular cardiomyopathy/dysplasia: a multicenter study. J Am Coll Cardiol 1997; 30:1512–1520.

275. Thiene G, Nava A, Corrado D, Rossi L, Pennelli N. Right ventricular cardiomyopathy and sudden death in young people. N Engl J Med 1988; 318:129–133.

276. McKenna WJ, Thiene G, Nava A, et al. Diagnosis of arrhythmogenic right ventricular dysplasia/cardiomyopathy. Br Heart J 1994; 71:215–218.

277. Corrado D, Basso C, Buja G, et al. Right bundle branch block, right precordial ST-segment elevation, and sudden death in young people. Circulation 2001; 103:710–717.

278. Tabib A, Loire R, Chalabreysse L, et al. Circumstances of death and gross and microscopic observations in a series of 200 cases of sudden death associated with arrhythmogenic right ventricular cardiomyopathy and/or dysplasia. Circulation 2003; 108:3000–3005.

279. Bluemke DA, Krupinski EA, Ovitt T, Gear K, Unger E, Axel L, Boxt LM, Casolo G, Ferrari VA, Funski B, Globits S, Higgins CB, Julsrud P, Lipton M, Mawson J, Nygren A, Pennell DJ, Stillman A, White RD, Wichter T, Marcus F. MR Imaging of arrhythmogenic right ventricular cardiomyopathy: morphologic findings and interobserver reliability. Cardiology 2003; 99:153–162.

280. Corrado D, Leoni L, Link MS, et al. Implantable cardioverter-defibrillator therapy for prevention of sudden death in patients with arrhythmogenic right ventricular cardiomyopathy/dysplasia. Circulation 2003; 108:3084–3091.

281. Nava A, Thiene G, Canciani B, et al. Familial occurrence of right ventricular dysplasia: a study involving nine families. J Am Coll Cardiol 1988; 12:1222–1228.

282. Coonar AS, Protonotarios N, Tsatsopoulou A, et al. Gene for arrhythmogenic right ventricular cardiomyopathy with diffuse nonepidermolytic palmoplantar keratoderma and wooly hair (Naxos disease) maps to 17q21. Circulation 1998; 97:2049–2058.

283. Carvajal-Huerta L. Epidermolytic palmoplantar keratoderma with woolly hair and dilated cardiomyopathy. J Am Acad Dermatol 1998; 44:309–311.

284. Rampazzo A, Nava A, Danieli GA, et al. The gene for arrhythmogenic right ventricular cardiomyopathy maps to chromosome 14q23–q24. Hum Mol Genet 1994; 3:959–962.

285. Rampazzo A, Nava A, Erne P, et al. A new locus for arrhythmogenic right ventricular cardiomyopathy (ARVD2) maps to chromosome 1q42–q43. Hum Mol Genet 1995; 4:2151–2154.

286. Severini GA, Krajinovic M, Pinamonti B, et al. A new locus for arrhythmogenic right ventricular dysplasia on the long arm of chromosome 14. Genomics 1996; 31:193–200.

287. Rampazzo A, Nava A, Miorin M, et al. A new locus for arrhythmogenic right ventricular cardiomyopathy (ARVD4) maps to chromosome 2q32. Genomics 1997; 45:259–263.

288. Li D, Ahmad F, Gardner MJ, et al. The locus of a novel gene responsible for arrhythmogenic right ventricular dysplasia characterized by early onset and high penetrance maps to chromosome 10p12–p14. Am J Hum Genet 2000; 66:148–156.

289. Ahmad F, Li D, Karibe A, et al. Localization of a gene responsible for arrhythmogenic right ventricular dysplasia to chromosome 3p23. Circulation 1998; 98:2791–2795.

290. McKoy G, Protonotarios N, Cosby A, et al. Identification of a deletion in plakoglobin in arrhythmogenic right ventricular cardiomyopathy with palmoplantar keratoderma and woolly hair (Naxos disease). Lancet 2000; 355:2119–2124.

291. Norgett EE, Hatsell SJ, Carvajal-Huerta L, et al. Recessive mutation in desmoplakin disrupts desmoplakin-intermediate filament interactions and causes dilated cardiomyopathy, woolly hair and ketatoderma. Hum Mol Genet 2000; 9:2761–2766.

292. Tiso N, Stephan DA, Nava A, et al. Identification of mutations in the cardiac ryanodine receptor gene in families with arrhythmogenic right ventricular cardiomyopathy type 2 (ARVD2). Hum Mol Genet 2001; 10:189–194.

293. Priori SG, Napolitano C, Tiso N, et al. Mutations in the cardiac ryanodine receptor gene (hRyR2) underlie catecholaminergic polymorphic ventricular tachycardia. Circulation 2001; 103:196–200.

294. Vatta M, Li H, Towbin JA. Molecular biology of arrhythmic syndromes. Curr Opin Cardiol 2000; 15:12–22.

295. Towbin JA. Cardiac arrhythmias: the genetic connection. J Cardiovasc Electrophysiol 2000; 11:601–602.

296. Rampazzo A, Nava A, Malacride S, et al. Mutation in human desmoplakin domain binding to plakaglobin causes a dominant form of arrhythmogenic right ventricular cardiomyopathy. Am J Hum Genet 2002; 71:1200–1206.

297. Bowles NE, Ni J, Marcus F, Towbin JA. The detection of cardiotropic viruses in the myocardium of patients with arrhythmogenic right ventricular dysplasia/cardiomyopathy. J Am Coll Cardiol 2002; 39:892–895.

298. Grumbach IM, Heim A, Vonhof S, et al. Coxsackievirus genome in myocardium of patients with arrhythmogenic right ventricular dysplasia/cardiomyopathy. Cardiology 1998; 89:241–245.

299. Wigle ED, Sasson Z, Henderson MA, et al. Hypertrophic cardiomyopathy. The importance of the site and the extent of hypertrophy. A review. Prog Cardiovasc Dis 1985; 28:1–83.

300. Maron BJ. Hypertrophic cardiomyopathy: a systemic review. JAMA 2002; 287:1308–1320.

301. Maron BJ, Gardin JM, Flack JM, et al. Prevalence of hypertrophic cardiomyopathy in a general population of young adults. Echocardiographic analysis of 411 subjects in the CARDIA study. Circulation 1995; 92:785–789.

302. Ommen SR, Nishimura RA. Hypertrophic cardiomyopathy. Curr Probl Cardiol 2004; 29:239–291.

303. Vulpian A. Contribution à l'étude des rétrécissements de l'orifice ventriculo-aortique. Arch Physiol 1868; 3:220–222.

304. Watkins H. Genetic clues to disease pathways in hypertrophic and dilated cardiomyopathies. Circulation 2003; 107:1344–1346.
305. Towbin JA, Lipshultz SE. Genetics of neonatal cardiomyopathy. Curr Opin Cardiol 1999; 14:250–262.
306. Moolman JC, Corfield VA, Posen G, et al. Sudden death due to troponin T mutations. J Am Coll Cardiol 1997; 29:549–555.
307. Watkins H, McKenna WJ, Thierfelder L, et al. Mutaitons in the genes for cardiac troponin T and α-tropomyosin in hypertrophic cardiomyopathy. N Engl J Med 1995; 332:1058–1064.
308. Kimura A, Harada H, Park JE, et al. Mutations in the cardiac troponin I gene associated with hypertrophic cardiomyopathy. Nat Genet 1997; 16:379–382.
309. Olson TM, Doan TP, Kishimoto NY, et al. Inherited and de novo mutations in the cardiac actin gene cause hypertrophic cardiomyopathy. J Mol Cell Cardiol 2000; 32:1687–1694.
310. Poetter K, Jiang H, Hassanzadeh S, et al. Mutations in either the essential or regulatory light chains of myosin are associated with a rare myopathy in human heart and skeletal muscle. Nat Genet 1996; 13:63–69.
311. Gollob MH, Green MS, Tang ASL, et al. Identification of a gene responsible for familial Wolff–Parkinson–White syndrome. N Engl J Med 2001; 344:1823–1831.
312. Blair E, Redwood C, Ashrafian H, et al. Mutations in the α2 subunit of AMP-activated protein kinase cause familial hypertrophic cardiomyopathy: evidence for a central role of energy compromise in disease pathogenesis. Hum Mol Genet 2001; 10:1215–1220.
313. McKenna WJ, Behr ER. Hypertrophic cardiomyopathy: management, risk stratification, and prevention of sudden death. Heart 2002; 87:169–176.
314. Frenneaux MP. Assessing the risk of sudden cardiac death in a patient with hypertrophic cardiomyopathy. Heart 2004; 90: 570–575.
315. Nimura H, Bachinski LL, Sangwatanaroj S, et al. Mutations in the gene for cardiac myosin-binding protein C and late-onset familial hypertrophic cardiomyopathy. N Engl J Med 1998; 338: 1248–1257.
316. Maron BJ, Carney KP, Lever HM, Lewis JF, Barac I, Casey SA, Sherrid MV. Relationship of race to sudden cardiac death in competitive athletes with hypertrophic cardiomyopathy. J Am Coll Cardiol 2003; 41:974–980.
317. Vikstrom KL, Leinwand LA. Contractile protein mutations and heart disease. Curr Opin Cell Biol 1996; 8:97–105.
318. Watkins H, Rosenweig A, Hwang DS, et al. Characteristics and prognostic implications of myosin missense mutations in familial hypertrophic cardiomyopathy. N Engl J Med 1992; 326:1108–1114.

319. Jarcho JA, McKenna W, Pare JAP, et al. Mapping a gene for familial hypertrophic cardiomyopathy to chromosome 14q1. N Engl J Med 1989; 321:1372–1378.
320. Solomon SD, Jarcho JA, McKenna WJ, et al. Familial hypertrophic cardiomyopathy is a genetically heterogeneous disease. J Clin Invest 1990; 86:993–999.
321. Watkins H, MacRae C, Thierfelder L, et al. A disease locus for familial hypertrophic cardiomyopathy maps to chromosome 1q3. Nat Genet 1993; 3:333–337.
322. Thierfelder L, MacRae C, Watkins H, et al. A familial hypertrophic cardiomyopathy locus maps to chromosome 15q2. Proc Natl Acad Sci USA 1993; 90:6270–6274.
323. Carrier L, Hengstenberg C, Beckmann JS, et al. Mapping of a novel gene for familial hypertrophic cardiomyopathy to chromosome 11. Nature Genet 1993; 4:311–313.
324. MacRae CA, Ghaisas N, Kass S, et al. Familial hypertrophic cardiomyopathy with Wolff–Parkinson–White Syndrome maps to a locus on chromosome 7q3. J Clin Invest 1995; 96:1216–1220.
325. Poetter K, Jiang H, Hassanzadeh S, et al. Mutation in either the essential regulatory light chains of myosin are associated with a rare myopathy in human heart and skeletal muscle. Nat Genet 1996; 13:63–69.
326. Kimura A, Harada H, Park JE, et al. Mutations in the cardiac troponin I gene associated with hypertrophic cardiomyopathy. Nature Genet 1997; 16:379–382.
327. Mogensen J, Klausen IC, Pederson AK, et al. α-Cardiac actin is a novel disease gene in familial hypertrophic cardiomyopathy. J Clin Invest 1999; 103:T39–R43.
328. Schiaffino S, Reggiani C. Molecular diversity of myofibrillar proteins: gene regulation and functional significance. Physiol Rev 1996; 76:371–423.
329. Geier C, Perrot A, Ozcelik C, et al. Mutations in the human muscle LIM protein gene in families with hypertrophic cardiomyopathy. 2003.
330. Blair E, Redwood C, de Jesus Oliveira M, et al. Mutations of the light meromyosin domain of the β-myosin heavy chain rod in hypertrophic cardiomyopathy. Circ Res 2002; 90:263–269.
331. Hofmann PA, Hartzell HC, Moss RL. Alterations in Ca^{2+} sensitive tension due to partial extraction of C-protein from rat skinned cardiac myocytes and rabbit skeletal muscle fibers. J Gen Physiol 1991; 97:1141–1163.
332. Lees-Miller JP, Helfman DM. The molecular basis for tropomyosin isoform diversity. Bioessays 1991; 13:429–437.
333. Mesnard L, Logeart D, Taviaux S, Diriong S, Mercadier JJ, Samson F. Human cardiac troponin T: cloning and expression of new isoforms in the normal and failing heart. Circ Res 1995; 76:687–692.

334. Townsend P, Barton P, Yacoub M, Farza H. Molecular cloning of human cardiac troponin T isoforms: expression in developing and failing heart. J Mol Cell Cardiol 1995; 27:2223–2236.

335. Hunkeler NM, Kullman J, Murphy AM. Troponin I isoform expression in human heart. Circ Res 1991; 69:1409–1414.

336. Watkins H, Rosenzweig T, Hwang DS, et al. Characteristic and prognostic implications of myosin missense mutations in familial hypertrophic cardiomyopathy. N Engl J Med 1992; 326:1106–1114.

337. Moolman JC, Corfield VA, Posen B, et al. Sudden death due to troponin T mutations. J Am Coll Cardiol 1997; 29:549–555.

338. Nakajima-Taniguchi C, Matsui H, Fujio Y, et al. Novel missense mutation in cardiac troponin T gene found in Japanese patient with hypertrophic cardiomyopathy. J Mol Cell Cardiol 1997; 29:839–843.

339. Bonne G, Carrier L, Bercovici J, et al. Cardiac myosin binding protein-C gene splice acceptor site mutation is associated with familial hypertrophic cardiomyopathy. Nat Genet 1995; 11:438–440.

340. Watkins H, Conner D, Thierfelder L, et al. Mutations in the cardiac myosin binding protein-C gene on chromosome 11 cause familial hypertrophic cardiomyopathy. Nature Genet 1995; 11:434–437.

341. Nimura H, Bachinski LL, Sangwatanaroh S, et al. Mutations in the gene for cardiac myosin-binding protein C and late-onset familial hypertrophic cardiomyopathy. N Engl J Med 1998; 33:1248–1257.

342. Charron P, Dubourg O, Desnos M, et al. Clinical features and prognostic implications of familial hypertrophic cardiomyopathy related to cardiac myosin binding protein C gene. Circulation 1998; 97:2230–2236.

343. Van Driest SL, Ackerman MJ, Ommen SR, et al. Prevalence and severity of "benign" mutations in the β-myosin heavy chain, cardiac troponin T, and α-tropomyosin genes in hypertrophic cardiomyopathy. Circulation 2002; 106:3085–3090.

344. Yonega K, Okamoto H, Machida M, et al. Angiotensin-converting enzyme gene polymorphism in Japanese patients with hypertrophic cardiomyopathy. Am Heart J 1995; 130:1089–1093.

345. Tesson F, Dufour C, Moolman JC, et al. The influence of the angiotensin I converting enzyme genotype in familial hypertrophic cardiomyopathy varies with the disease gene mutation. J Mol Cell Cardiol 1997; 29:831–838.

346. Ortlepp JR, Vosberg HP, Reith S, Ohme F, Mahon NG, Schroder D, Klues HG, Hanrath P, McKenna WJ. Genetic polymorphisms in the rennin–angiotensin–aldosterone system associated with expression of left ventricular hypertrophy in hypertrophic cardiomyopathy: a study of five polymorphic genes in a family with a disease causing mutation in the myosin binding protein C gene. Heart 2002; 87:270–275.

347. Doiuchi J, Hamada M, Ito T, Kokubu T. Comparative effects of calcium-channel blockers and beta-adrenergic blocker on early diastolic time intervals and A-wave ratio in patients with hypertrophic cardiomyopathy. Clin Cardiol 1987; 10:26–30.

348. Lorell BH. Use of calcium channel blockers in hypertrophic cardiomyopathy. Am J Med 1985; 78:43–54.

349. Moran AM, Colan SD. Verapamil therapy in infants with hypertrophic cardiomyopathy. Cardiol Young 1998; 8:310–319.

350. Nagueh SF, Ommen SR, Lakkis NM, Killip D, Zoghbi WA, Schaff HV, Danielson GK, Quinones MA, Tajik AJ, Spencer WH. J Am Coll Cardiol 2001; 38:1701–1706.

351. O'Rourke RA. Cardiac pacing. An alternative treatment for selected patients with hypertrophic cardiomyopathy and adjunctive therapy for certain patients with dilated cardiomyopathy. Circulation 1999; 100:786–788.

352. Maron BJ. Appraisal of dual-chamber pacing therapy in hypertrophic cardiomyopathy: too soon for a rush to judgment?. J Am Coll Cardiol 1996; 27:431–432.

353. Begley D, Mohiddin S, Fananapazir L. Dual chamber pacemaker therapy for mid-cavity obstructive hypertrophic cardiomyopathy. Pacing Clin Electrophysiol 2001; 24:1639–1644.

354. Chang SM, Lakkis NM, Franklin J, Spencer WH III, Nagueh SF. Predictors of outcome after alcohol septal ablation therapy in patients with hypertrophic obstructive cardiomyopathy. Circulation 2004; 109:824–827.

355. Nielsen CD, Killip D, Spencer WH III. Nonsurgical septal reduction therapy for hypertrophic obstructive cardiomyopathy: short-term results in 50 consecutive procedures. Clin Cardiol 2003; 26:275–279.

356. Park TH, Lakkis NM, Middleton KJ, Franklin J, Zoghbi WA, Quinones MA, Spencer WH III, Nagueh SF. Acute effect of nonsurgical septal reduction therapy on regional left ventricular asynchrony in patients with hypertrophic obstructive cardiomyopathy. Circulation 2002; 106:412–415.

357. Maron BJ. Hypertrophic cardiomyopathy and sudden death: new perspective on risk stratification and prevention with the implantable cardioverter-defibrillator. Eur Heart J 2000; 21:1979–1983.

358. Tam JW, Shaikh N, Sutherland E. Echocardiographic assessment of patients with hypertrophic and restrictive cardiomyopathy: imaging and echocardiography. Curr Opin Cardiol 2002; 17:470–477.

359. Rivenes SM, Towbin JA, Gajarski RJ, Price JK, Denfield SW. Sudden death and cardiovascular collapse in children with restrictive cardiomyopathies. Circulation 2000; 102:876–882.

360. Cetta F, O'Leary PW, Seward JB, Driscoll DJ. Idiopathic restrictive cardiomyopathy in childhood: diagnostic features and clinical course. Mayo Clin Proc 1995; 70:634–640.

361. Gewillig M, Mertens L, Moerman P, Dumoulin M. Idiopathic restrictive cardiomyopathy in childhood: a diastolic disorder characterized by delayed relaxation. Eur Heart J 1996; 17:1413–1420.

362. Denfield SW. Sudden death in children with restrictive cardiomyopathy. Card Electrophysiol Rev 2002; 6:163–167.

363. Chen SC, Balfour IC, Jureidini S. Clinical spectrum of restrictive cardiomyopathy in children. J Heart Lung Transplant 2001; 20: 90–92.

364. Lewis AB. Clinical profile and outcome of restrictive cardiomyopathy in children. Am Heart J 1992; 123:1589–1593.

365. Mogensen J, Kubo T, Duque M, Uribe W, Shaw A, Murphy R, Gimeno JR, Elliott P, McKenna WJ. Idiopathic restrictive cardiomyopathy is part of the clinical expression of cardiac troponin I mutations. J Clin Invest 2003; 111:209–216.

366. Perles Z, Bowles NE, Vatta M, Jimenez S, Szmuszkovicz J, Capetanaki Y, Towbin JA. Familial restrictive cardiomyopathy caused by a missense mutation in the desmin gene: possible role of apoptosis in disease pathogenesis. J Am Coll Cardiol 2002; 39:45A.

367. Wang X, Osinska H, Dorn GW II, Nieman M, Lorenz JN, Gerdes AM, Witt S, Kimball T, Gulick J, Robbins J. Circulation :2402–2407.

368. Wang X, Osinska H, Gerdes AM, Robbins J. Desmin filaments and cardiac disease: establishing causality. J Card Fail 2002; 8(6 suppl):S287–S292.

369. Mavroidis M, Capetanaki Y. Extensive induction of important mediators of fibrosis and dystrophic calcification in desmin-deficient cardiomyopathy. Am J Pathol 2002; 160:943–952.

370. Jacobson DR, Pan T, Kyle RA, Buxbaum JN. Transthyretin ILE20, a new variant associated with late-onset cardiac amyloidosis. Hum Mutat 1997; 9:83–85.

371. Hattori T, Takei Y, Koyama J, Nakazato M, Ikeda S. Clinical and pathological studies of cardiac amyloidosis in transthyretin type familial amyloid polyneuropathy. Amyloid 2003; 10:229–239.

372. Stollberger C, Finsterer J, Blazek G. Left ventricular hypertrabeculation/noncompaction and association with additional cardiac abnormalities and neuromuscular disorders. Am J Cardiol 2002; 90:899–902.

373. Stollberger C, Finsterer J. Left ventricular hypertrabeculation/noncompaction. J Am Soc Echocardiogr 2004; 17:91–100.

374. Chin TK, Perloff JK, Williams RG, Jue K, Mohrmann R. Isolated noncompaction of left ventricular myocardium. A study of eight cases. Circulation 1990; 82:507–513.

375. Ichida F, Tsubata S, Bowles KR, Haneda N, Uese K, Miyawaki T, Dreyer WJ, Messina J, Li H, Bowles NE, Towbin JA. Novel gene mutations in patients with left ventricular noncompaction or Barth syndrome. Circulation 2001; 103:1256–1263.

376. Chen Q, Kirsch GE, Zhang D, Brugada R, Brugada J, Brugada P, Potenza D, Moya A, Borggrefe M, Breithardt G, Ortiz-Lopez R, Wang Z, Antzelevitch C, O'Brien RE, Schultz-Bahr E, Towbin JA, Wang Q. Genetic basis and molecular mechanisms for idiopathic ventricular fibrillation. Nature 1998; 392:293–296.

10

Inflammatory Causes of Pediatric Heart Failure: Rheumatic Fever, Rheumatic Heart Disease, and Kawasaki Disease

LLOYD Y. TANI and ROBERT E. SHADDY

Division of Pediatric Cardiology, Primary
Children's Medical Center, University of Utah
School of Medicine, Salt Lake City, Utah, U.S.A.

RHEUMATIC FEVER

Rheumatic fever (RF) is a poststreptococcal inflammatory illness with multiorgan involvement commonly affecting the joints, brain, heart, or skin. Although most of the manifestations are self-limiting and resolve without sequelae, cardiac changes may persist and account for the majority of the morbidity and mortality associated with the acute illness. Acute rheumatic carditis varies in severity from very mild to severe

371

cases with significant acute mitral and/or aortic regurgitation resulting in heart failure. Of all patients with acute RF, severe carditis resulting in signs and symptoms of heart failure occurs in 13–64%, depending on the series reported and whether patients with recurrences are included (Table 1) (1–10). The acute rheumatic cardiac involvement may resolve or persist and evolve as chronic rheumatic valvular disease, with heart failure developing years after the initial episode in some cases (11).

Scope of the Problem

Worldwide, it has been estimated that 12 million people are affected by RF and rheumatic heart disease (RHD), with 400,000 deaths annually (12). Rheumatic fever is the most common cause of acquired cardiac disease in children in developing countries of the world (12–17) where the incidence has been reported as high as 100–200 per 100,000 (12,16,17). In these countries, RF and RHD account for 30–40% of all cardiac admissions (14,18) and the estimated prevalence of RHD ranges from 4.9 to 30 million with a mortality rate of 0.9–8.0 per 100,000 population (12,19,20). In contrast to industrialized countries, the initial episode of RF in developing countries occurs at a younger age, and often goes unnoticed. In fact, in some settings, more than 50% of patients are unaware of their disease and as many as 70% do not receive prophylaxis against recurrences (12), leading to a greater likelihood of chronic RHD. In these settings, chronic RHD occurs earlier, evolves more rapidly, and is of greater severity, eventually leading to heart failure with its associated morbidity and mortality (14,21–24). The cost of hospitalizations, the negative impact on work and productivity, the significant resources required to care for affected patients, and the patient suffering associated with RF and RHD remain high (25,26).

Compared with developing countries, the incidence of RF in industrialized countries is much lower and has been estimated at 0.5–3 per 100,000 population (27,28). In fact, the incidence of RF was so low during the 1960s and 1970s that the disease was thought to have "virtually disappeared"

Table 1 Rheumatic Fever, Carditis, and Heart Failure

Series (reference)	Years	Number of RF cases	Carditis (n)(%)	RF with CHF (n)(%)	Carditis with CHF (%)	Included recurrences
Giannoulia-Karantana et al.(1)	1980–1997	66	69.7 (46)	10.6 (7)	15.2	No
Sanyal et al.(10)	1967–1971	102	33.3 (34)	11.8 (12)	35.2	No
Ravisha et al.(6)	1971–2001	250	42.0 (105)	12.4 (31)	29.5	No
Feinstein et al.(4)	1950–1957	271	47.6 (129)	11.4 (31)	24.0	No
Bland and Jones(5)	1921–1931	1000	65.3 (653)	20.7 (207)	31.7	Not stated
Veasy et al.(3)	1985–1992	274	68.2 (187)	13.1 (36)	19.3	10%
Bitar et al.(2)	1980–1995	91	93.4 (85)	44.0 (40)	47.1	45%
Joshi et al.(9)	Not stated	337	74.2 (250)	41.8 (141)	56.4	Yes, many
Mota and Meira (8)	1976–1994	715	55.2 (395)	29.1 (208)	52.7	Yes, many
Chagani and Aziz (7)	1991–1994	104	96.1 (100)	31.7 (33)	33.0	All recurrences
Feinstein et al.(4)	1950–1957	170	51.2 (87)	25.9 (44)	50.6	All recurrences
Ravisha et al.(6)	1971–2001	224	79.5 (178)	63.8 (143)	80.3	All recurrences

by the early 1980s (29). However, in the mid-1980s, several sites around the United States reported focal outbreaks or resurgences of RF activity (30–35) and by 1988, a survey of pediatric cardiologists revealed an increased incidence of RF in 24 states (36).

Etiology and Pathogenesis

Although the relationship to a preceding streptococcal pharyngitis has been established and is well accepted, the pathogenesis of RF is still not completely understood. Complex interactions between the organism, the host, and the environment influence its occurrence.

Only pharyngitis caused by certain strains of group A streptococci lead to RF. Specifically, certain M types and heavily encapsulated or mucoid strains are more likely to lead to RF and are considered rheumatogenic (37–41). It has been estimated that 0.3% (during nonepidemic) to 3% (during streptococcal epidemics) of individuals who have not had RF will develop the illness following an untreated symptomatic or asymptomatic streptococcal pharyngitis. It is important to emphasize the fact that RF may follow a very mild or even asymptomatic streptococcal pharyngitis (3,30).

Rheumatic fever occurs approximately 1–5 weeks following a group A streptococcal pharyngitis in a susceptible host. Children between the ages of 5 and 15 years are most commonly affected, and with the exception that chorea is more common in girls, there is no gender predisposition (42–45). A number of sources support the importance of host factors in the pathogenesis of RF. First, only a small minority of patients with streptococcal pharyngitis develops RF, even during streptococcal epidemics. Second, the incidence of recurrent RF in patients with a previous history of RF with cardiac involvement is as high as 50% following a group A streptococcal pharyngitis (46–48). Third, studies indicate a familial incidence, a higher concordance rate between identical as compared to fraternal twins, and a higher incidence of RF in some ethnicities (Maori's and Samoans) (49–52). Last, although some have reported associations between human leukocyte antigen (HLA) subgroups and RF (53–56), consistent associations in different populations have not been found. Recently, a specific B cell alloantigen detected by monoclonal antibody has been reported to occur much more commonly in patients with RF than in the general population (57,58).

The environment and living conditions also play an important role in the pathogenesis of RF. Both RF and RHD continue to be major problems in developing countries where poverty, crowded living conditions, poor hygiene, and poor access to medical care are common (59,60). In fact, the reduction in the incidence of RF in the United States has been attributed in part to improved living conditions since the decline began before the introduction of penicillin (61).

Although RF follows group A streptococcal pharyngitis, the organism has not been isolated from any of the organ systems of affected individuals. Several studies have shown the immune response of affected individuals to be abnormal and important in the pathogenesis of RF. These findings have led to the hypothesis that the streptococcal breakdown products show molecular mimicry and are immunologically cross-reactive with host tissues, resulting in a humoral and cellular autoimmune response leading to tissue inflammation and damage in a susceptible host (62–67).

The prognosis and natural history of rheumatic carditis and heart disease is strongly influenced by the severity of the cardiac involvement that occurs with the initial RF illness as well as the number of recurrences (4,5,68–70). Mild carditis without recurrences is much more likely to show resolution than severe initial carditis and/or cases with recurrent episodes of RF. Both the severity of the initial carditis as well as the frequency and severity of recurrences are affected by the use of penicillin. The proportion of patients with RF who develop chronic RHD has decreased from 60% to 90% during the prepenicillin era to 35–65% (4,5,68,71,72). In industrialized countries, penicillin use decreased mortality attributed to rheumatic carditis from 8% to 30% to nearly 0 (61,71,73). In contrast, the mortality rate in developing countries continues to be significant for several reasons. Inadequate secondary prophylaxis results in recurrent episodes of RF and more severe RHD (9,14,23). Gender also influences prognosis, as acute rheumatic cardiac involvement resolves more frequently in boys (4,68). Finally, children presenting with RF before 5 years of age have more severe cardiac involvement and more commonly have persistent chronic RHD (74,75).

Diagnosis and Evaluation

Since there is no pathognomonic test, the diagnosis of RF is made using the modified Jones criteria. First proposed by Jones over 60 years ago in 1944 (76), these criteria have undergone four revisions or modifications, the latest in 1992 (77–81). The latest updated Jones criteria are intended to be used to establish the initial attack of acute RF and not for diagnosing recurrences (Table 2). The diagnosis of RF requires two major, or one major and two minor Jones criteria along with evidence of a preceding streptococcal infection. The major criteria are polyarthritis, carditis, chorea, a characteristic rash called erythema marginatum, and subcutaneous nodules. The minor criteria are fever, arthralgia, elevated acute phase reactants, and a prolonged PR interval on the electrocardiogram (ECG) (Table 2). The latest update allows the diagnosis of RF to be made without fulfilling the

Table 2   Updated Jones Criteria for Diagnosis of Rheumatic Fever

Major criteria	Minor criteria
Carditis	Fever
Chorea	Arthralgia
Polyarthritis	Elevated acute phase reactants
Erythema marginatum	Erythrocyte sedimentation rate
Subcutaneous nodules	C-reactive protein
	Prolonged PR interval (ECG)

Supporting evidence of antecedent group A streptococcal infection
   Positive throat culture or rapid streptococcal test
   Elevated or rising streptococcal antibody titer

Criteria for diagnosis: two major or one major and two minor criteria PLUS evidence of preceding streptococcal infection.

above criteria in patients who present with isolated chorea, indolent carditis (usually mitral regurgitation), or a prior history of RF or RHD (79).

Of the major Jones criteria, arthritis is most common, affecting 50–70% of cases. Classically a migratory polyarthritis involving the large joints (knees, ankles, elbows, and wrists), it is noteworthy that in some parts of the world, monoarthritis is a common mode of presentation (82). Even untreated, this polyarthritis usually resolves within 3 weeks and is not associated with residual abnormalities. Unfortunately, although arthritis is the most common major criteria, it is also the least definitive. The Jones criteria often fail to exclude other causes of febrile polyarthritis (43), and an alternative diagnosis may be made over the course of time as more chronic findings develop (i.e., chronic, recurrent arthritis). Although carditis and arthritis commonly occur together, the severity of the joint and heart involvement are inversely related (4). It is possible that joint involvement leads to earlier medical attention and initiation of anti-inflammatory treatment, thus preventing more severe cardiac involvement.

Patients may present with Sydenham chorea (15–30%), which is characterized by involuntary, purposeless movements, muscular incoordination and/or weakness, and emotional lability (43,44,83). These symptoms, which decrease with rest and sedation and increase with effort or excitement, resolve over a median of 15 weeks, and by 6 months in 75% of cases (84). The latency between the streptococcal pharyngitis and the onset of chorea is longer than for arthritis or carditis, ranging from 1 to 6 months. Because of this longer latency period, arthritis and chorea do not occur simultaneously in affected patients. When carditis and chorea are found in the same patient, it is often the chorea that prompts medical attention at which time rheumatic cardiac involvement is detected. Although the combination of chorea and carditis is common, occurring in 47% of patients with RF in a recent series (3), the cardiac involvement tends to be relatively mild and heart failure is uncommon (45). Even patients with "pure" chorea are at risk, however, as 20–44% of such patients go on to develop chronic RHD that may eventually result in heart failure (5,85–87).

Skin manifestations include a serpiginous, evanescent, erythematous, macular, mainly truncal rash called erythema marginatum and small painless subcutaneous nodules appearing on extensor surfaces are included in the Jones criteria; both are uncommon and almost always occur with carditis and/or arthritis (43,88).

Carditis, the only Jones criteria associated with long-term morbidity and mortality, occurs in 30–70% of initial RF illnesses. Despite traditionally being described as a pancarditis, the dominant and most important abnormality with acute rheumatic cardiac involvement is the valvulitis, specifically mitral and/or aortic regurgitation. The clinical presentation is quite variable, ranging from the asymptomatic patient with a characteristic heart murmur to a critically ill patient presenting in heart failure. Severe carditis and heart failure occur in 13–64% of RF cases and represent 15–80% of patients with carditis (Table 1) (1–8). Rheumatic carditis remains the major cause of acquired heart disease in children and young adolescents in developing countries. Approximately 80% of patients who develop carditis do so within the first two weeks of the RF illness. Therefore, if no cardiac involvement is detected in the first two weeks, the likelihood of subsequent cardiac involvement during the acute phase is low (89). Patients with acute carditis may improve as the inflammation subsides. If the cardiac involvement is mild, patients may show complete resolution of cardiac findings, but patients with more severe involvement are more likely to experience persistent and/or evolving RHD (4,5). Chronic RHD may include any combination of mitral regurgitation, mitral stenosis, aortic regurgitation, aortic stenosis, or less commonly, tricuspid stenosis or regurgitation.

Testing

There are no diagnostic tests for RF. With few exceptions, in addition to the major and/or minor Jones criteria, diagnosis of acute RF requires evidence of a preceding group

A streptococcal infection (positive throat culture, rapid streptococcal antigen test, or elevated or rising streptococcal antibody titers, most commonly antistreptolysin O (ASO) and antideoxyribonuclease B [anti-DNase b]). Acute phase reactants such as C-reactive protein and/or erythrocyte sedimentation rate help differentiate acute carditis from indolent RHD and may guide treatment with anti-inflammatory agents (90). The degree of inflammation at presentation is of prognostic importance since acute carditis is more likely than chronic RHD to resolve over time.

An ECG should be performed since first degree AV block, a minor Jones criterion, occurs in up to one-third of patients who have group A streptococcal infections, regardless of whether they develop RF (88). Though useful as a minor Jones criterion in support of the diagnosis of RF, first degree AV block is not associated with either the severity of the initial cardiac involvement or a greater likelihood of developing chronic RHD (4,91). In addition, much less commonly, the ECG may reveal other conduction abnormalities (92,93).

A chest radiograph may be valuable in assessing patients with acute or chronic RHD to evaluate cardiac size, configuration, and pulmonary venous markings. In the absence of a pericardial effusion, the radiographic heart size reflects the severity of valvular regurgitation.

Two-dimensional and Doppler echocardiography is central to the diagnosis and management of valvular disease, and should be performed in all patients with acute or chronic RHD. Echocardiography is valuable for evaluating the mechanism and severity of valvular regurgitation and/or stenosis, leaflet and chordal morphology, annular size, chamber sizes and function, pericardial effusion, and pulmonary artery pressure (94–98). In addition, echocardiography helps differentiate RHD from other entities such as innocent murmurs, congenitally abnormal valves, endocardial cushion defect, or myocarditis (99,100). Ventricular size and function are important in determining the timing of intervention for patients with chronic valvular heart disease and should be assessed in all patients with RHD (97).

Catheterization and angiography are rarely necessary for the management of patients with acute rheumatic valvular disease, including those who ultimately require surgery. Endomyocardial biopsy does not add to the diagnosis or management (101). Catheterization should be reserved for those in whom symptoms, clinical findings, and noninvasive imaging are discrepant, and for those in whom balloon valvuloplasty for mitral stenosis is being contemplated (102). In adults with RHD, catheterization and angiography may be indicated to evaluate the coronary vascular bed prior to surgical intervention (97).

RHEUMATIC HEART DISEASE

Mitral Regurgitation

Mitral regurgitation is the dominant cardiac abnormality in patients with RF, occurring in approximately 95% of patients with *acute* rheumatic carditis. Both echocardiographic and surgical studies have shown the mechanism of this to be a combination of annular dilatation and chordal elongation that results in abnormal coaptation, and in some cases, prolapse of the tip of the anterior mitral leaflet (Fig. 1) (103–105). Rarely, mitral valve chordae rupture, resulting in a flail mitral leaflet, severe mitral regurgitation, and acute congestive heart failure (87,106–108).

In most cases, acute mild mitral regurgitation does not cause symptoms. With acute moderate-to-severe mitral regurgitation, the left ventricular myocardium is unable to handle the significant volume overload and left heart filling pressures rise, leading to pulmonary venous congestion and pulmonary edema (109). Secondary pulmonary hypertension may develop and lead to tricuspid regurgitation and right heart failure. With acute severe mitral regurgitation, patients present with features of left heart failure, including dyspnea, orthopnea, paroxysmal nocturnal dyspnea, cough, and even hemoptysis. In contrast to older patients in whom joint symptoms occur frequently enough to bring them to the attention of physicians, children presenting with RF before age of

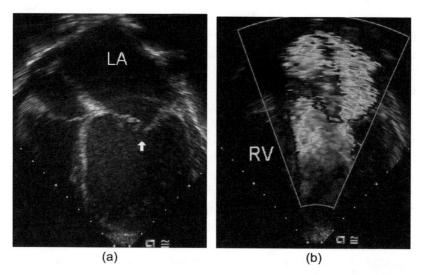

(a)   (b)

Figure 1 Acute rheumatic carditis. (a) Two-dimensional echocardiographic apical four-chamber image showing mitral prolapse, a regurgitant orifice (arrow), and left heart dilation. (b) Color Doppler demonstration of severe mitral regurgitation. LA = left atrium, RV = right ventricle.

5 years often have a more insidious onset, with fever, decreased appetite, lethargy, fatigue, and vague pains. Because of the more subtle symptoms, diagnosis may be delayed and some may present in heart failure (74,75).

On physical examination, tachycardia is often one of the earliest signs of carditis. In addition, patients with elevated left heart filling pressures and pulmonary venous congestion are often tachypneic with increased work of breathing. Precordial activity is increased in the setting of significant valvular regurgitation. A high-pitched, regurgitant, holosystolic murmur of mitral regurgitation is heard best at the apex, usually radiating into the left axilla. This murmur is best heard at end-expiration with the patient in the left lateral decubitus position. It is noteworthy that acute, severe mitral regurgitation may be present despite a fairly soft systolic murmur (110). Although mitral stenosis does not occur with the initial episode of acute rheumatic fever and carditis, an apical low-pitched mid-diastolic apical murmur (Carey Coombs murmur) due to increased flow across the mitral valve may be heard in the setting of significant mitral regurgitation (111). Contrary to some reports (79), this murmur is never heard in isolation (112).

In children and young adults, chronic mitral regurgitation is the most common form of RHD (68,69,113) while mitral stenosis is increasingly common in patients who are in the fourth to the sixth decade of life (53). In contrast to the acute changes occurring with acute rheumatic mitral valvulitis (chordal elongation and annular dilatation), chronic rheumatic mitral regurgitation results from shortening, rigidity, deformation, and retraction of mitral valve leaflets, often associated with fusion and shortening of the mitral valve chordae. In addition, left ventricular dilation may alter the position and orientation of the mitral valve papillary muscles, further impairing leaflet coaptation and resulting in a larger regurgitant orifice and regurgitant volume (114). However, as rheumatic mitral regurgitation becomes chronic, compensatory dilation of the left ventricle occurs, allowing for an increased total stroke volume that maintains forward flow. The combination of compensatory dilation of the left ventricle and the left atrium prevents the rise in left ventricular filling, left atrial, and pulmonary venous pressures that occur in the acute setting. Although patients may remain asymptomatic for years with this compensation, in many cases, the mitral regurgitation progresses over time (115). Eventually, the chronic volume overload may result in ventricular dysfunction with decreased ejection fraction and elevated end-systolic volume. Symptoms, most commonly exertional dyspnea or decreased exercise tolerance, may develop prior to, or with the onset of ventricular dysfunction (97,116,117).

In the setting of chronic mitral regurgitation, precordial activity is increased and the apical impulse is displaced because of ventricular dilation. The first heart sound is often softer than normal and the second heart sound may be widely split due to shortened aortic ejection and earlier aortic valve closure. If there is associated pulmonary hypertension, the pulmonary component of the second heart sound (P2) may be increased. A regurgitant systolic murmur is heard at the apex; subtle murmurs may be heard at end-expiration with the patient in the left lateral decubitus position. When the regurgitant volume is significant, an apical diastolic flow rumble may be heard in the absence of mitral stenosis.

The chest radiograph is usually normal in patients with mild mitral regurgitation. With increasing regurgitation, left atrial and left ventricular enlargement result in cardiomegaly. Pulmonary venous congestion and interstitial edema may be evident with severe mitral regurgitation and heart failure.

The ECG is normal in patients with mild mitral regurgitation but may show left atrial enlargement and/or left ventricular hypertrophy in patients with moderate-to-severe mitral valve incompetence. Right ventricular hypertrophy may be evident in cases with secondary pulmonary hypertension. Atrial fibrillation is rare in children.

The mitral valve may appear normal on two-dimensional echocardiographic imaging of patients with mild acute mitral regurgitation. In cases severe enough to result in heart failure, chordal elongation and annular dilatation may be seen, often resulting in anterior leaflet prolapse (103,118). Rarely, late chordal rupture results in a flail leaflet (106–108,119). The mitral valve prolapse seen in RF patients differs from that seen with mitral valve prolapse (Barlow) syndrome. In rheumatic carditis, only the coapting portion of the anterior leaflet prolapses, and there is no billowing of the medial portion or body of the leaflet (120). This results in abnormal leaflet coaptation, a regurgitant orifice, and a jet of mitral regurgitation that is typically posterolaterally directed (Fig. 1A and B) (121,122). Others have described focal nodular thickening of valve leaflets (thought to represent the verrucae seen at autopsy of patients who died with acute carditis) that disappear on follow-up (94). In addition to assessing left atrial and left ventricular size as indirect indicators, the severity of mitral regurgitation can be evaluated using a variety of methods including the size and extent of the color Doppler regurgitant jet in the left atrium (123), color Doppler proximal flow convergence (124), vena contracta width (125), pulmonary vein Doppler tracings (126), the intensity of the continuous wave Doppler mitral regurgitation signal, and by estimating regurgitant fraction (98,115,127).

Aortic Regurgitation

Aortic regurgitation occurs in approximately 20–25% of patients with acute rheumatic carditis, often in combination with mitral regurgitation. Approximately 5% of patients with rheumatic carditis will have isolated aortic regurgitation (3,11). Some have reported leaflet prolapse to be one of the mechanisms of this acute valvular dysfunction (95,105). Chronic changes include leaflet thickening and fibrosis with leaflet contracture, resulting in abnormal leaflet coaptation and a regurgitant orifice.

While patients with *acute* mild aortic regurgitation are usually asymptomatic, patients with acute severe aortic regurgitation, rare in the setting of acute RF, are quite ill. The large regurgitant volume imposed on a left ventricle that has not had time to compensate for the significant volume load results in a decreased forward stroke volume in conjunction with significant elevation of ventricular end-diastolic pressure, leading to a combination of low cardiac output (or even shock) and pulmonary edema (97). Patients with acute severe aortic regurgitation are tachycardic and tachypneic. Unlike chronic aortic regurgitation, the pulse pressure is often narrow so the increased or bounding pulses characteristic of significant chronic aortic regurgitation may not be present in the acute setting. Precordial activity is often increased, but the apical impulse may not be significantly displaced. On auscultation, the decrescendo diastolic murmur is softer, lower-pitched and shorter (ending before S1) than the murmur heard with chronic regurgitation. In some patients, this can be easily missed, especially with the tachycardia commonly present during the acute phase of the illness. A short systolic ejection murmur may be heard over the left ventricular outflow tract due to increased flow. A low-pitched mid-to-late diastolic rumbling murmur with presystolic accentuation may be heard at the apex, even with a nonstenotic mitral valve. If present, this "Austin Flint" murmur is softer and shorter in the setting of acute as compared to chronic severe aortic regurgitation. Acute rheumatic aortic regurgitation is less likely than mitral regurgitation to disappear with resolution of the acute inflammatory stage of the illness (4,5,128).

Chronic aortic regurgitation results in both volume and pressure overload of the left ventricle. During a compensatory phase, ventricular dilation occurs to maintain forward stroke volume and cardiac output, and ejection fraction remains normal. Similar to patients with chronic mitral regurgitation, patients with chronic severe aortic regurgitation may remain asymptomatic for years (97,109). Over time, decompensation may occur, resulting in decreased left ventricular ejection fraction and usually, symptoms of dyspnea on exertion or decreased exercise tolerance. On examination, a wide pulse pressure (elevated systolic and low diastolic pressures) and bounding pulses are typically evident. Precordial activity is increased, and the apical impulse is displaced laterally due to the dilated left ventricle. The typical murmur of aortic regurgitation is diastolic, relatively high-pitched, decrescendo, heard best along the left sternal border with the patient leaning forward at end-expiration. The duration of the murmur rather than the intensity correlates with the severity of regurgitation. A short systolic ejection murmur may be heard at the mid-left or upper right sternal border from increased flow across the left ventricular outflow tract or associated aortic valve stenosis. A low-pitched mid-to-late diastolic rumbling murmur in the absence of organic mitral stenosis (Austin Flint murmur) may be audible in patients with moderate-to-severe aortic regurgitation.

The chest radiograph is usually normal in mild aortic regurgitation and shows progressive cardiomegaly with increasing severity of aortic valve incompetence. With significant aortic regurgitation, a dilated ascending aorta may be evident.

The ECG is usually normal in cases with mild aortic regurgitation, but may show left ventricular hypertrophy with moderate-to-severe aortic valve incompetence.

Echocardiographic evaluation of acute rheumatic aortic regurgitation may reveal a normal appearing valve or leaflet prolapse (95). Chronic rheumatic aortic valve disease, however, often shows leaflet thickening, retraction, and variable degrees of commissural fusion. These changes may result in variable degrees of aortic regurgitation, sometimes in combination with stenosis. Fibrotic thickening and retraction of aortic valve leaflets without commissural fusion result in dominantly aortic regurgitation. Aortic regurgitation can be assessed using a variety of methods (98) including color Doppler jet height and width (129,130), vena contracta width (131,132), determination of regurgitant fraction and regurgitant orifice area, and diastolic flow reversal in the downstream aorta (130,133). Although useful in evaluating adults with chronic aortic regurgitation (134), the slope of the continuous wave Doppler tracing is less valuable for assessing the severity of aortic regurgitation in children (130).

Pericarditis

Pericarditis occurs in approximately 4–11% of patients with acute rheumatic carditis (2,3,7,11). When it occurs, the pericarditis of acute rheumatic carditis is invariably associated with significant left-sided valvular disease. In the absence of significant mitral and/or aortic regurgitation, pericarditis is unlikely related to RF, and other etiologies should be considered. Clinically, patients may have the typical positional chest and shoulder pain seen with pericarditis, and a friction rub may be heard on auscultation. Echocardiography allows detection and semiquantitation of pericardial effusions. However, unlike pericarditis associated with other etiologies, pericardial tamponade (135) and constrictive pericarditis (136) rarely occur.

Myocarditis

Although acute RHD has long been considered a pancarditis (137,138), the clinically important abnormalities are related to valvular pathology rather than myocardial dysfunction

(118). Biopsy and autopsy pathologic specimens have shown evidence of myocardial involvement (including the characteristic Aschoff bodies), but unlike other types of myocarditis, myocyte necrosis associated with lymphocytic infiltration does not occur (101) and troponin I levels are not elevated (139,140). Further, although there may be evidence of subtle abnormalities of contractility (141), several studies have shown that left ventricular ejection phase indices are normal in these patients (94,118,142). Thus, it is important to emphasize that *heart failure does not occur in acute or chronic RHD in the absence of significant valvular regurgitation* (21,104,118,143).

Mitral Stenosis

Although mitral stenosis does not occur with acute initial carditis, RF resulting in chronic RHD is the most common cause of mitral stenosis. "Pure" mitral stenosis occurs in about 25% of patients with RHD, and another 40% have combined stenosis and regurgitation of the mitral valve (144). Women are more likely than men to develop rheumatic mitral stenosis (68,145). In industrialized countries, the interval between the occurrence of RF and the onset of symptoms from mitral stenosis is usually 20–40 years, resulting in presentation in the fourth to the fifth decade of life (53). In contrast, symptomatic rheumatic mitral stenosis may occur in the second decade of life in children with chronic RHD from developing countries of the world (19,22,24). While both greater severity of cardiac involvement with the initial illness and multiple recurrences of RF likely contribute to the development of this more aggressive form of chronic RHD, it is also possible that the disease process itself is different in developing countries of the world (22).

Rheumatic mitral stenosis results from a combination of leaflet thickening, fusion of commissures, cusps and chordae, and chordal shortening, creating a funnel-shaped valve orifice. Over time, the valve may calcify, further impairing leaflet mobility. A continuous and usually (at least in industrialized countries) slowly progressive process, mitral stenosis results in left ventricular inflow obstruction and a diastolic gradient between the left atrium and ventricle. Patients with mild stenosis are usually minimally symptomatic. With increasing stenosis, however, left atrial, and pulmonary venous pressures rise, leading to pulmonary venous congestion and eventually, pulmonary hypertension. Many patients accommodate their lifestyle to the gradual development of symptoms and are unaware of their significant functional limitations (116). The most common early symptoms are dyspnea on exertion and decreased exercise tolerance, but cough, wheezing, shortness of breath, orthopnea, and paroxysmal nocturnal dyspnea occur as the patient's condition worsens and pulmonary edema develops. Although atrial fibrillation rarely occurs in children, when it does, it may result in atrial thrombi and systemic embolization. With severe obstruction, hemoptysis and symptoms of right heart failure including edema and abdominal distension may be present.

On examination, precordial activity may be abnormal with a tapping, palpable first heart sound, but the apical impulse is not usually displaced unless there is associated mitral and/or aortic regurgitation. Prominent a-waves may be visible in the jugular venous pulsations. On auscultation, the characteristic findings of mitral stenosis are an increased S1, an early diastolic opening snap, and a low-pitched, rumbling diastolic murmur are best heard at the apex with the patient in a left lateral decubitus position. The duration rather than the intensity of the murmur correlates with the severity of obstruction. In addition, the interval between S1 and the opening snap decreases with increased stenosis (elevated left atrial pressure results in earlier opening snap). Late diastolic or presystolic accentuation of the murmur may be audible due to the increased gradient associated with atrial contraction. With severe stenosis and a rigid, calcified mitral valve, the opening snap and S1 may be inaudible. When secondary pulmonary hypertension occurs, P2 increases, and a right ventricular impulse or lift may be noted. Tricuspid regurgitation due to a combination of rheumatic involvement and pulmonary hypertension may become clinically evident with a holosystolic murmur, pulsatile liver, and abnormal jugular venous pulsations.

Typically, the chest radiograph is normal if the mitral stenosis is mild, but shows left atrial enlargement with significant mitral valve obstruction. The left ventricle is not enlarged unless there is associated mitral or aortic regurgitation. The pulmonary artery and right ventricle may enlarge in cases with pulmonary hypertension.

The ECG is normal if the mitral stenosis is mild, but may show left atrial enlargement with significant stenosis or right ventricular hypertrophy if there is secondary pulmonary hypertension.

On echocardiography, patients with rheumatic mitral stenosis have thickened echo-dense leaflets, commissural and/or chordal fusion, and abnormal diastolic leaflet excursion. Mitral regurgitation and stenosis may coexist in such patients. The leaflets begin to open in diastole, and although the body of the leaflets may continue to move, commissural fusion limits the excursion of the leaflet tips resulting in the characteristic "bent-knee" or "hockey-stick" appearance of the anterior leaflet typical of rheumatic mitral stenosis (Fig. 2A and B). Over time, the valve may calcify, first at the leaflet tips and later extending toward the annulus. With increased thickness and calcification, the leaflets become less pliable and motion is further restricted. Although the left atrium is dilated with significant stenosis, the left ventricle is normal in size unless there is concomitant mitral and/or aortic regurgitation. The severity of the mitral stenosis may be assessed from Doppler peak and mean gradients (146), planimetry of the valve opening (147), pressure half-time (148,149), or proximal Doppler flow convergence (150–152). Studies have shown echocardiographic features of leaflet mobility, thickening, calcification, and subvalvular thickening are useful for identifying patients likely to be candidates for balloon valvotomy of mitral stenosis (153–155). When possible, pulmonary artery pressures should be estimated from the tricuspid and pulmonary regurgitation velocities. Both right and left ventricular function should be assessed in all patients with mitral stenosis.

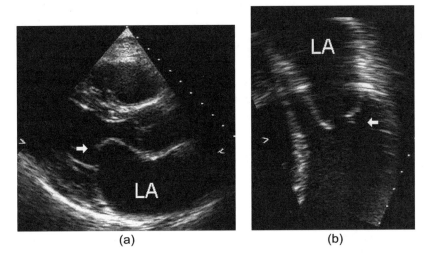

(a)   (b)

Figure 2 Chronic rheumatic mitral stenosis. (a) Two-dimensional echocardiographic parasternal long-axis image demonstrating "bent-knee" or "hockey-stick" configuration to thickened anterior mitral valve leaflet. Note restricted posterior leaflet. Combination results in restricted, stenotic orifice (arrow). (b) Apical four-chamber image showing thickened, echogenic leaflets, and restricted diastolic opening (arrow). LA = left atrium.

Aortic Stenosis

Like mitral stenosis, aortic valve stenosis is a form of chronic rather than acute RHD and occurs years after the acute illness as adhesions, leaflet thickening, fibrosis, commissural fusion, and calcific nodules may develop over time. These changes lead to a decrease in the aortic orifice size and stenosis. Rheumatic aortic stenosis and regurgitation often occur concurrently, usually along with rheumatic mitral valve disease. The increase in stenosis is gradual, allowing for ventricular compensation and the absence of symptoms. With time, compensation fails and symptoms develop (including angina, syncope, dyspnea on exertion and heart failure), most often in the fifth to the sixth decade of life (156).

With severe stenosis, the arterial pulse may be decreased, with a slow rate of rise. If there is associated aortic regurgitation, however, the pulses may be increased. Similar to congenital aortic valve stenosis, a thrill may be palpable at the upper right sternal border or in the suprasternal notch. In contrast to congenital aortic valve disease, an ejection click is uncommon with rheumatic aortic valve stenosis. An associated diastolic murmur is common if aortic regurgitation occurs in combination with stenosis.

On echocardiography, imaging often reveals thickened leaflets with variable degrees of commissural fusion and leaflet retraction, responsible for the variable degrees and combinations of aortic regurgitation and stenosis. Doming of the leaflets, increased echogenicity from calcification, and restricted motion develop as the stenosis progresses. The severity of aortic stenosis can be evaluated by measuring peak instantaneous and mean Doppler gradients or aortic valve area using the continuity equation (97,157,158). Left ventricular dimensions, volumes, wall thicknesses, mass, and function can be measured and contribute to clinical management decisions. The mitral valve should be carefully evaluated in any patient with chronic rheumatic aortic valve disease since coexistent mitral valve involvement is common.

Right Heart Involvement

The right heart valves may be involved secondary to left-sided valvular disease and pulmonary hypertension (functional) or from organic rheumatic valvular disease. The tricuspid valve is affected more often than the pulmonary valve by the rheumatic process, but significant involvement of either valve is uncommon. Rheumatic tricuspid valve disease (stenosis and/or regurgitation) virtually always occurs with significant mitral or aortic valve disease. In patients with chronic RHD, tricuspid regurgitation is more often functional than organic (159). Although histological evidence of rheumatic tricuspid valve involvement may be detectable in up to 15–40% of patients with RHD (159–162), significant tricuspid valve disease is detectable by echocardiography in only 7–9% (159,163), and clinically apparent in 3–5% of patients with RHD (162,164). Rheumatic tricuspid stenosis results from a combination of leaflet thickening, fusion of commissures and chordae, and chordal contraction that limits diastolic leaflet motion and creates a stenotic orifice. Tricuspid valve chordae may also fuse, with contraction and shortening. Leaflet contraction and annular dilation may result in tricuspid regurgitation.

In some cases, it may be difficult to determine whether a patient's symptoms (fatigue, exercise intolerance, peripheral edema) are from tricuspid stenosis or mitral stenosis. Features typical of tricuspid stenosis include prominent jugular venous a-wave pulsations, an opening snap, and a low-pitched diastolic rumbling murmur at the lower left or right sternal border (as opposed to the apex where mitral stenosis is characteristically heard) (165). If secondary pulmonary hypertension occurs, the pulmonary component of S2 will be louder than normal with a palpable right ventricular impulse. Right heart failure with hepatomegaly, tenderness on palpation of the right upper quadrant, edema, and ascites may be evident in advanced disease.

On echocardiography, patients with tricuspid regurgitation may have right ventricular enlargement and/or hypertrophy, right atrial enlargement, and tricuspid annular dilatation. Similar to the rheumatic stenotic mitral valve, thickened leaflets with doming and decreased motion are characteristic findings in rheumatic tricuspid stenosis (166). Doppler allows estimation of the severity of both the tricuspid regurgitation (167,168) and stenosis (166).

Although the pulmonary valve is rarely involved in either acute or chronic RHD, there is evidence of rheumatic involvement after the Ross procedure (pulmonary autograft replacement of the aortic valve) (169) that leads to significant neo-aortic regurgitation and, in some cases, the need for subsequent aortic valve replacement (170,171).

TREATMENT OF RHEUMATIC HEART DISEASE

Unfortunately, medical management of acute rheumatic carditis has not changed substantially since the mid-1950s, and treatment remains directed at both primary and secondary prophylaxis. Although anti-inflammatory treatment is widely accepted as an integral part of the treatment regimen of acute RF and provides symptomatic relief, there is little evidence that such treatment alters the natural history of RHD (19,68,172). Although it varies from patient to patient, the duration of an untreated case of RF has been reported as approximately 3 months, with the course for patients with carditis varying from that of complete recovery with no seque-lae to intractable heart failure requiring surgical interven-tion. The various forms of treatment of acute rheumatic carditis and chronic RHD are summarized in Table 3.

Table 3   Treatment of Acute Carditis and Chronic RHD

Acute rheumatic carditis
General management
  Restricted activity
  Anti-inflammatory agents (aspirin, steroids)
  Primary prophylaxis (eradicate streptococci)
  Initiate secondary prophylaxis (prevent recurrences)
Moderate-to-severe carditis
  Consider salt and fluid restriction, diuretics, afterload
    reduction as temporizing measures
  Surgery (valve repair or replacement)
Chronic RHD
Medical management
  Serial evaluation
  Recognition of progression, symptoms
  Echocardiography: LV size, function, pulmonary pressures; education:
    early recognition of symptoms, prevention of complications
  Secondary prophylaxis
  Infective endocarditis prophylaxis
  Afterload reduction for asymptomatic severe aortic regurgitation
    with preserved ventricular function
  Activity restrictions based on severity of valvular disease
Percutaneous mitral balloon valvotomy
  Indications: symptoms, pulmonary hypertension
  Selected patients (can be identified with echocardiography)
Surgery
  Indications: symptoms, ventricular dysfunction, marked ventricular
    enlargement, pulmonary hypertension, possibly arrhythmias
  Valve repair or replacement

Primary Prophylaxis

It is well established that appropriate treatment of streptococcal pharyngitis markedly decreases the risk of developing RF (27,28,61,173,174). Unfortunately, for many patients, the streptococcal pharyngitis is subclinical (3), precluding effective primary prevention. Even with a negative throat culture, all patients with acute RF should be treated to eradicate group A streptococci from the pharynx (27). A single intramuscular injection of benzathine penicillin is the most effective method, but oral penicillin is an alternative, requiring compliance with the full 10-day treatment course. Penicillin-allergic patients should receive erythromycin or a first-generation cephalosporin, although some patients allergic to penicillin may also be allergic to cephalosporins (175). Penicillin-resistant strains of group A streptococcus have not been reported (176), and follow-up cultures are not necessary.

Secondary Prophylaxis

Patients who have had RF, especially those with cardiac involvement, are at risk for recurrences. Some studies report that this risk is as high as 40–60% for patients with carditis early after an episode of RF (48,177,178). The pattern of clinical involvement with such recurrences is likely to follow the pattern of the initial episode, so patients who have carditis with their first episode of RF are likely to have cardiac involvement with recurrences. The recurrences result in more severe cardiac involvement and a greater likelihood of significant chronic RHD (45,179), so all patients who have had RF should receive prophylaxis against recurrences. In the absence of specific and effective treatment for RF, preventing recurrences is the most effective means of decreasing the likelihood and severity of long-term chronic RHD (180). Intramuscular benzathine penicillin (1.2 million units) every 4 weeks (every 3 weeks where RF is endemic) is the most effective secondary prophylaxis regimen. Oral penicillin (250 mg twice a day) or sulfadiazine/sulfisoxazole are alternatives, especially in low-risk cases (27,175). Recent reports emphasize the importance of

Table 4 Duration of Secondary Prophylaxis After Rheumatic Fever

Category	Duration
RHD (clinical or echocardiographic)	At least 10 years since last episode and at least until age 40 yrs; possibly lifelong
RF with carditis, but no RHD	Ten years or well into adulthood[a]
RF without carditis	Five years or until age 21 years[a]

[a]Whichever is longer.
Modified from Ref. 27.

noncompliance in the precipitation of congestive heart failure in an at-risk population (181).

The recommended duration of secondary prophylaxis is influenced by the presence of acute and chronic cardiac involvement, and by the time since the last episode of RF (Table 4) (27). In selected low-risk patients (e.g., no carditis or rheumatic heart disease) more than 5 years out from the RF illness, earlier discontinuation of prophylaxis may be justified (182). Some recommend that patients with persistent RHD receive such prophylaxis indefinitely (27,183), even after valve replacement (184), while others suggest that prophylaxis is unnecessary beyond age mid-20s (185).

Endocarditis Prophylaxis

Endocarditis continues to be a significant complication of RHD (186). Similar to patients with other forms of valvular heart disease, patients with rheumatic valvular disease should receive endocarditis prophylaxis (187). Since such patients on chronic penicillin are likely to be colonized with amoxicillin-resistant organisms, clindamycin, clarithromycin, or azithromycin are recommended for indicated procedures (175).

Medical Management of Acute Carditis

Management of acute rheumatic carditis should include bed rest (188,189) and anti-inflammatory treatment (176,183,190).

Some restriction of activity during the acute phase is warranted, but the prolonged strict bed rest practiced in the 1940s and 1950s is unnecessary (190). Although of unproven benefit, anti-inflammatory treatment with either aspirin or steroids is considered standard of care for patients with rheumatic carditis since a subset of patients with significant acute rheumatic mitral and/or aortic regurgitation will improve with medical management as the acute inflammation subsides (191). Although numerous studies have been performed, there is no clear-cut evidence that steroids are superior to aspirin in affecting long-term outcome. However, compared to aspirin, steroids do result in a more prompt resolution of inflammation (192,193), fewer new murmurs (194), and more rapid disappearance of existing murmurs (195). Many recommend aspirin (dose 80–100 mg/kg/day) for mild-to-moderate carditis and steroids (prednisone 2 mg/kg/day or equivalent) for moderate-to-severe carditis, including patients in mild congestive heart failure (137,145,177,196). Nonsteroidal anti-inflammatory agents may be an effective alternative to aspirin for patients with polyarthritis, but have not been evaluated for the treatment of carditis (197–199). Intravenous gamma globulin (199) and pentoxifylline (200) have not been found to be of benefit.

Medical Management of Acute Rheumatic Carditis and Heart Failure

Although some of the older literature suggest a role for digoxin (51,176,201), it should be emphasized that the underlying pathology is valvular incompetent rather than myocardial dysfunction. Diuretics and afterload reduction may be valuable as temporizing measures since the degree of valvular regurgitation may decrease significantly as the inflammation subsides. However, in cases with intractable heart failure, the surgical restoration of valvular competency (repair or replacement) may be life saving (108,185). In particular, patients with chordal rupture and a flail mitral valve leaflet are unlikely to respond to medical management and require surgery (106,119).

Medical Management of Chronic RHD

There are little data to guide the management of children with chronic valvular disease. In the absence of such data, many practitioners extrapolate from the adult literature and guidelines. Asymptomatic patients with rheumatic valvular disease can often be followed conservatively as most remain stable for years. In the absence of symptoms, medical management should include serial evaluation, prevention of complications (i.e., recurrent RF, endocarditis, or embolic events), early detection of ventricular dysfunction, and the early recognition of symptoms. Anticoagulation is recommended for patients with mitral stenosis who have a history of a prior embolic event and for those in atrial fibrillation (97).

Afterload reduction (calcium-channel blockers or angiotensin-converting enzyme inhibitors) has been shown to be of value for asymptomatic patients with chronic, severe aortic regurgitation, and preserved left ventricular function (97,202). The role of afterload reduction in the management of asymptomatic patients with chronic severe mitral regurgitation and preserved left ventricular function remains unclear and is not currently recommended (97,203). In the absence of symptoms, indications for intervention include ventricular dysfunction, marked ventricular enlargement, pulmonary hypertension, or atrial fibrillation (97). Once symptoms develop, medical management of mitral or aortic regurgitation has little role except as a temporizing measure, and surgical intervention is indicated.

Unfortunately, there are even less data to guide management of patients with combined mitral and aortic regurgitation. Although symptoms are an indication for surgical intervention, there is evidence suggesting that by the time such patients are symptomatic, the likelihood that left and right ventricular function are compromised is greater than in similar patients with isolated mitral or aortic regurgitation. Since right ventricular function is a valuable predictor of postoperative mortality in patients with combined left-sided valvular regurgitation, detection of decreased right or left ventricular function should prompt referral for surgical intervention (204).

Heart Failure in Chronic RHD

There is no role for long-term medical management of patients with symptomatic chronic mitral and/or aortic regurgitation; such patients should be referred for surgery (97,203).

Patients with mitral stenosis and mild symptoms of dyspnea on exertion related to higher heart rates may benefit from negative chronotropic agents, such as beta-blockers or calcium-channel blockers. Judicious use of diuretics and/or sodium restriction may be valuable in cases with pulmonary venous congestion (97). With significant disease and symptoms, both catheter-based balloon valvuloplasty (205,206) and surgical intervention have been effective. An echocardiographically determined mitral valve morphology score combining assessment of leaflet mobility, subvalvular thickening, leaflet thickening, and leaflet calcification has been found to be a predictor of outcome after balloon valvuloplasty for mitral stenosis (153,155). Symptomatic patients who are not candidates for percutaneous balloon valvuloplasty should be referred for surgery.

There is no effective medical therapy for symptomatic aortic valve stenosis. Unlike congenital aortic valve stenosis in children, balloon valvuloplasty is not effective and has a limited role in the treatment of symptomatic calcific aortic valve stenosis (207,208). In this setting, it should be reserved for patients who are unacceptable surgical candidates (97).

Similarly, medical management of symptomatic rheumatic tricuspid valve disease is unlikely to be successful. Diuretics may be useful as a temporizing measure in symptomatic patients, but optimal treatment is surgical commissurotomy, usually at the time of concomitant mitral valve surgery (209).

Surgical Treatment of RHD

Acute Carditis

Although some patients with significant acute mitral or aortic regurgitation improve with time as the inflammation subsides, others have intractable or progressive heart failure that is unresponsive to medical therapy. Surgical intervention with valvuloplasty or valve replacement during the acute illness can be life-saving because valvular regurgitation rather than myocardial dysfunction is the underlying problem, and restoration of valvular competence results in significant clinical improvement (118). Despite earlier reports of higher reoperation rates and surgical mortality for repair performed during the acute period (210,211), more recent investigators have shown no relationship to rheumatic activity, with mortality rates <5% (118,177,211,212). Because acute rheumatic mitral changes are annular dilatation and chordal elongation resulting in poor leaflet coaptation, surgical annuloplasty and/or chordal shortening have been performed with good results (103,118).

Chronic RHD

The development of heart failure in patients with established RHD may occur due to a recurrent RF illness with carditis, or with time due to the chronic hemodynamic burden of the underlying and often progressive valvular disease (90).

As previously stated, the primary indications for surgical intervention for chronic severe mitral regurgitation are symptoms and/or left ventricular dysfunction. Additional indications include marked ventricular enlargement, atrial fibrillation, and pulmonary hypertension (97,117). Recently, some have advocated surgery in asymptomatic patients with severe mitral regurgitation and preserved ventricular function if valve repair rather than replacement is likely and can be performed with low morbidity and mortality (213). The rheumatic mitral valve can be repaired using techniques including commissuroplasty, debridement or thinning of the anterior leaflet along with an annuloplasty if the annulus is near adult size (214–217). In some cases, the mitral valve cannot be repaired and must be replaced with a prosthetic valve (2,218).

Indications for surgical intervention for chronic aortic regurgitation are similar to those for mitral regurgitation and include symptoms, ventricular dysfunction, and marked ventricular enlargement (97). When surgery is indicated, the valve may be repaired or replaced. Although historically most aortic valves warranting intervention have been replaced, there is increasing experience with valve repair techniques including commissuroplasty, leaflet shortening, and aortic cusp extension (210,219,220). Similar to the case with mitral valves, some valves are not amenable to repair and must be replaced. Although the pulmonary autograft (Ross) procedure has been performed on some patients with rheumatic aortic valve disease, the autograft has been shown to be susceptible to rheumatic involvement with an increased risk of valve failure and reoperation (169,221). Symptomatic chronic rheumatic aortic stenosis should be treated with aortic valve replacement.

The surgical approach to rheumatic tricuspid valve disease is based on the underlying abnormality. A tricuspid annuloplasty may be performed for tricuspid regurgitation due to annular dilation. Tricuspid commissurotomy is the preferred approach to rheumatic tricuspid stenosis (159,161,164,209). It is now routine to inspect and evaluate the tricuspid valve at the time of surgery for rheumatic mitral valve disease.

KAWASAKI DISEASE

Kawasaki disease (KD), or mucocutaneous lymph node syndrome, is an acquired, self-limiting vasculitis of unknown etiology with multiorgan involvement. Males of any age and children of both sexes under age 4–5 years are most commonly affected. First described in the late 1960s in Japan, KD is now known to occur throughout the world and is one of the leading causes of acquired heart disease in children. Although the vasculitis may result in a pancarditis during the acute phase of KD, the most important sequelae involve the coronary arteries. Untreated, approximately 25% of children with KD develop coronary artery aneurysms with an associated risk of myocardial ischemia/infarction, heart failure, or sudden death. Long-term morbidity occurs mainly related to coronary artery abnormalities and ischemic heart disease. This section will review the etiologies of heart failure in KD and the treatment options currently available for the treatment of heart failure in patients with KD.

Etiologies and Pathogenesis of Heart Failure in KD

Although the epidemiology of the illness suggests an infectious cause, the etiology of KD remains unknown. The vasculitis results in acute cardiovascular manifestations of KD that can lead to heart failure, including acute perivasculitis and vasculitis of the cardiac microvessels and small arteries, acute perivasculitis and endarteritis of the major coronary arteries, pericarditis, myocarditis, inflammation of the conduction system, endocarditis, and valvulitis (222).

Myocarditis

Endomyocardial biopsies obtained from children during the acute phase of KD have shown myocarditis to be universal. The cellular infiltrate includes lymphocytes, plasma cells, histiocytes, and some mast cells; myocardial edema and necrosis have also been noted (223,224). Although the exact mechanism of this myocarditis is poorly understood, multiple immunologic abnormalities have been noted in association with KD, including elevated serum IgM antibodies (225), antihuman cardiac myosin IgM autoantibodies (226), elevated IgA and IgM anticardiolipin antibodies (227), and abnormal circulating levels of tumor necrosis factor, interleukin-2, interleukin-6, interferon-gamma, vascular endothelial growth factor, and T cell subsets (228–232). There is also evidence for superantigen involvement from the finding that there is expansion of T cells expressing $V\beta_2$ gene segments (233). Activation of these cytokines and T cells may play an important role in the pathogenesis of vascular endothelial cell injury during the acute phase of KD by eliciting proinflammatory and prothrombotic responses. Chronic abnormalities seen on biopsy have included fibrosis with myocyte hypertrophy and degeneration with architectural disruption of the myocardium, abnormalities associated with cardiomyopathies of other etiologies (223,234,235).

The degree of actual myocardial injury that occurs as a result of this myocardial inflammation is controversial as evidenced by the conflicting findings with regard to circulating cardiac troponin I levels in patients with acute KD. Some investigators have demonstrated elevations whereas others have not (236–238). In addition, although B-type natriuretic peptide levels (a functional plasma marker of ventricular dysfunction) have been shown to be elevated in the acute phase of KD, there is no correlation between these levels and echocardiographic left ventricular fractional shortening (239).

Valvular Dysfunction

Mitral, aortic, and tricuspid valve regurgitation are relatively uncommon occurrences in patients with acute or chronic KD, although when present can be a cause of heart failure. Mitral and aortic regurgitation have been described as presenting either during the acute phase or presenting months or years later. During the acute phase, valvular regurgitation may be secondary to acute valvular, myocardial, or papillary muscle inflammation. Conversely, the development of valve regurgitation (particularly mitral) late after KD is usually related to associated coronary artery abnormalities and ischemic heart disease (240–246). Mitral regurgitation occurs in about 1% of children with Kawasaki disease (247). Nakano et al.(243) found a 4.6% incidence of angiographic aortic regurgitation in a group of children who were 6 weeks to one year after the onset of KD. The degree of mitral and aortic regurgitation is variable, and the outcomes vary from complete resolution to the need for valve replacement or death. At least some of the aortic valve abnormalities seen in patients after KD may be related to mild aortic root dilation seen early after KD (248). Pathological tricuspid regurgitation has also rarely been described during the acute phase of KD (249).

Coronary Artery Disease

By far, the most common and most serious cause of heart failure after KD is coronary artery disease resulting in myocardial ischemia. Although the administration of intravenous immunoglobulin (IVIG) has greatly reduced the incidence of aneurysms, coronary abnormalities may still occur and can lead to thrombosis and/or stenosis of the coronary arteries after KD. Coronary artery ectasia or aneurysms occur in 20–25% of untreated children with KD (250). Newburger et al.(251,252) have shown that IVIG significantly reduces this incidence to less than 5%. Risk factors for the development of aneurysms include male gender, age under 1 year, prolonged or recrudescent fever, anemia, high white blood and/or neutrophil counts, hypoalbuminemia, a low initial platelet count, and markedly elevated acute phase reactants (250,253,254). The long-term sequelae for those who develop aneurysms are becoming well defined. About one-half to two-thirds of aneurysms will resolve over time without sequelae, with the smaller aneurysms having a higher likelihood of resolution (255,256). Larger or giant (>8 mm) aneurysms are likely to be associated with persistent and progressive coronary artery disease. Heart failure as a result of these aneurysms is usually related to the ischemic left ventricular abnormalities that result from the stenoses of previously ectatic or aneurysmal coronary arteries. Complete coronary artery occlusion from thrombosis has been reported to occur in as many as 16% of patients with coronary artery lesions after KD, with myocardial infarction occurring in up to 1/3 of these patients (257). "Segmental stenosis" has been defined as severe narrowing over a long segment of a coronary artery, and is thought to be the result of recanalization of a thrombosed aneurysm (258). Prior to the use of IVIG for treatment of KD, ischemic heart failure developed in 4.7%, myocardial infarction in 1.9%, and death in 0.8% of patients (247).

Diagnosis and Evaluation

Acute KD

Since the etiology of KD remains unclear and there is no single diagnostic test, clinical criteria are used to establish the diagnosis (259). These criteria include fever for at least five days and at least four of the following five criteria: (1) rash (polymorphous), (2) conjunctivitis (without exudates), (3) oral and mucous membrane changes,(4) extremity changes (palmar or solar erythema and/or edema), and (5) cervical adenopathy (>1.5 cm in diameter). These criteria are not specific, however, and other diseases with similar features should be excluded. Other clinical findings seen in some patients with KD include marked irritability, joint symptoms (arthralgia/arthritis), or gastrointestinal symptoms. Since some patients who do not fulfill the above criteria have been subsequently diagnosed with KD ("incomplete" or "atypical" KD), the diagnosis should be considered in the differential diagnosis for children with prolonged fever and some of the above features (260,261). The reader is referred to other sources for detailed discussion of the diagnostic and clinical features of KD (259,260,262).

Clinical cardiac findings often include a resting tachycardia, a gallop rhythm, and flow murmurs. A systolic regurgitant murmur may be heard in children with significant mitral regurgitation, and a pericardial friction rub may be audible if there is associated pericarditis. Although uncommon, clinical heart failure and low cardiac output may occur during the acute phase of the illness.

Laboratory tests usually reveal elevated white blood cell count and acute phase reactants (erythrocyte sedimentation rate, C-reactive protein). Platelet counts are usually elevated during the second–third week of the illness. Other abnormalities may also be present and include anemia, sterile pyuria, hypoalbuminemia, elevated serum transaminases, and aseptic meningitis.

Electrocardiographic abnormalities are not uncommon, and include P–R interval prolongation, QT_c prolongation, low amplitude R wave in lead V_1 or V_6, and nonspecific ST and/or T wave changes.

Echocardiography (often requiring sedation in younger, irritable children) should be performed on all patients with suspected KD. Studies have shown echocardiography to be both sensitive and specific for the detection of proximal coronary artery abnormalities (ectasia, aneurysm, perivascular echogenicity). Left main, anterior descending, circumflex, and right coronary arteries should be imaged from multiple views with measurement of the internal lumen diameters (263). In addition to using the Japanese Ministry of Health criteria classifying coronaries as abnormal if the diameter is >3 mm in children <5 years of age or >4 mm in children >5 years of age, measurements should be compared to normals for body size (z-scores) (264). Echocardiography also allows assessment of left ventricular function, detection of pericardial effusions, and the detection and semiquantitation of valvular regurgitation. Careful echocardiographic examination of patients with acute KD has demonstrated larger systolic and diastolic LV dimensions, and decreased LV fractional shortening and rate-adjusted mean velocity of shortening compared to controls (265). For patients diagnosed with KD, this echocardiographic evaluation should be performed at diagnosis and at 2 and 6–8 weeks after disease onset (first day of fever). If the 6–8 week echocardiogram is normal, further echocardiography is unlikely to demonstrate coronary abnormalities (266,267). Patients with persistent fever or cardiac abnormalities may warrant more frequent evaluation and echocardiographic imaging.

Other noninvasive imaging studies have demonstrated the presence of white blood cells in the myocardium of patients with acute KD (268–271), and treatment with IVIG has been shown to reduce the number of these white blood cells (269).

It is noteworthy that there is no correlation between either the severity of biopsy findings or the findings on white blood cell scans and the severity of coronary artery involvement (272,273).

Heart Failure

Heart failure during the acute phase of KD may occur due to myocarditis and decreased myocardial contractility. In most cases, this ventricular dysfunction reverses rapidly with IVIG treatment (265,274). Less commonly, pericarditis or valvulitis may contribute to compromised cardiac output. In the absence of ischemic heart disease, persistent LV dysfunction after the acute phase of KD is uncommon (274). Heart failure after the acute phase of KD is almost invariably due to ischemic changes to the myocardium from coronary artery abnormalities (265,274). These ischemic changes may result in myocardial dysfunction, valvular regurgitation, and heart failure.

Coronary artery stenosis can be diagnosed by invasive and noninvasive means. Coronary angiography is the definitive method for diagnosing coronary artery stenoses, although the physiologic consequences of these stenoses (e.g., coronary flow reserve) may not be easily defined by angiography alone (275). Intravascular ultrasound during cardiac catheterization has demonstrated a persistently thickened but smooth intima in regions of regressed coronary aneurysms (276). There are several noninvasive methods of assessing coronary artery abnormalities after KD and the physiologic consequences of those abnormalities. Vogel et al. (277) described LV regional wall motion abnormalities as occurring in two of 18 KD patients (11%) with echocardiographic evidence of coronary artery enlargement, although these abnormalities showed no correlation with the extent of the coronary artery enlargement. Stress echocardiography is another adjunctive diagnostic tool for following patients with coronary artery abnormalities after an episode of KD. Pahl et al. (278) performed treadmill exercise stress echocardiography in 28 children 1–10 years old, after an acute episode of KD, and found a 50% incidence of postexercise regional wall motion abnormalities in a group of four patients with severe coronary artery abnormalities (278). Dipyridamole-loading cineventriculography has been shown to detect abnormal LV wall motion in 42% of KD patients within 6 months of the disease with coronary lesions >4 mm, and in 70% of KD patients >6 months after the disease with stenosis or obstruction of the coronary arteries (279). This method provides information regarding regional areas of ischemia affected by stenotic coronary arteries. Single-photon emission computed tomographic (SPECT) imaging performed at rest and at peak exercise in patients after KD can demonstrate stress-induced myocardial perfusion defects. Paridon et al. (280) studied KD patients at least 6 months after the disease and found perfusion defects in 37% with no objective evidence of coronary artery lesions, 63% with resolved aneurysms, and 100% with persistent coronary aneurysms. More subtle abnormalities of altered myocardial flow reserve and endothelial dysfunction in patients late after KD suggest that significant minor abnormalities exist in these patients even in the absence of obvious anatomic or stress-induced ischemic changes. Dhillon et al. (281) found markedly reduced flow-mediated endothelial-dependent brachial artery dilation in asymptomatic KD patients > 5 years after the disease, when compared to controls. Using positron emission tomography, Furuyama et al. (282) found impaired myocardial flow reserve in KD patients, regardless of the presence or absence of objective evidence of residual coronary artery abnormalities.

TREATMENT OF HEART FAILURE IN PATIENTS WITH KD

Acute Phase of KD

In the absence of a known etiology, the goals of treatment are to reduce inflammation and minimize the cardiac sequelae of KD. Studies have shown the combination of IVIG and high dose aspirin to be effective in reducing the risk of coronary artery abnormalities in KD (251,252). Although the exact mechanisms by which IVIG produces these dramatic changes is unclear, possibilities include Fc receptor blockage, a direct neutralizing effect on a possible as yet undefined etiologic agent, an antitoxic effect, an immunomodulatory effect possibly mediated by either anti-idiotypic antibodies or by induction of suppressor T cells, or downregulation of cytokine production by activated immune cells (283). High dose aspirin (80–100 mg/kg/day) is recommended until the patient is afebrile (or alternatively, until the 14th day of illness) (259).

It has been estimated that 5–15% of patients with KD fail to respond to the first does of IVIG (persistent or recrudescent fever >36 hr after initial dose). In such cases, a second course of IVIG (2 g/kg) is recommended (259). For refractory cases, corticosteroids may be considered (284–286).

In addition to IVIG, the precise therapy directed against the development of coronary artery ectasia, aneurysms, thromboses, and stenoses is controversial. Antiplatelet therapy with low-dose aspirin remains the mainstay of antithrombotic therapy and should be continued for approximately 6–8 weeks after the illness onset in those without evidence of coronary artery involvement, and indefinitely in those with coronary artery involvement (263). Other antiplatelet agents such as dipyridamole or clopidogrel can be substituted in those who have a contraindication to aspirin (250). In those with giant or complex coronary artery aneurysms, the best chronic antithrombotic regimen is yet to be determined, since no prospective data exist to guide therapy. Since this group is at greatest risk for stenosis and thrombosis, some experts recommend a combination of warfarin plus aspirin (250). Thrombolytic agents such as streptokinase, urokinase, and tissue plasminogen activator have been used with varying degrees of success in acute KD patients with coronary thromboses (287–289). Preliminary data from our institution suggest that inhibition of the platelet glycoprotein IIb/IIIa receptor with a monoclonal antibody such as abciximab may have a role in reducing the size of coronary artery aneurysms during the acute phase of KD (290,291), although further study is needed before this therapy can be routinely recommended.

The treatment of heart failure in patients with acute or a history of KD depends upon the cause of the heart failure. As discussed above, heart failure can occur in the acute phase of KD due to acute perivasculitis and vasculitis of the cardiac microvessels and small arteries, acute perivasculitis and endarteritis of the major coronary arteries, pericarditis, myocarditis, inflammation of the conduction system, endocarditis, and valvulitis (222). Initial treatment of the acute phase of KD with anti-inflammatory medications in addition to IVIG will reduce inflammation and therefore reduce the immediate cardiovascular manifestations of the acute inflammatory process. Administration of IVIG in the acute phase of KD also appears to have a direct beneficial effect on LV systolic performance, an effect not seen in KD patients treated only with aspirin. In a prospective, randomized trial comparing aspirin alone to aspirin plus IVIG in patients with acute KD, IVIG resulted in improvement in LV fractional shortening and rate-corrected velocity of circumferential fiber shortening (265,274).

Overt congestive heart failure requiring intravenous pressor support during the acute phase of KD is rare. In this setting, one should suspect either a more severe inflammatory myocarditis or a more severe coronary artery abnormality that has resulted in ischemia or infarction. Therapy is then directed toward the abnormality. If there is significant LV dysfunction, then pressor support should be acutely administered as needed. Options for management of acute heart failure include inotropic support with dobutamine, milrinone, or, if hypotension is a problem, then dopamine, epinephrine and/or vasopressin or other pressors. See also Chapters 9 and 20 in this book for more detailed analysis of the acute management of heart failure due to LV dysfunction. If coronary artery abnormalities are suspected, then coronary angiography may be warranted and therapy then directed (as described below) toward the specific abnormality. Valvular insufficiency may rarely cause heart failure in the acute phase, and diuretics, pressors, and afterload reducing agents may be necessary (see the section on treatment of acute rheumatic heart disease).

Chronic Phase of KD

In the absence of ischemic heart disease, it is very uncommon to have persistent abnormalities of LV function after the acute phase of KD (274). Heart failure after the acute phase of KD is almost invariably due to ischemic myocardial changes secondary to coronary artery abnormalities. The diagnosis of the coronary artery abnormalities is discussed above. Many treatment options have been used to palliate patients with heart failure due to coronary artery abnormalities after KD. Transcatheter intervention has been successfully used to treat coronary artery stenoses due to KD (292). The Research Committee of the Ministry of Health, Labor and Welfare "Study of treatment and long-term management in Kawasaki disease" has published guidelines for catheter intervention in coronary artery lesion in KD (293). Indications for intervention include: (1) ischemic symptoms; (2) ischemic findings on noninvasive testing; (3) greater than 75% angiographic stenosis in the left anterior descending coronary artery; and (4) severe LV dysfunction with coronary artery disease. Recommended interventional procedures include percutaneous transluminal coronary balloon angioplasty, stent implantation (in older children), and rotational ablation. Due to the increased stiffness and frequent calcification of chronic stenotic coronary artery lesions in KD compared with atheromatous lesions in adults, results of transcatheter interventions are generally not as effective as in other lesions (250).

Surgical management of chronic coronary artery lesions after KD has also been successfully performed. Saphenous vein grafts have been described as patent as long as 22 years after placement in both a 5-year-old and 7-year-old child (294). Follow-up in 105 KD patients with internal thoracic artery coronary artery bypass has reported 98% survival and 78% freedom from cardiac events 20 years after bypass (295). The authors compared this to a 39% patency rate of saphenous vein grafts 15 years after surgery, with the finding that patency of saphenous vein grafts in children under 5 years of age was "almost hopeless."

Chronic heart failure due to systolic LV dysfunction after KD requires evaluation of the coronary vascular bed as described above. If these coronary artery abnormalities are amenable to pharmacologic, transcatheter interventional or surgical intervention, these should be undertaken. However, if these coronary artery abnormalities are not amenable to direct treatment, or if treatment does not correct the underlying dysfunction, then pharmacologic therapy can be directed toward the ischemic LV dysfunction. There are no studies of treatment of chronic heart failure in patients who have had KD. However, it is reasonable to attempt treatments that have been shown to be successful in adults with ischemic cardiomyopathy. These treatments are discussed in detail in previous chapters of this book and include diuretics, digoxin, angiotensin-converting enzyme inhibitors, and β-adrenergic receptor blockers. In situations where pharmacologic, transcatheter, or surgical options are unsuccessful in reversing severe symptoms, then cardiac transplantation can be performed with good outcomes in patients after KD (296,297).

REFERENCES

1. Giannoulia-Karantana A, Anagnostopoulos G, Kostaridou S, Georgakopoulou T, Papadopoulou A, Papadopoulos G. Childhood acute rheumatic fever in Greece: experience of the past 18 years. Acta Paediatr 2001; 90:809–812.
2. Bitar FF, Hayek P, Obeid M, Gharzeddine W, Mikati M, Dbaibo GS. Rheumatic fever in children: a 15-year experience in a developing country. Pediatr Cardiol 2000; 21:119–122.
3. Veasy LG, Tani LY, Hill HR. Persistence of acute rheumatic fever in the intermountain area of the United States [see comments]. J Pediatr 1994; 124:9–16.
4. Feinstein AR, Stern EK, Spagnuolo M. The prognosis of acute rheumatic fever. Am Heart J 1964; 68:817–834.
5. Bland EF, Jones TD. Rheumatic fever and rheumatic heart disease: a twenty year report on 1000 patients followed since childhood. Circulation 1951; 4:836–843.
6. Ravisha MS, Tullu MS, Kamat JR. Rheumatic fever and rheumatic heart disease: clinical profile of 550 cases in India. Arch Med Res 2003; 34:382–387.
7. Chagani HS, Aziz K. Clinical profile of acute rheumatic fever in Pakistan. Cardiol Young 2003; 13:28–35.
8. Mota CC, Meira ZM. Rheumatic fever. Cardiol Young 1999; 9: 239–248.
9. Joshi MK, Kandoth PW, Barve RJ, Kamat JR. Rheumatic fever. Clinical profile of 339 cases with long term follow up. Indian Pediatr 1983; 20:849–853.
10. Sanyal SK, Thapar MK, Ahmed SH, Hooja V, Tewari P. The initial attack of acute rheumatic fever during childhood in North India; a prospective study of the clinical profile. Circulation 1974; 49:7–12.
11. Arora R, Subramanyam G, Khalilullah M, Gupta MP. Clinical profile of rheumatic fever and rheumatic heartdisease: a study of 2,500 cases. Indian Heart J 1981; 33:264–269.
12. Strategy for controlling rheumatic fever/rheumatic heart disease, with emphasis on primary prevention: memorandum from a joint WHO/ISFC meeting. Bull World Health Organ 1995; 73:583-587.
13. Steer AC, Carapetis JR, Nolan TM, Shann F. Systematic review of rheumatic heart disease prevalence in children in developing

countries: the role of environmental factors [see comments]. J Paediatr Child Health 2002; 38:229–234.

14. Agarwal BL. Rheumatic heart disease unabated in developing countries. Lancet 1981; 2:910–911.

15. Mendez GF, Cowie MR. The epidemiological features of heart failure in developing countries: a review of the literature. Int J Cardiol 2001; 80:213–219.

16. Olivier C. Rheumatic fever—is it still a problem? Journal of Antimicrobial Chemotherapy 2000; 45(Suppl):13–21.

17. Ibrahim A, Rahman AR. Rheumatic heart disease: how big is the problem? Med J Malaysia 1995; 50:121–124.

18. Soler-Soler J, Galve E. Worldwide perspective of valve disease. Heart 2000; 83:721–725.

19. Rheumatic fever and rheumatic heart disease. Report of a WHO Study Group. World Health Organ Tech Rep Ser 1988; 764:1–58.

20. Gibofsky A, Kerwar S, Zabriskie JB. Rheumatic fever. The relationships between host, microbe, and genetics. Rheum Dis Clin North Am 1998; 24:237–759.

21. Barlow JB. Aspects of active rheumatic carditis. Aust NZJ Med 1992; 22:592–600.

22. Marcus RH, Sareli P, Pocock WA, Barlow JB. The spectrum of severe rheumatic mitral valve disease in a developing country. Correlations among clinical presentation, surgical pathologic findings, and hemodynamic sequelae [see comments]. Ann Intern Med 1994; 120: 177–183.

23. Carapetis JR, Currie BJ. Mortality due to acute rheumatic fever and rheumatic heart disease in the Northern Territory: a preventable cause of death in aboriginal people. ANZ J Public Health 1999; 23:159–163.

24. Roy SB, Bhatia ML, Lazaro EJ, Ramalingaswami V. Juvenile Mitral Stenosis in India. Lancet 1963; 41:1193–1195.

25. WHO programme for the prevention of rheumatic fever/rheumatic heart disease in 16 developing countries: report from Phase I (1986–90). WHO Cardiovascular Diseases Unit and principal investigators. Bull World Health Organ 1992; 70:213–218.

26. Terreri MT, Ferraz MB, Goldenberg J, Len C, Hilario MO. Resource utilization and cost of rheumatic fever. J Rheumatol 2001; 28: 1394–1397.

27. Dajani A, Taubert K, Ferrieri P, Peter G, Shulman S. Treatment of acute streptococcal pharyngitis and prevention of rheumatic fever: a statement for health professionals. Committee on rheumatic fever, endocarditis, and Kawasaki disease of the Council on Cardiovascular Disease in the Young, the American Heart Association. Pediatrics 1995; 96:758–764.

28. Markowitz M. The decline of rheumatic fever: role of medical intervention. Lewis W. Wannamaker Memorial Lecture.J Pediatr 1985; 106:545–550.
29. Gordis L. The virtual disappearance of rheumatic fever in the United States: lessons in the rise and fall of disease. T. Duckett Jones memorial lecture. Circulation 1985; 72:1155–1162.
30. Veasy LG, Wiedmeier SE, Orsmond GS, Ruttenberg HD, Boucek MM, Roth SJ, Tait VF, Thompson JA, Daly JA, Kaplan EL. Resurgence of acute rheumatic fever in the intermountain area of the United States. N Engl J Med 1987; 316:421–427.
31. Hosier DM, Craenen JM, Teske DW, Wheller JJ. Resurgence of acute rheumatic fever. Am J Diseases Child 1987; 141:730–733.
32. Congeni B, Rizzo C, Congeni J, Sreenivasan VV. Outbreak of acute rheumatic fever in northeast Ohio. J Pediatr 1987; 111:176–179.
33. Wald ER, Dashefsky B, Feidt C, Chiponis D, Byers C. Acute rheumatic fever in western Pennsylvania and the tristate area. Pediatrics 1987; 80:371–374.
34. Westlake RM, Graham TP, Edwards KM. An outbreak of acute rheumatic fever in Tennessee. Pediatr Infect Dis J 1990; 9:97–100.
35. Leggiadro RJ, Birnbaum SE, Chase NA, Myers LK. A resurgence of acute rheumatic fever in a mid-South children's hospital. South Med J 1990; 83:1418–1420.
36. Kavey RE, Kaplan EL. Resurgence of acute rheumatic fever. Pediatrics 1989; 84:585–586.
37. Stollerman GH. Rheumatogenic streptococci and autoimmunity. Clin Immunol Immunopathol 1991; 61:131–142.
38. Stollerman GH. Rheumatogenic group A streptococci and the return of rheumatic fever. Adv Intern Med 1990; 35:1–25.
39. Johnson DR, Stevens DL, Kaplan EL. Epidemiologic analysis of group A streptococcal serotypes associated with severe systemic infections, rheumatic fever, or uncomplicated pharyngitis. J Infect Dis 1992; 166:374–382.
40. Smoot JC, Korgenski EK, Daly JA, Veasy LG, Musser JM. Molecular analysis of group A Streptococcus type emm18 isolates temporally associated with acute rheumatic fever outbreaks in Salt Lake City, Utah. J Clin Microbiol 2002; 40:1805–1810.
41. Miner LJ, Petheram SJ, Daly JA, Korgenski EK, Selin KS, Firth SD, Veasy LG, Hill HR, Bale JF Jr. Molecular characterization of Streptococcus pyogenes isolates collected during periods of increased acute rheumatic fever activity in Utah. Pediatr Infect Dis J 2004; 23:56–61.
42. Stollerman GH. Rheumatic fever [see comments]. Lancet 1997; 349: 935–942.
43. Bisno AL. Noncardiac Manifestations of rheumatic fever. In: Narula J, Virmani R, Reddy KS, Tandon R, eds. Rheumatic Fever. Washington, DC: American Registry of Pathology, 1999:245–256.

44. Nausieda PA, Grossman BJ, Koller WC, Weiner WJ, Klawans HL. Sydenham chorea: an update. Neurology 1980; 30:331–334.

45. Feinstein AR, Spagnuolo M. The clinical patterns of acute rheumatic fever: a reappraisal. Medicine 1962; 41:279–305.

46. Taranta A, Wood HF, Feinstein AR, Simpson R, Kleinberg E. Rheumatic fever in children and adolescents. IV. Relation of the rheumatic fever recurrence rate per streptococcal antibodies. Ann Intern Med 1964; 60(suppl 5):47–86.

47. Rammelkamp CH. Epidemiology of streptococcal infections. Harvey Lect 1956; 51:113–142.

48. Massell BF. Factors in the pathogenesis of rheumatic fever recurrences. J Maine Med Assoc 1962; 53:88–93.

49. Ayoub EM. The search for host determinants of susceptibility to rheumatic fever: the missing link. T. Duckett Jones Memorial Lecture. Circulation 1984; 69:197–201.

50. Chun LT, Reddy V, Rhoads GG. Occurrence and prevention of rheumatic fever among ethnic groups of Hawaii. Am J Dis Child 1984; 138:476–478.

51. DiSciascio G, Taranta A. Rheumatic fever in children. Am Heart J 1980; 99:635–658.

52. Kurahara D, Tokuda A, Grandinetti A, Najita J, Ho C, Yamamoto K, Reddy DV, Macpherson K, Iwamuro M, Yamaga K. Ethnic differences in risk for pediatric rheumatic illness in a culturally diverse population. J Rheumatol 2002; 29:379–383.

53. Horstkotte D, Niehues R, Strauer BE. Pathomorphological aspects, aetiology and natural history of acquired mitral valve stenosis. Eur Heart J 1991; 12(suppl B):55–60.

54. Ayoub EM, Barrett DJ, Maclaren NK, Krischer JP. Association of class II human histocompatibility leukocyte antigens with rheumatic fever. J Clin Invest 1986; 77:2019–2026.

55. Guedez Y, Kotby A, El-Demellawy M, Galal A, Thomson G, Zaher S, Kassem S, Kotb M. HLA class II associations with rheumatic heart disease are more evident and consistent among clinically homogeneous patients. Circulation 1999; 99:2784–2790.

56. Gerbase-DeLima M, Scala LC, Temin J, Santos DV, Otto PA. Rheumatic fever and the HLA complex. A cosegregation study. Circulation 1994; 89:138–141.

57. Khanna AK, Buskirk DR, Williams RC, Jr, Gibofsky A, Crow Mk, Menon A, Fotino M, Reid Hm, Poon-King T, Rubinstein P, et al. Presence of a non-HLA B cell antigen in rheumatic fever patients and their families as defined by a monoclonal antibody. J Clin Invest 1989; 83:1710–1716.

58. Zabriskie JB, Lavenchy D, Williams RC Jr, Fu SM, Yeadon CA, Fotino M, Braun DG. Rheumatic fever-associated B cell alloantigens as identified by monoclonal antibodies. Arthritis Rheum 1985; 28: 1047–1051.

59. Kumar RK, Rammohan R, Narula J, Kaplan EL. Epidemiology of streptococcal pharyngitis, rheumatic fever, and rheumatic heart disease. In: Narula J, Virmani R, Reddy KS, Tandon R, eds. Rheumatic Fever. Washington, DC: American Registry of Pathology, 1999; 41–68.
60. Bisno AL. Group A streptococcal infections and acute rheumatic fever. N Engl J Med 1991; 325:783–793.
61. Massell BF, Chute CG, Walker AM, Kurland GS. Penicillin and the marked decrease in morbidity and mortality from rheumatic fever in the United States. N Engl J Med 1988; 318:280–286.
62. Cunningham MW, McCormack JM, Talaber LR, Harley JB, Ayoub EM, Muneer RS, Chun LT, Reddy DV. Human monoclonal antibodies reactive with antigens of the group A streptococcus and human heart. J Immunol 1988; 141:2760–2766.
63. Zabriskie JB, Hsu KC, Seegal BC. Heart-reactive antibody associated with rheumatic fever: characterization and diagnostic significance. Clin Exp Immunol 1970; 7:147–159.
64. Dale JB, Beachey EH. Epitopes of streptococcal M proteins shared with cardiac myosin. J Exp Med 1985; 162:583–591.
65. Cunningham MW. Molecular mimicry between group A streptococci and myosin in the pathogenesis of acute rheumatic fever. In: Narula J, Virmani R, Reddy KS, Tandon R, eds. Rheumatic Fever. Washington, DC: American Registry of Pathology, 1999:135–165.
66. Carreno-Manjarrez R, Visvanathan K, Zabriskie JB. Immunogenic and genetic factors in rheumatic fever. Curr Infect Dis Rep 2000; 2:302–307.
67. Kaplan MH, Meyeserian M. An immunological cross-reaction between group-A streptococcal cells and human heart tissue. Lancet 1962; 1:706–710.
68. The natural history of rheumatic fever and rheumatic heart disease. Ten-year report of a cooperative clinical trial of ACTH, cortisone, and aspirin. Circulation 1965, 32: 457–476.
69. Sanyal S, Berry A, Duggal S, Hooja V, Ghosh S. Sequelae of the initial attack of acute rheumatic fever in children from north India. A prospective 5-year follow-up study. Circulation 1982; 65:375–379.
70. Feinstein AR, Stern EK. Clinical effects of recurrent attacks of acute rheumatic fever: a prospective epidemiologic study of 105 episodes. J Chronic Dis 1967; 20:13–27.
71. Majeed HA, Batnager S, Yousof AM, Khuffash F, Yusuf AR. Acute rheumatic fever and the evolution of rheumatic heart disease: a prospective 12 year follow-up report. J Clin Epidemiol 1992; 45: 871–875.
72. Thomas GT. Five-year follow-up on patients with rheumatic fever treated by bed rest, steroids, or salicylate. Br Med J 1961; 5240: 1635–1639.

73. Sanyal SK. Acute rheumatic fever and its sequelae during childhood: historical perspective and a global overview. Indian Pediatr 1987; 24:275–294.

74. Tani LY, Veasy LG, Minich LL, Shaddy RE. Rheumatic fever in children younger than 5 years: is the presentation different? Pediatrics 2003; 112:1065–1068.

75. Rosenthal A, Czoniczer G, Massell BF. Rheumatic fever under 3 years of age. A report of 10 cases. Pediatrics 1968; 41:612–619.

76. Jones TD. Diagnosis of rheumatic fever. JAMA 1944; 126:481–484.

77. Stollerman GH et al. Jones criteria (revised) for guidance in the diagnosis of rheumatic fever. Circulation 1965; 32:664–668.

78. Shulman ST et al. Jones Criteria (revised) for guidance in the diagnosis of rheumatic fever. Circulation 1984; 69:204A–208A.

79. Dajani AS et al. Guidelines for the diagnosis of rheumatic fever. Jones criteria, 1992 update. Special Writing Group of the Committee on Rheumatic Fever, Endocarditis, and Kawasaki Disease of the Council on Cardiovascular Disease in the Young of the American Heart Association [see comments]. [erratum appears in JAMA 1993; 269(4):476]. JAMA 1992; 268:2069–2073.

80. Rutstein DD, Bauer, Dorfman A, Gross RE, Lichty JA, Taussig HB, Whittemore R, Hagberg K, Parker ME. Jones criteria (modified) for guidance in the diagnosis of rheumatic fever. Mod Concepts Cardiovasc Dis 1955; 24:291–293.

81. Shiffman RN. Guideline maintenance and revision. 50 years of the Jones criteria for diagnosis of rheumatic fever [see comments]. Arch Pediatr Adolescent Med 1995; 149:727–732.

82. Carapetis JR, Currie BJ. Rheumatic fever in a high incidence population: the importance of monoarthritis and low grade fever. Arch Dis Childhood 2001; 85:223–227.

83. Goldenberg J, Ferraz MB, Fonseca AS, Hilario MO, Bastos W, Sachetti S. Sydenham chorea: clinical and laboratory findings. Analysis of 187 cases. Rev Paul Med 1992; 110:152–157.

84. Lessof MH, Bywaters EG. The duration of chorea. Br Med J 1956; 4982:1520–1523.

85. Bland EF. Chorea as a manifestation of rheumatic fever: a long-term perspective. Trans Am Clin Climatol Assoc 1961; 73:209–213.

86. Carapetis JR, Currie BJ. Rheumatic chorea in northern Australia: a clinical and epidemiological study. Arch Dis Childhood 1999; 80: 353–358.

87. Aron AM, Freeman JM, Carter S. The natural history of Sydenham's chorea. Review of the literature and long-term evaluation with emphasis on cardiac sequelae. Am J Med 1965; 38:83–95.

88. Feinstein AR. The natural histories of acute rheumatic fever. Bull Rheum Dis 1966; 17:423–428.

89. Massell BF, Fyler DC, Roy SB. The clinical picture of rheumatic fever. Diagnosis, immediate prognosis, course and therapeutic implications. Am J Cardiol 1958; 1:436–449.

90. Spagnuolo M, Feinstein AR. Congestive heart failure and rheumatic activity in young patients with rheumatic heart disease. Pediatrics 1964; 33:653–660.

91. Massell BF, Fyler DC, Roy SB. The clinical picture of rheumatic fever: diagnosis, immediate prognosis, course, and therapeutic implications. Am J Cardiol 1958; 1:436–449.

92. Mirowski M, Rosenstein BJ, Markowitz M. A comparison of atrioventricular conduction in normal children and in patients with rheumatic fever, glomerulonephritis, and acute febrile illnesses. A quantitative study with determination of the P–R index. Pediatrics 1964; 33:334–340.

93. Lenox CC, Zuberbuhler JR, Park SC, Neches WH, Mathews RA, Zoltun R. Arrhythmias and Stokes–Adams attacks in acute rheumatic fever. Pediatrics 1978; 61:599–603.

94. Vasan RS, Shrivastava S, Vijayakumar M, Narang R, Lister BC, Narula J. Echocardiographic evaluation of patients with acute rheumatic fever and rheumatic carditis. Circulation 1996; 94:73–82.

95. Tomaru T, Uchida Y, Mohri N, Mori W, Furuse A, Asano K. Postinflammatory mitral and aortic valve prolapse: a clinical and pathological study. Circulation 1987; 76:68–76.

96. Minich LL, Tani LY, Veasy LG. Role of echocardiography in the diagnosis and follow-up evaluation of rheumatic carditis. In: Narula J, Virmani R, Reddy KS, Tandon R, eds. Rheumatic Fever. Washington, DC: American Registry of Pathology, 1999:307–318.

97. Bonow RO, Carabello B, de Leon AC Jr, Edmunds LH Jr, Fedderly BJ, Freed MD, Gaasch WH, McKay CR, Nishimura RA, O'Gara PT, O'Rourke RA, Rahimtoola SH, Ritchie JL, Cheitlin MD, Eagle KA, Gardner TJ, Garson A Jr, Gibbons RJ, Russell RO, Ryan TJ, Smith SC Jr. Guidelines for the management of patients with valvular heart disease: executive summary. A report of the American College of Cardiology/American Heart Association Task Force on Practice Guidelines (Committee on Management of Patients with Valvular Heart Disease). Circulation 1998; 98:1949–1984.

98. Zoghbi WA, Enriquez-Sarano M, Foster E, Grayburn PA, Kraft CD, Levine RA, Nihoyannopoulos P, Otto CM, Quinones MA, Rakowski H, Stewart WJ, Waggoner A, Weissman NJ. Recommendations for evaluation of the severity of native valvular regurgitation with two-dimensional and Doppler echocardiography. J Am Soc Echocardiogr 2003; 16:777–802.

99. Regmi PR, Pandey MR. Prevalence of rheumatic fever and rheumatic heart disease in school children of Kathmandu city. Indian Heart J 1997; 49:518–520.

100. Grover A, Dhawan A, Iyengar SD, Anand IS, Wahi PL, Ganguly NK. Epidemiology of rheumatic fever and rheumatic heart disease in a rural community in northern India. Bull World Health Organ 1993; 71:59–66.

101. Narula J, Chopra P, Talwar KK, Reddy KS, Vasan RS, Tandon R, Bhatia ML, Southern JF. Does endomyocardial biopsy aid in the diagnosis of active rheumatic carditis? Circulation 1993; 88: 2198–2205.

102. Krishnamoorthy KM, Tharakan JA. Balloon mitral valvulotomy in children aged < or = 12 years. J Heart Valve Dis 2003; 12:461–468.

103. Marcus RH, Sareli P, Pocock WA, Meyer TE, Magalhaes MP, Grieve T, Antunes MJ, Barlow JB. Functional anatomy of severe mitral regurgitation in active rheumatic carditis. Am J Cardiol 1989; 63:577–584.

104. Barlow JB, Marcus RH, Pocock WA, Barlow CW, Essop R, Sareli P. Mechanisms and management of heart failure in active rheumatic carditis. S Afr Med J 1990; 78:181–186.

105. Zhou LY, Lu K. Inflammatory valvular prolapse produced by acute rheumatic carditis: echocardiographic analysis of 66 cases of acute rheumatic carditis. Int J Cardiol 1997; 58:175–178.

106. de Moor MM, Lachman PI, Human DG. Rupture of tendinous chords during acute rheumatic carditis in young children. Int J Cardiol 1986; 12:353–357.

107. Oliveira DB, Dawkins KD, Kay PH, Paneth M. Chordal rupture. I: aetiology and natural history. Br Heart J 1983; 50:312–327.

108. Kalangos A, Beghetti M, Vala D, Jaeggi E, Kaya G, Karpuz V, Murith N, Faidutti B. Anterior mitral leaflet prolapse as a primary cause of pure rheumatic mitral insufficiency. Ann Thorac Surg 2000; 69:755–761.

109. Greenberg BH. Congestive heart failure as a consequence of valvular heart disease. In: Hosenpud JD, Greenberg BH, eds. Congestive Heart Failure: Pathophysiology, Diagnosis, and Comprehensive Approach to Management. New York: Springer-Verlag, 1994: 234–245.

110. Sutton GC, Craige E. Clinical signs of severe acute mitral regurgitation. Am J Cardiol 1967; 20:141–144.

111. Coombs CF. Rheumatic Heart Disease. New York: William Woods, 1924.

112. Veasy LG. Rheumatic fever—T. Duckett Jones and the rest of the story. Cardiol Young 1995; 5:293–301.

113. The Evolution of Rheumatic Heart Disease in Children. Five-year report of a cooperative clinical trial of ACTH, cortisone, and aspirin. Circulation 1960; 22:503–515.

114. Otsuji Y, Handschumacher MD, Schwammenthal E, Jiang L, Song JK, Guerrero JL, Vlahakes GJ, Levine RA. Insights from three-dimensional echocardiography into the mechanism of functional

mitral regurgitation: direct in vivo demonstration of altered leaflet tethering geometry. Circulation 1997; 96:1999–2008.

115. Enriquez-Sarano M, Basmadjian AJ, Rossi A, Bailey KR, Seward JB, Tajik AJ. Progression of mitral regurgitation: a prospective Doppler echocardiographic study. J Am Coll Cardiol 1999; 34:1137–1144.

116. Otto CM. Mitral regurgitation. In: Otto CM, ed. Valvular Heart Disease. Philadelphia: Saunders, 2004:336–367.

117. Otto CM. Timing of surgery in mitral regurgitation. Heart 2003; 89:100–105.

118. Essop MR, Wisenbaugh T, Sareli P. Evidence against a myocardial factor as the cause of left ventricular dilation in active rheumatic carditis. J Am Coll Cardiol 1993; 22:826–829.

119. Hwang WS, Lam KL. Case reports. Rupture of chordae tendineae during acute rheumatic carditis. Br Heart J 1968; 30:429–431.

120. Barlow JB. Idiopathic (degenerative) and rheumatic mitral valve prolapse: historical aspects and an overview. J Heart Valve Dis 1992; 1:163–174.

121. Zucker N, Goldfarb BL, Zalzstein E, Silber H, Rovner M, Goldbraich N, Wanderman KL. A common color flow doppler finding in the mitral regurgitation of acute rheumatic fever. Echocardiography 1991; 8:627–631.

122. Minich LL, Tani LY, Pagotto LT, Shaddy RE, Veasy LG. Doppler echocardiography distinguishes between physiologic and pathologic "silent" mitral regurgitation in patients with rheumatic fever. Clinical Cardiol 1997; 20:924–926.

123. Wu YT, Chang AC, Chin AJ. Semiquantitative assessment of mitral regurgitation by Doppler color flow imaging in patients aged < 20 years. Am J Cardiol 1993; 71:727–732.

124. Schwammenthal E, Chen C, Benning F, Block M, Breithardt G, Levine RA. Dynamics of mitral regurgitant flow and orifice area. Physiologic application of the proximal flow convergence method: clinical data and experimental testing. Circulation 1994; 90:307–322.

125. Zhou X, Jones M, Shiota T, Yamada I, Teien D, Sahn DJ. Vena contracta imaged by Doppler color flow mapping predicts the severity of eccentric mitral regurgitation better than color jet area: a chronic animal study. J Am Coll Cardiol 1997; 30:1393–1398.

126. Klein AL, Obarski TP, Stewart WJ, Casale PN, Pearce GL, Husbands K, Cosgrove DM, Salcedo EE. Transesophageal Doppler echocardiography of pulmonary venous flow: a new marker of mitral regurgitation severity. J Am Coll Cardiol 1991; 18:518–526.

127. Irvine T, Li XK, Sahn DJ, Kenny A. Assessment of mitral regurgitation. Heart 2002; 88(suppl 4):iv11–19.

128. Tompkins DG, Boxerbaum B, Liebman J. Long-term prognosis of rheumatic fever patients receiving regular intramuscular benzathine penicillin. Circulation 1972; 45:543–551.

129. Perry GJ, Helmcke F, Nanda NC, Byard C, Soto B. Evaluation of aortic insufficiency by Doppler color flow mapping. J Am Coll Cardiol 1987; 9:952–959.

130. Tani LY, Minich LL, Day RW, Orsmond GS, Shaddy RE. Doppler evaluation of aortic regurgitation in children. Am J Cardiol 1997; 80:927–931.

131. Shiota T, Jones M, Agler DA, McDonald RW, Marcella CP, Qin JX, Zetts AD, Greenberg NL, Cardon LA, Sun JP, Sahn DJ, Thomas JD. New echocardiographic windows for quantitative determination of aortic regurgitation volume using color Doppler flow convergence and vena contracta. Am J Cardiol 1999; 83:1064–1068.

132. Tribouilloy CM, Enriquez-Sarano M, Bailey KR, Seward JB, Tajik AJ. Assessment of severity of aortic regurgitation using the width of the vena contracta: a clinical color Doppler imaging study. Circulation 2000; 102:558–564.

133. Takenaka K, Dabestani A, Gardin JM, Russell D, Clark S, Allfie A, Henry WL. A simple Doppler echocardiographic method for estimating severity of aortic regurgitation. Am J Cardiol 1986; 57: 1340–1343.

134. Labovitz AJ, Ferrara RP, Kern MJ, Bryg RJ, Mrosek DG, Williams GA. Quantitative evaluation of aortic insufficiency by continuous wave Doppler echocardiography. J Am Coll Cardiol 1986; 8: 1341–1347.

135. Tan AT, Mah PK, Chia BL. Cardiac tamponade in acute rheumatic carditis. Ann Rheum Dis 1983; 42:699–701.

136. Przybojewski JZ. Rheumatic constrictive pericarditis. A case report and review of the literature. S Afr Med J 1981; 59:682–686.

137. Burge DJ, DeHoratius RJ. Acute rheumatic fever. Cardiovasc Clin 1993; 23:3–23.

138. Stollerman G. Rheumatic Fever And Streptococcal Infection. New York: Grune & Stratton, 1975:127–131.

139. Kamblock J, Payot L, Iung B, Costes P, Gillet T, Le Goanvic C, Lionet P, Pagis B, Pasche J, Roy C, Vahanian A, Papouin G. Does rheumatic myocarditis really exists? Systematic study with echocardiography and cardiac troponin I blood levels. Eur Heart J 2003; 24:855–862.

140. Williams RV, Minich LL, Shaddy RE, Veasy LG, Tani LY. Evidence for lack of myocardial injury in children with acute rheumatic carditis. Cardiol Young 2002; 12:519–523.

141. Gentles TL, Colan SD, Wilson NJ, Biosa R, Neutze JM. Left ventricular mechanics during and after acute rheumatic fever: contractile dysfunction is closely related to valve regurgitation. J Am Coll Cardiol 2001; 37:201–207.

142. Vardi P, Markiewicz W, Weiss Y, Levi J, Benderly A. Clinical-echocardiographic correlations in acute rheumatic fever. Pediatrics 1983; 71:830–834.

143. Veasy LG. Time to take soundings in acute rheumatic fever. Lancet 2001; 357:1994–1995.
144. Braunwald E. Valvular heart disease. Braunwald E, Zipes DP, Libby P, eds. Heart Disease. Philadelphia: W.B. Saunders Company, 2001:1643–1722, .
145. Stollerman GH. Rheumatic fever in the 21st century. Clin Infect Dis 2001; 33:806–814.
146. Nishimura RA, Rihal CS, Tajik AJ, Holmes DR Jr. Accurate measurement of the transmitral gradient in patients with mitral stenosis: a simultaneous catheterization and Doppler echocardiographic study. J Am Coll Cardiol 1994; 24:152–158.
147. Martin RP, Rakowski H, Kleiman JH, Beaver W, London E, Popp RL. Reliability and reproducibility of two dimensional echocardiograph measurement of the stenotic mitral valve orifice area. Am J Cardiol 1979; 43:560–568.
148. Wranne B, Ask P, Loyd D. Analysis of different methods of assessing the stenotic mitral valve area with emphasis on the pressure gradient half-time concept. Am J Cardiol 1990; 66:614–620.
149. Hatle L, Brubakk A, Tromsdal A, Angelsen B. Noninvasive assessment of pressure drop in mitral stenosis by Doppler ultrasound. Br Heart J 1978; 40:131–140.
150. Rifkin RD, Harper K, Tighe D. Comparison of proximal isovelocity surface area method with pressure half-time and planimetry in evaluation of mitral stenosis. J Am Coll Cardiol 1995; 26:458–465.
151. Rodriguez L, Thomas JD, Monterroso V, Weyman AE, Harrigan P, Mueller LN, Levine RA. Validation of the proximal flow convergence method. Calculation of orifice area in patients with mitral stenosis. Circulation 1993; 88:1157–1165.
152. Lee TY, Tseng CJ, Chiao CD, Chiou CW, Mar GY, Liu CP, Lin SL, Chiang HT. Clinical applicability for the assessment of the valvular mitral stenosis severity with doppler echocardiography and the proximal isovelocity surface area (PISA) method. Echocardiography 2004; 21:1–6.
153. Wilkins GT, Weyman AE, Abascal VM, Block PC, Palacios IF. Percutaneous balloon dilatation of the mitral valve: an analysis of echocardiographic variables related to outcome and the mechanism of dilatation. Br Heart J 1988; 60:299–308.
154. Reid CL, Chandraratna PA, Kawanishi DT, Kotlewski A, Rahimtoola SH. Influence of mitral valve morphology on double-balloon catheter balloon valvuloplasty in patients with mitral stenosis. Analysis of factors predicting immediate and 3-month results. Circulation 1989; 80:515–524.
155. Iung B, Cormier B, Ducimetiere P, Porte JM, Nallet O, Michel PL, Acar J, Vahanian A. Immediate results of percutaneous mitral commissurotomy. A predictive model on a series of 1514 patients. Circulation 1996; 94:2124–2130.

156. Kennedy KD, Nishimura RA, Holmes DR Jr, Bailey KR. Natural history of moderate aortic stenosis. J Am Coll Cardiol 1991; 17:313–319.
157. Snider AR, Serwer GA, Ritter SB. Abnormalities of ventricular outflow. Snider AR, Serwer GA, Ritter SB, eds. Echocardiography in Pediatric Heart Disease. St. Louis: Mosby-Year Book, Inc., 1997: 408–451.
158. Shavelle DM, Otto CM. Aortic stenosis. In: Otto CM, ed. The Practice of Clinical Echocardiography. Philadelphia: W.B. Saunders Company, 2002:469–499.
159. Roguin A, Rinkevich D, Milo S, Markiewicz W, Reisner SA. Long-term follow-up of patients with severe rheumatic tricuspid stenosis. Am Heart J 1998; 136:103–108.
160. Chopra P, Bhatia ML. Chronic rheumatic heart disease in India: a reappraisal of pathologic changes. J Heart Valve Dis 1992; 1:92–101.
161. Duran CM. Tricuspid valve surgery revisited. J Card Surg 1994; 9: 242–247.
162. Kitchin A, Turner R. Diagnosis and treatment of tricuspid stenosis. Br Heart J 1964; 26:354–379.
163. Goswami KC, Rao MB, Dev V, Shrivastava S. Juvenile tricuspid stenosis and rheumatic tricuspid valve disease: an echocardiographic study. Int J Cardiol 1999; 72:83–86.
164. Carpentier A, Deloche A, Hanania G, Forman J, Sellier P, Piwnica A, Dubost C, McGoon DC. Surgical management of acquired tricuspid valve disease. J Thorac Cardiovasc Surg 1974; 67:53–65.
165. Wooley CF, Fontana ME, Kilman JW, Ryan JM. Tricuspid stenosis. Atrial systolic murmur, tricuspid opening snap, and right atrial pressure pulse. Am J Med 1985; 78:375–384.
166. Guyer DE, Gillam LD, Foale RA, Clark MC, Dinsmore R, Palacios I, Block P, King ME, Weyman AE. Comparison of the echocardiographic and hemodynamic diagnosis of rheumatic tricuspid stenosis. J Am Coll Cardiol 1984; 3:1135–1144.
167. Tribouilloy CM, Enriquez-Sarano M, Bailey KR, Tajik AJ, Seward JB. Quantification of tricuspid regurgitation by measuring the width of the vena contracta with Doppler color flow imaging: a clinical study. J Am Coll Cardiol 2000; 36:472–478.
168. Shapira Y, Porter A, Wurzel M, Vaturi M, Sagie A. Evaluation of tricuspid regurgitation severity: echocardiographic and clinical correlation. J Am Soc Echocardiogr 1998; 11:652–659.
169. Choudhary SK, Mathur A, Sharma R, Saxena A, Chopra P, Roy R, Kumar AS. Pulmonary autograft: should it be used in young patients with rheumatic disease? J Thorac Cardiovasc Surg 1999; 118:483–90. Discussion 490–491.
170. Pieters FA, Al-Halees Z, Hatle L, Shahid MS, Al-Amri M. Results of the Ross operation in rheumatic versus non-rheumatic aortic valve disease. J Heart Valve Dis 2000; 9:38–44.

171. Pieters FA, al-Halees Z, Zwaan FE, Hatle L. Autograft failure after the Ross operation in a rheumatic population: pre- and postoperative echocardiographic observations. J Heart Valve Dis 1996; 5:404–408. Discussion 408–409.

172. Czoniczer G, Amezcua F, Pelargonio S, Massell BF. Therapy of severe rheumatic carditis. Comparison of adrenocortical steroids and aspirin. Circulation 1964; 29:813–819.

173. Denny FW, Wannamaker LW, Brink WR, Rammelkamp CH Jr, Custer EA. Landmark article May 13, 1950: prevention of rheumatic fever. Treatment of the preceding streptococcic infection. By Floyd W. Denny, Lewis W. Wannamaker, William R. Brink, Charles H. Rammelkamp Jr., Edward A. Custer. JAMA 1985; 254:534–537.

174. Gerber MA, Markowitz M. Management of streptococcal pharyngitis reconsidered. Pediatr Infect Dis 1985; 4:518–526.

175. Pediatrics AAO. Group A Streptococcal Infections. Elk Grove Village, IL: American Academy of Pediatrics, 2003.

176. Thatai D, Turi ZG. Current guidelines for the treatment of patients with rheumatic fever. Drugs 1999; 57:545–555.

177. Chandrashekhar Y, Narula J. Rheumatic fever. Alpert JS, Dalen JE, Rahimtoola SH, eds. Valvular Heart Disease. Philadelphia: Lippincott Williams & Wilkins, 2000:41–73.

178. Spagnuolo M, Pasternack B, Taranta A. Risk of rheumatic-fever recurrences after streptococcal infections. Prospective study of clinical and social factors. N Engl J Med 1971; 285:641–647.

179. Kuttner AG, Mayer FE. Carditis during second attacks of rheumatic fever. N Engl J Med 1963; 268:1259–1261.

180. Lue HC, Wu MH, Wang JK, Wu FF, Wu YN. Three- versus four-week administration of benzathine penicillin G: effects on incidence of streptococcal infections and recurrences of rheumatic fever. Pediatrics 1996; 97:984–988.

181. Joshi PP, Mohanan CJ, Sengupta SP, Salkar RG. Factors precipitating congestive heart failure—role of patient non-compliance. J Assoc Physicians India 1999; 47:294–295.

182. Majeed HA, Khuffash FA, Bhatnagar S, Farwana S, Yusuf AR, Yousof AM. Acute rheumatic polyarthritis. The duration of secondary prophylaxis. Am J Dis Child 1990; 144:831–833.

183. da Silva NA, Pereira BA. Acute rheumatic fever. Still a challenge. Rheum Dis Clin North Am 1997; 23:545–568.

184. Hodes RM. Recurrence of rheumatic fever after valve replacement. Cardiology 1989; 76:465–468.

185. Kalangos A, Beghetti M, Baldovinos A, Vala D, Bichel T, Mermillod B, Murith N, Oberhansli I, Friedli B, Faidutti B. Aortic valve repair by cusp extension with the use of fresh autologous pericardium in children with rheumatic aortic insufficiency. J Thorac Cardiovasc Surg 1999; 118:225–236.

186. Deshpande J, Vaideeswar P, Amonkar G, Vasandani S. Rheumatic heart disease in the past decade: an autopsy analysis. Indian Heart J 2002; 54:676–680.

187. Dajani AS, Taubert KA, Wilson W, Bolger AF, Bayer A, Ferrieri P, Gewitz MH, Shulman ST, Nouri S, Newburger JW, Hutto C, Pallasch TJ, Gage TW, Levison ME, Peter G, Zuccaro G Jr. Prevention of bacterial endocarditis. Recommendations by the American Heart Association. JAMA 1997; 277:1794–1801.

188. Taran LM. The treatment of acute rheumatic fever and acute rheumatic heart disease. Am J Med 1947; 2:285–295.

189. Bywaters EG, Thomas GT. Bed rest, salicylates, and steroid in rheumatic fever. Br Med J 1961; 5240:1628–1634.

190. Lendrum BL, Simon AJ, Mack I. Relation of duration of bed rest in acute rheumatic fever to heart disease present 2 to 14 years later. Pediatrics 1959; 24:389–394.

191. Combined Rheumatic Fever Study Group. A COMPARISON of the effect of prednisone and acetylsalicylic acid on the incidence of residual rheumatic heart disease. N Engl J Med 1960; 262:895–902.

192. TREATMENT of acute rheumatic fever in children a co-operative clinical trial of A.C.T.H., cortisone, aspirin; a joint report by the Rheumatic Fever Working Party of the Medical Research Council of Great Britain and the Subcommittee of Principal Investigators of the American Council on Rheumatic Fever and Congenital Heart Disease, American Heart Association. Br Med J 1995; 4913:555–574.

193. Saxena A. Treatment of rheumatic carditis. Indian J Pediatr 2002; 69:513–516.

194. Rothman PE. Treatment of rheumatic carditis. A critical evaluation. Clin Pediatr (Phila) 1965; 4:619–625.

195. Markowitz M, Kuttner G. Treatment of acute rheumatic fever. Am J Dis Child 1962; 104:313–320.

196. Albert DA, Harel L. The treatment of rheumatic fever and rheumatic carditis. In: Narula J, Virmani R, Reddy KS, Tandon R, eds. Rheumatic Fever. Washington, DC: American Registry of Pathology, 1999:359–370.

197. Hashkes PJ, Tauber T, Somekh E, Brik R, Barash J, Mukamel M, Harel L, Lorber A, Berkovitch M, Uziel Y. Naproxen as an alternative to aspirin for the treatment of arthritis of rheumatic fever: a randomized trial. J Pediatr 2003; 143:399–401.

198. Uziel Y, Hashkes PJ, Kassem E, Padeh S, Goldman R, Wolach B, Vollach B. The use of naproxen in the treatment of children with rheumatic fever. J Pediatr 2000; 137:269–271.

199. Voss LM, Wilson NJ, Neutze JM, Whitlock RM, Ameratunga RV, Cairns LM, Lennon DR. Intravenous immunoglobulin in acute rheumatic fever: a randomized controlled trial. Circulation 2001; 103:401–406.

200. Nanna M, Chandraratna PA, Reid C, Nimalasuriya A, Rahimtoola SH. Value of two-dimensional echocardiography in detecting tricuspid stenosis. Circulation 1983; 67:221–224.

201. Stollerman GH. Rheumatic fever. AMA Arch Intern Med 1956; 98:211–220.

202. Scognamiglio R, Rahimtoola SH, Fasoli G, Nistri S, Dalla Volta S. Nifedipine in asymptomatic patients with severe aortic regurgitation and normal left ventricular function. N Engl J Med 1994; 331: 689–694.

203. Borer JS, Bonow RO. Contemporary approach to aortic and mitral regurgitation. Circulation 2003; 108:2432–2438.

204. Niles N, Borer JS, Kamen M, Hochreiter C, Devereux RB, Kligfield P. Preoperative left and right ventricular performance in combined aortic and mitral regurgitation and comparison with isolated aortic or mitral regurgitation. Am J Cardiol 1990; 65:1372–1378.

205. Shrivastava S, Dev V, Vasan RS, Das GS, Rajani M. Percutaneous balloon mitral valvuloplasty in juvenile rheumatic mitral stenosis. Am J Cardiol 1991; 67:892–894.

206. Gamra H, Betbout F, Ben Hamda K, Addad F, Maatouk F, Dridi Z, Hammami S, Abdellaoui M, Boughanmi H, Hendiri T, Ben Farhat M. Balloon mitral commissurotomy in juvenile rheumatic mitral stenosis: a ten-year clinical and echocardiographic actuarial results. Eur Heart J 2003; 24:1349–1356.

207. Lieberman EB, Bashore TM, Hermiller JB, Wilson JS, Pieper KS, Keeler GP, Pierce CH, Kisslo KB, Harrison JK, Davidson CJ. Balloon aortic valvuloplasty in adults: failure of procedure to improve long-term survival. J Am Coll Cardiol 1995; 26:1522–1558.

208. Otto CM, Mickel MC, Kennedy JW, Alderman EL, Bashore TM, Block PC, Brinker JA, Diver D, Ferguson J, Holmes DR Jr, et al. Three-year outcome after balloon aortic valvuloplasty. Insights into prognosis of valvular aortic stenosis. Circulation 1994; 89:642–650.

209. Revuelta JM, Garcia-Rinaldi R, Duran CM. Tricuspid commissurotomy. Ann Thorac Surg 1985; 39:489–491.

210. Duran CM, Gometza B, De Vol EB. Valve repair in rheumatic mitral disease. Circulation 1991; 84(5 Suppl):III125–132.

211. Skoularigis J, Sinovich V, Joubert G, Sareli P. Evaluation of the long-term results of mitral valve repair in 254 young patients with rheumatic mitral regurgitation. Circulation 1994; 90(5 Pt 2):II167–174.

212. Gometza B, al-Halees Z, Shahid M, Hatle LK, Duran CM. Surgery for rheumatic mitral regurgitation in patients below twenty years of age. An analysis of failures. J Heart Valve Dis 1996; 5:294–301.

213. Enriquez-Sarano M. Timing of mitral valve surgery. Heart 2002; 87:79–85.

214. Rumel WR, Vaughn CC, Guibone RA. Surgical reconstruction of the mitral valve. Ann Thorac Surg 1969; 8:289–296.

215. Chauvaud S, Perier P, Touati G, Relland J, Kara SM, Benomar M, Carpentier A. Long-term results of valve repair in children with acquired mitral valve incompetence. Circulation 1986; 74(3 Pt 2):I104–109.

216. Sulayman R, Mathew R, Thilenius OG, Replogle R, Arcilla RA. Hemodynamics and annuloplasty in isolated mitral regurgitation in children. Circulation 1975; 52:1144–1151.

217. Kitamura N, Uemura S, Kunitomo R, Utoh J, Noji S. A new technique for debridement in rheumatic valvular disease: the rasping procedure. Ann Thorac Surg 1975; 69:121–125.

218. John S, Ravikumar E, Jairaj PS, Chowdhury U, Krishnaswami S. Valve replacement in the young patient with rheumatic heart disease. Review of a twenty-year experience. J Thorac Cardiovasc Surg 1990; 99:631–638.

219. Grinda JM, Latremouille C, Berrebi AJ, Zegdi R, Chauvaud S, Carpentier AF, Fabiani JN, Deloche A. Aortic cusp extension valvuloplasty for rheumatic aortic valve disease: midterm results. Ann Thorac Surg 2002; 74:438–443.

220. Kalangos A, Beghetti M, Baldovinos A, Vala D, Bichel T, Mermillod B, Murith N, Oberhansli I, Friedli B, Faidutti B. Aortic valve repair by cusp extension with the use of fresh autologous pericardium in children with rheumatic aortic insufficiency. J Thorac Cardiovasc Surg 1999; 118:225–236.

221. al-Halees Z, Kumar N, Gallo R, Gometza B, Duran CM. Pulmonary autograft for aortic valve replacement in rheumatic disease: a caveat. Ann Thorac Surg 1995; 60:S172–S175. Discussion S176.

222. Fujiwara H, Hamashima Y. Pathology of the heart in Kawasaki disease. Pediatrics 1978; 61:100–107.

223. Yutani C, Go S, Kamiya T, Hirose O, Misawa H, Maeda H, Kozuka T, Onishi S. Cardiac biopsy of Kawasaki disease. Arch Pathol Lab Med 1981; 105:470–473.

224. Yutani C, Okano K, Kamiya T, Oguchi K, Kozuka T, Ota M, Onishi S. Histopathological study on right endomyocardial biopsy of Kawasaki disease. Br Heart J 1980; 43:589–592.

225. Leung DY, Collins T, Lapierre LA, Geha RS, Pober JS. Immunoglobulin M antibodies present in the acute phase of Kawasaki syndrome lyse cultured vascular endothelial cells stimulated by gamma interferon. J Clin Invest 1986; 77:1428–1435.

226. Cunningham MW, Meissner HC, Heuser JS, Pietra BA, Kurahara DK, Leung DY. Anti-human cardiac myosin autoantibodies in Kawasaki syndrome. J Immunol 1999; 163:1060–1065.

227. Gupta M, Johann-Liang R, Bussel JB, Gersony WM, Lehman TJ. Elevated IgA and IgM anticardiolipin antibodies in acute Kawasaki disease. Cardiology 2002; 97:180–182.

228. Lang BA, Silverman ED, Laxer RM, Lau AS. Spontaneous tumor necrosis factor production in Kawasaki disease. J Pediatr 1989; 115: 939–943.

229. Lang BA, Silverman ED, Laxer RM, Rose V, Nelson DL, Rubin LA. Serum-soluble interleukin-2 receptor levels in Kawasaki disease. J Pediatr 1990; 116:592–596.

230. Matsubara T, Furukawa S, Yabuta K. Serum levels of tumor necrosis factor, interleukin 2 receptor, and interferon-gamma in Kawasaki disease involved coronary-artery lesions. Clin Immunol Immunopathol 1990; 56:29–36.

231. Maeno N, Takei S, Masuda K, Akaike H, Matsuo K, Kitajima I, Maruyama I, Miyata K. Increased serum levels of vascular endothelial growth factor in Kawasaki disease. Pediatr Res 1998; 44: 596–599.

232. Terai M, Kohno Y, Niwa K, Toba T, Sakurai N, Nakajima H. Imbalance among T-cell subsets in patients with coronary arterial aneurysms in Kawasaki disease. Am J Cardiol 1987; 60:555–559.

233. Abe J, Kotzin BL, Jujo K, Melish ME, Glode MP, Kohsaka T, Leung DY. Selective expansion of T cells expressing T-cell receptor variable regions V beta 2 and V beta 8 in Kawasaki disease. Proc Natl Acad Sci USA 1992; 89:4066–4070.

234. Yonesaka S, Nakada T, Sunagawa Y, Tomimoto K, Naka S, Takahashi T, Matubara T, Sekigami I. Endomyocardial biopsy in children with Kawasaki disease. Acta Paediatr Jpn 1989; 31: 706–711.

235. Yonesaka S, Takahashi T, Matubara T, Nakada T, Furukawa H, Tomimoto K, Oura H. Histopathological study on Kawasaki disease with special reference to the relation between the myocardial sequelae and regional wall motion abnormalities of the left ventricle. Jpn Circ J 1992; 56:352–358.

236. Kim M, Kim K. Changes in cardiac troponin I in Kawasaki disease before and after treatment with intravenous gammaglobulin. Jpn Circ J 1998; 62:479–482.

237. Checchia PA, Borensztajn J, Shulman ST. Circulating cardiac troponin I levels in Kawasaki disease. Pediatr Cardiol 2001; 22:102–106.

238. Kim M, Kim K. Elevation of cardiac troponin I in the acute stage of Kawasaki disease. Pediatr Cardiol 1999; 20:184–188.

239. Kawamura T, Wago M, Kawaguchi H, Tahara M, Yuge M. Plasma brain natriuretic peptide concentrations in patients with Kawasaki disease. Pediatr Int 2000; 42:241–248.

240. Akagi T, Kato H, Inoue HK, Sato N. Valvular heart disease in Kawasaki syndrome—incidence and natural history. Kurume Med J 1989; 36:137–149.

241. Takao A, Niwa K, Kondo C, Nakanishi T, Satomi G, Nakazawa M, Endo M. Mitral regurgitation in Kawasaki disease. Prog Clin Biol Res 1987; 250:311–323.

242. Akagi T, Kato H, Inoue O, Sato N, Imamura K. Valvular heart disease in Kawasaki syndrome: incidence and natural history. Am Heart J 1990; 120:366–372.

243. Nakano H, Nojima K, Saito A, Ueda K. High incidence of aortic regurgitation following Kawasaki disease. J Pediatr 1985; 107: 59–63.

244. Gidding SS, Shulman ST, Ilbawi M, Crussi F, Duffy CE. Mucocutaneous lymph node syndrome (Kawasaki disease): delayed aortic and mitral insufficiency secondary to active valvulitis. J Am Coll Cardiol 1986; 7:894–897.

245. Fuse S, Tomita H, Ohara T, Iida K, Takamuro M. Severely damaged aortic valve and cardiogenic shock in an infant with Kawasaki disease. Pediatr Int 2003; 45:110–113.

246. Takahashi T, Taniguchi K, Matsuda H. Surgical treatment for aortic regurgitation and left ventricular dysfunction caused by Kawasaki disease. Cardiol Young 1998; 8:123–125.

247. Kato H, Sugimura T, Akagi T, Sato N, Hashino K, Maeno Y, Kazue T, Eto G, Yamakawa R. Long–term consequences of Kawasaki disease. A 10- to 21-year follow-up study of 594 patients. Circulation 1996; 94:1379–1385.

248. Ravekes WJ, Colan SD, Gauvreau K, Baker AL, Sundel RP, van der Velde ME, Fulton DR, Newburger JW. Aortic root dilation in Kawasaki disease. Am J Cardiol 2001; 87:919–922.

249. Shinohara T, Tanihira Y. A patient with Kawasaki disease showing severe tricuspid regurgitation and left ventricular dysfunction in the acute phase. Pediatr Cardiol 2003; 24:60–63.

250. Newburger JW, Burns JC. Kawasaki disease. Vasc Med 1999; 4: 187–202.

251. Newburger JW, Takahashi M, Beiser AS, Burns JC, Bastian J, Chung KJ, Colan SD, Duffy CE, Fulton DR, Glode MP, et al. A single intravenous infusion of gamma globulin as compared with four infusions in the treatment of actue Kawasaki syndrome. N Engl J Med 324:1633-1639, 1991.

252. Newburger JW, Takahashi M, Burns JC, Beiser AS, Chung KJ, Duffy CE, Glode MP, Mason WH, Reddy V, Sanders SP, et al. The treatment of Kawasaki syndrome with intravenous gamma globulin. N Engl J Med 1986; 315:341–347.

253. Beiser AS, Takahashi M, Baker AL, Sundel RP, Newburger JW, US Multicenter Kawasaki Disease Study Group. A predictive instrument for coronary artery aneurysms in Kawasaki disease. Am J Cardiol 1998; 81:1116–1120.

254. Saavedra WF, Tunin RS, Paolocci N, Mishima T, Suzuki G, Emala CW, Chaudhry PA, Anagnostopoulos P, Gupta RC, Sabbah HN, Kass DA. Reverse remodeling and enhanced adrenergic reserve from passive external support in experimental dilated heart failure. J Am Coll Cardiol 2002; 39:2069–2076.

255. Takahashi M, Mason W, Lewis AB. Regression of coronary aneurysms in patients with Kawasaki syndrome. Circulation 1987; 75:387–394.

256. Nakano H, Ueda K, Saito A, Nojima K. Repeated quantitative angiograms in coronary arterial aneurysm in Kawasaki disease. Am J Cardiol 1985; 56:846–851.

257. Suzuki A, Kamiya T, Ono Y, Kohata T, Okuno M. Myocardial ischemia in Kawasaki disease: follow-up study by cardiac catheterization and coronary angiography. Pediatr Cardiol 1988; 9:1–5.

258. Suzuki A, Kamiya T, Kuwahara N, Ono Y, Kohata T, Takahashi O, Kimura K, Takamiya M. Coronary arterial lesions of Kawasaki disease: cardiac catheterization findings of 1100 cases. Pediatr Cardiol 1986; 7:3–9.

259. Dajani AS, Taubert KA, Gerber MA, Shulman ST, Ferrieri P, Freed M, Takahashi M, Bierman FZ, Karchmer AW, Wilson W, et al. Diagnosis and therapy of Kawasaki disease in children. Circulation 1993; 87:1776–1780.

260. Rowley AH: Incomplete (atypical) Kawasaki disease. Pediatr Infect Dis J 2002; 21:563–565.

261. Witt MT, Minich LL, Bohnsack JF, Young PC. Kawasaki disease: more patients are being diagnosed who do not meet American Heart Association criteria. Pediatrics 1999; 104:e10.

262. Newburger JW. Kawasaki disease. Curr Treat Options Cardiovasc Med 2000; 2:227–236.

263. Dajani As, Taubert KA, Takahashi M, Bierman FZ, Freed MD, Ferrieri P, Gerber M, Shulman ST, Karchmer AW, Wilson W, et al. Guidelines for long-term management of patients with Kawasaki disease. Report from the Committee on Rheumatic Fever, Endocarditis, and Kawasaki Disease, Council on Cardiovascular Disease in the Young, American Heart Association. Circulation 1994; 89:916–922.

264. de Zorzi A, Colan SD, Gauvreau K, Baker AL, Sundel RP, Newburger JW. Coronary artery dimensions may be misclassified as normal in Kawasaki disease. J Pediatr 1998; 133:254–258.

265. Newburger JW, Sanders SP, Burns JC, Parness IA, Beiser AS, Colan SD. Left ventricular contractility and function in Kawasaki syndrome. Effect of intravenous gamma-globulin. Circulation 1989; 79:1237–1246.

266. McMorrow Tuohy AM, Tani LY, Cetta F, Lewin MB, Eidem BW, Van Buren P, Williams RV, Shaddy RE, Tuohy RP, Minich LL. How many echocardiograms are necessary for follow-up evaluation of patient with Kawasaki disease? Am J Cardiol 2001; 88:328–330.

267. Scott JS, Ettedgui JA, Neches WH. Cost-effective use of echocardiography in children with Kawasaki disease. Pediatrics 1999; 104:e57.

268. Kao CH, Hsieh KS, Wang YL, Wang SJ, Yeh SH. The detection of ventricular dysfunction and carditis in children with Kawasaki disease using equilibrium multigated blood pooling ventriculography

and 99Tcm-HMPAO-labelled WBC heart scans. Nucl Med Commun 1993; 14:539–543.

269. Kao CH, Hsieh KS, Wang YL, Chen CW, Liao SQ, Wang SJ, Yeh SH. Tc-99m HMPAO WBC imaging to detect carditis and to evaluate the results of high-dose gamma globulin treatment in Kawasaki disease. Clin Nucl Med 1992; 17:623–626.

270. Kao CH, Hsieh KS, Wang YL, Chen CW, Liao SQ, Wang SJ, Yeh SH. Tc-99m HMPAO labeled WBC scan for the detection of myocarditis in different phases of Kawasaki disease. Clin Nucl Med 1992; 17: 185–190.

271. Matsuura H, Ishikita T, Yamamoto S, Umezawa T, Ito R, Hashiguchi R, Saji T, Matsuo N, Takano M. Gallium-67 myocardial imaging for the detection of myocarditis in the acute phase of Kawasaki disease (mucocutaneous lymph node syndrome): the usefulness of single photon emission computed tomography. Br Heart J 1987; 58: 385–392.

272. Kao CH, Hsieh KS, Chen YC, Wang YL, Wang SJ. Relationships between coronary artery dilatation and severity of carditis detected by two-dimensional echocardiography and [99mTc]HMPAO-labeled white blood cell heart scan in children with Kawasaki disease. Pediatr Radiol 1994; 24:41–44.

273. Hiraishi S, Yashiro K, Oguchi K, Kusano S, Ishii K, Nakazawa K. Clinical course of cardiovascular involvement in the mucocutaneous lymph node syndrome. Relation between clinical signs of carditis and development of coronary arterial aneurysm. Am J Cardiol 1981; 47:323–330.

274. Moran AM, Newburger JW, Sanders SP, Parness IA, Spevak PJ, Burns JC, Colan SD. Abnormal myocardial mechanics in Kawasaki disease: rapid response to gamma-globulin. Am Heart J 2000; 139: 217–223.

275. Pahl E, Ettedgui J, Neches WH, Park SC. The value of angiography in the follow-up of coronary involvement in mucocutaneous lymph node syndrome (Kawasaki disease). J Am Coll Cardiol 1989; 14: 1318–1325.

276. Sugimura T, Kato H, Inoue O, Fukuda T, Sato N, Ishii M, Takagi J, Akagi T, Maeno Y, Kawano T, et al. Intravascular ultrasound of coronary arteries in children. Assessment of the wall morphology and the lumen after Kawasaki disease. Circulation 1994; 89: 258–265 .

277. Vogel M, Smallhorn JF, Freedom RM. Serial analysis of regional left ventricular wall motion by two-dimensional echocardiography in patients with coronary artery enlargement after Kawasaki disease. J Am Coll Cardiol 1992; 20:915–919.

278. Pahl E, Sehgal R, Chrystof D, Neches WH, Webb CL, Duffy CE, Shulman ST, Chaudhry FA. Feasibility of exercise stress echocardio-

graphy for the follow-up of children with coronary involvement secondary to Kawasaki disease. Circulation 1995; 91:122–128.

279. Kosuda T, Sone K. Assessment of left ventricular function in Kawasaki disease by dipyridamole-loading cineventriculography. Am J Cardiol 1992; 70:863–868.

280. Paridon SM, Galioto FM, Vincent JA, Tomassoni TL, Sullivan NM, Bricker JT. Exercise capacity and incidence of myocardial perfusion defects after Kawasaki disease in children and adolescents. J Am Coll Cardiol 1995; 25:1420–1424.

281. Dhillon R, Clarkson P, Donald AE, Powe AJ, Nash M, Novelli V, Dillon MJ, Deanfield JE. Endothelial dysfunction late after Kawasaki disease. Circulation 1996; 94:2103–2106.

282. Furuyama H, Odagawa Y, Katoh C, Iwado Y, Ito Y, Noriyasu K, Mabuchi M, Yoshinaga K, Kuge Y, Kobayashi K, Tamaki N. Altered myocardial flow reserve and endothelial function late after Kawasaki disease. J Pediatr 2003; 142:149–154.

283. Shulman ST. IVGG therapy in Kawasaki disease: mechanism(s) of action. Clin Immunol Immunopathol 1989; 53:S141–S146.

284. Williams RV, Minich LL, Tani LY. Pharmacological therapy for patients with Kawasaki disease. Paediatr Drugs 2001; 3:649–660.

285. Sundel RP, Baker AL, Fulton DR, Newburger JW. Corticosteroids in the initial treatment of Kawasaki disease: report of a randomized trial. J Pediatr 2003; 142:611–616.

286. Onouchi Z, Kawasaki T. Overview of pharmacological treatment of Kawasaki disease. Drugs 1999; 58:813–822.

287. Cheatham JP, Kugler JD, Gumbiner CH, Latson LA, Hofschire PJ. Intracoronary streptokinase in Kawasaki disease: acute and late thrombolysis. Prog Clin Biol Res 1987; 250:517–518.

288. Kato H, Ichinose E, Inoue O, Akagi T. Intracoronary thrombolytic therapy in Kawasaki disease: treatment and prevention of acute myocardial infarction. Prog Clin Biol Res 1987; 250:445–454.

289. Levy M, Benson LN, Burrows PE, Bentur Y, Strong DK, Smith J, Johnson D, Jacobson S, Koren G. Tissue plasminogen activator for the treatment of thromboembolism in infants and children. J Pediatr 1991; 118:467–472.

290. Williams RV, Wilke VM, Tani LY, Minich LL. Does Abciximab enhance regression of coronary aneurysms resulting from Kawasaki disease? Pediatrics 2002; 109:E4

291. Etheridge SP, Tani LY, Minich LL, Revenaugh JR. Platelet glycoprotein IIb/IIIa receptor blockade therapy for large coronary aneurysms and thrombi in Kawasaki disease. Cathet Cardiovasc Diagn 1998; 45:264–268.

292. Negoro N, Nariyama J, Nakagawa A, Katayama H, Okabe T, Hazui H, Yokota N, Kojima S, Hoshiga M, Morita H, Ishihara T, Hanafusa T. Successful catheter interventional therapy for acute coronary

syndrome secondary to Kawasaki disease in young adults. Circ J 2003; 67:362–365.

293. Ishii M, Ueno T, Akagi T, Baba K, Harada K, Hamaoka K, Kato H, Tsuda E, Uemura S, Saji T, Ogawa S, Echigo S, Yamaguchi T. Guidelines for catheter intervention in coronary artery lesion in Kawasaki disease. Pediatr Int 2001; 43:558–562.

294. Suda Y, Takeuchi Y, Ban T, Ichikawa S, Higashita R. Twenty-two-year follow-up of saphenous vein grafts in pediatric Kawasaki disease. Ann Thorac Surg 2000; 70:1706–1768.

295. Kitamura S. The role of coronary bypass operation on children with Kawasaki disease. Coron Artery Dis 2002; 13:437–447.

296. Travaline JM, Hamilton SM, Ringel RE, Laschinger JC, Ziskind AA. Cardiac transplantation for giant coronary artery aneurysms complicating Kawasaki disease [see comments]. Am J Cardiol 1991; 68: 560–561.

297. Checchia PA, Pahl E, Shaddy RE, Shulman ST. Cardiac transplantation for Kawasaki disease. Pediatrics 1997; 100:695–699.

11

Arrhythmias and Sudden Cardiac Death in Pediatric Heart Failure

MICHAEL J. SILKA and JACQUELINE R. SZMUSZKOVICZ

Division of Cardiology, Children's Hospital, The Keck School of Medicine, University of Southern California, Los Angeles, California, U.S.A.

INTRODUCTION

Cardiac arrhythmias are significant risk factors for morbidity and mortality in children and adolescents with heart failure. Arrhythmias may result in diverse clinical symptoms, adversely affect ventricular function and have prognostic implications. However, conventional treatments for cardiac arrhythmias may not favorably or even adversely influence the clinical course of the disease process in heart failure patients. Therefore, decisions regarding the evaluation and treatment of arrhythmias must consider both hemodynamic and electrophysiologic factors.

There are several problems in assessing the prevalence of arrhythmias in pediatric heart failure patients. These include the lack of uniform definitions of heart failure and ventricular dysfunction as well as the transient nature of most cardiac arrhythmias. Although patients with advanced heart failure may die suddenly, the cause of death is often uncertain and incorrectly presumed to be due to a primary ventricular arrhythmia (1). Given the efficacy of implantable cardioverter-defibrillators (ICD) in the prevention of sudden death in well-defined subsets of patients, an accurate definition of the causal relationship between the ventricular arrhythmias and sudden death has assumed greater importance (2,3). To date, the very limited data in pediatric heart failure patients regarding both arrhythmias and sudden death have prevented attempts to establish risk-stratification and define appropriate treatment strategies (4).

Clinical trials in adult heart failure may have limited relevance to pediatric patients, in whom either right or left ventricular dysfunction may predominate, the etiologies of heart failure are diverse and the clinical course may be variable. It is also important that in the interpretation and application of adult studies to children, one considers the primary ascertainment variable. The randomized clinical trials have focused on arrhythmias in patients with left ventricular systolic dysfunction, whereas epidemiologic studies have used clinical signs and symptoms of circulatory insufficiency as the primary endpoints for analysis (5).

This chapter will discuss the proposed cause and effect relationships between ventricular dysfunction and cardiac arrhythmias. With this background, the published literature regarding cardiac arrhythmias in children with heart failure will be reviewed, followed by an analysis of treatment options for children in the context of large-scale adult epidemiologic and randomized controlled trials of heart failure patients. Based on this evaluation, general treatment guidelines and recommendations will be offered.

PATHOPHYSIOLOGY OF ARRHYTHMIAS
AND SUDDEN DEATH IN HEART FAILURE

Dilated Cardiomyopathies: Cause or Effect?

During the past 20 years, a variety of inotropic, diuretic, and vasodilator drugs have been introduced that have improved the symptoms and enhanced the functional capacity of patients with chronic heart failure. Despite these advances, the prognosis of patients with congestive heart failure remains guarded, with an annual mortality rate between 5% and 25%, depending on the severity of the underlying disease (6,7). As many of these patients die suddenly, an arrhythmic cause often is presumed in the absence of a defined cause.

Patients with chronic heart failure have electrophysiologic abnormalities that often develop and progress in parallel with their mechanical dysfunction. This has given rise to the concept that cardiac arrhythmias and ventricular dysfunction are manifestations of the same fundamental myocardial abnormality (8). At the cellular level, it has been proposed that a fundamental abnormality in calcium uptake and release may be the cause of both ventricular dysfunction and cardiac arrhythmias (9):

Prolonged action potential duration → Cardiac arrhythmias

↑

Abnormal calcium release and uptake

↓

Down regulation of calcium cycling → Impaired systolic and
diastolic function

Clinically, in the captopril–digoxin multicenter trial of *mild to moderate* heart failure, high-grade ventricular ectopy was the primary predictor of progression to advanced heart failure during follow-up, irrespective of the treatment arm during the study. Of note, no patient with high-grade ectopy in this study died suddenly or required resuscitation (10). Other investigators have also noted that in heart failure patients, those with nonsustained ventricular tachycardia are more likely to die of progressive heart failure than sudden death (11).

In patients with an idiopathic (nonischemic) dilated cardiomyopathy, sudden death is often the result of a bradyarrhythmia or electromechanical dissociation (EMD) (1). In studies of adult pretransplant patients, a bradyarrhythmia or EMD was the terminal event in 80–100% of patients with idiopathic dilated cardiomyopathy, but in only 20–36% of patients with advanced coronary artery disease (ischemic heart disease). Therefore, it is critical to consider arrhythmias in the setting of advanced heart failure as a manifestation of a global cardiovascular disorder, rather than as an expression of a specific arrhythmogenic substrate.

These findings have brought into question the routine use of antiarrhythmic drugs or implantable cardioverter-defibrillator (ICD) therapy for primary treatment of heart failure patients with nonsustained ventricular arrhythmias. The converse would appear to apply for ischemic/postinfarc-postinfarction heart failure patients, where most sudden deaths are due to ventricular tachycardia/fibrillation. In these patients, a specific arrhythmic focus or substrate related to prior myocardial infarction/scarring may provide a logical target for pharmacologic suppression or catheter ablative therapy. As will be discussed later, the benefit of an ICD on all-cause mortality has been not been demonstrated in adult heart failure patients with idiopathic dilated cardiomyopathy (12).

Beyond the presence of a fundamental myocardial abnormality, several physiologic responses may also promote the development of cardiac arrhythmias in the setting of heart failure. These include a generalized state of neurohumoral sympathetic activation and cardiac remodeling and dilation due to myocardial hypertrophy, fibrosis, and cell death (13,14). Additional factors such as local myocardial ischemia, electrolyte abnormalities and drug toxicity may further promote the development of cardiac arrhythmias (15). When possible, reversal of these factors provides a more rationale strategy for the treatment of ventricular arrhythmias in the heart failure patient, rather than the empiric use of antiarrhythmic medications for the suppression of simple or complex ventricular ectopy.

As stated earlier, the application of the findings of studies of adult patients with idiopathic dilated cardiomyopathies to young patients with a similar disorder of myocardial function must be made cautiously and critically. However, beyond the first 2 years of life, when cardiomyopathies may at times be considered uniquely reversible, there would appear to be enough commonalities to allow some inference and extension of adult studies to younger patients. This is discussed further in the section on treatment of arrhythmias.

Tachycardia-Related Cardiomyopathies

Persistent tachycardia is a common clinical finding in pediatric patients with heart failure. Although tachycardia may be a physiologic response to impaired ventricular function, it may also be the cause, rather than the consequence of heart failure (16). This distinction is critically important, as correction of a chronic nonphysiologic tachycardia may result in improvement or even complete resolution of ventricular dysfunction. Thus, in the patient with a persistently elevated heart rate and either ventricular systolic dysfunction or clinical congestive heart failure, it is imperative to carefully evaluate cardiac rhythm with careful attention to the P wave axis and P–QRS relationship.

In 1962, Whipple et al. (17) first demonstrated that a cardiomyopathy due to systolic dysfunction could be produced in large mammals if the heart was persistently paced at a rapid rate. Furthermore, this model of biventricular failure was reversible upon the termination of rapid atrial pacing. This model has been repeated by multiple investigators, and has stressed the importance of controlling tachycardia in the overall management of heart failure.

The reasons for the development of myocardial contractile dysfunction in patients with chronic tachycardias are multiple and complex. Deterioration of ventricular function may be due to myocardial energy depletion or impaired energy use, regional ischemia (typically subendocardial), abnormalities of myocyte calcium flux and finally myocyte and interstitial matrix remodeling (18–20). Several studies of chronic rapid pacing in animals have demonstrated reductions in creatine, phosphocreatine, and adenosine triphosphate. Alterations in subendocardial–subepicardial blood flow ratios, with impaired coronary flow reserve in models of chronic rapid pacing, may contribute to myocyte dysfunction due to relative ischemia. Downregulation of calcium cycling, with the ultimate result of decreased availability of this ion for myocyte contractility may provide the final basis to explain the systolic dysfunction that occurs in this syndrome. The additional observations of myocyte hypertrophy and extracellular matrix deposition with resultant stiffening may explain the diastolic dysfunction noted in models of chronic tachycardia (21). Collectively, these pathophysiologic effects result in low cardiac output, elevated filing pressures and dilation and hypertrophy of the heart.

The electrophysiologic mechanisms of chronic tachycardias in children and adolescents include atrial and junctional automatic tachycardias, the permanent form of junctional reciprocating tachycardia and intra-atrial re-entrant tachycardia (atrial flutter). This is in contrast to adult heart failure patients, where atrial fibrillation is the most common cause of tachycardia-induced cardiomyopathy (22). These arrhythmias and their clinical presentations are discussed in subsequent sections in this chapter.

ARRHYTHMIAS IN SPECIFIC CONDITIONS ASSOCIATED WITH PEDIATRIC HEART FAILURE

Dilated Cardiomyopathy

As discussed, cardiac arrhythmias are common in patients with ventricular dysfunction and clinical heart failure. As a consequence of a generalized myopathic process, electrophysiologic abnormalities may include not only atrial and ventricular tachyarrhythmias, but also conduction abnormalities, such as AV nodal or bundle branch block and repolarization abnormalities with QT prolongation and dispersion (Fig. 1).

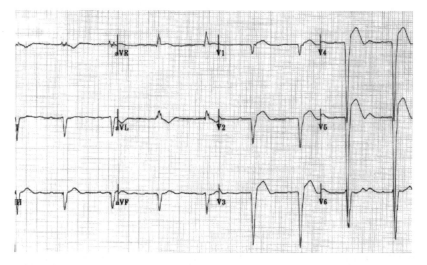

Figure 1 Electrocardiographic findings in a patient with severe dilated cardiomyopathy. There is prolongation of conduction (P–R interval 220 msec), delayed ventricular depolarization (QRS complex = 130 msec), and abnormal repolarization (QT interval = 620 msec in lead V5).

Ventricular Arrhythmias

The prognostic implications of ventricular arrhythmias in the context of heart failure have been studied extensively in adults, with new-onset ventricular arrhythmias often viewed as a manifestation of progressive ventricular dysfunction as much as a risk factor for sudden death (8,10). Nonsustained VT (NSVT) is demonstrated in 30–80% of adult heart failure patients who do not have symptoms of arrhythmia during 24 hr Holter monitoring (23,24). However, there is no evidence that suppression of NSVT has a favorable influence on prognosis in asymptomatic patients with heart failure. Therefore, pharmacologic treatment of asymptomatic NSVT is not advocated in adults with heart failure (25).

To date, ventricular arrhythmias and sudden death have not been studied systematically in pediatric patients with ventricular dysfunction due to idiopathic dilated cardiomyopathy. However, pooled analysis (26–36) of the pediatric

studies which have been published (Table 1) allows the following conclusions: (1) of 456 pediatric patients with dilated
cardiomyopathy, the cumulative mortality was 172 patients
(39%), with the highest mortality during the first year post-
diagnosis; (2) of the deaths, 46 (27%), were classified as
sudden and thus potentially arrhythmic, whereas 126 (73%)
were attributed to progressive heart failure.

Cardiac arrhythmias were specifically identified as risk
factors for sudden or total mortality in only three studies
(27,30,31), and in these studies, ventricular arrhythmias were
associated with other factors, such as an age >2 years at initial
diagnosis or a left ventricular end-diastolic pressure >25 mm
Hg. The prevalence of arrhythmias was not specifically stated
in each study, but where reported, ventricular ectopy or
arrhythmias were identified in only 73 of 270 patients (27%).
Of note, ventricular arrhythmias were uncommon in the
youngest patients (age < 2 years). A cautious interpretation
must be made of these data, however, due to nonuniform methods of arrhythmia ascertainment and frequency of monitoring.
Some studies have suggested a correlation between ventricular
arrhythmias and total mortality, but as in adults, the events
may reflect advanced ventricular dysfunction rather than mortality directly attributable to a cardiac arrhythmia.

Similar to adults, when nonsustained ventricular
arrhythmias occur in pediatric heart failure patients, consideration must be made regarding the need for and type of treatment. Other than isolated PVCs, one of the more common
ventricular arrhythmias in pediatric heart failure is an accelerated ventricular rhythm (Fig. 2). This arrhythmia is defined as
having an origin below the bundle of His and a rate no faster
than 20% of the basic sinus cycle length. This arrhythmia is
usually transient and not associated with hemodynamic compromise. The occurrence of new-onset arrhythmias in pediatric
heart failure patients should prompt a re-evaluation of cardiac
function, with an attempt to improve hemodynamics before
initiating the use of antiarrhythmic medications.

The use of conventional antiarrhythmic drugs for treatment of ventricular arrhythmias in the setting of advanced
ventricular dysfunction must be done with a great deal of

Table 1 Sudden Heart Failure and Total Mortality in Pediatric Series of Dilated Cardiomyopathy

Ref.	Year	No. of patients	No. of deaths	Mortality, %	Mean f/u (months)	1-year mortality, %	5-year mortality, %	No. of sudden deaths	No. of CHF deaths	Risk factors for mortality	Arrhythmic risk factor
Ref. 26	1985	24	12	63	33	37	63	1	11	Severe MR	No
Ref. 27	1988	32	17	53	36	15	25	7	10	Age > 2	Yes
Ref. 28	1990	23	11	48	43	30	44	4	7	Low EF, EFE family history	No
Ref. 29	1991	25	18	72	12	60	80	1	17	CT ratio > 65%, EF < 30%	
Ref. 30	1991	36	12	33	59	25	33	4	8	Undefined	Yes
Ref. 31	1991	81	30	37	42	20	64	11	19	LVEDP > 25 mm Hg	Yes
Ref. 32	1991	63	10	16	48	11	20	3	7	Persistent CHF	No
Ref. 33	1994	19	7	37	39	21	36	3	4	Undefined	No
Ref. 34	1994	63	17	27	19	21	61	7	10	Age > 2; no improvement	
Ref. 35	1995	28	9	32	49	11	22	4	5	Undefined	No
Ref. 36	1998	62	29	47	47	38	50	1	28	EFE, RHF	No
Total		456	172	38				46 27%	126 73%		

CHF, Congestive Heart Failure; CT, Cardiothoracic Ratio on Chest Roentgenogram; EF, Ejection Fraction; EFE, Endocardial Fibroelastosis; LVEDP, Left Ventricular End-Diastolic Pressure; MR, Mitral Regurgitation; RHF, Right Heart Failure.

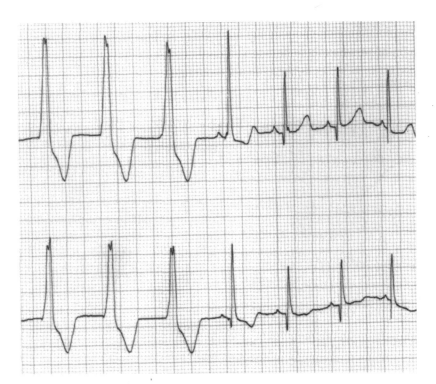

Figure 2 Leads II and aVF demonstrating an accelerated idioventricular rhythm. The first three QRS complexes are wide and not preceded by P waves. The fourth QRS is preceded by a P wave and has an intermediate morphology (fusion) between the first three beats and the subsequent three sinus beats. The cycle length of the idioventricular rhythm (700 msec) is comparable to the sinus rate (760 msec). This rhythm should prompt re-evaluation of hemodynamics and ventricular function. Antiarrhythmic treatment is rarely effective and generally not indicated.

caution, due to the potential for further impairment of ventricular function and drug toxicities due to impaired hepatic metabolism and renal clearance (37,38). Beyond improvement of hemodynamics, acute suppression of sustained ventricular arrhythmias may be achieved with either intravenous lidocaine or amiodarone (39). However, these effects are likely to be temporary at best, and may have unpredictable effects on cardiac conduction and ventricular function.

The use of programed electrical stimulation has limited predictive value in patients with ventricular arrhythmias and dilated cardiomyopathy. Wilber (40) reported a pooled analysis of six studies of DCM patients, with similar protocols and follow-up interval. Of the 288 patients, sustained monomorphic VT was inducible in only 31 (11%). The 2-year risk of sudden death or sustained VT was 32% (10 of 31 patients) with inducible VT vs. 12% (30 of 257) in the noninducible patients, suggesting that patients with a positive response to programed stimulation may represent a higher risk group. However, a negative test had poor predictive value and failed to identify 75% of patients with sudden death or arrhythmic events.

Supraventricular tachycardias may occur in the setting of heart failure, often the consequence of atrial dilation and stretch, resulting in nonuniform conduction and increased automaticity (41). Due to the lack of myocardial reserve and potential for worsening myocardial ischemia and ventricular arrhythmias, sustained supraventricular arrhythmias should be treated promptly. AV reciprocating and nodal re-entrant tachycardias should be treated with adenosine, although prolonged circulation times may prevent therapeutic effect due to the short half-life of adenosine. New-onset atrial re-entrant arrhythmias (flutter, fibrillation) should be treated with synchronized DC cardioversion. Although pharmacologic treatment of atrial flutter/fibrillation with ibutelide may be effective in the setting of "normal" hemodynamics, the potential for QT prolongation and proarrhythmia in advanced ventricular dysfunction must be recognized (42).

Automatic atrial tachycardias may develop in pediatric heart failure patients as a consequence of atrial pressure overload and dilation. At times, the cause and effect relationship between the atrial tachycardia and heart failure may not be clear; however, when the dilated cardiomyopathy antedates the atrial tachycardia, the arrhythmia is likely the consequence, rather than cause, of the cardiomyopathy.

Conduction Abnormalities

Recently, attention has focused on abnormalities of cardiac conduction and repolarization as electrophysiological manifestation of the same intrinsic myocardial disease also resulting in advanced ventricular dysfunction. Conduction system disease most often manifests as a wide QRS complex that may or may not correspond to a specific bundle branch block pattern. The finding of bundle branch block has taken on new importance as criteria are developed to define patients who may benefit from ventricular resynchronization therapy (43,44).

New-onset AV block in association with acute heart failure may be a manifestation of acute myocarditis rather than a chronic dilated cardiomyopathy (45). Ventricular rate support and stabilization with temporary pacing is recommended when acute myocarditis is suspected, with a relatively high rate of recovery of AV conduction within 48–72 hr.

Both prolongation and dispersion of the QT interval are sequelae of abnormal depolarization and repolarization processes which occur in the setting of intrinsic myocardial disease. Martin et al. (46) have reported that compared to other groups of pediatric patients with various causes of heart failure, prolongation of the QT interval (defined as > 0.45 sec) was most common in patients with dilated cardiomyopathy. Furthermore, Dubin et al. (47) reported a strong correlation between the dispersion of the QT interval, which reflects heterogeneity of repolarization times in the ventricular myocardium, and the subsequent development of ventricular arrhythmias in pediatric patients awaiting heart transplantation. QT dispersion of >90 msec provided a 78% sensitivity and 70% sensitivity for pediatric heart failure patients who subsequently developed ventricular arrhythmias. These authors concluded that the finding of this degree of QT dispersion may help identify patients at a higher risk of developing ventricular arrhythmias and who may warrant more frequent monitoring.

Tachycardia-Induced Cardiomyopathies

The initial clinical evaluation of all children with a new diagnosis of cardiomyopathy should include a careful evaluation of the P wave axis and P–QRS relationship. The ECG findings of atrial ectopic tachycardias or chronic AV re-entrant tachycardias may be subtle, due to the subtle variations in P wave axis and P–QRS relationship that may occur. For example, when there is an ectopic tachycardia focus is in the upper right atrium (usually related to the crista terminalis) or right upper pulmonary vein, which is immediately posterior to the location of the sinus node, the P wave axis may be within the normal (0–90°) frontal plane axis (48). The P–R interval may provide some guidance, as a long P–R interval will be more likely in an ectopic atrial tachycardia, whereas a short P–R interval more probable in a sinus tachycardia (49) (Fig. 3). At times, catheter mapping of the sequence of atrial activation may be required to make this differentiation (50). It has been suggested that a persistent heart rate >140 per min is the threshold for development of a tachycardia-related cardiomyopathy in children (51) (Fig. 4).

Definitive treatment of atrial ectopic tachycardia and related cardiomyopathy is usually achieved with RF catheter ablation. However, a high incidence of recurrence of tachycardia following ablation has been reported, most often when the focus is located in the atrial appendages

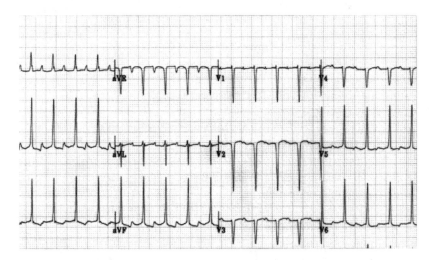

Figure 3 Right atrial ectopic tachycardia associated with a prolonged P–R interval. The P waves are superimposed on the T waves, but the constant rate of tachycardia and P–R prolongation favor diagnosis of an automatic tachycardia rather than sinus tachycardia.

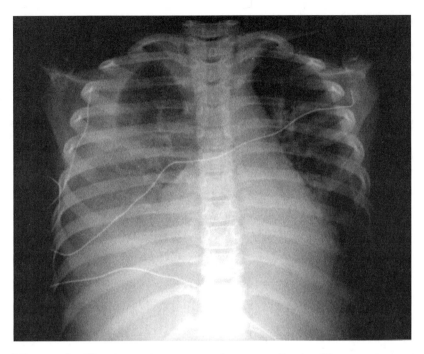

Figure 4 Chest roentgenogram from a patient with recent-onset (<1 week) atrial ectopic tachycardia, rate 220 per min and 1:1 AV conduction. There are bilateral pleural effusions and pulmonary edema. There was resolution of the pleural effusions and pulmonary edema with 36 hr of restoration of sinus rhythm following catheter ablation of the automatic tachycardia focus.

(52). Surgical excision/ablation remains an alternate therapy, particularly when multiple atrial foci are present (53).

A variant of AET presenting as heart failure in the infant is chaotic atrial tachycardia. The electrocardiographic hallmarks are variances in the P wave morphology and axis, accompanied by variable AV conduction (Fig. 5)(54). This arrhythmia is most common in the infant, and unlike the other chronic tachycardias, is amenable to treatment with antiarrhythmic medications. The clinical course of this arrhythmia is one of nonrecurrence beyond the first 6 months of life.

The permanent form of junctional reciprocating tachycardia is also a common cause of tachycardia-induced cardiomyopathy

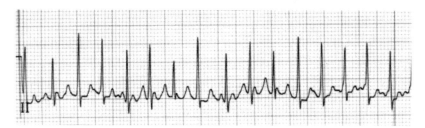

Figure 5 Chaotic atrial tachycardia. This lead II rhythm strip demonstrates an atrial tachycardia in a newborn with variable P wave morphology and an average ventricular rate of 218 per min. Neonatal heart failure commonly occurs within 48 hr of onset of this arrhythmia. The goal of therapy in treatment of chaotic atrial tachycardia is termination of the arrhythmia, rather than control of the ventricular response rate.

in children and adolescents. The electrophysiologic basis is a concealed (retrograde conducting only) accessory connection with properties of decremental retrograde conduction (55). This allows recovery of the AV node for antegrade conduction which allows the tachycardia to persist (or be permanent). This results in the long R–P and normal P–R intervals, the ECG hallmarks of PJRT (Fig. 6). These accessory AV connections may be located at any aspect of the tricuspid or mitral annulus, although most commonly at the posterior septal regions (56). These pathways are highly amenable to definitive treatment with RF catheter ablation, which many have advocated as primary treatment upon diagnosis of PJRT. The arrhythmia may present in infancy, childhood, or adolescence.

Junctional ectopic tachycardia (nonsurgical) may also result in ventricular dysfunction and heart failure. Due to the synchronous ventricular and atrial activation, there tends to be rapid development of pulmonary and systemic venous circulatory congestion. Catheter ablation may offer definitive cure, but is associated with a significant risk of permanent AV block (57).

The degree and time course to recovery of ventricular function following development of a tachycardia-related cardiomyopathy is not clearly defined. This is due to the small numbers of patients at any one medical center, the variety of

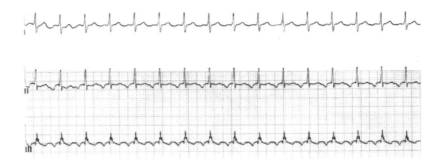

Figure 6 Electrocardiographic features of the permanent form of junctional reciprocating tachycardia with an R–P interval > P–R interval and negative P waves in leads II and III. Although the rate is only 110 per min, this 16-year-old patient presented with severe right heart failure and markedly diminished left ventricular function. The history suggested that tachycardia had been present for several months. Gradual improvement in ventricular function occurred over a 6-month period following ablation of the accessory pathway.

mechanisms of tachycardia and variations in the ventricular rates and duration of tachycardia. The studies of tachycardia-induced cardiomyopathies in children reported to date are listed in Table 2, noting the types of arrhythmias, ages of patients and time to recovery (53,58–61). It is important to note that complete recovery of ventricular function does not always occur, although some improvement in function generally occurs in weeks to months following elimination of the chronic tachycardia.

Cardiomyopathy in Association with Isolated Congenital Complete AV Block

Prior to the development of pacemakers and lead systems which could be safely implanted in young children, the mortality rate associated with congenital complete AV block (CCAVB) was 30–40% (62). With the development of smaller and more reliable pacing systems, this mortality rate improved significantly as the chronic bradycardia resulting in ventricular dilation and mitral insufficiency were

Table 2 Incidence and Time Course to Improvement or Recovery of Left Ventricular Systolic Function in Chronic Tachycardia

Ref.	Year	Number of patients	Number of atrial ectopic tachycardia	Number of permanent junctional tachycardia	Number with ventricular dysfunction	Number of ventricular function recovery	Time to recover (months)
Ref. 51	1985	16	16		10	9	2–6
Ref. 52	2004	30	30		11	11	N.A.
Ref. 58	1992	12	12		12	12	1–6
Ref. 59	1997	8	6	2	8	8	0–6
Ref. 60	2002	4		4	4	4	< 1
Ref. 61	2003	7	6	1	7	7	< 6

eliminated. However, it has become appreciated that some patients with CCAVB may develop a severe form of dilated cardiomyopathy, in whom ventricular function does not improve despite cardiac pacing. The histology in these patients demonstrates a combination of cellular hypertrophy, interstitial fibrosis, and myocyte degeneration (63).

There appear to be three distinct presentations of dilated cardiomyopathy in association with CCAVB. The first are neonates with an in utero or newborn diagnosis of dilated cardiomyopathy associated with CCAVB; these patients appear to have a guarded prognosis, as improvement in ventricular function often does not occur (64). The second are patients who appear to have normal ventricular function and an adequate rate at birth, who may or may not require pacing during the first year of life. These patients develop progressive deterioration of ventricular function during the first 24 months of life (63). Once there is development of a dilated cardiomyopathy, the prognosis also appears poor, with most patients either dying due to congestive heart failure or undergoing heart transplantation (Table 3) (Fig. 10).

The third subset is somewhat older patients with CCAVB who did not require pacing during the first 10–20 years of life. A significant number of these patients develop progressive left ventricular dilation with subsequent mitral insufficiency, which in turn results in further ventricular dilation (65,66).

Table 3 Incidence of Transplantation or Mortality in Patients with Dilated Cardiomyopathy (DCM) Associated with Congenital Complete Heart Block

Ref.	Year	Number of CCAVB patients	Number of DCM	Number of deaths (DCM)	Number of transplants
Ref. 63	2001		16	4	8
Ref. 64	2000	91	21	13	
Ref. 65	2001	149	9	3	6
Ref. 66	2000	34		3	
Ref. 67	1994	55		7	

This presentation has been noted most commonly in the third or fourth decade, and again, once left ventricular dysfunction has occurred, does not appear reversible with conventional pacing methods.

The cause and effect relationship between the arrhythmia and left ventricular dysfunction may differ in these clinical presentations. For example, in the newborn with CCAVB and DCM, active immune-mediated carditis maybe a factor in the early development of ventricular dysfunction (67). Conversely, it has not been proven whether pacing will prevent the delayed-onset DCM in older patients. Regardless, ventricular function should be evaluated on a regular basis in patients with CCAVB, regardless of pacing status. Also, a greater awareness of the poor prognosis for the infant or young child with CCAVB and advanced ventricular dysfunction needs to be emphasized.

Arrhythmias and Sudden Death in Restrictive Cardiomyopathy

Restrictive cardiomyopathy (RCM) is a rare disorder in children and is generally considered to have a poor prognosis, with a reported 2-year survival rates less than 50% (68–70). This is in contrast to adults, where RCM may have a relatively benign and prolonged course, occurring secondary to other disease processes, such as amyloidosis. Ventricular diastolic dysfunction, which is the hallmark of RCM, may result in overt right or left heart failure at initial presentation in children.

Unexpected sudden death has been frequently reported in pediatric series of RCM patients, which has been attributed to arrhythmic events (71). Most sudden deaths appear to occur in patients either with marked elevation of pulmonary vascular resistance or ECG findings of myocardial ischemia. In spite of the marked atrial dilation that is characteristic of RCM, Weller et al. noted atrial arrhythmias in only 3 of 18 patients. Rivenes *et al* also noted conduction defects or the need for pacemaker implantation in 4 of 16 RCM patients. In the later series, ventricular tachycardia or fibrillation was documented in three patients who expired, with the arrhythmias interpreted as secondary to myocardial ischemia.

Similar to DCM, arrhythmias in RCM may reflect a general-ized myocardial disorder—of impaired ventricular perfusion dur-ing diastole or atrial distention due to the elevated end-diastolic pressures. Treatment options are limited, although β-adrenergic receptor blockade has been suggested as having a potentially beneficial effect on both ischemia and catecholamine-related ven-tricular arrhythmias (71). The role of the ICD must be carefully considered, due to the risk of thrombo embolism related to the indwelling defibrillation lead(s) and low-output states. Given the poor prognosis, several authors have advocated preferential listing for heart transplantation upon diagnosis of RCM in children (71,72).

Arrhythmogenic Right Ventricular Cardiomyopathy (ARVC)

Arrhythmogenic right ventricular cardiomyopathy (ARVC) is a progressive myocardial disease characterized by fibrofatty replacement of the myocardium, primarily involving the right ventricle (73,74). Clinically, the manifestations may be either life-threatening ventricular arrhythmias or progressive heart failure (Fig. 7). The diagnosis remains difficult, because the disease often only involves patchy areas of the right ventricle, and many of the electrocardiographic changes mimic patterns seen in normal children. Imaging modalities for diagnosis of ARVC have remained suboptimal, at best. These include echo-cardiography, angiography, and magnetic resonance imaging (75). In part, this reflects the patchy or focal nature of right ventricular involvement in ARVC and in part the thin wall of the RV, resulting in insufficient spacial resolution to adequately quantify freewall myocardial thickness, in addition to the normal presence of epicardial fat.

ARVC is typically inherited as an autosomal dominant trait with variable penetrance and incomplete expression. At this time, the genes responsible for ARVC have not been identified, but seven loci have been mapped to chromosome 14. The cardiac ryanodine receptor gene (RyR2) has also been recently implicated in ARVC and may offer insight into the mechanisms of the adrenergically mediated ventricular

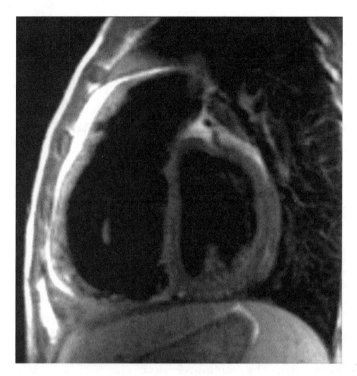

Figure 7 Lateral view of a cardiac magnetic resonance image in a 12-year-old patient with arrhythmogenic right ventricular cardiomyopathy. There is global dilation of the right ventricle, most notable in the right ventricular outflow region. The patient presented with both atrial and ventricular tachyarrhythmias. Fibrofatty replacement of the right ventricular myocardium was confirmed following heart transplantation.

arrhythmias in this disease (76). In addition to genetic causes, degenerative, inflammatory, and apoptotic theories have been proposed as either the cause of ARVC or factors facilitating gene expression (73).

ARVC should be considered in young patients presenting with unexplained syncope, ventricular tachycardia or unexplained cardiac arrest (76). In older patients (>40 years of age), congestive heart failure may be a more common presentation. Heart failure is due to progressive replacement of the right and later the septal and left ventricular myocytes by fibrofatty tissue.

The definitive diagnosis of ARVC requires histologic demonstration of transmural fibrofatty replacement of right ventricular myocardium at autopsy, surgery, or biopsy. Because of the risks of biopsy, an expert consensus group has proposed clinical criteria for the diagnosis of ARVC, with two major or one major and two minor criteria required for diagnosis (Table 4).

Similar to ARVC, patients with idiopathic right ventricular outflow tract (RVOT) tachycardia may also demonstrate mild enlargement of the right ventricle. Programed ventricular stimulation may allow distinction as monomorphic sustained ventricular tachycardia in usually inducible in ARVC (97%) , whereas idiopathic RVOT tachycardia is most often not inducible with timed programed ventricular stimulation, but may be initiated with rapid atrial pacing or isoproterenol, reflecting the triggered mechanism of the arrhythmia (77).

The management of asymptomatic patients with ARVC remains empiric, with the use of β-adrenergic receptor blockade a reasonable concept to reduce the risk of adrenergically

Table 4 Arrhythmogenic Right Ventricular Cardiomyopathy Diagnostic Criteria: Expert Consensus Panel

Major criteria	Minor criteria
Severe isolated RV dilation or dysfunction	Mild RV dilation or dysfunction
Localized RV aneurysm(s) or segmental RV dilation	Regional RV hypokinesia
Transmural fibrofatty replacement	Inverted T waves (V2–V3) without RBBB
Epsilon wave or isolated QRS >110 msec in V1–V3	LBBB-VT or >1,000 PVCs/24 hr
Confirmed familial ARVC	Probable familial ARVC or SD <35 years

LBBB-VT, left bundle branch QRS morphology ventricular tachycardia; RV, right ventricular; SD, unexplained sudden death.
From Ref. 73.

mediated arrhythmias. In patients with sustained or inducible VT, Wichter et al. (78) reported that sotalol was the most effective medication in preventing VT during programed stimulation, with an efficacy of 68%. Class I drugs were effective in <5% of patients. In noninducible patients, sotalol resulted in significant reduction of PVCs in 83% of patients.

Catheter ablation has limited success in ARVC, in part reflecting the progressive nature of the process and multiple foci of arrhythmia. Fontaine et al. (79) have reported sequential success rates of 32%, 45%, and 66% in patients with ARVC after one, two, and three ablation procedures with a mean follow-up of 5.4 years. In the current era, patients who have been resuscitated or considered to be at high risk for sudden death should receive an ICD. Lead placement may be difficult as the sensed ventricular electrograms may be of very low amplitude due to fibrofatty tissue replacement of the myocardium along with the theoretical risk of perforation of the freewall due to thinning of the myocardium.

Congenital Heart Disease

Patients with congenital heart disease may develop both cardiac arrhythmias and symptomatic heart failure as the result of ventricular dysfunction. Similar to other cardiomyopathies, the two findings may be manifestations of the same fundamental myocardial disorder. Multiple factors, including hypertrophy, chamber dilation and postoperative scarring are potential factors in the development of postoperative arrhythmias.

The roles of volume and pressure overload in the development of arrhythmias and subsequent deterioration of cardiac function are well established (80,81). An example of this is the patient with an atrial septal defect with right atrial and right ventricular dilation who develops atrial fibrillation. If chronic, the atrial fibrillation will lead to further deterioration of ventricular function (tachycardia-related cardiomyopathy) with further atrial dilation and remodeling resulting in perpetuation of atrial fibrillation (82). Therefore, a more aggressive approach to ASD closure has been advocated, at least in patients less than 40 years of age (83).

Myocardial dilation (distention) has been demonstrated to be arrhythmogenic, both in isolated tissue as well as in vivo studies (41). Acute distention results in shortening of the action potential duration, which results in after-depolarizations, manifest clinically as PVCs. Chronic volume overload results in prolongation and dispersion of refractoriness, which may facilitate the development of re-entrant arrhythmias. Chronic volume overload thus may result in either QRS prolongation or QTc dispersion. The postoperative tetralogy of Fallot patient with right ventricular volume overload secondary to pulmonary insufficiency is a well-recognized model of this phenomenon. Pulmonary valve placement has been associated with reduction in ectopy and arrhythmia inducibility, although the long-term benefit remains to be proven (84,85).

Intra-atrial re-entrant tachycardia (IART) represents an arrhythmia unique to the postoperative congenital heart disease population. Most common in postoperative Fontan patients, IART may also result in a tachycardia-induced cardiomyopathy. Most often, there is 2:1 AV block that results in atrial and venous pressure elevation, resulting in right as well as left heart failure (Fig. 8). IART or atrial fibrillation may also be a consequence of pulmonary embolism in the post-Fontan patient, which may be another cause of heart failure in this patient group (86). Several studies have suggested that abnormal hemodynamic factors in postoperative congenital heart disease patients including AV valve insufficiency, ventricular failure, or baffle obstruction facilitate the development of IART (87–89).

Whether atrial or ventricular in origin, the hemodynamic significance of an arrhythmia is often accentuated by coexisting ventricular dysfunction. In a meta-analysis of 4627 postoperative tetralogy of Fallot patients, Garson (90) reported that the combination of ventricular dysfunction and spontaneous ventricular arrhythmias was the strongest predictor of patients at risk for sudden death. Sudden death

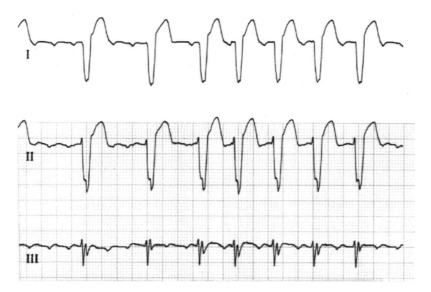

Figure 8 Intra-atrial re-entrant tachycardia with variable conduction. The atrial cycle length is 270 msec (rate 222 per min) in this teenage patient who presented in heart failure 15 years following a Mustard procedure. Inappropriate tachycardia in a patient with prior extensive atrial surgery for congenital heart disease should suggest the possibility of an atrial tachycardia, which may not be obvious on the routine electrocardiogram.

in patients with IART has also been documented, with 1:1 AV conduction resulting in ventricular ischemia or dysfunction that degenerates to ventricular fibrillation (91).

Bradyarrhythmias (either sinus or AV node dysfunction) may result in marked reduction of cardiac output in patients with impaired ventricular function. Bradyarrhythmias may also result in marked dispersion of ventricular refractoriness, resulting in secondary ventricular arrhythmia (Fig.9). Pacemaker devices and indications continue to evolve, but must include restoration of atrioventricular synchrony, when possible in the patient with heart failure (92). Loss of AV conduction may be an intermittent event in patients with AV discordance, but may present as otherwise unexplained heart failure in the presence of ventricular dysfunction (93). In the

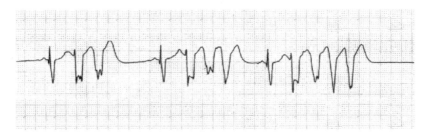

Figure 9 Bradycardia-dependent polymorphic nonsustained ventricular tachycardia in a patient with dilated cardiomyopathy. The long sinus cycle length results in both prolongation and dispersion of ventricular refractoriness, which favor development of the arrhythmia. Atrial pacing at 800 msec (75 per min) resulted in complete suppression of a ventricular ectopy.

post-Fontan patient, restoration of atrial (sinus) rhythm by atrial pacing in patients with a persistent junctional rhythm has been reported to result in resolution of protein-losing enteropathy (94).

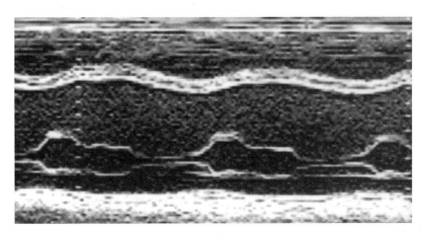

Figure 10 M-mode echocardiographic findings in dilated cardiomyopathy associated with congenital complete heart block. There is marked dilation of the left ventricle with minimal systolic movement of the left ventricular freewall. The infant was born with a ventricular rate of 43 per min, and as demonstrated by this image, there was no objective improvement in ventricular function following DDD pacing.

TREATMENT OF ARRHYTHMIAS IN PEDIATRIC HEART FAILURE

In patients with heart failure, the primary objectives in the treatment of cardiac arrhythmias are to reduce the risk of sudden death, improve hemodynamics, and to alleviate symptoms. However, it is the patient with heart failure in whom the risk of all-cause mortality is highest and the hemodynamic consequences of the arrhythmia may be greatest. The treatment of arrhythmias in these patients must be based on addressing the fundamental defect in physiology, which may be ionic or ischemic, or related to myocardial stretch, or tachycardia-induced cardiomyopathy.

Anticongestive Measures

An initial goal in the acute treatment of arrhythmias is to reverse any recent-onset correctable factors: these may include synchronized cardioversion of an atrial tachycardia or correction of electrolyte disturbance, such as hypokalemia, secondary to diuretic usage. Beyond these obvious issues, improvement in hemodynamics (cardiac output) is often the crucial factor required for control of ventricular arrhythmias in heart failure patients, which may be triggered by mechanical stretch or ischemic causes.

Diverse approaches to sustained ventricular arrhythmia management in the setting of heart failure have been advocated, often with conflicting results. This reflects the physiologic complexities and diverse causes of arrhythmias in these patients. For example, the short-term use of inotropic agents may improve ventricular function and myocardial perfusion resulting in resolution of ventricular arrhythmias—conversely, the same therapy may aggravate the arrhythmias due to increased myocardial oxygen consumption and increased wall stress.

Similar disparate results have been observed with the use of β-adrenergic receptor blockade. This class of drugs may result in further initial compromise of ventricular function due to altered β-adrenergic receptor responsiveness—which may result in further increases in wall stress, myocardial oxygen consumption and arrhythmias; or they may result in resolution of ventricular arrhythmias due to neurohormonal blockade and slowing of ventricular rate allowing for improved perfusion during diastole. The above conflicting results emphasize the uncertainties and caution that must be exercised in the treatment of ventricular arrhythmias, and the need for objective clinical trials to address these complex physiologic issues.

Two recently completed randomized clinical trials of the use of selective β-adrenergic receptor blockade in moderate–severe heart failure have demonstrated significant improvements in overall and sudden cardiac mortality, and make compelling arguments for the use of these agents in heart failure patients, regardless whether the effect is due to anticongestive or antiarrhythmic effect (95,96). The randomized intervention trial in heart failure trial (MERIT-HF) involved 3991 patients randomized to placebo or metoprolol in addition to standard therapy for heart failure. Significant reductions in both heart failure and sudden death were demonstrated in the metoprolol treated group. Similar reductions in all-cause and sudden mortality were reported in the Cardiac Insufficiency Bisoprolol Study-II (CIBIS-II), with 2547 patients randomized either to bisoprolol or placebo. The cumulative survival and antiarrhythmic effects of selective β-blockade in children with heart failure have not been established, but warrant study in a randomized clinical trial.

Carvedilol has complex cardiovascular effects including neurohormonal modulation due to alpha and nonselective β-blockade (97). The hemodynamic studies of carvedilol are discussed elsewhere in this book (see Chapter 15, Medical Management of Chronic Left Ventricular Dysfunction in Children). More recently, it has been appreciated that carvedilol may directly inhibit the HERG potassium channels, thereby altering cardiac action potentials (98). Conceptually, this may result in more homogeneous cardiac repolarization and reduction in QTc dispersion, an effect not seen in a group of children with heart failure treated with β-adrenergic receptor blockers (99).

The effects of carvedilol on complex ventricular arrhythmias in dilated cardiomyopathy may vary, based on the specific disease substrate. In a study of 168 patients with ischemic or idiopathic dilated cardiomyopathy and complex ventricular arrhythmias, the early antiarrhythmic effects of carvedilol were significantly greater in patients with ischemic cardiomyopathy (100). However, after 3 months, when the ejection fraction was significantly improved in both groups, the efficacy of carvedilol was similar in the two groups. The antiarrhythmic efficacy of carvedilol was paralleled by improvement in ventricular function, independent of the etiology of heart failure. Therefore, it is not certain whether the observed benefits were a direct antiarrhythmic effect or secondary to improved hemodynamics, due to decreased stretch or ventricular remodeling.

The potential antiarrhythmic effect of carvedilol will be difficult to assess in children with heart failure, due to the limited population and lower frequency of sustained arrhythmias. This is further compromised by the fact that sustained or symptomatic ventricular arrhythmias were defined as exclusion criteria from the ongoing pediatric randomized carvedilol trial; thus, this question will not be addressed by this study (101).

Class I Antiarrhythmic Agents

In the 1980s, the observation was made that ventricular ectopy after myocardial infarction was predictive of increased mortality, independent of left ventricular function (102). This resulted in the widespread development and use of antiarrhythmic drugs for the suppression of PVCs in all forms of heart disease (103). However, the cardiac arrhythmic suppression trial (CAST) was then performed to test the hypothesis that suppression of ventricular ectopy following myocardial infarction with type IC agents (flecainide and encainide) would improve survival (37). The results of the trial, published in 1991, reported an excess of sudden deaths in the active treatment group compared to the placebo group, and the CAST study was discontinued. A subsequent trial (CAST II) with moricizine demonstrated similar findings in the treatment group and this study was closed in 1992 (104). The survival with oral D-sotalol (SWORD) was a third study that demonstrated an adverse drug effect in patients with impaired ventricular function (105). Based on these randomized clinical trials, the routine use of antiarrhythmic medications for the suppression of PVCs and nonsustained ventricular arrhythmias has been largely abandoned.

Several studies have subsequently reported that the use of class IA or IC antiarrhythmic agents in patients with impaired ventricular function may be particularly deleterious, due to a combination of negative inotrophic effects and unpredictable effects on the processes of cardiac depolarization and repolarization (106,107). Based on the unfavorable risk–benefit ratio in adult heart failure patients, the use of the routine use of class IA or 1C antiarrhythmic drugs in pediatric heart failure patients with nonsustained ventricular arrhythmias would appear to be inadvisable.

Amiodarone

In contrast to other antiarrhythmic agents, the clinical studies of amiodarone in heart failure patients have been more encouraging (12,108). The empiric use of low-dose amiodarone (2–2.5 mg/kg/day) may be preferred for sustained or symptomatic arrhythmias because of absence of significant negative hemodynamic effects and low proarrhythmic potential in heart failure patients (109). The GESICA trial randomized 516 patients, with predominately nonischemic dilated cardiomyopathy (mean LVEF = 20%) to amiodarone vs. placebo (110). The study was terminated at 13 months due to a 28% overall mortality reduction in the amiodarone treated group compared to the controls. Reduction in mortality was observed within 30 days of treatment onset, with persistent benefit beyond 2 years. Conversely, the CHF-STAT (survival trial of antiarrhythmic therapy in CHF) randomized 674 ischemic cardiomyopathy patients with impaired ventricular function and > 10 PVCs per hour to placebo or low-dose amiodarone (111). At 2 years, no significant benefit on survival was observed and there was no significant difference in mortality between those patients with suppression of PVCs vs. those with persistent ventricular arrhythmias treated with amiodarone.

These disparate results may reflect the differences in disease substrate (ischemic vs. nonischemic cardiomyopathy). While amiodarone has not been definitively shown to improve survival, the low incidence of proarrhythmia and side effects suggest it may be the preferred antiarrhythmic agent in this patient population. Furthermore, low-dose amiodarone combined with β-adrenergic receptor blockade may have a synergistic effect, with a greater beneficial effect than either agent alone (109). Similar results have previously been reported in the treatment of pediatric patients with atrial ectopic tachycardia (112).

Implantable Devices

Major advances in design technology and implant techniques have allowed implantable devices to increasingly offer effective therapies for patients with advanced heart failure. These include cardiac resynchronization therapy (CRT) with biventricular pacemakers, ICDs and devices that incorporate the capabilities of both. The optimal indications for both types of devices are topics of intense clinical investigation.

It is estimated that 33% of adults with advanced heart failure have left bundle branch block (LBBB). In some patients with symptomatic heart failure due to systolic dysfunction and LBBB, resynchronization of left ventricular contraction may be achieved with simultaneous stimulation(pacing) of the right ventricular septal apex and basal left ventricle via the coronary sinus branch veins. The concept is to restore "systolic synchrony" of left ventricular contraction with simultaneous apical septal and freewall basal stimulation (44,113). However, clinical investigations have suggested that additional benefits of CRT may also occur due to increasing the interval for diastolic mitral inflow and by prevention of deleterious remodeling due to asynchronous left ventricular contraction (114).

Cardiac resynchronization therapy may provide a secondary antiarrhythmic effect due to improvement in heart failure status, the prevention of ventricular remodeling or reduction in basal sympathetic tone. The COMPANION trial was a randomized clinical trial of CRT in adults with advanced heart failure, LBBB and no ICD indication (115). The patients were randomized in a 1:2:2 sequence to medical therapy, CRT device, or CRT therapy combined with an ICD. The primary endpoints of the study were all-cause mortality and all-cause hospitalization. The study was terminated prematurely at enrollment of 1520 of the planned 2200 patents following the recommendation of the data safety monitoring board. Compared with the control patients (medical therapy alone), the primary endpoints were significantly reduced in both treatment groups, 18.6% in the CRT alone and 19.3% in the combined CRT–ICD group ($p = 0.015$ vs. control). It should be noted that 85% of patients enrolled in this study were classified as New York Heart Association (NYHA) class III.

To date, there have been limited data regarding long-term CRT in pediatric heart failure patients. Several investigators have reported improved ventricular systolic function in the acute postoperative period following surgery for congenital heart disease (116–118). Cardiac resynchronization therapy was accomplished with epicardial pacing wires, and the patients were studied as their own controls comparing right ventricular apical vs. simultaneous biventricular stimulation. Short-term improvements in function and reduced inotropic support were demonstrated in the biventricular paced group.

Dubin et al. (119) have reported acute improvement in right ventricular systolic function in patients with congenital heart disease. Multiple single sites of bipolar stimulation were tested in this series of patients, with right ventricular systolic performance evaluated in response to pacing at various sites. The authors demonstrated acute improvement in right ventricular systolic function with pacing at certain sites compared to others; however, the exact site resulting in optimal stimulation was not consistent and appeared to be patient specific.

Cardiac resynchronization therapy is in early stages of development and the long-term benefit of this approach remains to be demonstrated. It is currently recommended that this therapy should be reserved for patients who remain symptomatic despite optimal medical therapy, who have a wide QRS (>120 msec) and LV systolic dysfunction and dilation (44). Furthermore, the benefit in adult patients with NYHA class II heart failure has not been consistent. An important question, particularly for pediatric patients, will be the benefit of CRT for the large number of late survivors after cardiac surgery with right bundle branch block (RBBB) and right or left ventricular systolic dysfunction.

The technical challenges of coronary sinus lead placement for CRT have not been completed solved. In the randomized clinical trials, failure to implant a functioning lead occurred in 8–12% of all cases (120). Optimal hemodynamic benefit from CRT also involves optimization of the atrioventricular interval and timing or sequence between the right and left ventricle, which again, are variables that remain to be defined. In spite of the novel status of this therapy, CRT offers great promise for many, but not all heart failure patients.

Clinicians should be aware that the pacing nomenclature has been updated to include a fifth character to indicate whether multisite pacing is present (121). The code indicates the chamber where multisite pacing is present: (0) = not present; A = atrial multisite pacing and V = ventricular multisite pacing. Hence, the patient with dual chamber, rate responsive pacing with biventricular stimulation would be coded as DDDRV.

Implantable Cardioverter-Defibrillators (ICDs)

Randomized clinical trials in the 1990s clearly established that the ICD provided a significant survival benefit in well-defined subsets of patients who had a prior myocardial infarction or had impaired ventricular function and sustained ventricular arrhythmias (122). Subsequently, the MADIT II trial demonstrated that improved survival could also be demonstrated in patients with impaired ventricular function (ejection fraction <35%) with no identified ventricular arrhythmias (123,124). This has resulted in considerable debate regarding the prophylactic use of ICDs for prevention of sudden death in diverse subsets of heart failure patients with and without ischemic heart disease. The relative benefits of other therapies such as amiodarone or CRT remain under study (12,115).

The ICD has been shown to be superior to amiodarone for *secondary* prevention of ventricular tachycardia and fibrillation in several large randomized clinical trials where the majority of patients had coronary artery disease (125–127). However, in subgroup analysis, those with dilated cardiomyopathy derived similar benefited from ICD therapy compared to those with coronary disease (128). Therefore, ICD implantation is indicated for the patient with dilated cardiomyopathy and sustained ventricular arrhythmias or aborted sudden cardiac death.

The role of the ICD in primary prophylaxis for dilated cardiomyopathy patients has not been established. The CArdiomyopathy Trial (CAT) evaluated patients with recently diagnosed dilated cardiomyopathy (128). This study was discontinued early due to futility largely due to a lower than expected incidence of all-cause mortality (33). This was a relatively small study (50 ICD patients and 54 controls) with the five-year follow-up reporting 13 deaths in the ICD group vs. 17 in the control cohort ($p = $ ns).

In the AMIOVERT study (12), 103 patients with dilated cardiomyopathy, ejection fraction less than 35% and nonsustained VT were randomized to amiodarone or ICD. The primary endpoint was total mortality and the study was concluded prematurely due to a lower than expected event rate. No differences were observed between the amiodarone and ICD group with respect to outcome.

The sudden cardiac death in heart failure trial (SCD-Heft) is a large ongoing trial comparing amiodarone, ICD, and optimal medical therapy with an endpoint of total mortality (129). It includes patients with both coronary artery disease and nonischemic cardiomyopathy who are in New York Heart Association (NYHA) class II or III heart failure and with ejection fraction less than 35%. The final results of this trial are pending.

There are limited data regarding the use of ICDs in pediatric patients with heart failure or dilated cardiomyopathy. The 1993 report of the Pediatric Electrophysiology Society was a retrospective study of the use of ICDs for young patients with prior ventricular tachycardia or aborted sudden death (130). This study included patients with congenital heart disease, primary electrical disorders, and various cardiomyopathies. Perhaps the most important finding of this study was that the primary risk for all-cause mortality post-ICD implant was impaired ventricular function, irrespective of disease substrate.

In pediatric patients with advanced heart failure awaiting heart transplantation, it is estimated that the risk of sudden death or major morbidity due to a cardiac arrhythmia is 25% (131). Given the increased survival of patients with complex congenital heart disease and those supported with mechanical devices, and the lack of corresponding increase in donor availability, the waiting times and thus risk of an adverse arrhythmic event will increase.

The results of a multicenter study of 27 pediatric heart failure patients (median age 14.5 years) who underwent ICD implantation while awaiting heart transplantation were recently reported (132). Diagnoses included cardiomyopathy ($n = 19$) and congenital heart disease ($n = 7$). Among the 27 patients, there were 51 appropriate therapies in 13 patients and 10 spurious therapies in four patients. The mean time to the first appropriate ICD therapy was 7.7 months postimplant. Two patients developed electromechanical dissociation following ICD discharge. It should be noted that this was a highly selected group of patients, with a mean echocardiographic shortening fraction $7 \pm 5\%$ among the cardiomyopathy patients. The conclusions of this study were that since 50% of patients experienced an appropriate ICD rescue while awaiting transplant and that given the 25% arrhythmic mortality while awaiting transplant, the ICD represents a potential therapy to significantly improve survivorship of those with advanced ventricular dysfunction awaiting transplant. The authors also conclude that methods to risk-stratify young patients while awaiting transplant are needed.

CONCLUSIONS

There are complex mechanistic relationships between heart failure, ventricular dysfunction, and cardiac arrhythmias. It is important to consider the arrhythmias in the context of the underlying disease process and to direct therapy at the fundamental cause, if possible. At times, there may be a primary arrhythmic cause of heart failure, such as a tachycardia-related cardiomyopathy or advanced atrioventricular block. In other scenarios, ventricular arrhythmias may be a manifestation of a fundamental abnormality in myocyte function or impaired myocardial perfusion. Regardless, attempts to restore sinus rhythm and improve hemodynamics may provide significant benefits in allowing sustained arrhythmia control.

Therapies for arrhythmia prevention and treatment are rapidly evolving, with a growing role for device-based therapy. Those therapies that improve hemodynamic status, such as CRT, offer great promise for reducing the morbidity and mortality associated with advanced heart failure. Further advances in the management of heart failure and clinical trials in the next decade will better define those patients who are candidates for long-term device therapy and those who will require heart transplantation.

REFERENCES

1. Luu M, Stevenson WG, Stevenson LW, Baron K, Walden J. Diverse mechanisms of unexpected cardiac arrest in advanced heart failure. Circulation 1989; 80:1675–1680.
2. Buxton AE, Lee KL, Hafley GE, Wyse DG, Fisher JD, Lehmann MH, Pires LA, Gold MR, Packer DL, Josephson ME, Prystowsky EN, Talajic MR; MUSTT Investigators. Relation of ejection fraction and inducible ventricular tachycardia to mode of death in patients with coronary artery disease: an analysis of patients enrolled in the multicenter unsustained tachycardia trial. Circulation 2002; 106(19):2466–2472.

3. Moss AJ, Hall WJ, Cannom DS, Daubert JP, Higgins SL, Levine JH, Saksena S, Waldo AL, Wiiber D, Brown MW, Heo M. Improved survival with an implanted defibrillator in patients with coronary disease at high risk for ventricular arrhythmia. N Engl J Med 1996; 335:1933–1940.

4. Lipshultz, SE. Ventricular dysfunction clinical research in infants, children and adolescents. Prog Pediatr Cardiol 2000; 12:1–28.

5. Cleland JGF, Chattopadhyay S, Khand A, Houghton T, Kaye GC. Prevalence and incidence of arrhythmias and sudden death in heart failure. Heart Fail Rev 2002; 7:229–242.

6. Young JB. Sudden cardiac death syndrome and pump dysfunction: the link. J Heart Lung Transplant 2000; 19:S27–S31.

7. Huikiri HV, Castennalos A, Myerburg RJ. Sudden death due to cardiac arrhythmias. N Engl J Med 2001; 345:1473–1482.

8. Packer M. Lack of relation between ventricular arrhythmias and sudden death in patients with chronic heart failure. Circulation 1992; 85(suppl 1):I-50–I-56.

9. Mishra S, Gupta RC, Tiwari N, Sharov VG, Sabbah HN. Molecular mechanisms of reduced sarcoplasmic reticulum Ca(2+) uptake in human failing left ventricular myocardium. J Heart Lung Transplant 2002; 21:366–373.

10. Gradman A, Deedwania P, Cody R, Massie B, Packer M, Pitt B, Goldstein S. Predictors of total mortality and sudden death in mild to moderate heart failure. Captopril–Digoxin Study Group. J Am Coll Cardiol 1989; 14:564–570.

11. Wilson JR, Schwartz JS, Stoon MS, Ferrero N, Horowitz LN, Reichek N, Josephson ME. Prognosis in severe heart failure: relation to hemo-dynamic measurements and ventricular ectopic activity. J Am Coll Cardiol 1983; 2:403–410.

12. Strickberger SA, Hummel JD, Bartlett TG, Frumin HI, Schuger CD, Beau SL, Bitar C, Morady F. AMIOVIRT Investigators. Amiodarone versus implantable cardioverter-defibrillator: randomized trial in patients with nonischemic dilated cardiomyopathy and asympto-matic nonsustained ventricular tachycardia—AMIOVIRT. J Am Coll Cardiol 2003; 41:1707–1712.

13. Stevenson WG, Stevenson LW, Middlekauff HR, Saxon LA. Sudden death prevention in patients with advanced ventricular dysfunction. Circulation 1993; 88:2953–2961.

14. Floras J. Clinical aspects of sympathetic activation and parasympa-thetic withdrawal in heart failure. J Am Coll Cardiol 1992; 22(suppl A):72A–84A.

15. Eisenhofer G, Friberg P, Rundqvist B, Quyyumi AA, Lambert G, Kaye DM, Kopin IJ, Goldstein DS, Esler MD. Cardiac sympathetic nerve function in congestive heart failure. Circulation 1996; 93:1667–1676.

16. Umana E, Solares A, Alpert MA. Tachycardia-induced cardiomyopathy. Am J Med 2003; 114:51–55.
17. Whipple GH, Sheffield LT, Woodman EG, Theophilis C, Friedman S. Reversible congestive heart failure due to chronic rapid stimulation of the normal heart. Proc N Engl Cardiovasc Soc 1962; 20:39–40.
18. Spinale FG, Hendrick DA, Crawford FA, Smith AC, Hamada Y, Carabello BA. Chronic supraventricular tachycardia casues ventricular dysfunction and subendocardial injury in swine. Am J Physiol 1990; 259:H218–H229.
19. Spinale FG, Grine RC, Tempel GE. Alterations in myocardial capillary vasculature accompany tachycardia-induced cardiomyopathy. Basic Res Cardiol 1992; 87:65–79.
20. O'Brien PJ, Ianuzzo CD, Moe GW. Rapid ventricular pacing in dogs to heart failure: biochemical and physiological studies. Can J Physiol Pharmacol 1990; 68:34–39.
21. Balijepalli RC, Lokuta AJ, Maertz NA, Buck JM, Haworth RA, Valdivia HH, Kamp TJ. Depletion of T-tubules and specific subcellular changes in sarcolenunal proteins in tachycardia-induced heart failure. Caridovasc Res 2003; 59:67–77.
22. Shinbane JS, Wood MA, Jensen DN, Ellenbogen KA, Fitzpatrick AP, Scheinman MM. Tachycardia-induced cardiomyopathy: a review of animal models and clinical studies. J Am Coll Cardiol 1997; 29:709–715.
23. Singh SN, Fisher SG, Carson PE, Fletcher RD. Prevalence and significance of nonsustained ventricular tachycardia in patients with premature ventricular contractions and heart failure treated with vasodilator therapy. Department of Veterans Affairs CHF STAT Investigators. J Am Coll Cardiol 1998; 32:942–947.
24. Doval HC, Nul DR, Grancelli HO, Varini SD, Soifer S, Corrado G, Dubner S, Scapin O, Perrone SV. Nonsustained ventricular tachycardia in severe heart failure. Independent marker of increased mortality due to sudden death. GESICA-GEMA Investigators. Circulation 1996; 94:3198–3203.
25. Singh SN, Fletcher RD, Fisher SG, Singh BN, Lewis HD, Deedwania PC, Massie BM, Colling C, Lazzeri D. Amiodarone in patients with congestive heart failure and asymptomatic ventricular arrhythmia. Survival trial of antiarrhythmic therapy in congestive heart failure. N Engl J Med 1995; 333:77–82.
26. Taliercio CP, Seward JB, Driscoll DJ, Fisher LD, Gersh BJ, Tajik AJ. Idiopathic dilated cardiomyopathy in the young: clinical profile and natural history. J Am Coll Cardiol 1985; 6:1126–1131.
27. Griffin ML, Hernandez A, Martin TC. Dilated cardiomyopathy in infants and children. J Am Coll Cardiol 1988; 11:39–44.
28. Chen S-C, Nouri S, Balfour I, Jureidini S, Appleton RS. Clinical profile of congestive cardiomyopathy in children. J Am Coll Cardiol 1990; 15:189–193.

29. Akagi T, Benson LN, Lightwood NE, Chin K, Wilson G, Freedom RM. Natural history of dilated cardiomyopathy in children. Am Heart J 1991; 121:1502–1506.
30. Wiles HB, McArthur PD, Taylor AB. Prognostic features of children with idiopathic dilated cardiomyopathy. Am J Cardiol 1991; 68: 1372–1376.
31. Lewis AB, Chabot M. Outcome of infants and children with dilated cardiomyopathy. Am J Cardiol 1991; 68:365–369.
32. Friedman RA, Moak JP, Garson A. Clinical course of idiopathic dilated cardiomyopathy in children. J Am Coll Cardiol 1991; 18:152–156.
33. Ciszewski A, Bilinska ZT, Lubiszewska B, Ksiezycka E, Poplawska W, Walczak ME, Walczak E, Wlaczak F, Ruzyllo W. Dilated cardiomyopathy in children: clinical course and prognosis. Pediatr Cardiol 1994; 15:121–126.
34. Burch M, Siddiqi SA, Celermajer DS, Scott C, Bull C, Deanfield JE. Dilated cardiomyopathy in children: determinants of outcome. Br Heart J 1994; 72:246–250.
35. Muller G, Ulmer HE, Hagel KJ, Wolf D. Cardiac dysrhythmias in children with idiopathic dilated or hypertrophic cardiomyopathy. Pediatr Cardiol 1995; 16:56–60.
36. Arola A, Tuominen J, Ruuskanen O, Jokinen E. Idiopathic dilated cardiomyopathy in children: prognostic indicators and outcome. Pediatrics 1998; 101:369–376.
37. Echt DS, Liebson PR, Mitchell LB, Peters RW, Obias-Manno D, Barker AH, Arensberg D, Baker A, Friedman L, Greene HL. Mortality and morbidity in patients receiving encainide, flecainide or placebo. The cardiac arrhythmia suppression trial. N Engl J Med 1991; 324:781–788.
38. Roden DM. Antiarrhythmic drugs: past, present and future. PACE 2003; 26:2340–2349.
39. Atkins DL, Dorian P, Gonzalez ER, Gorgels AP, Kudenchuk PJ, Lurie BD, Morley PT, Robertson C, Samson RA, Silka MJ, Singh BN. Revised American Heart Association/Emergency Care Committee guidelines for resuscitative procedures: treatment of tachyarrhythmias. Ann Emerg Med 2001; 37:S91–S107.
40. Wilber D. Evaluation and treatment of nonsustained ventricular tachycardia. Curr Opin Cardiol 1996; 11:23–31.
41. Franz MR, Cima R, Wang D, Profitt D, Kurz R. Electrophysiological effects of myocardial stretch and mechanical determinants of stretch-activated arrhythmias. Circulation 1992; 86:968–978.
42. Chugh SS, Johnson SB, Packer DL. Altered response to ibutilide in a heart failure model. Cardiovasc Res 2001; 49:94–102.
43. Bristow MR, Feldman AM, Saxon LA. Heart failure management using implantable devices for ventricular resynchronization:

comparison of medical therapy, pacing and defibrillation in chronic heart failure (COMPANION) trial. J Card Fail 2000; 6:276–285.

44. Abraham WT, Hayes DL. Cardiac resynchronization therapy for heart failure. Circulation 2003; 108:1596–2603.

45. Batra AJ, Epstein D, Silka MJ. Clinical course of acquired atriventricular block in children with acute myocarditis. Pediatr Cardiol 2003; 24:495–497.

46. Martin AB, Garson A Jr, Perry JC. Prolonged QT interval in hypertrophic and dilated cardiomyopathy in children. Am Heart J 1994; 127:64–70.

47. Dubin AM, Rosenthal DN, Chin C, Bernstein D. QT dispersion predicts ventricular arrhythmia in pediatric cardiomyopathy patients referred for heart transplantation. J Heart Lung Transplant 1999; L18:781–785.

48. Hegbom F, Hoff PI, Rossvoll R, Ohm OJ. Atypical P wave morphology in incessant atrial tachycardia originating from the right upper pulmonary vein. Scand Cardiovasc J 2000; 34:277–280.

49. Gelb BD, Garson A Jr. Noninvasive discrimination of right atrial ectopic tachycardia from sinus tachycardia in "dilated cardiomyopathy". Am Heart J 1990; 120:886–891.

50. Gillette PC, Smith RT, Garson A Jr, Mullins CE, Gutgesell HP, Goh TH, Cooley DA, McNamara DG. Chronic supraventricular tachycardia. A curable cause of congestive cardiomyopathy. JAMA 1985; 253:391–392.

51. Gillette PC, Wampler DG, Garson A Jr, Zinner A,Ott D, Cooley D. Treatment of atrial automatic tachycardia by ablation procedures. J Am Coll Cardiol 1985; 6:404–409.

52. Salerno JC, Kertesz NJ, Friedman RA, Fenrich AL, Jr. Clinical course of atrial ectopic tachycardia is age-dependent: results and treatment in children < 3 or ≥3 years of age. J Am Coll Cardiol 2004; 43: 438–444.

53. Ott DA, Gillette PC, Garson AT, et al. Surgical management of refractory supraventricular tachycardia in infants and children. J Am Coll Cardiol 1985; 5:124–129.

54. Salim MA, Case CL, Gillette PC. Chaotic atrial tachycardia in children. Am Heart J 1995; 129:831–833.

55. Dorostkar P, Silka MJ, Morady F, Dick M. Clinical course of persistent junctional reciprocating tachycardia. J Am Coll Cardiol 1999; 33:366–376.

56. Ticho BS, Saul JP, Hulse JE, De W, Lulu J, Walsh EP. Variable location of accessory pathways associated with the permanent form of junctional reciprocating tachycardia and confirmation with radiofrequency ablation. Am J Cardiol 1992; 70:1559–1564.

57. Hamdan M, Van Hare GF, Fisher W, Gonzalez R, Dorostkar P, Lee R, Lesh M, Saxon L, Kalman J, Scheinman M. Selective catheter

ablation of the tachycardia focus in patients with nonreentrant junctional tachycardia. Am J Cardiol 1996; 78:1292–1297.

58. Walsh EP, Saul JP, Hulse E. Transcatheter ablation of ectopic atrial tachycardia in young patients using radiofrequency current. Circulation 1992; 86:139–146.

59. Lashus AG, Case CL, Gillette PC. Catheter ablation treatment of supraventricular tachycardia-induced cardiomyopathy. Arch Pediatr Adolesc Med 1997; 151:264–266.

60. Noe P, Van Driel V, Wittkampf F, Sreeram N. Rapid recovery of cardiac function after catheter ablation of persistent junctional reciprocating tachycardia in children. PACE 2002; 25:191–194.

61. Horenstein MS, Saarel E, Dick M, Karpawich PP. Reversible symptomatic dilated cardiomyopathy in older children and young adolescents due to primary non-sinus supraventricular tachyarrhythmias. PACE 2003; 24:274–279.

62. Michaelsson M, Engle MA. Congenital complete heart block: an international study of the natural history. In: Brest AN, Engle MA, eds. Cardiovascular Clinics. Philadelphia: FA Davis, 1972:85–101.

63. Moak JP, Barron KS, Hougen TJ, Wiles HB, Balaji S, Sreeram N, Cohen MH, Nordenberg A, Van Hare GF, Friedman RA, Perez M, Cecchin F, Schneider DS, Nehgme RA, Buyon JP. Congenital heart block: development of late-onset cardiomyopathy, a previously underappreciated sequela. J Am Coll Cardiol 2001; 37:238–242.

64. Eronen M, Siren MK, Ekblad H, Tikanoja T, Julkunen H, Paavilainen T. Short- and long-term outcome of children with congenital complete heart block diagnosed in utero or as a newborn. Pediatrics 2000; 106:86–91.

65. Udink ten Cate FE, Breur JM, Cohen MI, Boramanand N, Kapusta L, Crosson JE, Brenner JI, Lubbers LJ, Friedman AH, Vetter VL, Meijboom EJ. Dilated cardiomyopathy in isolated congenital complete atrioventricular block: early and long-term risk in children. J Am Coll Cardiol 2001; 37:1129–1134.

66. Villian E, Martelli H, Bonnet D, Iserin L, Butera G, Kachaner J. Characteristics and results of epicardial pacing in neonates and infants. PACE 2000; 23:1052–2056.

67. Waltuck J, Buyon JP. Autoantibody-associated congenital heart block: outcome in mothers and children. Ann Intern Med 1994; 120:544–551.

68. Lewis AB. Clinical profile and outcome of restrictive cardiomyopathy in children. Am Heart J 1992; 123:1589–1593.

69. Weller RJ, Weintraub R, Addonizio LJ, Chrisant MRK, Gersony WM, Hsu DT. Outcome of idiopathic restrictive cardiomyopathy in children. Am J Cardiol 2002; 90:501–506.

70. Chen SC, Balfour IC, Jureidini S. Clinical spectrum of restrictive cardiomyopathy in children. J Heart Lung Transplant 2001; 20:90–92.

71. Rivenes SM, Kearney DL, Smith EO, Towbin JA, Denfield S. Sudden death and cardiovascular collapse in children with restrictive cardiomyopathy. Circulation 2000; 102:876–882.

72. Kimberling MT, Balzer DT, Hirsch R, Mendeloff E, Huddleston CB, Canter CE. Cardiac transplantation for pediatric restrictive cardiomyopathy: presentation, evaluation and short-term outcome. J Heart Lung Transplant 2002; 21:455–459.

73. Gemayel C, Pelliccia A, Thompson PD. Arrhythmogenic right ventricular cardiomyopathy. J Am Coll Cardiol 2001; 38:1773–1781.

74. Marcus FI, Fontaine G. Arrhythmogenic right ventricular dysplasia/cardiomyopathy. A review. PACE 1995; 18:1298–1314.

75. Bluemke DA, Krupinski EA, Ovitt T, Gear K, Unger E, Axel L, Boxt LM, Casolo G, Ferrari VA, Funaki B, Globits S, Higgins CB, Julsrud P, Lipton M, Mawson J, Nygren A, Pennell DJ, Stillman A, White RD, Wichter T, Marcus F. MR Imaging of arrhythmogenic right ventricular cardiomyopathy: morphologic findings and interobserver reliability. Cardiology 2003; 99:153–162.

76. Tabib A, Loire R, Chalabreysse L, Meyronnet D, Miras A, Malicier D, Thivolet F, Chevalier P, Bouvagnet P. Circumstances of death and gross and microscopic observations in a series of 200 cases of sudden death associated with arrhythmogenic right ventricular cardiomyopathy and/or dysplasia. Circulation 2003; 108:3000–3005.

77. O'Donnell D, Cox D, Bourke J, Mitchell L, Furniss S. Clinical and electrophysiological differences between patients with arrhythmogenic right ventricular dysplasia and right ventricular outflow tract tachycardia. Eur Heart J 2003; 24:801–810.

78. Wichter T, Hindricks G, Lerch H, Bartenstein P, Borggrefe M, Schober O, Breithardt G. Regional myocardial sympathetic dysinnervation in arrhythmogenic right ventricular cardiomyopathy. An analysis using 1231-meta-iodobenzylguanidine scintigraphy. Circulation 1994; 89:667–683.

79. Fontaine G, Tonet J, Gallais Y, Lascault G, Hidden-Lucet F, Aouate P, Halimi F, Poulain F, Johnson N, Charfeddine H, Frank R. Ventricular tachycardia catheter ablation in arrhythmogenic right ventricular dysplasia: a 16-year experience. Curr Cardiol Rep 2000; 2:498–506.

80. Beuckelmann DJ, Nabauer M, Erdmann E. Alterations of K^+ currents in isolated human ventricular myocytes from patients with terminal heart failure. Circ Res 1993; 73:379–385.

81. Aronson RS, Ming Z. Cellular mechanisms of arrhythmias in hypertrophied and failing myocardium. Circulation 1993; 87:VII-76–VII-83.

82. Perloff JK. Surgical closure of atrial septal defects in adults. N Engl J Med 1995; 333:513–4.

83. Gatzoulis MA, Freeman MA, Sui SC, Webb GD, Harris L. Atrial arrhythmia after surgical closure of atrial septal defects in adults. N Engl J Med 1999; 340:839–846.

84. Zahka KG, Horneffer PJ, Rowe SA, Neill CA, Manolio TA, Kidd L, Gardner TJ. Long-term valvular function after total repair of tetralogy of Fallot. Relation to ventricular arrhythmias. Circulation 1988; 78:III-14–III-19.

85. Therrien J, Siu SC, Harris L, Dore A, Niwa K, Janousek J, Williams WG, Webb G, Gatzoulis MA. Impact of pulmonary valve replacement on arrhythmia propensity late after repair of tetralogy of Fallot. Circulation 2001; 103:2489–2494.

86. Peters NS, Somerville J. Arrhythmias after the Fontan procedure. Br Heart J 1992; 68:199–204.

87. Weipert J, Noebauer C, Schreiber C, Kostolny M, Zrenner B, Wacker A, Hess J, Lange R. Occurrence and management of atrial arrhythmia after long-term Fontan circulation. J Thorac Cardiovasc Surg 2004; 127:457–464.

88. Fishberger SB, Wernovsky G, Gentles TL, Gauvreau K, Burnett J, Mayer JE Jr, Walsh EP. Factors that influence the development of atrial flutter after the Fontan operation. J Thorac Cardiovasc Surg 1997; 113:80–86.

89. Mavroudis C, Backer CL, Deal BJ, Johnsrude C, Strasburger J. Total cavopulmonary conversion and maze procedure for patients with failure of the Fontan operation. J Thorac Cardiovasc Surg 2001; 122:863–871.

90. Garson A Jr. Ventricular arrhythmias after repair of congenital heart disease: who needs treatment? Cardiol Young 1991; 1:177–181.

91. Silka MJ, Kron J, McAnulty JH. Supraventricular tachycardia, congenital heart disease, and sudden cardiac death. Pediatr Cardiol 1992; 13:116–118.

92. Nicod P, Hillis LD, Winniford MD, Firth BG. Importance of the "atrial kick" in determining the effective mitral valve orifice area in mitral stenosis. Am J Cardiol 1986; 57:403–407.

93. Huhta JC, Danielson GK, Ritter DG, Ilstrup DM. Survival in atrioventricular discordance. Pediatr Cardiol 1985; 6:57–60.

94. Cohen MI, Rhodes LA, Wernovsky G, Gaynor JW, Spray TL, Rychik J. Atrial pacing: an alternative treatment for protein-losing enteropathy after the Fontan operation. J Thorac Cardiovasc Surg 2001; 121:542–543.

95. Hjalmarson A, Goldstein S, Fagerberg B. Effect of metoprolol CR/XL in chronic heart failure: metoprolol CR/XL randomised intervention trial in congestive heart failure (MERIT-HF). Lancet 1999; 353: 2001–2007.

96. Leizorovicz A, Lechat P, Cucherat M, Bugnard F, McMurray J. Bisoprolol for the treatment of chronic heart failure: a meta-analysis on individual data of two placebo-controlled studies—CIBIS and CIBIS II. Cardiac insufficiency bisoprolol study. Am Heart J 2002; 143: 301–307.

97. Giardini A, Formigari R, Bronzetti G, Prandstraller D, Donti A, Bonvicini M, Picchio FM. Modulation of neurohormonal activity after treatment of children in heart failure with carvedilol. Cardiol Young 2003; 13:333–336.

98. Karle CA, Kreye VA, Thomas D, Rockl K, Kathofer S, Zhang W, Kiehn J. Antiarrhythmic drug carvedilol inhibits HERG potassium channels. Cardiovasc Res 2001; 49:361–370.

99. Etheridge SP, Shaddy RE. QT dispersion after beta-blocker therapy (carvedilol or metoprolol) in children with heart failure. Am J Cardiol 2003; 91:1497–1500.

100. Di Lenarda A, Sabbadini G, Salvatore L, Sinagra G, Mestroni L, Pinamonti B, Gregori D, Ciani F, Muzzi A, Klugmann S, Camerini F. Long-term effects of carvedilol in idiopathic dilated cardiomyopathy with persistent left ventricular dysfunction despite chronic metoprolol. The Heart-Muscle Disease Study Group. J Am Coll Cardiol 1999; 33:1926–1934.

101. Shaddy RE, Curtin EL, Sower B, Tani LY, Burr J, LaSalle B, Boucek MM, Mahony L, Hsu DT, Pahl E, Burch GH, Schlencker-Herceg R. The pediatric randomized carvedilol trial in children with heart failure: rationale and design. Am Heart J 2002; 144:383–389.

102. Bigger JT Jr, Fleiss JL, Kleiger R, Miler JP, Rolnitzky LM. The relationships among ventricular arrhythmias, left ventricular dysfunction and mortality in the 2 years after myocardial infarction. Circulation 1984; 54:31–36.

103. Wilber DJ, Olshansky B, Moran JR, Scanlon PJ. Electrophysiological testing and nonsustained ventricular tachycardia. Use and limitations in patients with coronary artery disease and impaired ventricular function. Circulation 1990; 82:350–358.

104. Epstein AE, Bigger JT Jr, Wyse DG, Romhilt DW, Reynolds-Haertle RA, Hallstrom AP. Events in the cardiac arrhythmia suppression trial (CAST): mortality in the entire population enrolled. J Am Coll Cardiol 1991; 18:14–19.

105. Waldo AL, Camm AJ, deRuyter H, Friedman PL, MacNeil DJ, Pauls JF, Pitt B, Pratt CM, Schwartz PJ, Veltri EP. Effect of D-sotalol on mortality in patients with left ventricular dysfunction after recent and remote myocardial infarction. The SWORD Investigators. Survival With Oral D-Sotalol. Lancet 1996; 348:7–12.

106. Levy MN, Wiseman MN. Electrophysiologic mechanisms for ventricular arrhythmias in left ventricular dysfunction: electrolytes, catecholamines and drugs. J Clin Pharmacol 1991; 31:1053–1060.

107. Gillis AM. Effects of antiarrhythmic drugs on QT interval dispersion—relationship to antiarrhythmic action and proarrhythmia. Prog Cardiovasc Dis 2000; 42:385–396.

108. Amiodarone Trials Meta-analysis Investigators. The effect of prophylactic amiodarone on mortality after acute myocardial infarction and in congestive heart failure: meta-analysis of individual patient data

on 6500 patients from randomized trials. Lancet 1997; 350: 1417–1424.

109. Suzuki T, Shiga T, Wakaumi M, Matsuda N, Ishizuka N, Kasanuki H. Hemodynamics during chronic amiodarone administration in Japanese patients with idiopathic dilated cardiomyopathy and ventricular arrhythmia: a retrospective study. J Cardiol 2003; 41:169–173.

110. Doval HC, Nul DR, Grancelli HO, Perrone SV, Bortman GR, Curiel R. Randomised trial of low-dose amiodarone in severe congestive heart failure. Grupo de Estudio de la Sobrevida en la Insuficiencia Cardiaca en Argentina (GESICA). Lancet 1994; 344:493–498.

111. Deedwania PC, Singh BN, Ellenbogen K, Fisher S, Fletcher R, Singh SN. Spontaneous conversion and maintenance of sinus rhythm by amiodarone in patients with heart failure and atrial fibrillation: observations from the Veterans Affairs congestive heart failure survival trial of antiarrhythmic therapy (CHF-STAT). The Department of Veterans Affairs CHF-STAT Investigators. Circulation 1998; 98:2574–2579.

112. Pongiglione G, Strasburger JF, Deal BJ, Benson DW Jr. Use of amiodarone for short-term and adjuvant therapy in young patients. Am J Cardiol 1991; 68:603–608.

113. Cazeau S, Leclercq C, Lavergne T. Effects of multisite biventricular pacing in patients with heart failure and intraventricular conduction delay. N Engl J Med 2001; 344:873–880.

114. Saxon LA, Ellenbogen KA. Resynchronization therapy for the treatment of heart failure. Circulation 2003; 108:1044–1048.

115. Bristow MR, Feldman AM, Saxon LA. Heart failure management using implantable devices for ventricular resynchronization: comparison of medical therapy, pacing, and defibrillation in chronic heart failure (COMPANION) trial. COMPANION Steering Committee and COMPANION Clinical Investigators. J Card Fail 2000; 6:276–285.

116. Janousek J, Vojtovic P, Hucin B, TIaskal T, Gebauer RA, Gebauer R, Matejka T, Marek J, Reich O. Resynchronization pacing is a useful adjunct to the management of acute heart failure after surgery for congenital heart defects. Am J Cardiol 2001; 88:145–152.

117. Zimmerman FJ, Starr JP, Koenig PR, Smith P, Hijazi ZM, Bacha EA. Acute hemodynamic benefit of multisite ventricular pacing after congenital heart surgery. Ann Thorac Surg 2003; 75:1775–1780.

118. Roofthooft MT, Blom NA, Rijlaarsdarn ME, Bokenkamp R, Ottenkamp J, Schalij MJ, Bax JJ, Hazekamp MG. Resynchronization therapy after congenital heart surgery to improve left ventricular function. PACE 2003; 26:2042–2044.

119. Dubin AM, Feinstein JA, Reddy VM, Hanley FL, Van Hare GF, Rosenthal DN. Electrical resynchronization: a novel therapy for the failing right ventricle. Circulation 2003; 107:2287–2289.

120. Daoud EG, Kalbfleisch SJ, Hummel JD, Weiss R, Augustini RS, Duff SB, Polsinelli G, Castor J, Meta T. Implantation techniques and chronic lead parameters of biventricular pacing dual-chamber defibrillators. J Cardiovasc Electrophysiol 2002; 13:964–970.

121. Bernstein AD, Daubert JC, Fletcher RD, Hayes DL, uderitz B, Reynolds DW, Schoenfeld MH, Sutton R. The revised NASPE/BPEG BPEG generic code for antibradycardia, adaptive-rate, and multisite pacing. North American Society of Pacing and Electrophysiology/British Pacing and Electrophysiology Group. PACE 2002; 25: 260–264.

122. Lee DS, Green LD, Liu PP, Dorian P, Newman DM, Grant FC, Tu JV, Alter DA. Effectiveness of implantable defibrillators for preventing arrhythmic events and death: a meta-analysis. J Am Coll Cardiol 2003; 41:1573–1582.

123. Moss AJ, Zareba W, Hall WJ. Prophylactic implantation of a defibrillator in patients with myocardial infarction and reduced ejection fraction. N Engl J Med 2002; 346:877–883.

124. Reynolds MR, Josephson ME. MADIT II (second multicenter automated defibrillator implantation trial) debate: risk stratification, costs, and public policy. Circulation 2003; 108:1779–1783.

125. Moss AJ, Jackson Hall W, Cannom DS, Daubert JP, Higgins SL, Klein H, Levine JH, Saksena S, Waldo AL, Wilber D, Brown MW, Heo M. Improved survival with an implanted defibrillator in patients with coronary disease at high risk for ventricular arrhythmia. N Engl J Med 1996; 335:1933–1940.

126. Lee KL, Hafley G, Fisher JD, Gold MR, Prystowsky EN, Talajic M, Josephson ME, Packer DL, Buxton AE. Multicenter Unsustained Tachycardia Trial Investigators. Effect of implantable defibrillators on arrhythmic events and mortality in the multicenter unsustained tachycardia trial. Circulation 2002; 106:233–238.

127. Owens DK, Sanders GD, Heidenreich PA, McDonald KM, Hlatky MA. Effect of risk stratification on cost-effectiveness of the implantable cardioverter defibrillator. Am Heart J 2002; 144:440–448.

128. Rankovic V, Karha J, Passman R, Kadish AH, Goldberger JJ. Predictors of appropriate implantable cardioverter-defibrillator therapy in patients with idiopathic dilated cardiomyopathy. Am J Cardiol 2002; 89:1072–1076.

129. Klein H, Auricchio A, Reek S, Geller C. New primary prevention trials of sudden cardiac death in patients with left ventricular dysfunction: SCD-HEFT and MADIT. Sudden cardiac death in heart failure trial. Multicenter automatic defibrillator implantation trial. Am J Cardiol 1999; 83:91D–97D.

130. Silka MJ, Kron J, Dunnigan A, Dick M. for the Pedaitric Electrophysiology Society: Sudden cardiac death the use of implantable cardioverter defibrillators in young patients. Circulation 1993; 87:800–807.

131. Rosenthal DN, Dubin AM, Chin C, Falco D, Gamberg P, Bernstein D. Outcome while awaiting heart transplantation in children: a comparison of congenital heart disease and cardiomyopathy. J Heart Lung Transplant 2000; 19:751–755.

132. Dubin AM, Berul CI, Bevilacqua LM, Collins KK, Ethendge SP, Fenrich AL, Friedman RA, Hamilton RM, Schaffer MS, Shah M, Silka MJ, Van Hare GF, Kertesz NJ. The use of implantable cardioverter-defibrillators in pediatric patients awaiting heart transplantation. J Card Fail 2003; 9:375–379.

12

Single Ventricle Lesions

CHARLES E. CANTER

Washington University School of Medicine,
St. Louis, Missouri, U.S.A.

Congenital heart disease associated with only one effective pumping chamber, or single ventricle, comprises about 2% of all congenital heart disease (1). However, there are a wide diversity of structural heart defects where there is only one effective single ventricle. Variations are defined by the morphology of the ventricle, number and type of AV valves, orientation of the great vessels, associated lesions leading to obstruction of flow into or out of the single ventricle, and dependence of pulmonary or systemic flow upon a patent ductus arteriosus. Heart failure is a common complication of single ventricle lesions and may occur from the newborn period into adulthood.

The natural history of patients with single ventricles is extremely poor and most patients die in infancy and childhood without some sort of surgical intervention. Rare cases (2–4) can survive into adulthood, but they generally have associated congestive heart failure and/or pulmonary vascular disease (5). The majority of patients (6,7) do not survive to adulthood without multiple surgical interventions.

HEART FAILURE IN THE NEWBORN PERIOD

Most patients with single ventricle lesions present in infancy either with cyanosis from decreased pulmonary blood flow or congestive heart failure from left-to-right shunting associated with unrestricted pulmonary blood flow. Within the many anatomic variants of a single ventricle circulatory system, there are five pathophysiologic factors that are associated with heart failure in single ventricle patients in the newborn period: (1) unobstructed pulmonary blood flow; (2) obstruction to systemic flow; (3) obstruction to pulmonary venous return; (4) insufficiency of the atrio-ventricular valve(s); and (5) coronary hypoperfusion. Figure 1 illustrates that these factors can occur by themselves or in various combinations in multiple single ventricle lesions.

With the normal decrease in pulmonary vascular resistance that occurs after birth, infants with single ventricles without obstruction to pulmonary blood flow will develop increasing pulmonary overcirculation, volume overloading of the single ventricle, and congestive heart failure. Banding of the main pulmonary artery to restrict pulmonary blood flow has been the traditional technique used to relieve heart failure symptoms from pulmonary overcirculation and prevent subsequent elevation of pulmonary vascular resistance which can preclude later palliative procedures. Effective relief of heart failure symptoms is generally obtained when pulmonary pressures are reduced to one-third to one-half systemic and arterial oxygen saturations to 75–90% (8).

Pulmonary artery banding results in a reduction of ventricular volume overload, but also leads to ventricular hypertrophy proximal to the pulmonary artery band. In patients with single ventricles where outflow to the aorta is through a ventricular septal defect (or bulboventricular foramen) both

Pathophysiology	Anatomic Lesion
Unobstructed Pulmonary Blood Flow	
	Double inlet left ventricle
	Hypoplastic left heart syndrome
	Tricuspid atresia (some types)
	Mitral atresia
	Heterotaxies
Systemic Ventricular Outflow Obstruction	
	Any single ventricle with coarctation of the aorta
	Single ventricle with Bulbo-ventricular outflow chamber
	Tricuspid atresia (some types)
	Hypoplastic left heart syndrome
Obstruction of Pulmonary Venous Return	
	Heterotaxies
	Hypoplastic left heart syndrome
	Mitral atresia
Atrioventricular Valve Insufficiency	
	Unbalanced atrioventricular canal
	Double inlet left ventricle with tricuspid left
	atrioventricular A̶V̶ valve
	Heterotaxies
Decreased Coronary Perfusion	
	Hypoplastic left heart syndrome
	Pulmonary atresia with intact septum

Figure 1 Pathophysiologic factors and associated single ventricle lesions producing heart failure in the newborn period.

ventricular volume reduction (9) and increasing ventricular hypertrophy (10) after pulmonary artery banding may result in a decrease in the size of the ventricular septal defect (or bulboventricular foramen) and lead to acquired subaortic stenosis. These complications have made the routine use of pulmonary artery banding in this subgroup of patients controversial (10–13). Pulmonary artery banding still has its advocates (11,12) when the ventricular septal defect (or bulboventricular foramen) is large, but is a less attractive surgical option when the ventricular septal defect (or bulboventriculr foramen) is either restrictive in size or is thought to have the potential for the development of restriction to flow (12,13).

Hypoplastic left heart syndrome is the most common single ventricle lesion where heart failure occurs with the combination of pulmonary overcirculation and systemic ventricular outflow obstruction. The pioneering infant palliation of Norwood et al. (14) for this fatal lesion provided aortic arch reconstruction and relief of ventricular outflow obstruction and limitation of pulmonary blood flow through disconnection of the pulmonary arteries from the heart and provision of pulmonary flow by an aorto-pulmonary or Blalock-Taussig shunt. Recently (15,16) a new strategy to relieve ventricular outflow obstruction and limit pulmonary flow has utilized interventional catheterization techniques to stent the ductus arteriosus and band the pulmonary arteries. A totally interventional catheterization-based technique has been devised to combine stenting of the ductus arteriosus to provide unobstructed ventricular outflow and limit pulmonary flow by internal pulmonary artery partial obstruction (17).

A similar strategy for relief of systemic ventricular outflow obstruction and limitation of pulmonary flow is increasingly being employed to palliate heart failure in other single ventricle lesions with unobstructed pulmonary blood flow who have pre-existing subaortic stenosis, and are felt to be either at high risk for developing subaortic stenosis, or have concomitant aortic arch hypoplasia (18–20). In these cases, systemic ventricular outflow obstruction is relieved by connecting the unobstructed pulmonary trunk to the ascending aorta (Damus-Kaye-Stansel procedure). Distal obstructions if present, such as coarctation of the aorta, must also be relieved.

Recent models (21) of single ventricle physiology where pulmonary blood flow is provided by a flow-limiting connection (artificial aorto-pulmonary shunt) off of the aorta suggest that systemic vascular resistance exerts more of an effect on hemodynamics than pulmonary vascular resistance. In these models, large aorto-pulmonary connections (shunts) tend to reduce systemic oxygen delivery by diverting an increased proportion of cardiac output to the lungs. The optimal pulmonary-to-systemic blood flow ratio for the best systemic oxygen delivery over a variety of physiologic states for a single ventricle with pulmonary flow supplied by a connection from the aorta appears to be 1:1 (21,22).

Obstruction to pulmonary venous return leads to pulmonary venous hypertension and pulmonary edema. Single ventricle patients with heterotaxia, especially right-sided isomerism, or asplenia, frequently have anomalously draining pulmonary venous return that is often obstructed (23). As these patients may also have associated pulmonary stenosis or atresia, pulmonary venous obstruction may be occult and only cause heart failure after initial palliative surgery to increase pulmonary blood flow is performed. Pulmonary venous obstruction is one of the major risk factors for a poorer prognosis in single ventricle patients with heterotaxy syndromes, especially in the newborn period when it generally needs to be corrected (24–27).

Pulmonary venous obstruction with (28) or without anomalous drainage of pulmonary venous return may also occur in single ventricle patients who have a severely restrictive atrial septal defects or foramen ovale associated with an atretic or severely stenotic atrioventricular valve from the left atrium. This problem is generally observed in some patients with hypoplastic left heart syndrome or mitral atresia with double outlet right ventricle. Pulmonary venous obstruction from a restrictive atrial communication in patient with single ventricles is generally treated with balloon or blade atrial septostomy via interventional cardiac catheterization (15,16,28), but may require a surgical atrial septectomy. Hypoplastic left heart syndrome patients with severely restrictive foramen ovale or intact atrial septum are subgroup with a particularly poor prognosis (29). In these patients, pulmonary venous obstruction often leads to pathologic evidence of changes in the lymphatics and pulmonary venous microvasculature as a result of pulmonary veno-occlusive disease (30–32).

Atrioventricular valve regurgitation may occur in the newborn period in single ventricle patients with a common atrioventricular valve, tricuspid valve dysplasia (Ebstein's or non-Ebstein's), and in hypoplastic left heart syndrome. Moderate to severe regurgitation will exacerbate symptoms of congestive heart failure in single ventricle patients in the newborn period.

Severe abnormalities of coronary artery anatomy leading to dependence on the right ventricle for myocardial perfusion occur in 7–10% of patients with pulmonary—atresia with intact ventricular septum (33,34). These patients are at risk for myocardial ischemia and sudden death in the newborn period. Careful delineation of the coronary artery anatomy and the pattern of myocardial perfusion via cardiac catheterization and angiography is an important part of the initial evaluation of all patients with pulmonary atresia with intact septum. In instances where there is true right ventricular-dependent coronary circulation, decompression of the right ventricle can exacerbate left ventricular dysfunction (35,36) and should be avoided. However, sudden death may occur even without right ventricular decompression (35,37).

Hypoplastic left heart syndrome is generally not associated with gross abnormalities of coronary artery anatomy, but myocardial infarction and ischemia are frequently observed in infants with hypoplastic left ventricles dying before and after palliative surgery (38,39). Studies of coronary flow and coronary flow reserve by positron emission tomography have found that infants after a Norwood palliation for hypoplastic left heart syndrome have less coronary perfusion and oxygen delivery to the systemic ventricle than infants studied after a 2 ventricular repair of congenital heart disease

(40). The use of an aorto-pulmonary shunt to provide pulmonary blood flow in patients with hypoplastic left heart syndrome and other similarly palliated single ventricle lesions may lower aortic diastolic pressure and thus decrease coronary flow. A recent modification of the Norwood procedure has used a small right-ventricular-to-pulmonary-artery conduit for pulmonary artery perfusion instead of the more classic aorto-pulmonary shunt. Initial experience with this technique appears favorable, with higher diastolic aortic pressures and a pulmonary to systemic blood flow ratio closer to 1:1 compared to use of the classic Norwood technique with an aorto-pulmonary shunt (41,42).

ESTABLISHMENT OF A SERIES CONNECTION OF THE SYSTEMIC AND PULMONARY CIRCUIT IN THE SINGLE VENTRICLE PATIENT—FONTAN PHYSIOLOGY

Palliation of the infant with a single ventricle lesion combines augmenting or reducing pulmonary blood flow, relieving systemic outflow obstruction of the single ventricle, and eliminating obstruction of pulmonary venous return. In this situation, the pulmonary and systemic circulation are not in their normal series connection (Fig. 2A) but are in a parallel circuit (Fig. 2B) with resultant ventricular volume overload of the one pump that depends on the degree of pulmonary blood flow and valvular regurgitation. Average ventricular volume of single ventricles palliated in this fashion ranges from 110% to 140% of a normal left or right ventricle (43–45). Associated with this volume overload can be inappropriate increases in ventricular mass and ventricular mass/volume ratios (46,47), as well as increases in ventricular afterload (48). The ejection fraction of single ventricles with this palliation is low, averaging in the low to mid-50% range (43–48), and tends to decrease with increasing volume load because of increasing atrioventricular valve insufficiency. Abnormalities of systolic function exist independent of ventricular preload and afterload (49).

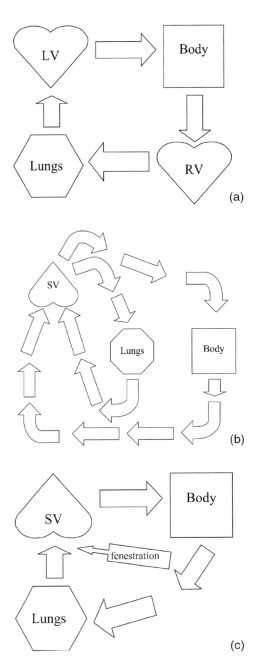

(a)

(b)

(c)

Figure 2 (*Caption on facing page*)

These ongoing abnormalities in ventricular size and function are associated with an ongoing attrition rate from progressive heart failure and death with age (5–7). Franklin et al. (50) found these risks often occurred prior to 4 years of age. Thus, palliations performed in infancy are of only short-term benefit.

In the early 1970s, Fontan and Baudet (51) and Kreutzer et al. (52) applied a new concept of placing the pulmonary and systemic circulation back in a series connection in the single ventricle patient (Fig. 2C). The series connection was accomplished by connecting the systemic venous return directly to the pulmonary arteries without a ventricular pump. With what has been ultimately termed "Fontan physiology," systemic venous pressure becomes markedly elevated and drives the pulmonary flow. This circulatory system can only succeed if (1) the pulmonary vascular resistance is low, and (2) the left atrial pressure is low, which requires good function of the systemic ventricular system of atrioventricular and semilunar valves, ventricular pump, and ventricular outflow tract. If successful, Fontan physiology leads to resolution of systemic hypoxemia and ventricular volume overload.

With short-term follow-up, conversion of single ventricle patients to Fontan physiology has been associated with an improved cardiac status. Driscoll et al. (53) found improved exercise tolerance and capacity in tricuspid atresia patients after the Fontan procedure compared to a group of tricuspid

---

Figure 2 (*Facing page*) (a) Normal circulatory circuit with systemic and pulmonary vascular beds in a series circuit separated by two ventricular pumping chambers. (b) Single ventricle circulatory circuit. Systemic and pulmonary vascular beds are in a parallel circuit with one pumping chamber for both circuits. (c) Single ventricle circuit after the Fontan procedure. Systemic and pulmonary circulatory beds are returned to a series circuit with only one pumping chamber. A connection (fenestration) of the systemic venous return to the pumping chamber is often created to improve pumping chamber filling.

atresia patients studied prior to the procedure. When the same patients were studied before the procedure and a mean of 1.8 years after the Fontan procedure, he noted an approximately 10% increase in predicted maximal oxygen consumption and 25% increase in predicted exercise duration (54). Sluysmans et al. (48) reported improvements in left ventricular wall stress and contractility in single ventricle patients when the Fontan procedure was performed prior to 10 years of age. Short-term improvements in ventricular contractility were also observed by Gewillig et al. (55).

While these studies demonstrated improvement in cardiovascular status after the Fontan procedure, it has become clear that single ventricle patients continue to have evidence of progressive cardiovascular insufficiency years after a successful Fontan procedure. While some patients after the Fontan procedure have normal exercise tolerance (56), most patients have mild-moderate exercise impairment. Predicted maximal oxygen consumption on average is only 55–65% of normal (53,54,57) and cardiac output, ejection fraction, and stroke volume response to exercise is reduced (53,54,57,58). Exercise capacity is also limited by a decrease in maximal heart rate (57).

A number of alterations in cardiovascular function can also be detected at rest in single ventricle patients after the Fontan procedure. Abnormalities of diastolic dysfunction can be detected with decreased peak filling rates (45,59) and longer isovolumic relaxation times (60,61) consistent with impaired ventricular relaxation and an augmentation of ventricular compliance (62,63). Ejection fraction and other measures of systolic function of the single ventricle after the Fontan procedure are decreased in comparison to normal values of a left or right ventricle (48,62–65). Ventricular afterload is elevated (45,66) as the one ventricle pumps to both the systemic and pulmonary circulations sequentially. Furthermore, these patients have a limited preload reserve (67,68) and concomitant decreased β-adrenergic reserve. This combination of a decrease in preload with increasing afterload may account for the observed abnormalities in systolic and diastolic function. Finally, chronotropic deficiencies frequently occur with sinus node dysfunction and an abnormal heart rate response to exercise (57,69).

With increasing follow-up and longer duration of observation, single ventricle patients undergoing the Fontan procedure continue to deteriorate in terms of ventricular performance and functional status. The risk of deterioration in terms of New York Heart Association class and risk of heart failure increase and accelerate five years after performance of the Fontan procedure (70,71). (Figure 3A and 3B). Driscoll et al. (72) found that only 34.7% of patients continued to have a higher New York Heart Association class than their preoperative class 5 years after the Fontan procedure. Performance on exercise tests and resting ventricular ejection fractions is decreased in adult patients after the Fontan procedure compared to children and adolescents (73). Cardiac arrhythmias require anti-arrhythmic medications and/or a pacemaker in at least 20% of patients 5 years after Fontan operation (72). Other serious complications, such as protein-losing enteropathy, occur in approximately 10% of long-term Fontan survivors (74) and are in part related to chronic venous congestion. These relatively disappointing long-term results in the single ventricle patient have led to the Fontan procedure being considered more of a palliation for the single ventricle patient as opposed to a reparative or curative procedure.

While the long-term morbidity of single ventricle patients is sobering, the progress made in the surgical palliation of these patients should not be understated. The relative success in combining initial infantile stabilizing surgical procedures with eventual Fontan palliation has dramatically improved the short-term outlook for infants born with single ventricle. As long-term survival can now be reasonably anticipated for single ventricle patients, ongoing efforts have focused on modification and revision of treatment strategies to optimize and extend survival of these patients into adulthood with best possible functional status and attempt to decrease the risk of disability and heart failure with increasing age.

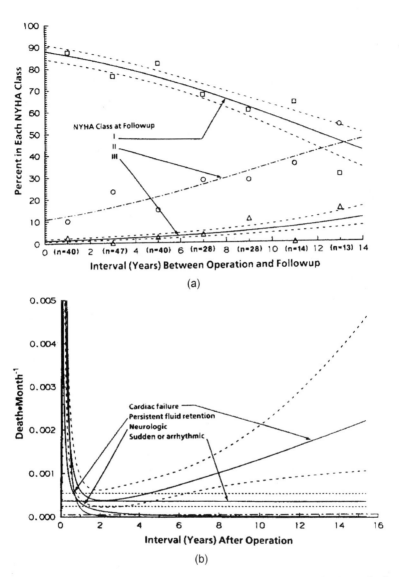

(a)

(b)

Figure 3 (a) Graph of a nomogram of a specific solution of a logistic regression equation depicting time-related functional status of surviving patients with Fontan physiology. (Reproduced with permission from Ref. 70.) (b) Graph showing instantaneous risk of death by most prevalent modes of death after the Fontan procedure over time. (Reproduced with permission from Ref. 70.)

OPTIMIZATION OF CARDIAC FUNCTION—THE TIMING AND MECHANISM OF VENTRICULAR VOLUME UNLOADING

Single ventricles that eject blood to the systemic and pulmonary circulations are chronically volume overloaded with secondary hypertrophy and become progressively dysfunctional with both diastolic and systolic dysfunction. Even partial volume unloading such as that provided by making superior vena caval flow the sole source of pulmonary flow (the Glenn shunt, bidirectional cavopulmonary anastomosis, or hemi-Fontan procedure) results in long-term benefits to ventricular function. In a study comparing a group of adult single ventricle patients palliated with the Glenn vs. aorto-pulmonary shunts, Gatzoulis et al. (75) found that over an average period of 12 years, ventricular function declined in the aorto-pulmonary shunt group, but remained stable in the group with superior-vena-cava-to pulmonary-artery anastomosis.

The degree of benefit of volume unloading single ventricle lesions appears to be age-dependent. Volume unloading operations (Glenn shunt or Fontan procedure) performed prior to 10 years of age show benefits of reduction of ventricular volume and mass with preserved ejection fraction, afterload, and contractility (48,76). However, these benefits are not observed in patients undergoing these procedures at greater than 10 years of age. In many of this older subgroup of patients ventricular ejection fraction not only did not improve, it actually decreased (76). Milanesi et al. (62) found that ventricular volume, mass, and ejection fraction were not significantly different between single ventricle patients who underwent volume unloading surgery at less than 12 months of age compared to normal controls. Single ventricle patients undergoing volume-unloading surgery at greater than 12 months of age had significantly greater ventricular volume and mass and lower ejection fractions when compared to patients undergoing volume unloading in the first year of life.

Exercise performance has also been shown to be influenced by age of volume unloading. In a study of preadolescent single ventricle patients, younger age at volume unloading was associated with increased aerobic capacity. Patients who underwent volume unloading surgery at less than 2 years of age achieved a mean percentage predicted maximal oxygen consumption (88.6 ± 24.1%) that was within normal limits for age (77).

Any type of partial or total cavopulmonary anastomosis will succeed only if there is a low pulmonary vascular resistance and a reasonably functioning ventricle. While volume unloading surgery has been demonstrated to ultimately improve the function of the single ventricle, acute reduction of volume in these lesions may exacerbate cardiac dysfunction in the immediate postoperative period. Immediately after single ventricle volume unloading surgery cardiac failure frequently occurs, leading to marked elevation of central venous pressures and secondary pleural effusions and ascites. Cardiac bypass can initiate an inflammatory cascade that will transiently elevate pulmonary vascular resistance. Myocardial dysfunction may also occur with this inflammatory response as well as the associated myocardial cellular damage and necrosis which may be associated with aortic cross-clamping (8). Myocardial dysfunction will lead to elevation of end-diastolic pressure which combined with even small elevations of pulmonary resistance will result in marked elevation of central venous pressure to maintain the transpulmonary gradient needed for pulmonary flow.

With the immediate decrease in the size of the ventricle cavity, ventricular wall thickness is increased, leading to a disproportionate amount of wall thickness for cavity size (55,78). This alteration in ventricular geometry appears to be more severe in infants than in older children (79). Animal studies indicate that with immediate removal of this chronic volume overload, the resultant increase in wall thickness-to-volume ratio does not appear to impair ventricular relaxation, but the viscosity and inertia from the increased ventricular mass/volume ratio leads to an acute impairment of early ventricular filling (80). Over the course of the first month after surgery, this relative hypertrophy will regress, and indices of early ventricular filling return to baseline control values. Absolute increases in myocardial mass further increasing the immediate postoperative mass/volume ventricular ratio can also occur as a result of myocardial edema from cardiopulmonary bypass and/or impaired myocardial lymphatic drainage from the acute rise in central venous pressure.

The bidirectional Glenn shunt, or bidirectional cavopulmonary anastomosis leads to a milder reduction of volume unloading compared to the Fontan or total cavopulmonary shunt. Similarly, the acute changes in mass/volume ratio immediately after surgery are less pronounced after completion of the bidirectional cavopulmonary anastomosis compared to a total cavopulmonary anastomosis with the Fontan procedure (79,81). Bidirectional cavopulmonary anastomosis can be performed with low mortality in infants less than 6 months of age (82,83). After initial stabilization surgery in single ventricle infants, the bidirectional cavopulmonary anastomosis provides the attractive option of increasing pulmonary blood flow and thus improving systemic arterial oxygen saturation while also volume unloading the ventricle.

Bidirectional cavopulmonary anastomosis can be successfully performed in patients whose anatomy and hemodynamics may be considered prohibitive for performance of a total cavopulmonary anastomosis (84). A potential benefit of a "staged" volume reduction of initial bidirectional cavopulmonary anastomosis followed by subsequent total cavopulmonary anastomosis is that partial volume unloading may improve cardiac status and improve the feasibility and outcome of a total cavopulmonary anastomosis. Besides the volume reduction achieved by diverting superior vena cava flow to the pulmonary arteries, the subsequent ventricular volume reduction has been demonstrated to be associated with a reduction in subsequent atrioventricular valve insufficiency that is sustained (85,86). Recent work by Tanoue et al. (87) has compared ventricular performance in single ventricle patients who underwent a primary total cavopulmonary connection to patients who underwent a staged procedure with a bidirectional cavopulmonary shunt. In the staged group, smaller ventricular volumes were associated with better

ventricular contractility when compared to group who underwent total cavopulmonary anastomosis with one procedure.
While ventricular afterload was increased in both groups,
the increment increase was smaller in the staged group.

AORTOPULMONARY COLLATERALS

After initial, palliative surgery for single ventricle lesions,
accessory sites of pulmonary blood flow may develop via dilation of aorto-pulmonary collateral vessels. Angiographically
apparent aortopulmonary collaterals occur in approximately
35–40% of patients after bidirectional Glenn or total cavopulmonary anastomosis (88,89). They can be suspected by either
the presence of increasing or very high arterial oxygen
saturations after completion of the bidirectional Glenn cavopulmonary anastomosis or at time of catheterization by a
step-up in arterial oxygen saturation between the superior
vena cava and distal pulmonary arteries. Many of these collaterals originate from the internal mammary arteries and
thyrocervical trunk and may require selective angiography
in the brachiocephalic, subclavian, or branch arteries as they
may not be visualized with aortography alone (88).

The presence of these aortopulmonary collateral vessels
has been associated with an exacerbation of fluid retention
and pleural effusions early after the Fontan procedure (89,90).
They have also been associated with refractory heart failure in
postoperative Fontan patients with long-term follow-up. These
findings have led to strong recommendations (89–91) for an
aggressive search for aortopulmonary collaterals in patients
prior to the Fontan procedure and the use of interventional coil
occlusion catheterization techniques to eliminate them prior to
surgery. Cardiac catheterization after the Fontan operation
may also be necessary to look for these collateral vessels.

ATRIOVENTRICULAR VALVE REGURGITATION

Atrioventricular valve regurgitation is another cause of
volume overload in single ventricle patients independent of

pulmonary blood flow. Atrioventricular valve regurgitation most frequently occurs in patients where the tricuspid valve is the primary systemic atrioventricular valve, such as in hypoplastic left heart syndrome, or where there is a common atrioventricular valve as is often seen in patients with heterotaxy syndromes. Atrioventricular valve insufficiency may occur in nearly one-third of patients undergoing the Fontan procedure (43,72). Over time, it frequently becomes progressively more severe in single ventricle patients (92) and eventually can contribute to ventricular dysfunction. The presence of high grade atrioventricular valve insufficiency in single ventricle patients increases the risk of early failure of the Fontan procedure in patients with hypoplastic left heart syndrome (93), heterotaxies (94), and other single ventricle lesions (72,95). Persistent atrioventricular valve regurgitation after the Fontan procedure has also been associated with poorer exercise capacity in long-term survivors (57).

In infants with single ventricle lesions and atrioventricular valve insufficiency, early volume unloading surgery with the bidirectional Glenn cavopulmonary connection may lead to a decrease in the severity of valvar regurgitation (85,86). In addition to indirect reduction of atrioventricular regurgitation with reduction of ventricular volume overload, additional atrioventricular valvuloplasty at the time of the Fontan procedure can be performed (25,96). As a result of these interventions, the risk of early failure after the Fontan procedure due to atrioventricular valve regurgitation has decreased. In the past, atrioventricular valve replacement in single ventricle patients carried a high mortality, but it is too currently being applied with increasing success (97) in these patients in an attempt to intervene prior to the development of ventricular dysfunction and/or atrial dysrhythmias.

OPTIMIZATION OF CARDIAC FUNCTION—THE MANIPULATION OF VENTRICULAR PRELOAD

Patients undergoing the Fontan procedure have an acute reduction in ventricular preload. Patients with elevated pulmonary blood flow may experience a 30–50% reduction in ventricular end-diastolic volume (55,79,81,87), while patients who have had a previous bidirectional Glenn cavopulmonary anastomosis have an approximately 15% (87) reduction in ventricular volume. Reduction of preload may contribute to abnormalities of resting ventricular systolic and diastolic function (62,98). Exercise studies (67,68) also demonstrate a limited preload reserve in single ventricle patients after the Fontan procedure. Besides intrinsic myocardial diastolic performance, filling of the single ventricle within Fontan physiology is also dependent upon pulmonary vascular resistance. Both pulmonary resistance and myocardial dysfunction may transiently increase after completion of a Fontan procedure leading to an exacerbation of the automatic reduction in preload that occurs with volume unloading surgery.

Over 10 years ago, it was hypothesized (99) that preload could be improved and cardiac performance increased in the immediate postoperative period by creating a small right-to-left shunting communication, or fenestration, from the vena cavae to the atrial chamber communicating with the ventricle as a modification of the Fontan procedure (Fig. 2C). An obligatory, residual right-to-left shunt leads to arterial oxygen desaturation, but the fenestration is small, usually only 3–4 mm in diameter. Initial experience with adding a fenestration modification to the Fontan procedure occurred in patients considered to be "high risk" for early failure because of increased pulmonary vascular resistance, atrioventricular valve insufficiency, complex anatomy, or pre-operative elevated ventricular end-diastolic pressure. In these patients, the increase in cardiac output with the fenestration more than compensated for the residual arterial oxygen desaturation as systemic oxygen delivery was greater with fenestration opened as opposed to closed (100,101). Furthermore, fenestration led to improved survival, a shorter duration of postoperative pleural effusions and shorter hospital stays after surgery in high risk patients (100–102). A recent (103) trial where all single ventricle patients regardless of perceived risk were prospectively randomized to receive a fenestrated or non-fenestrated Fontan procedure demonstrated a decrease in the duration of pleural effusion and shorter hospital stays even in standard risk patients.

Fenestration within a Fontan procedure has often been a temporary condition. Frequently, these small communications close spontaneously or are closed after the initial postoperative period with a transcatheter occlusion device (99) or via an adjustable suture (102) to leave the patient with no chronic intracardiac right-to-left shunt. However, diastolic filling properties in the single ventricle patient remain persistently abnormal months after the Fontan procedure (104). A substantial minority of fenestrated Fontan patients when their fenestration are test-occluded in the catheterization laboratory within 6 months after the procedure will have significant decreases in cardiac output and systemic oxygen delivery as well as significant increases in central venous pressure with their fenestration closed vs. open, suggesting that their long-term cardiac performance may be optimized by a persistent augmentation of ventricular filling from the right-to-left shunt from the patent fenestration (105). Some have suggested that a persistent fenestration should be maintained in all single ventricle patients after total cavopulmonary anastomosis to optimize preload reserve and cardiac performance (106).

Patients with poor functional outcomes after the Fontan procedure typically have higher central venous pressures than patients with good outcomes. Very high central venous pressures may lead to chronic pleural effusions and ascites. Within Fontan physiology, hepatic venous flow depends more on inspiration than hepatic flow with normal circulatory physiology. With increasing central venous pressures and decreasing functional status portal venous flow loses its normal expiratory augmentation, the adverse influence of gravity is enhanced, splanchnic venous pressures are higher, and the trans-hepatic venous gradient from the portal venous system to the inferior vena cava is lower (107). These circulatory phenomena may contribute to the development of protein-losing enteropathy which occurs in approximately10–15% of patients after the Fontan procedure (74) and can exacerbate fluid retention and fatigability.

Augmentation of cardiac preload and reduction of central venous pressure by creation of a fenestration late after the Fontan procedure has been performed in patients with protein-losing enteropathy or chronic effusions either surgically (108) or in the catheterization laboratory by transeptal puncture (109). Stenting of the fenestration can be utilized to prevent its spontaneous closure. Normalization of serum proteins and resolution of edema and ascites occurs in most, but not all of the patients providing a large enough right-to-left shunt was created to lower arterial oxygen saturations into the 80–85% range. Protein-losing enteropathy may occur even in the presence of relatively low central venous pressures and preserved cardiac output (110), and sometimes responds to medical anticongestive therapies, corticosteroids, or heparin (110–112). Despite the use of multiple therapies, development of protein-losing enteropathy generally portends a poor prognosis for survival (74,110).

OPTIMIZATION OF CARDIAC FUNCTION—THE INFLUENCE OF AFTERLOAD

When the pulmonary and systemic circulations are in a parallel arrangement prior to volume unloading with a cavopulmonary connection, systemic vascular resistance is on the average somewhat lower than normal values seen in normal patients with two ventricles (45,113). Completion of the Fontan procedure places the pulmonary and systemic circulations in a series connection (Fig. 3C). This arrangement theoretically increases afterload on the single ventricle (114,115), at least in part by a decrease in vascular cross-sectional area and an increase in vascular length (99). Systemic vascular resistance is increased in patients after the Fontan procedure (45,113). Neurohormonal activation occurs after the Fontan procedure with elevations of vasoconstrictors endothelin-1, renin, angiotensin II, and vasopressin occurring acutely as well as chronically after total cavopulmonary connection (116–118). Other evidence for peripheral vasoconstriction includes increased forearm vascular resistance (119) and diminished vascular endothelial function (120).

Elevation of vasoconstrictors like endothelin-1 will increase pulmonary as well as systemic vascular resistances (117). Increased pulmonary vascular resistance will necessarily increase afterload on the single ventricle after total cavopulmonary connection. However, increases in pulmonary vascular resistance will also decrease ventricular preload, as ventricular filling is dependent on pulmonary venous return. Fontan physiology in experimental models (106) and in patients (67,87) is characterized by a mismatch in ventricular contractility and afterload that leads to disadvantageous ventricular power, reduced mechanical efficiency, and limited ventricular functional reserve. With a normal heart, an increase in ventricular afterload generally leads to an increase in ventricular contractility (121,122). In patients after the Fontan procedure, there is little change in contractility (55,87,99). This phenomenon may be related to the negative effects on contractility that occur with a concomitant decrease in ventricular preload (123) that accompanies the increase in afterload in patients after Fontan palliation.

Many single ventricle lesions (Fig. 1) are associated with obstruction in the arterial tree or in the outflow of the single ventricle to the aorta. Anatomic increases in afterload from coarctation and/or recoarction can occur and this lesion, when present, continues to have an adverse long-term effect on outcome in the single ventricle patient even after repair (124). In many situations ventricular outflow must pass through a ventricular septal defect (or bulboventricular foramen) to a rudimentary ventricle and then to the aorta. These defects may decrease in size spontaneously, or as a result of increasing hypertrophy from pulmonary outflow tract obstruction or as a result of volume unloading surgery (9–13). Progressive decrease in size of the ventricular septal defect (or bulboventricular foramen) may progress after the Fontan procedure and prophylactic rerouting of systemic outflow via a Damus-Kaye-Stansel procedure has been advocated to avoid this additional increase in afterload (125).

Increased afterload and the associated neurohormonal activation after the Fontan procedure would make the use of afterload reduction with angiotensin-converting enzyme (ACE) inhibitors a tempting theoretical way to improve cardiac performance in single ventricle patients. Recent (126,127) outcome studies have reported that 17–42% of single ventricle patients are maintained on chronic ACE inhibitor therapy, whereas earlier (72) studies report lower rates of use. Despite the theoretical advantages of ACE inhibition, the only (128) randomized, double-blind, placebo-controlled trial assessing the effect of ACE inhibition in single ventricle patients 4–19 years after the Fontan procedure found that ACE inhibition did not alter abnormal systemic vascular resistance, resting cardiac index, diastolic function, or exercise capacity. However, limitation of this study included the small number of patients studied, the primary endpoint (exercise) and the fact that these patients were not clinically in heart failure.

PULMONARY VASCULAR RESISTANCE

Fontan physiology places the systemic and pulmonary vascular bed in series without a pump to aid in pulmonary blood flow as occurs in patients with two ventricles (Fig. 2). Pulmonary vascular resistance becomes a component of ventricular afterload in addition to systemic vascular resistance. Experimental studies mimicking Fontan physiology have documented the importance of pulmonary vascular resistance on ventricular afterload and have suggested it may be a more important factor than systemic vascular resistance on afterload in the single ventricle after the Fontan procedure (106,129,130). Pulmonary vascular resistance also is a critical factor determining ventricular preload in Fontan physiology (130).

The importance of pulmonary artery pressure and vascular resistance in outcomes after the Fontan procedure is well established. The initial criteria for successful direction of systemic venous return to the pulmonary arteries mandated a low pulmonary artery pressure and resistance (51,52).

Subsequent outcome studies have confirmed the importance of preoperative pulmonary artery pressures and resistance on long-term outcome (72,95,96). In addition to pulmonary arteriolar resistance, increased vascular resistance from distortion in large pulmonary arteries also increases the risk of a poor outcome (131). Earlier experience suggested that absolute size or cross-sectional area of the pulmonary arteries impacted the outcome for the Fontan procedure (132,133), but these findings have been questioned and not confirmed in other studies (134,135).

Experimental models (106,129) and clinical studies (136,117) have observed an acute rise in pulmonary vascular resistance immediately after completion of a Fontan procedure. Loss of pulsatility in the pulmonary arterial circulation may increase pulmonary vascular resistance (137). Postoperative pulmonary vascular resistance has been correlated with levels of endothelin-1 (117). This acute rise in pulmonary vascular resistance after surgery can be attenuated by performance of dilutional ultrafiltration/modified ultrafiltration which suppresses the increase in plasma concentrations of endothelin-1 after cardiopulmonary bypass (138). The connections between the venous conduit and the pulmonary architecture are another potential area for obstruction to pulmonary blood flow. In patients with heart failure after the Fontan procedure elevated central venous pressures have been shown to be related to pressure drops and increased resistance at the cavopulmonary connection (139), implying that these connections should be free of any obstruction or pressure gradients. Similarly, postoperative problems affecting pulmonary ventilation, such as hemidiaphragmatic paralysis, also may increase postoperative pulmonary pulmonary vascular resistance and exacerbate symptoms of fluid accumulation and/or low cardiac output (140).

The importance of pulmonary vascular resistance changes for the cardiac performance of single ventricle patients is further supported by the significant decline in exercise tolerance experienced by these patients at high altitudes (141). The pulmonary circuit is under ongoing risk of acquired obstruction and increased resistance from the

development of thrombi which may develop after performance
of the Fontan procedure. Abnormalities of venous blood flow,
elevated venous pressure, intravascular prosthetic material,
arrhythmia, and low cardiac output that can be observed with
Fontan palliation may predispose single ventricle patients
to develop venous thrombi. In addition, abnormalities of
hemostasis including diminished levels of Protein C, Protein
S, factor VII, anti-thrombin III activity, and plasminogen
have been observed as well as increased platelet reactivity
(142–145). Evidence for thrombosis has been detected in
17–33% of patients in recent series (146–148). The true prevalence of thrombosis is difficult to ascertain due to difficulties
in detection. Thrombosis can lead to acute reduction in pulmonary flow and venous return (149), but occult pulmonary
thrombosis can be observed with ventilation-perfusion
scanning (148) which has the potential to lead to a slow,
cumulative increase in pulmonary vascular resistance. Current strategies to minimize the risk of thrombosis have
included low dose aspirin and warfarin. In children, aspirin
has been reported to be efficacious in minimizing the incidence of thrombosis (150). However, other centers routinely
administer warfarin to their adult patients with Fontan
palliation to achieve a target INR of 2.5 by extrapolation for
prophylaxis of other systemic venous thrombosis syndromes
(151).

OPTIMIZATION OF CARDIAC FUNCTION—THE DESIGN OF THE PATHWAY OF SYSTEMIC VENOUS RETURN TO THE PULMONARY ARTERIES

The initial concept of separating systemic and pulmonary circulations in single ventricle patients involved the use of the
atrium and/or a hypoplastic ventricle to provide a source of
pulsatile ejection for the pulmonary circulation (51,152,153).
Valves were frequently utilized in these connections, but their
progressive calcification and tendency to cause flow obstruction and a need for reoperation (154) made these types of

pathways relatively untenable. Valves were eliminated and the pulmonary arteries were connected to the posterior side of the systemic venous atrium as an "atriopulmonary connection."(155,156) (Fig. 4).

Early experience also suggested that atrial contraction was not critical to the maintenance of an effective pulmonary blood flow with these connection (157). Satisfactory connections of systemic venous return to the pulmonary arteries were found to be successfully performed by constructing cavopulmonary tunnels in patients with complex single ventricle lesions that were not amenable to a simple atriopulmonary connection (158). Investigation of the hemodynamics of a pulsatile valveless chamber in a simple continuous flow circuit by de Leval et al.(159) suggested that an atriopulmonary connection generated undue turbulence and increased

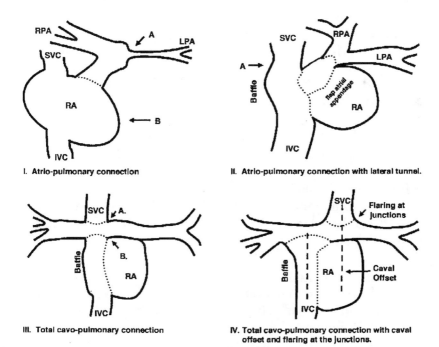

I. Atrio-pulmonary connection

II. Atrio-pulmonary connection with lateral tunnel.

III. Total cavo-pulmonary connection

IV. Total cavo-pulmonary connection with caval offset and flaring at the junctions.

Figure 4 Schematic representation of the common types of connections utilized for a Fontan procedure. (Reproduced with permission from Ref. 164.)

resistance to forward flow. Increasing dilatation of a systemic venous atrium as was observed after atriopulmonary connection combined with angulation and obstruction of the conduit led to dissipation of the energy for forward flow in the incoming caval streams. These observations led to modifications of the cavopulmonary connection (Fig. 4) from an atriopulmonary anastomosis to a more streamlined cavopulmonary connection by incorporating part of the atrium with prosthetic material to form a lateral tunnel (159) or by the use of an entirely external prosthetic conduit to channel inferior vena cava flow to the pulmonary arteries (160). Combined with variations of bidirectional superior vena cava pulmonary anastomosis, these procedures created a total cavopulmonary connection. More recently, fluid dynamic studies have confirmed the advantages of streamlined cavopulmonary connections for minimizing energy loss. These investigations (161–164) suggest that cavopulmonary connections are optimized if superior and inferior vena caval flows are offset and do not directly intersect in the pulmonary arteries; the cavo-pulmonary anastomoses are flared at the anastomotic site; and care is taken to avoid abrupt changes in cross-sectional area and flow direction (Fig. 4).

Magnetic resonance imaging studies of flow dynamics in vivo have confirmed in vitro findings, demonstrating more organized and uniform flow in patients with total pulmonary venous connections compared to patients with atriopulmonary connections (165). The advantages of offsetting caval flow into the pulmonary artery and flaring the anastomotic sites have been observed in vivo (166). Exercise studies have found that children with total cavopulmonary connections have a greater increase in stroke volume and reduced arterio-venous oxygen difference with exercise compared to children with atriopulmonary connections (167). Both groups had a similar exercise capacity, which was reduced compared to normal controls. Pulmonary blood flow in these connections is generated with negative intrathoracic pressure (168) and the increased pulmonary flow with exercise occurred with an increase in respiratory rate that allowed the blood to be "sucked" into the lungs.

With long-term follow-up, patients with the atriopulmonary connection may develop other problems aside from less efficient flow. Increasing systemic atrial distention over time may result in compression of the right pulmonary veins compromising pulmonary venous return and ventricular output and exacerbating heart failure (169–171). An atriopulmonary connection leads to elevated coronary sinus venous pressures which can potentially exacerbate ventricular dysfunction from decreased coronary flow gradients in patients with very high central venous pressures (172,173). Atrial arrhythmias are associated with dilated atria with multiple suture lines and chronic pressure elevation (174). Multiple centers (169–171,174–176) have demonstrated that conversion of the Fontan connection from an atriopulmonary to total cavopulmonary anastomosis will improve symptoms of heart failure, exercise tolerance, ventricular function, and protein-losing enteropathy in many but not all patients with circulatory insufficiency after the Fontan procedure. Conversion to a total cavopulmonary connection can be combined with atrial arrhythmia surgeries including the Maze procedure to control refractory atrial arrhythmias (176,177). The extracardiac total cavopulmonary anastomosis can be performed without cardiac bypass or with only a limited amount of cardiac bypass, which can be beneficial in patients with a history of multiple cardiac procedures and coexisting ventricular dysfunction.

OPTIMIZATION OF CARDIAC FUNCTION-ASSOCIATED DISTURBANCES OF CARDIAC RHYTHM

Supraventricular abnormalities of cardiac rhythm are a common long-term problem after the Fontan procedure. Elevation of atrial pressures from the Fontan connection exacerbated by atrioventricular valve regurgitation or ventricular dysfunction increases the risk for atrial arrhythmias with Fontan physiology. Atrial surgeries have the potential to injure the sinus node and compromise its vascular supply and atrial suture lines can participate in arrhythmia circuits (178).

Both brady- and tachyarrhythmias may occur and the risk of developing these arrhythmias increases with increasing time after performance of a Fontan procedure (72,95).

SINUS NODE DYSFUNCTION

Sinus node dysfunction may contribute to cardiac failure by limiting the heart's ability to appropriately increase heart rate with increasing metabolic demands and limiting stroke volume due to loss of atrial systole synchronized with the ventricular cardiac cycle. Sinus node dysfunction may occur in single ventricle patients prior to any surgical procedure (179). However, the prevalence of sinus node dysfunction increases after volume unloading surgery, with prevalences of 20% to over 40% with long-term follow-up (179,180). Sinus node dysfunction will frequently occur in the immediate postoperative period, and at times appear to resolve with time, only to recur years after surgery. Early postoperative sinus node dysfunction increases the risk for late sinus node dysfunction. A strategy of staged volume unloading with a bidirectional Glenn shunt followed by the Fontan procedure appears to increase the risk of early and late sinus node dysfunction (179,180). Some studies have suggested that a cavopulmonary anastomosis with an extracardiac conduit reduces the risk of sinus node dysfunction (181), but other studies (182) have found no difference with the prevalence of sinus node dysfunction with an extracardiac conduit compared to a lateral tunnel cavopulmonary anastomosis.

Besides sinus node dysfunction, high-grade atrioventricular block may occur in single ventricle patients before and after surgery. A need for pacing prior to the Fontan procedure may increase the likelihood of long-term cardiac disability (95). However, bradyarrhythmias requiring pacing occur in approximately 10% of single ventricle patients with time after the Fontan procedure (76,183,184). Pacing modes (DDD, AAI) which allow for synchronous atrial and ventricular systole are associated with survivals similar to single ventricle patients that do not require pacing (183).

The frequent coexistence of atrial tachyarrhythmias with bradyarrhythmias can be addressed by insertion of pacemakers with antitachycardia capabilities. Given the risk of thromboembolic phenomena in postoperative Fontan patients and the lack of a pulmonary ventricle, transvenous pacing is problematic and even older single ventricle patients have a need for epicardial pacing implantation (185).

INTRA-ATRIAL REENTRANT TACHYCARDIA (IART)/ATRIAL FLUTTER

Atrial tachyarrhythmias occurring after the Fontan procedure generally are due to an intra-atrial reentrant tachycardia (IART) that is similar to atrial flutter except it is generally slightly slower and has an abnormal P wave morphology instead of the classic "sawtooth" flutter waves (Fig. 5) IART

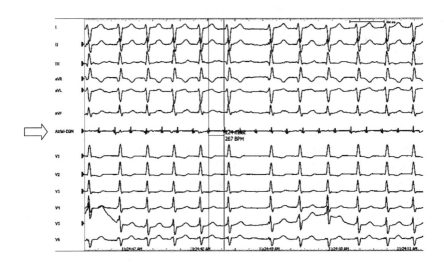

Figure 5 Intra-atrial tachycardia (IART) in single ventricle patient after the Fontan procedure with chronic severe heart failure. Ventricular rate is 136 bpm and the QRS complexes are not associated with classic sawtooth waves of atrial flutter. Atrial electrogram (arrow) demonstrates the reentrant circuit proceeding at a rate of 267 bpm.

may occur early after operation, but perhaps more significantly tends to become increasingly prevalent with increasing age after the Fontan procedure. Pediatric studies have demonstrated an approximately 20% prevalence rate of IART 5 years after the Fontan procedure (184,186,187), but studies in adult patients have found prevalence rates of approximately 40% (188). Cardiac dysfunction and IART coexist in Fontan patients and conditions that exacerbate dysfunction like atrioventricular regurgitation increase the risk of IART. Sinus node dysfunction and IART often coexist. The relationship of IART to the type of cavopulmonary connection is unclear. There is conflicting evidence whether the risk of IART is decreased with atriopulmonary connections vs. lateral tunnel connections vs. extracardiac cavopulmonary anastomosis (184,186,187,189). Advantages of the newer connections over the older connections are confounded by the overall shorter duration of follow-up observed with newer connections.

IART is poorly tolerated and can precipitate acute heart failure in single ventricle patients. Control of IART is difficult. Drug therapy is effective in only about 50% of patients (190). Amiodarone (191) and sotalol (192) appear to be the most effective anti-arrhythmics. Antitachycardia pacing can be utilized, especially if there is associated bradyarrhythmias. Ablation of the reentrant circuit can lead to an acute success, but IART frequently recurs with long-term follow-up (193,194). Newer ablation catheters in addition to newer electroanatomic mapping systems may decrease the risk of IART recurrence after ablation (195). For some cases, Mavroudis et al. (177) have successfully treated IART with a variation of the MAZE procedure combined with conversion of the atriopulmonary connection to an extracardiac conduit.

OPTIMIZATION OF CARDIAC FUNCTION— MYOCARDIAL ISSUES

The single ventricle of right ventricular morphology does not respond to volume loading with the same increase in muscular hypertrophy for a given increase in volume that is observed in the single morphologically left ventricle (59,196). Geometric alterations are similar after volume unloading in single right and single left ventricles (79), but decreased mass for ventricular volume observed in the single right ventricle leads to a relative increased afterload in single right ventricles (66) which may lead to a relatively poorer performance for single right ventricles compared to single morphologic left ventricles. Right ventricular morphology has been correlated to poorer exercise performance in single ventricle patients (57) and an increased risk for protein-losing enteropathy late after the Fontan procedure (197). Studies in adult single ventricle patients show a high prevalence of heart failure in those patients with morphologic right ventricles (198).

Single right ventricles tend to have prolonged activation times (63). Single ventricle patients irregardless of morphology frequently show wall motion abnormalities which can lead to uncoordinated and prolonged diastolic relaxation (60,199,200). This dysynchronous ventricular activation can be associated with prolonged ventricular conduction times. Cardiac performance has been improved in adults with heart failure and interventricular conduction delay with multisite ventricular pacing. Multisite ventricular pacing has been applied to single ventricle patients in the immediate postoperative period with some improvement in cardiac index in one relatively small series of patients (201). Its utility for chronic cardiac dysfunction in single ventricle patients remains unexplored.

Myocardial edema, damage, and necrosis accompany prolonged aortic cross-clamping and cardiopulmonary bypass. Signs of acute ischemic injury in hypertrophied hearts have been observed in patients who died after the Fontan procedure (202). Avoidance of excessive hypertrophy in single ventricle patients by eliminating congenital and acquire ventricular outflow obstruction from coarctation of the aorta, aortic stenosis, and subaortic stenosis from restrictive ventricular septal defects (or bulboventricular foramina) is an important part of management of the single ventricle patient (9,10). Over time, experience from multiple institutions (96,131,203,204) has found decreasing aortic cross-clamp and cardiopulmonary bypass times to correlate with reduction in early mortality and postoperative cardiac morbidity after the Fontan procedure. The effects of long bypass and cross-clamp time on late cardiac dysfunction are not well established. However, one study (197) found that the risk for protein-losing enteropathy increased with longer cardiopulmonary bypass time with the Fontan procedure.

TREATMENT OF CARDIAC FAILURE IN THE SINGLE VENTRICLE PATIENT

Failure of the single, systemic ventricle is a common problem with increasing age in the single ventricle patient. Systemic ventricular failure is the leading cause of late failure after Fontan palliation (95). Moderate-severe ventricular dysfunction has been noted in approximately 10% of long-term survivors after Fontan palliation in one series (71) and elevated (>12 mm Hg) end-diastolic ventricular pressure has been noted in approximately 50% of long-term survivors in another series (72). Restrictive physiology is especially troublesome after Fontan palliation as the lack of a pulmonary ventricle makes it impossible to compensate for the obligatory rise in pulmonary artery pressures that occurs with elevations of systemic ventricular end-diastolic pressure.

The high prevalence of late ventricular failure is reflected in the frequent use of anti-congestive medications such as digoxin, diuretics, and/or vasodilators in series of long-term survivors of Fontan palliation (71,72,127). More recently, the initial experience in pediatric heart failure centers with β-blockers such as carvedilol has included a substantial proportion of single ventricle patients with heart failure (205,206) with a similar short-term success with improving ejection and symptoms as has been observed in adult heart failure. These findings are limited to a handful of patients, and the utility and efficacy of β-blocker therapy in single ventricle patients should be better clarified by the currently ongoing double-blind, placebo-controlled trial of the use of carvedilol for pediatric heart failure (207).

CARDIAC TRANSPLANTATION

Cardiac transplantation has been used for decades as therapy for single ventricle lesions. The first pediatric heart transplant was performed on an infant with tricuspid atresia (208). The development of improved long-term immunosuppression with calcineurin inhibitors such as cyclosporine led to the work of Bailey et al.(209) utilizing primary transplantation for hypoplastic left heart syndrome. Early and mid-term survival were encouraging and appeared to offer a better chance of survival than staged, palliative surgery leading to a Fontan procedure (210). The success of primary infant transplantation for hypoplastic left heart syndrome led to its use for other "high-risk" single ventricle patients such as heterotaxies (211) and patients with pulmonary atresia—with intact ventricular septum and right ventricular-dependent coronary circulation (212). Infant cardiac transplantation, however, is handicapped by a very limited donor supply, which leads to a higher mortality rate waiting for transplantation in infants than is observed in older children (213). This problem, along with the steadily improving survival with palliative surgery in infant single ventricle patients (8,96,214), has led to a decrease in the use of primary transplantation in infants for single ventricle lesions (215).

Single ventricle lesions, however, comprise the greatest proportion of lesions in series of cardiac transplantation for congenital heart disease in older children, adolescents, and adults (216–218). Successful transplantation leads to a reversal of symptoms of heart failure in these patients. The particularly disabling complication of protein-losing enteropathy after the Fontan procedure appears to be quickly reversible in a large majority, but not all, single ventricle patients with protein-losing enteropathy undergoing heart transplantation (219,220). Transplantation after congenital heart disease surgery is complicated by longer donor ischemic times and postoperative bleeding (216–218) due to the technical challenges offered by adhesions and complicated anatomy of systemic and pulmonary venous return as well as position of the heart and great vessels observed in many patients with single ventricle. These patients may also be at greater risk for having a high titer of anti-HLA antibodies from past transfusions and the use of valved or nonvalved material in previous repairs, which increases the risk of rejection after transplantation (221,222). Cardiac transplantation after Fontan palliation has a survival comparable to other congenital heart diagnoses leading to transplant when it is performed for cardiac failure late after Fontan palliation. Survival after cardiac transplantation for heart failure in the early postoperative procedure after a Fontan procedure is significantly poorer than when it is performed for late failure (219).

REFERENCES

1. Kreutzer EA, Kreutzer J, Kreutzer GO. Univentricular heart. In: Moller JH, Hoffman JIE, eds. Pediatric Cardiovascular Medicine. New York: Churchill Livingstone, 2000:469–498.
2. Moodie DS, Ritter DG, Tajik AJ, O'Fallon WM. Long-term follow-up in the unoperated univentricular heart. Am J Cardiol 1984;53:1124–1128.
3. Ammash NM, Warnes CA. Survival in adulthood of patients with unoperated single ventricle. Am J Cardiol 1996; 77:542–544.
4. Hager A, Kaemmerer H, Eicken A, Fratz S, Hess J. Long-term survival of patients with univentricular heart not treated surgically. J Thorac Cardiovasc Surg 2002; 123:1214–1217.
5. Moodie DS, Ritter DG, Tajik AH, McGoon DC, Danielson GK, O'Fallon WM. Long-term follow-up after palliatle operation for univentricular heart. Am J Cardiol 1984; 53:1648–1651.
6. Franklin RCG, Spiegelhalter DJ, Anderson RH, Macartney FJ, Rossi Filho RI, Rigby ML, Deanfield JE. Double-inlet ventricle presenting in infancy. II. Results of palliative operations. J Thorac Cardiovasc Surg 1991; 101:917–923.
7. Dick M, Fyler DC, Nadas AS. Tricuspid atresia: clinical course in 101 patients. Am J Cardiol 1975; 36:327–337.
8. Tweddell JS, Litwin SB, Thomas JP, Mussatto K. Recent advances in the surgical management of the single ventricle patient. Pediatr Clin N America 1999; 46:465–479.
9. Donofrio MT, Jacobs ML, Norwood WI, Rychik J. Early changes in ventricular septal defect size and ventricular geometry in the single left ventricle after volume-unloading surgery. J Am Coll Cardiol 1995; 26:1008–1015.
10. Freedom RM, Benson LN, Smallhorn JF, Williams WG, Trusler GA, Rowe RD. Subaortic stenosis, the univentricular heart, and banding

of the pulmonary artery: an analysis of the courses of 43 patients with univentricular heart palliated by pulmonary artery banding. Circulation 1986; 73:758–764.

11. Jensen RA, Williams RG, Laks H, Drinkwater D, Kaplan S. Usefulness of banding of the pulmonary trunk with single ventricle physiology at risk of subaortic obstruction. Am J Cardiol 1996; 77: 1089–1093.

12. Lan YT, Chang RK, Drant S, Odim J, Laks H, Wong Al, Allada V. Outcome staged surgical approach to neonates with single left ventricle and moderate size bulboventricular foramen. Am J Cardiol 2002; 89:959–963.

13. Matitiau A, Geva T, Colan SD, Sluysmans T, Parness IA, Spevak PJ, Van der Velde M, Mayer JE, Sanders SP. Bulboventricular foramen size in infants with double-inlet left ventricle or tricuspid atresia with transposed great arteries: influence on initial palliative operation and rate of growth. J Am Coll Cardiol 1992; 19:142–148.

14. Norwood WI, Lang P, Hansen DD. Physiologic repair of aortic atresia-hypoplastic left heart syndrome. N Engl J Med 1983; 308:23–26.

15. Gibbs JL, Wren C, Watterson KG, Hunter S, Hamilton JRL. Stenting of the arterial duct combined with banding of the pulmonary arteries and atrial septectomy or septostomy: a new approach to palliation for the hypoplastic left heart syndrome. Br Heart J 1993; 69:551–555.

16. Akinturerk H, Michel-Behnke I, Valeske K, Mueller M, Thul J, Bauer J, Hagel K-J, Kreuder J, Vogt P, Schranz D. Stenting of the arterial duct and banding of the pulmonary arteries. Circulation 2002; 105:1099–1103.

17. Boucek MM, Chan KC, Pietra BA, Mashburn C, Mitchell MB, Campbell DN. Primary and total interventional stage I palliation for hypoplastic left heart syndrome (abstract). Circulation 2002; 106(suppl 2):II–522.

18. Kanter KR, Miller BE, Cuadrado AG, Vincent RN. Successful application of the Norwood procedure for infants without hypoplastic left heart syndrome. Ann Thorac Surg 1995; 59:301–304.

19. Serraf A, Conte S, Lacour Gayat F, Bruniaux J, Sousauva M, Roussin R, Planche C. Systemic obstruction in univentricular hearts—surgical options for neonates. Ann Thorac Surg 1995; 60:970–977.

20. Tchervenkov CI, Shum-Tim D, Beland MJ, Jutras L, Platt R. Single ventricle with systemic obstruction in early life: comparison of initial pulmonary artery banding versus the Norwood operation. Eur J Cardiothorac Surg 2001; 19:671–677.

21. Bradley SM, Simsic JM, Atz AM, Dorman BH. The infant with single ventricle and excessive pulmonary blood flow: results of a strategy of pulmonary artery division and shunt. Ann Thorac Surg 2002; 74:805–810.

22. Migliavacca F, Pennati G, Dubini G, Fumero R, Pietrasbissa R, Urcelay G, Bove EL, Hsia TY, de Leval MR. Modeling of the Norwood

circulation: effects of shunt size, vascular resistances, and heart rate. Am J Physiol Heart Circ Physiol 2001; 280:H2076–H2086.

23. Kitaichi T, Chikugo F, Kawahito T, Hori T, Masuda Y, Kitagawa T. Suitable shunt size for regulation of pulmonary blood flow in a canine model of univentricular parallel circulations. J Thorac Cardiovasc Surg 2003; 125:71–78.

24. Jacobs ML. Complications associated with heterotaxy in Fontan patients. Sem Thorac Cardiovasc Surg 2002; 5:25–35.

25. Stamm C, Friehs I, Duebener LF, Zurakowski D, Mayer JE, Jonas RA, del Nido PJ. Improving results of the modified Fontan operation in patients witk heterotaxy syndrome. Ann Thorac Surg 2002; 74:1967–1978.

26. Cheung YF, Cheung VY, Chau Ak, Chiu Cs, Yung TC, Leung MP. Outcome of infants with right atrial isomerism: is prognosis better with normal pulmonary venous drainage. Heart 2002; 87:146–152.

27. McElhinney DB, Reddy VM. Anomalous pulmonary venous return in the staged palliation of functional univentricular heart defects. Ann Thorac Surg 1998; 66:683–687.

28. Seliem MA, Chin AJ, Norwood WI. Patterns of anomalous pulmonary venous connection/drainage in hypoplastic left heart syndrome: diagnostic role of Doppler color flow mapping and surgical implications. J Am Coll Cardiol 1992; 19:135–141.

29. Seliem MA, Lang P, Keane JF, Joans RA, Saunders SP, Lock JE. Creation and maintenance of an adequate interatrial communication in left atrioventricular valve atresia or stenosis. Am J cardiol 1986; 58:622–626.

30. Collins MH, Darragh RK, Caldwell RL, Turrentine MW, Brown JW. Short-term survivors of pediatric heart transplantation: an autopsy study of their pulmonary vascular disease. J Heart Lung Transplant 1995; 14:1116–1125.

31. Rychik J, Rome JJ, Collins MH, DeCampli WM, Spray TL. The hypoplastic left heart syndrome with intact atrial septum: atrial morphology, pulmonary vascular histopatho logy, and outcome. J Am Coll Cardiol 1999; 34:554–560.

32. Graziano JN, Heidelberger KP, Ensing GJ, Gomez CA, Ludomirsky A. The influence of a restrictive atrial septal defect on pulmonary vascular morphology in patients with hypoplastic left heart symdrome. Pediatr Cardiol 2002; 23:146–151.

33. Daubeney PEF, Delany DJ, Anderson RH, Sandor GGS, Slavik Z, Keeton BR, Webber SA. Pulmonary atresia with intact ventricular septum. Range of morphology in population-based study. J Am Coll Cardiol 2002; 39:1670–1679.

34. Hanley FL, Sade RM, Blackstone EH, Kirklin JW, Freedom RM, Nanda NC. Outcomes in neonatal pulmonary atresia with intact ventricular septum. A multiinstitutional study. J Thorac Cardiovasc Surg 1993; 105:406–427.

35. Fyfe DA, Edwards WD, Driscoll DJ. Myocardial ischemia in patients with pulmonary atresia and intact septum. J Am Coll Cardiol 1986; 8:402–406.

36. Gentles TL, Colan SD, Giglia TM, Mandell VS, Mayer JE, Sanders SP. Right ventricular decompression and left ventricular function in pulmonary atresia with intact ventricular septum. Circulation 1993; 88 [part 2]:183–188.

37. Powell AJ, Mayer JE, Lang P, Lock JE. Outcome in infants with pulmonary atresia, intact ventricular septum, and right ventricle-dependent coronary circulation. Am J Cardiol 2000; 86:1272–1274.

38. Lloyd TR, Marvin WJ. Age at death in the hypoplastic left heart syndrome: multivariate analysis and importance of the coronary arteries. Am Heart J 1989; 117:1337–1343.

39. Bartram U, Grünen felder J, Van Praagh R. Causes of death after the modified Norwood procedure: a study of 122 postmortem cases. Ann Thorac Surg 1997; 64:1795–1802.

40. Donnelly JP, Raffel DM, Shulkin BL, Corbett JR, Bove EL, Mosca RS, Kulik TJ. Resting coronary flow and coronary flow reserve in human infants after repair or palliation of congenital heart defects as measured by positron emission tomography. J Thorac Cardiovasc Surg 1998; 115:103–110.

41. Pizzaro C Malec E, Maher KO, Januszewska K, Gidding SS, Norwood WI. Right ventricle to pulmonary artery conduit improves outcome after Norwood procedure for hypoplastic left heart syndrome (abstract). Circulation 2002; 106(suppl 2):II–394.

42. Maher KO, Pizarro C, Gidding SS, Murphy J, Januszewska K, Malec E, Norwood W. Improved hemodynamic profile following the Norwood procedure with right ventricle to pulmonary artery conduit (abstract). Circulation 2002; 106(suppl 2):II–522.

43. Shimazaki Y, Kawashima Y, Mori T, Kitamura S, Matsuda H, Yokota K. Ventricular volume characteristics of single ventricle before corrective surgery. Am J Cardiol 1980; 45:806–810.

44. Kitamura S, Kawashima Y, Shimazaki Y, Mori T, Nakano S, Beppu S, Kozuka T. Characteristics of ventricular function in single ventricle. Circulation 1979; 60:849–855.

45. Akagi T, Benson LN, Green M, Ash J, Gilday DL, Williams WG, Freedom RM. Ventricular performance before and after Fontan repair for univentricular atrioventricular connection: angiographic and radionuclide assessment. J Am Coll Cardiol 1992; 20:920–926.

46. Kuroda O, Sano T, Matsuda H, Nakano S, Hirose H, Shimazaki Y, Kato H, Taniguchi K, Ogawa M, Kawashima Y. Analysis of the effects of the Blalock-Taussig shunt on ventricular function and the prognosis in patients with single ventricle. Circulation 1987; 76(suppl III):24–28.

47. Seliem M, Muster AJ, Paul MH, Benson DW. Relation between preoperative left ventricular muscle mass and outcome of the Fontan

procedure in patients with tricuspid atresia. J Am Coll Cardiol 1989; 14:750–755.

48. Sluysmans T, Sanders SP, van der Velde M, Matitiau A, Parness IA, Spevak PJ, Mayer JE, Colan SD. Natural history and patterns of recovery of contractile function in single left ventricle after Fontan operation. Circulation 1992; 86:1753–1761.

49. Sandor GGS, Patterson MWH, LeBlanc JG. Systolic and diastolic function in tricuspid valve atresia before the Fontan operation. Am J Cardiol 1994; 73:292–297.

50. Franklin RCG, Spiegelhalter DJ, Filho RI, Macartney FJ, Anderson RH, Rigby ML, Deanfield JE. Double-inlet ventricle presenting in infancy. III. Outcome and potential for definitive repair. J Thorac Cardiovasc Surg 1991; 101:924–934.

51. Fontan F, Baudet E. Surgical repair of tricuspid atresia. Thorax 1971; 26:240–248.

52. Kreutzer G, Galindez E, Bono H, DePalma C, Laura JP. An operation for the correction of tricuspid atresia. J Thorac Cardiovasc Surg 1973; 66:613–621.

53. Driscoll DJ, Danielson GK, Puga FJ, Schaff HV, Heise CT, Staats BA. Exercise tolerance and cardiorespiratory response to exercise after the Fontan operation for tricuspid atresia or functional single ventricle. J Am Coll Cardiol 1986; 7:1087–1094.

54. Zellers TM, Driscoll DJ, Mottram CD, Puga FJ, Schaff HV, Danielson GK. Exercise tolerance and cardiorespiratory response to exercise before and after the Fontan operation. Mayo Clin Proc 1989; 64:1489–1497.

55. Gewillig MH, Lundström UR, Deanfield JE, Bull C, Franklin RC, Graham TP, Wyse RK. Impact of Fontan operation on left ventricular size and contractility in tricuspid atresia. Circulation 1990; 81: 118–127.

56. Gewillig MH, Lundström UR, Bull C, Wyse RK, Deanfield JE. Exercise responses in patients with congenital heart disease after Fontan repair: patterns and determinants of performance. J Am Coll Cardiol 1990; 15:1424–1432.

57. Ohuchi H, Yasuda K, Hasegawa S, Miyazaki A, Takamuro M, Yamada O, Ono Y, Uemura H, Yagihara T, Echigo S. Influence of ventricular morphology on aerobic exercise capacity after the Fontan operation. J Am Coll Cardiol 2001; 37:1967–1974.

58. Del Torso S, Kelly MJ, Kalff V, Venables AW. Radionuclide assessment of ventricular contraction at rest and during exercise following the Fontan procedure for either tricuspid atresia or single ventricle. Am J Cardiol 1985; 55:1127–1132.

59. Akagi T, Benson LN, Gilday DL, Ash J, Green M, Williams WG, Freedom RM. Influence of ventricular morphology on diastolic filling performance in double-inlet ventricle after the Fontan procedure. J Am Coll Cardiol 1993; 22:1948–1952.

60. Penny DJ, Rigby ML, Redington AN. Abnormal patterns of intraventricular flow and diastolic filling after the Fontan operation: evidence for incoordinate ventricular wall motion. Br Heart J 1991; 66: 375–378.

61. Frommelt PC, Snider AR, Melinones JN, Vermilion RP. Doppler assessment of the pulmonary artery flow patterns and ventricular function after Fontan operation. Am J Cardiol 1991; 68:1211–1215.

62. Milanesi O, Stellin G, Colan SD, Facchin P, Crepaz R, Biffanti R, Zacchello F. Systolic and diastolic performance late after the Fontan procedure for a single ventricle and comparison of those undergoing operation at <12 months of age and at >12 months of age. Am J Cardiol 2002; 89:276–280.

63. Mahle WT, Coon PD, Wernovsky G, Rychik J. Quantitative echocardiographic assessment of the performance of the functionally single right ventricle after the Fontan operation. Cardiol Young 2001; 11:399–406.

64. Parikh SR, Hurwitz RA, Caldwell RL, Girod DA. Ventricular function in the single ventricle before and after Fontan surgery. Am J Cardiol 1991; 67:1390–1395.

65. Williams RV, Ritter S, Tani LY, Pagoto LT, Minich LL. Quantitative assessment of ventricular function in children with single ventricles using the Doppler myocardial performance index. Am J Cardiol 2000; 86:1106–1110.

66. Sano T, Ogawa M, Taniguchi K, MatusudaH, Nakajima T, Arisawa J, Yasuhisa S, Nakano S, Kawashima Y. Assessment of ventricular contractile state and function in patients with univentricular heart. Circulation 1989; 79:1247–1256.

67. Senazi H, MasutaniS, Kobayashi T, Sasaki N, AsanoH, Kyo S, Yokote Y, Ishizawa A. Ventricular afterload and ventricular work in Fontan circulation. Circulation 2002; 105:2885–2892.

68. Gewillig M, Kallis N. Pathophysiological aspects after cavopulmonary anatomosis. Thorac Cardiovasc Surg 2000; 48:336–341.

69. Kürer C, Tanner CS, Vetter VL. Electophysiologic findings after Fontan repair of functional single ventricle. J Am Coll Cardiol 1991; 17:174–181.

70. Fontan F, Kirklin JW, Fernandez G, Coast F, Naftel DC, Tritto F, Blackstone EH. Outcome after a "perfect" Fontan operation. Circulation 1990; 81:1520–1536.

71. Gentles TL, Gauvreau K, Mayer JE, Fishberger SB, Burnett J, Colan Sd, Newburger JW, Wernovsky G. Functional outcome after the Fontan operation: factors influencing late morbidity. J Thorac Cardiovasc Surg 1997; 114:392–403.

72. Driscoll DJ, Offord KP, Feldt RH, Schaff HV, Puga FJ, Danielson GK. Five-to fifteen-year follow-up after Fontan operation. Circulation 1992; 85:469–496.

73. Harrison DA, Liu P, Walters JE, Goodman JM, Siu SC, Webb GD, Williams WG, McLaughlin PR. Cardiopulmonary function in adult patients late after Fontan repair. J Am Coll Cardiol 1995; 26: 1016–1021.

74. Feldt RH, Driscoll DJ, Offord KP, Cha RH, Perrault J, Schaff HV, Puga FJ, Danielson GK. Protein-losing enteropathy after the Fontan operation. J Thorac Cardiovasc Surg 1996; 112:672–680.

75. Gatzoulis MA, Munk M-D, Williams WG, Webb GD. Definitive palliation with cavopulmonary or aortopulmonary shunts for adults with single ventricle physiology. Heart 2000; 83:51–57.

76. Forbes TJ, Gajarski R, Johnson GL, Reul GJ, Ott DA, Drescher K, Fisher DJ. Influence of age on the effect of bidirectional cavopulmonary anastomosis on left ventricular volume, mass, and ejection fraction. J Am Coll Cardiol 1996; 28:1301–1307.

77. Mahle WT, Wernovsky G, Bridges ND, Linton AB, Paridon SM. Impact of early ventricular unloading on exercise performance in preadolescents with single ventricle Fontan physiology. J Am Coll Cardiol 1999; 34:1637–1643.

78. Donofrio, MT, Jacobs ML, Spray TL, Rychik J. Acute changes in preload, afterload, and systolic functions after superior cavopulmonary connection. Ann Thorac Surg 1998; 65:503–508.

79. Chin AJ, Franklin WH, Andrews AA, Norwood WJ. Changes in ventricular geometry after Fontan operation. Ann Thorac Surg 1993; 56:1359–1565.

80. Gewillig M, Daenen W, Aubert A, Van der Hauwaert L. Abolishment of chronic volume overload. Implications for diastolic function of the systemic ventricle immediately after Fontan repair. Circulation 1992; 86(suppl II):93–99.

81. Fogel MA, Weinberg PM, Chin AJ, Fellows KE, Hoffman EA. Late ventricular geometry and performance changes of functional single ventricle throughout staged Fontan reconstruction assessed by magnetic resonance imaging. J Am Coll Cardiol 1996; 28:212–221.

82. Chang AC, Hanley FL, Wernovsky G, Rosenfeld HM, Wessel DL, Jonas RA, Mayer JE, Locke JE, Castaneda AR. Early bidirectional cavopulmonary shunt in young infants. Postoperative course and early results. Circulation 1993; 88[part 2]:149–158.

83. Bradley Sm, Mosca RS, Hennein HA, Crowley DC, Kulik TJ, Bove EL. Bidirectional superior cavopulmonary connection in young infants. Circulation 1996; 94(suppl 2):5–11.

84. Bridges ND, Jonas RA, Mayer JE, Flanagan MF, Keane JF, Castaneda AR. Bidirectional cavopulmonary anastomosis as interim palliation for high-risk Fontan candidates. Circulation 1990; 82(suppl IV):170–176.

85. Michelfelder EC, Kimball TR, Pearl JM, Manning PB, Beekman RH. Effect of superior cavopulmonary anastomosis on the rate of tricuspid

annulus dilation in hypoplastic left heart syndrome. Am J Cardiol 2002; 89:96–99.

86. Mahle WT, Cohen MS, Spray TL, Rychik J. Atriventricular valve regurgitation in patients with single ventricle: impact of the bidirectional cavopulmonary anastomosis. Ann Thorac Surg 2001; 72: 831–835.

87. Tanoue Y, Sese A, Ueno Y, Kunitaka J, Hijii T. Bidirectional Glenn procedure improves the mechanical efficiency of a total cavopulmonary connection in high-risk Fontan candidates. Circulation 2001; 103:2176–2180.

88. Triedman JK, Bridges ND, Mayer JE, Lock JE. Prevalence and risk factors for aortopulmonary collateral vessels after Fontan and bidirectional Glenn procedures. J Am Coll Cardiol 1993; 22:207–215.

89. Kanter, KR, Vincent RN, Raviele AA. Importance of acquired systemic-to-pulmonary collaterals after the Fontan operation. Ann Thorac Surg 1999; 68:969–975.

90. Spicer RL, Uzark KC, Moore JW, Mainwaring RD, Lamberti JJ. Aortopulmonary collateral vessels and prolonged pleural effusions after modified Fontan procedures. Am Heart J 1996; 131:1164–1168.

91. Ichikawa H, Yagihara T, Kishimoto H, Isobe F, Yamamoto F, Nishigaki K, Matsuki O, Fujita T. Extent of aortopulmonary collateral blood-flow as a risk factor for Fontan operations. Ann Thorac Surg 1995; 59:433–437.

92. Moak JP, Gersony WM. Progressive atrioventricular valvular regurgitation in single ventricle. Am J Cardiol 1987; 59:656–658.

93. Chang AC, Farrell PE, Murdison KA, Baffa JM, Barber G, Norwood WI, Murphy JD. Hypoplastic left heart syndrome: hemodynamic and angiographic assessment after initial reconstructive surgery and relevance to modified Fontan procedure. J Am Coll Cardiol 1991; 17:1143–1149.

94. Michielon G, Gharagozloo F, Julsrud PR, Danielson GK, Puga FJ. Modified Fontan operation in the presence of anomalies of systemic and pulmonary connection. Circulation 1993; 88[part 2]:141–148.

95. Gentles TL, Mayer JE, Gauvreau K, Newburger JW, Lock JE, Kupferschmid JP, Burnett J, Jonas RA, Castaneda AR, Wernovsky G. Fontan operation in five hundred consecutive patients: factors influencing early and late outcome. J Thorac Cardiovasc Surg 1997; 114:376–391.

96. Mosca RS, Kulik TJ, Goldberg CS, Vermilion RP, Charpie JR, Crowley DC, Bove EL. Early results of the Fontan procedure in one hundred consecutive patients with hypoplastic left heart syndrome. J Thorac Cardiovasc Surg 2000; 119:1110–1118.

97. Mahle WT, Gaynor JW, Spray TL. Atrioventricular valve replacement in patients with a single ventricle. Ann Thorac Surg 2001; 72:182–186.

98. Colan SD. Systolic and diastolic function of the univentricular heart. Prog Pediatr Cardiol 2002; 16:79–87.

99. Bridges ND, Lock JE, Cataneda AR. Ballfe fenestration with subsequent transcatheter closure. Modification of the Fontan operation for patients at increased risk. Circulation 1990; 82:1681–1689.

100. Mavroudis C, Zales VR, Backer CL, Muster AJ, Latson LA. Fenestrated Fontan with delayed catheter closure. Effects of volume loading and baffle fenestration on cardiac index and oxygen delivery. Circulation 1992; 86(suppl II):85–92.

101. Harake B, Kuhn MA, Jarmakani JM, Laks H, Al-Khatib Y, Elami A, Williams RG. Acute hemodynamic effects of adjustable atrial septal defect closure in the later tunnel Fontan procedure. J Am Coll Cardiol 1994; 23:1671–1676.

102. Bridges ND, Mayer JE, Locke JE, Jonas RA, Hanley FL, Keane JF, Perry SB, Castaneda AR. Effect of baffle fenestration on outcome of the modified Fontan operation. Circulation 1992; 86:1762–1769.

103. Lemler MS, Scott WA, Leonard SR, Stromberg D, Ramaciotti C. Fenestration improves clinical outcome of the Fontan procedure. A prospective, randomized study. Circulation 2002; 105:207–212.

104. Cheung YF, Penny DJ, Redington AN. Serial assessment of left ventricular diastolic function after Fontan procedure. Heart 2000; 83:420–424.

105. Bridges ND, Lock JE, Mayer JE, Burnett J, Castaneda AR. Cardiac catheterization and test occlusion of the interatrial communication after the fenestrated Fontan operation. J Am Coll Cardiol 1995; 25:1712–1717.

106. Szabó G, Buhman V, Graf A, Melnitschuk S, Bährle S, Vahl C, Hagl S. Ventricular energetics after the Fontan operation: contractility-afterload mismatch. J Thorac Cardiovasc Surg 2003; 125:1061–1069.

107. Hsia T-Y, Khambadkone S, Deanfield JE, Taylor JFN, Migliavacca F, de Leval MR. Subdiaphragmatic venous hemodynamics in the Fontan circulation. J Thorac Cardiovasc Surg 2001; 121:436–447.

108. Rychik JE, Rome JJ, Jacobs ML. Late surgical fenestration for complications after the Fontan operation. Circulation 1997; 96:33–36.

109. Mertens L, Dumoulin M, Gewillig M. Effect of percutaneous fenestration of the atrial septum on protein-losing enteropathy after the Fontan operation. Br Heart J 1994; 72:591–592.

110. Mertens L, Hagler DJ, Sauer U, Somerville J, Gewillig M. Protein losing enteropathy after the Fontan operation: an international multicenter study. J Thorac Cardiovasc Surg 1998; 115:1063–1073.

111. Rychik J, Piccoli D, Barber G. Usefulness of corticosteroid therapy for protein-losing enteropathy after the Fontan procedure. Am J Cardiol 1991; 121:618–619.

112. Donnelly JP, Rosenthal A, Castle VP, Holmes RD. Reversal of protein-losing enteropathy with heparin therapy in three patients with univentricular hearts and Fontan palliation. J Pediatr 1997; 130:474–478.

113. Buchhorn R, Bartmus D, Buhre W, Bursch J. Pathogenetic mechanisms of venous congestion after the Fontan procedure. Cardiol Young 2001; 11:161–168.

114. Magosso E, Cavalcanti S, Ursino M. Theoretical analysis of rest and exercise hemodynamics with total cavopulmonary anastomosis. Am J Physiol 2002; 282:H1018–H1034.

115. Nogaki M, Senzaki H, Masutani S, Kobayashi J, Kobayashi T, Sasaki N. Ventricular energetics in Fontan circulation: evaluation with a theoretical model. Pediatr Int 2000; 42:651–657.

116. Mainwaring RD, Lamberti JJ, Moore JW, Billman GF, Nelson JC. Comparison of the hormonal response after bidirectional Glenn and Fontan procedures. Ann Thorac Surg 1994; 57:59–64.

117. Hiramatsu T, Imai Y, Takanashi Y, Seo K, Terada M, Aoki M, Nakazawa M. Time course of endothelin-1 and adrenomedullin after the Fontan procedure. Ann Thorac Surg 1999; 68:169–172.

118. Hjortdal VE, Stenbøg HB Ravn, Emmertsen K, Jensen KT, Pedersen EB, Olsen KH, Hansen OK, Sørensen KE. Neurohormonal activation late after cavopulmonary connection. Heart 2000; 83:439–443.

119. Kelley JR, Mack GW, Fahey JT. Diminished venous capacitance in patients with univentricular hearts after the Fontan procedure. Am J Cardiol 1995; 76:158–163.

120. Mahle WT, Todd K, Fyfe DA. Endothelial function following the Fontan operation. Am J Cardiol 2003; 91:1286–1288.

121. Suga H, Sagawa K, Kostiuk DP. Controls of ventricular contractility assessed by pressure–volume raio, E_{max}. Cardiovasc Res 1976; 10:582–592.

122. Klautz RJM, Teitel DF, Steendijk P, Van Bel F, Baan J. Interaction between afterload and contractility in the newborn heart: evidence of homeometric autoregulation in the intact circulation. J Am Coll Cardiol 1995; 25:1428–1435.

123. Crozatier B. Stretch-induced modifications of myocardial performance: from ventricular function to cellular and molecular mechanisms. Cardiovasc Res 1996; 32:25–37.

124. Stamm C, Friehs I, Mayer JE, Zurakowski JK, Moran AM, Walsh EP, Lock JE, Jonas RA, del Nido PJ. Long-term results of the lateral tunnel Fontan procedure. J Thorac Cardiovasc Surg 2001; 121:28–41.

125. Hiramatsu T, Imai Y, Kurosawa H, Takanashi Y, Aoki M, Sin'oka T, Sakamoto T. Midterm results of surgical treatment of systemic ventricular outflow obstruction in Fontan patients. Ann Thorac Surg 2002; 73:855–861.

126. Mahle WT, Clancy RR, Moss Em, Gerdes M, Jobes DR, Wernovsky G. Neurodevelopmental outcome and lifestyle assessment in school-aged and adolescent children with hypoplastic left heart syndrome. Pediatrics 2000; 105:1082–1089.

127. Goff DA, Blume ED, Gauvreau K, Mayer JE, Locke JE, Jenkins KJ. Clinical outcome of fenestrated Fontan patients after closure. Circulation 2000; 102:2094–2099.

128. Kouatli AA, Garcia JA, Zellers TM, Weinstein EM, Mahony L. Enalapril does not enhance exercise capacity in patients after Fontan procedure. Circulation 1997; 96:1507–1512.

129. Nawa S, Irie H, Takata K, Sugawara E, Teramoto S. Development of a new experimental model for total exclusion of the right heart without the aid of cardiopulmonary bypass. J Thorac Cardiovasc Surg 1989; 97:130–134.

130. Macé L, Dervanian P, Bourriez A, Mazmanian, Lambert V, Losay J, Neveux J. Changes in venous return parameters associated with univentricular Fontan circulations. Am J Physiol 2000; 279: H2335–H2343.

131. Mayer JE, Bridges ND, Locke JE, Hanley FL, Jonas RA, Castaneda AR. Factors associated with marked reduction in mortality for Fontan operations in patients with single ventricle. J Thorac Cardiovasc Surg 1992; 103:444–452.

132. Nakazawa M, Nojima K, Okuda H, Imai Y, Nakanishi T, Kurosawa H, Takao A. Flow dynamics in the main pulmonary artery after the Fontan procedure in patients with tricuspid atresia or single ventricle. Circulation 1987; 75:1117–1123.

133. Fontan F, Fernandez G, Costa F, Naftel DC, Tritto F, Blackstone EH, Kirklin JW. The size of the pulmonary arteries and the results of the Fontan operation. J Thorac Cardiovasc Surg 1989; 98:711–724.

134. Knott-Craig CJ, Julsrud PR, Schaff HV, Puga FJ, Danielson GK. Pulmonary artery size and clinical outcome after the modified Fontan operation. Ann Thorac Surg 1993; 55:646–651.

135. Bridges ND, Farrell PE, Pigott JD, Norwood WI, Chin AJ. Pulmonary artery index. A nonpredictor of operative survival in patients undergoing modified Fontan repair. Circulation 1989; 80:1216–1221.

136. Serraf A, Houyel L, Nicolas F, Lacdour-Gayet F, Bruniawx J, Petit J, Uva M, Roux D, Planche C. Pulmonary circulation evaluation before cavopulmonary connections: the cavopulmonary bypass. Ann Thorac Surg 1994; 58:1096–1102.

137. Tamaki S, kawazoe K, Yagihara T, Abe T. A model to simulate the hemodynamic effects of right heart pulsatile flow after modified Fontan procedure. Br Heart J 1992; 67:177–179.

138. Hiramatsu T, Imai Y, Kurosawa H, Takanashi Y, Aoki M, Shin'oka T, Nakazawa M. Effects of dilutional and modified ultrafiltration in plasma endothelin-1 and pulmonary vascular resistance after the Fontan procedure. Ann Thorac Surg 2002; 73:82–85.

139. Cavalcanti S, Gnudi G, Masetti P, Ussia GP, Marcelletti CF. Analysis by mathematical model of haemodynamic data in the failing Fontan circulation. Physiol Measurement 2001; 22:209–222.

140. Amin Z, McElhinney DB, Strawn JK, Kugler JD, Duncan KF, Reddy VM, Petrossian E, Hanley FL. Hemidiaphragmatic paralysis increases postoperative morbidity after a modified Fontan operation. J Thorac Cardiovasc Surg 2001; 122:856–862.

141. Day RW, Orsmund GS, Sturtevant JE, Hawkins JA, Doty DB, McGough EC. Early and intermediate results of the Fontan procedure at moderately high altitude. Ann Thorac Surg 1994; 57:170–176.

142. Van Nierwenhuizen RC, Peters M, Lubbers LJ, Trip MD, Tijssen JG, Mulder BJ. Abnormalities in liver function and coagulation profile following the Fontan procedure. Heart 1999; 82:40–46.

143. Rauch R, Ries M, Hofbeck M, Buheitel G, Singer H, Klinge J. Hemostatic changes following the modified Fontan operation (total cavopulmonary connection). Thromb Haemost 2000; 83:678–682.

144. Ravn HB, Hjortdal VE, Stenbog EV. Increased platelet reactivity and significant changes in coagulation markers after cavopulmonary connection. Heart 2001; 85:61–65.

145. Jahangiri M, Kreutzer J, Zurakowski D, Bacha E, Jonas RA. Evaluation of hemostatic and coagulation factor abnormalities in patients undergoing the Fontan operation. J Thorac Cardiovasc Surg 2000; 120:778–782.

146. Rosenthal DN, Friedman AH, Kleinman CS, Kopf GS, Rosenfeld LE, Hellenbrand WE. Thromboembolic complications after Fontan operations. Circulation 1995; 92(suppl II):287–293.

147. Balling G, Vogt M, Kaemmerer H, Eicken A, Meisner H, Hess J. Intracardiac thrombus formation after the Fontan operation. J Thorac Cardiovasc Surg 2000; 119:745–752.

148. Varma C, Warr MR, Hendler AL, Paul NS, Webb GE, Therrien J. Prevalence of "silent" pulmonary emboli in adults after the Fontan operation. J Am Coll Cardiol 2003; 41:2252–2258.

149. Hedrick M, Elkins RC, Knott-Craig J, Razook JD. Successful thrombectomy for thrombosis of the right side of the heart after the Fontan operation. J Thorac Cardiovasc Surg 1993; 105:297–301.

150. Jacobs ML, Pourmoghadam KK, Geary EM, Reyes AT, Madan N, McGrath LB, Moore JW. Fontan's operation: Is aspirin enough? Is Coumadin too much? Ann Thorac Surg 2002: 73:64–8.

151. O'Donnell, Landzberg MJ. The "failing" Fontan circulation. Prog Pediatr Cardiol 2002; 16:105–114.

152. Björk V, Olin CL, Bjarke BB, Thorén CA. Right atrial-right ventricular anastomosis for correction of tricuspid atresia. J Thorac Cardiovasc Surg 1979; 77:452–458.

153. Bull C, de Leval MR, Stark J, Taylor JFN, Macartney FJ. Use of a subpulmonary ventricular chamber in the Fontan circulation. J Thorac Cardiovasc Surg 1983; 85:21–31

154. Bull C, Macartney FJ, Horvath P, Almeida R, Merill W, Douglas J, Taylor JFN, de Leval MR, Stark J. Evaluation of long-term results

of homograft valves in extracardiac conduits. J Thorac Cardiovasc Surg 1987; 94:12–19.

155. Kreutzer G. Atriopulmonary anastomosis. J Thorac Cardiovasc Surg 1982; 83:427–436.

156. Molina J, Wang Y, Lucas R, Moller J. The technique of the Fontan procedure with posterior right atrium-pulmonary artery connections. Ann Thorac Surg 1985; 39:371–379.

157. Matsuda H, Kawashima Y, Takano H, Miyamoto K, Mori T. Experimental evaluation of atrial function in right atrium-pulmonary artery conduit operation for tricuspid atresia. J Thorac Cardiovasc Surg 1981; 81:762–767.

158. Puga FJ, Chiavarelli M, Hagler DJ. Modifications of the Fontan operation applicable to patients with left atrioventricular valve atresia or single atrioventricular valve. Circulation 1987; 76(suppl III):53–60.

159. de Leval M, Kilner P, Gewillig M, Bull C. Total cavopulmonary connection: a logical alternative to atriopulmonary connection for complex Fontan operations. J Thorac Cardiovasc Surg 1988; 96: 682–685.

160. Giannico S, Corno A, Marino B, Cicini MP, Gagliardi MG, Amodeo A, Picardo S, Marcelletti C. Total extracardiac right heart bypass. Circulation 1992; 86(suppl II):110–117.

161. de Leval MR, Dubini G, Migliavacca F, JalaliH, Camporini G, Redington A, Pietrabissa R. Use of computational fluid dynamics in the design of surgical procedures: application to the study of competitive flows in cavopulmonary connections. J Thorac Cardiovasc Surg 1996; 111: 502–513.

162. Ensley AE, Lynch P, Chatzimavroudis P, Lucas C, Sharma S, Yoganathan AP. Toward designing the optimal total cavopulmonary connection: an in vitro study. Ann Thorac Surg 1999; 68:1384–1390.

163. Lardo AC, Webber SA, Friehs I, del Nido PJ, Cape EG. Fluid dynamic comparison of intra-atrial and extracardiac total cavopulmonary connections. J Thorac Cardiovasc Surg 1999; 117:697–704.

164. Ascuitto RJ, Kydon DW, Ross-Ascuitto NT. Streamlining fluid pathways lessens flow energy dissipation: relevance to atriocavopulmonary connections. Pediatr Cardiol 2003; 24:249–258.

165. Be'eri E, Maier SE, Landzberg MJ, Chung T, Geva T. In vivo evaluation of Fontan pathway flow dynamics by multidimensional phase-velocity magnetic resonance imaging. Circulation 1998; 98: 2873–2882.

166. Sharma S, Ensley AE, Hopkins K, Chatzimzvroudis GP, Healy TM, Tam VKH, Kanter KR, Yoganathan AP. In vivo flow dynamics of the total cavopulmonary connection from three-dimensional multislice magnetic resonance imaging. Ann Thorac Surg 2001; 71: 889–898.

167. Rosenthal M, Bush A, Deanfield J, Redington A. Comparison of cardiopulmonary adaptation during exercise in children after the

atriopulmonary and total cavopulmonary connection Fontan procedures. Circulation 1995; 91:372–378.

168. Redington AN, Penny D, Shinebourne EA. Pulmonary blood flow after total cavopulmonary connection. Br Heart J 1991; 65:213–217.
169. Vitullo DA, DeLeon SY, Berry TE, Bonilla JJ, Chhangani SV, Cetta F, Quinones JA, Bell TJ, Fisher EA. Clinical improvement after revision in Fontan patients. Ann Thorac Surg 1996; 61:1797–1804.
170. Kreutzer J, Keane JF, Lock JE, Walsh EP, Jonas RA, Castañeda AR, Mayer JE. Conversion of modified Fontan procedure to lateral atrial tunnel cavopulmonary anastomosis. J Thorac Cardiovasc Surg 1996; 111:1169–1176.
171. McElhinney DB, Reddy VM, Moore P, Hanley FL. Revision of previous Fontan connections to extracardiac or interatrial conduit cavopulmonary anastomosis. Ann Thorac Surg 1996; 62:1276–1283.
172. Ilbawi MN, Idriss FS, Muster AJ, DeLeon SY, Berry TE, Duffy CE, Paul MH. Effects of elevated coronary sinus pressure on left ventricular function after the Fontan operation. J Thorac Cardiovasc Surg 1986; 92:231–237.
173. Miura T, Hiramatsu T, Forbess JM, Mayer JE. Effects of elevated coronary sinus pressure on coronary blood flow and left ventricular function. Circulation 1995; 92(suppl II):298–303.
174. Mavroudis C, Backer CL, Deal BJ, Johnsrude CL. Fontan conversion to cavopulmonary connection and arrhythmiz circuit cryoablation. J Thorac Cardiovasc Surg 1998; 115:547–556.
175. Marcelletti CF, Hanley FL, Mavroudis C, McElhinney DB, Abella RF, Marianeschi SM, Reddy VM, Petrossian E, de la Torre T, Colagrande L, Backer CL, Cipriani A, Iorio FS, Fontan F. Revision of previous Fontan connections to total extracardiac cavopulmonary anastomosis: a multicenter experience. J Thorac Cardiovasc Surg 2000; 119:340–346.
176. Agnoletti G, Borghi A, Vignati G, Crupi GC. Fontan conversion to total cavopulmonary connection and arrhythmia ablation: clinical and functional results. Heart 2003; 89:193–198.
177. Mavroudis C, Backer DL, Deal BJ, Johnsrude C, Strasburger J. Total cavopulmonary conversion and maze procedure for patients with failure of the Fontan operation. J Thorac Cardiovasc Surg 2001; 122:863–871.
178. Rodefeld LE, Bromberg BI, Schuessler RB, Boineau JP, Cox JL, Huddleston CB. Atrial flutter after lateral tunnel construction in the modified Fontan operation: a canine model. J Thorac Cardiovasc Surg 1996; 111:514–526.
179. Cohen MI, Wernovsky G, Vetter VL, Wienand TS, Gaynor JW, Jacobs ML, Spray TL, Rhodes LA. Sinus node function after a systemically staged Fontan procedure. Circulation 1998; 98:II-352–359.

180. Manning PB, Mayer JE, Wernovsky G, Fishberger SB, Walsh EP. Staged operation to Fontan increases the incidence of sinoatrial node dysfunction. J Thorac Cardiovasc Surg 1996; 111:833–840.

181. Laschinger JC, Redmond JM, Cameron DE, Kan JS, Ringel RE. Intermediate results of the extracardiac conduit Fontan procedure. Ann Thorac Surg 1996; 62:1261–1267.

182. Cohen MI, Bridges ND, Gaynor JM, Hoffman TM, Wernovsky G, Vetter VL, Spray TL, Rhodes LA. Modifications to the cavopulmonary anastomosis do not eliminate early sinus node dysfunction. J Thorac Cardiovasc Surg 2000; 120:891–901.

183. Fishberger SB, Wernovsky G, Gentles TL, Gamble WJ, Gauvreau K, Burnett J, Mayer JE, Walsh EP. Long-term outcome in patients with pacemakers following the Fontan operation. Am J Cardiol 1996; 77:887–889.

184. Gelatt M, Hamilton RM, McCrindle BW, Gow RM, Williams WG, Trusler GA, Freedom RM. Risk factors for atrial tachyarrhythmias after the Fontan operation. J Am Coll Cardiol 1994; 24:1735–1741.

185. Cohen MI, Vetter VL, Wernovsky G, Bush DM, Gaynor JW, Iyer VR, Spray TL, Tanel RE, Rhodes LA. Epicardial pacemaker implantation and follow-up in patients with a single ventricle after the Fontan operation. J Thorac Cardiovasc Surg 2001; 121:804–811.

186. Durongpisitkul K, Porter EJ, Cetta F, Offord KP, Slezak JM, Puga FJ, Schaff HV, Danielson GK, Driscoll DJ. Predictors of early- and late-onset supraventricular tachyarrhythmias after Fontan operation. Circulation 1998; 98:1099–1107.

187. Fishberger SB, Wernovsky G, Gentles TL, Gauvreau K, Burnett J, Mayer JE, Walsh EP. Factors that influence the development of atrial flutter after the Fontan operation. J Thorac Cardiovasc Surg 1997; 113:80–86.

188. Ghai A, Harris L, Harrison DA, Webb GD, Siu SC. Outcomes of late atrial tachyarrhythmias in adults after the Fontan operation. J Am Coll Cardiol 2001; 37:585–592.

189. Pearl JM, Laks H, Stein DG, Drinkwater DC, George BL, Williams RG. Total cavopulmonary anastomosis versus conventional modified Fontan procedure. Ann Thorac Surg 1991; 52:189–196.

190. Balaji S, Johnson TB, Sade EM, Case CL, Gillette PC. Management of arial flutter after the Fontan procedure. J Am Coll Cardiol 1994; 23:1209–1215.

191. Guccione P, Paul T, Garson A. Long-term follow-up of amiodarone therapy in the young: continued efficacy, unimpaired growth, moderate side effects. J Am Coll Cardiol 1990; 15:1118–1124.

192. Beaufort-Krol GCM, Bink-Boelkens MTE. Effectiveness of sotalol for atrial flutter in children after surgery for congenital heart disease. Am J Cardiol 1997; 79:92–94.

193. Kalman JM, Van Hare GF, Olgin JE, Saxon LA, Stark SI, Lesh MD. Ablation of "incisional" reentrant atrial tachycardia complicating surgery for congenital heart disease. Circulation 1996; 93:502–512.
194. Triedman JK, Bergau DM, Saul JP, Epstein MR, Triedman JK. Efficacy of radiofrequency ablation for control of intraatrial reentrant tachycardia in patients with congenital heart disease. J Am Coll Cardiol 1997; 30:1032–1038.
195. Nakagawa H, Shah N, Matsudaira K, Overholt E, Chandrasekaran K, Beckman KJ, Spector P, Calame JD, Rao A, Hasdemir C, Otomo K, Wang Z, Lazzara R, Jackman WM. Characterization of reentrant circuit in macroreentrant right atrial tachycardia after surgical repair of congenital heart disease. Circulation 2001; 103:699–709.
196. Sano T, Ogawa M, Yabuuchi H, Matsuda H, Nakano, Shimazaki Y, Tankguchi K, Arisawa J, Hirose H, Kawashima Y. Quantitative cineangiographic analysis of ventricular volume and mass in patients with single ventricle: relation to ventricular morphologies. Circulation 1988; 77:62–69.
197. Powell AJ, Gauvreau K, Jenkins KJ, Blume ED, Mayer JE, Lock JE. Perioperative risk factors for development of protein-losing enteropathy following a Fontan procedure. Am J Cardiol 2001; 88: 1206–1209.
198. Piran S, Veldtman G, Siu S, Webb GD, Liu PP. Heart failure and ventricular dysfunction in patients with single or systemic right ventricles. Circulation 2002; 105:1189–1194.
199. Akagi T, Benson LN, Williams WG, Freedom RM. Regional ventricular wall-motion abnormalities in tricuspid-atresia after the Fontan procedure. J Am Coll Cardiol 1993; 22:1182–1188.
200. Fogel MA, Gupta KB, Weinberg PM, Hoffman EA. Regional wall motion and strain analysis across stages of Fontan reconstruction by magnetic resonance imaging. Am J Physiol Heart Circ Physiol 1995; 269:H1132–H1152.
201. Zimmerman FJ, Starr JP, Koenig PR, Smith P, Hijazi ZM, Bacha EA. Acute hemodynamic benefit of multisite ventricular pacing after congenital heart surgery. Ann Thorac Surg 2003; 75:1775–1780.
202. Caspi J, Coles JG, Rabinovich M, Cohen D, Trusler GA, Williams WG, Wilson GJ, Freedom RM. Morphological findings contributing to a failed Fontan procedure. Circulation 1990; 82(suppl IV):177–182.
203. Knott-Craig CJ, Danielson GK, Schaff HV, Puga FJ, Weaver AL, Driscoll DD. The modified Fontan operation. An analysis of risk factors for early postoperative death or takedown in 702 consecutive patients from one institution. J Thorac Cardiovasc Surg 1995; 109:1237–1243.
204. Van Arsdell GS, McCrindle BW, Einarson KD, Lee K, Oag I, Caldarone CA, Williams WG. Interventions associated with minimal Fontan mortality. Ann Thorac Surg 2000; 70:568–574.

205. Bruns LA, Kichuk Chrisant M, Lamour JM, Shaddy RE, Pahl E, Blume ED, Hallowell S, Addonizio LJ, Canter CE. Carvedilol as therapy in pediatric heart failure: an initial multicenter experience. J Pediatr 2001; 138:505–511.

206. Blume ED, Canter CE, Colan SD, Marcus EM, Gauvreau K, Spicer RL, Jenkins K. Prospective trial of adjunct carvedilol in pediatric patients with moderate ventricular dysfunction (abstract). Circulation 2002; 106(suppl 2):361.

207. Shaddy RE, Curtin EL, Sower B, Tani LY, Burr J, LaSalle B, Boucek MM, Mahony L, Hsu DT, Pahl E, Burch GH, Schlencker-Herceg R. The pediatric randomized carvedilol trial in children with chronic heart failure: rationale and design. Am Heart J 2002; 144:383–389.

208. Kantrowitz A, Haller JD, Joos H, Cerruti MM, Carstensen HE. Transplantation of the heart in an infant and an adult. Am J Cardiol 1968; 22:782–790.

209. Bailey LL, Gundry SR, Razzouk AJ, Wang N, Sciolaro Cm, Chiavarelli M. Bless the babies: one hundred fifteen late survivors of heart transplantation during the first year of life. J Thorac Cardiovasc Surg 1993; 105:805–815.

210. Jenkins PC, Flanagan MF, Jenkins KJ, Sargent JD, Canter CE, Chinnock RE, Vincent RN, Tosteson AN, O'Connor GT. Survival analysis and risk factors for mortality in transplantation and staged surgery for hypoplastic left heart syndrome. J Am Coll Cardiol 2000; 36:1178–1185.

211. Bailey LL. Heart transplantation techinques in complex congenital heart disease. J Heart Lung Transplant 1993; 12:S–168–175.

212. Rychik J, Levy H, Gaynor JW, DeCampli WM, Spray TL. Outcome after operations for pulmonary atresia with intact ventricular septum. J Thorac Cardiovasc Surg 1998; 116:924–931.

213. McGiffin DC, Naftel DC, Kirklin JK, Morrow WR, Towbin J, Shaddy R, Alejos J, Rossi A. Predicting outcome after listing for heart transplantation in children: comparison of Kaplan-Meier and parametric and competing risk analysis. J Heart Lung Transplant 1997; 16:713–722.

214. Azakie A, Merklinger SL, McCrindle BW, Van Arsdell GS, Lee K, Benson LN, Coles JG, Williams WG. Evolving strategies and improving outcomes of the modified Norwood procedure: a 10-year single-institution experience. Ann Thorac Surg 2001; 72:1349–1353.

215. Boucek MM, Edwards LB, Keck BM, Trulock EP, Taylor DO, Mohacsi PJ, Hertz MI. The Registry of the International Society for Heart and Lung Transplantation: sixth official pediatric report—2003. J Heart Lung Transplant 2003; 22:636–652.

216. Webber SA, Fricker FJ, Michaels M, Pickering RM, del Nido PJ, Griffith BP, Armitage JM. Orthotopic heart transplantation in children with congenital heart disease. Ann Thorac Surg 1994; 58: 1664–1669.

217. Hsu DT, Quaegebeur JM, Michler RE, Smith CR, Rose EA, Kichuk MR, Gersony WM, Douglas JF, Addonizio LJ. Heart transplantation in children with congenital heart disease. J Am Coll Cardiol 1995; 26:743–749.

218. Chugh R, Marelli D, Child JS, Patel B, Perloff JK, Miner PD, Kobashigawa JA, George BL, Laks H. Heart transplanatation in adolescents and adults with congenital heart disease. (abstract) J am Coll Cardiol 2002; 40:401A.

219. Bernstein D, Naftel DT, Hsu DT, Addonizio LJ, Blume ED, Gamberg PL, Kirklin JK, Morrow WR. Outcome of listing for cardiac transplantation for failed Fontan: a multi-institutional study (abstract) J Heart Lung Transplant 1999; 18:69.

220. Mertens LL, Hagler DJ, Canter CE, Goldberg SJ, Parisi F, Pahl E, Wilkinson J, Gewillig M. The outcome of heart transplanatation for protein-losing enteropathy after the Fontan operation. (abstract) Circulation 1999; 100(suppl II):II-602.

221. Itescu S, Tung TC, Burke EM, Weinberg A, Moazami N, Artrip JH, Suciu-Foca N, Rose EA, Oz MC, Michler RE. Preformed IgG antibodies against major histocompatibility complex class II antigens are major risk factors for high-grade cellular rejection in recipients of heart transplantation. Circulation 1998; 98:786–793.

222. Shaddy RE, Hunter DD, Osborn KA, Lambert LM, Minich LL, Hawkins JA, McGough EC, Fuller TC. Prospective analysis of HLA immunogenecity of cryopreserved valved allografts used in pediatric heart surgery. Circulation 1996; 94:1063–1067.

13

Right-Sided Heart Failure

**ERIKA BERMAN ROSENZWEIG and
ROBYN J. BARST**

Columbia University, College of Physicians and
Surgeons, New York, New York, U.S.A.

Right-sided heart failure is a common problem among
pediatric patients due to the prevalence of congenital heart
defects and the association with pulmonary hypertension.
Approximately 90% of general adult cardiology focuses on
the integrity of the left heart structure and function. In the
field of pediatric cardiology, more attention is focused on
the structure of the right heart particularly in association
with congenital heart defects and chronic lung disease. While
there is extensive literature on the pathophysiology and treatment of left heart failure, the data for right-sided heart
failure is scarce. When added to the complex nature of some
of the associated congenital heart defects, right-sided heart
failure can be challenging to manage. An understanding of
right ventricular physiology and hemodynamics will lead to

a better understanding of current and future treatment strategies for right heart failure. This chapter will review right-sided heart failure among the pediatric population.

ETIOLOGY

Pediatric conditions associated with right heart dysfunction and right ventricular failure include certain congenital heart defects, cardiomyopathy, chronic lung disease (cor pulmonale), idiopathic pulmonary arterial hypertension (IPAH) (primary pulmonary hypertension), pulmonary thrombo-embolic disease, and myocardial infarction (Table 1) (1). In children, thrombo-embolic disease and myocardial infarction are rarely-seen. However, cor pulmonale or right ventricular dysfunction secondary to congenital heart defects are not uncommon. Cor pulmonale is defined as right ventricular hypertrophy secondary to parenchymal lung disease, pulmonary vascular disease or secondary to abnormalities of pulmonary function (2).

   Certain congenital heart defects are more commonly associated with right heart failure and deserve mention. Congenital heart defects with pure increase in afterload such as severe pulmonic stenosis can be associated with right ventricular failure. Single right ventricle, congenitally corrected transposition of the great vessels, and transposition of the great vessels following Senning or Mustard repair are a few of the lesions in which the right ventricle is also exposed to increased afterload (i.e., systemic pressures) and may fail over time. This may not occur until adulthood or may not occur at all in some cases. As longer follow up becomes available for hypoplastic left heart syndrome patients following Fontan surgery, we may gain a better understanding of the right ventricle's capacity to act as a systemic ventricle. Lesions of pure increase in preload, e.g., atrial septal defect (ASD), may be associated with preserved right ventricular function at the expense of right ventricular dilatation for many years. Patients may not present clinically until adulthood when systemic arterial hypertension or coronary artery disease cause impairment of left ventricular diastolic function

Table 1 Causes of Right Heart Failure in Pediatrics

Congenital heart disease
Hyperkinetic pulmonary arterial hypertension—congenital systemic to
    pulmonary communications with increased pulmonary blood flow
    (e.g.,ventricular septal defect, patent ductus arteriosus)
Pulmonary venous hypertension—disorders of left heart filling (e.g.,
    mitral stenosis, pulmonary vein obstruction, or left ventricular failure)
Uhl's disease
Acquired heart disease
Post cardiopulmonary bypass (usually transient)
Coronary disease (e.g., Kawasaki disease)
Lung disease—hypoxia
Parenchymal lung disease
    Obstructive (e.g., cystic fibrosis)
    Restrictive (e.g., interstitial pneumonitis, diffuse interstitial fibrosis)
Bronchopulmonary dysplasia
Hyaline membrane disease
Pulmonary hypoplasia
Diminished ventilatory drive (e.g., Ondine's curse)
Congenital anomalies (e.g., congenital diaphragmatic hernia)
Extrinsic Factors
Upper airway obstruction
Neuromuscular disorders
Thoracic cage deformities
Respiratory center dysfunction
High altitude (hypoxia induced)
Thromboembolic disease
Connective tissue and granulomatous diseases
Scleroderma
Systemic lupus erythematosus
Mixed connective tissue disease
Rheumatoid arthritis
Sarcoidosis
Overlap syndrome
Conditions associated with pulmonary arterial hypertension
Exogenous substances
    Anorexic agents
    Toxic rapeseed oil
    Psychotropic drugs (e.g., L-tryptophan or cocaine)
Portal hypertension
    Portal vein thrombosis
    Liver disease
    HIV infection
        Sickle cell disease

(Continued)

Table 1   Causes of Right Heart Failure in Pediatrics (*Continued*)

Primary pulmonary hypertension or idiopathic pulmonary arterial hypertension (IPAH)
Persistent pulmonary hypertension of the newborn
Pulmonary veno-occlusive disease
Pulmonary capillary hemangiomatosis
Alveolar capillary dysplasia

Adapted from Ref. 1.

leading to increased systemic to pulmonary shunting. This may not be well tolerated by the already dilated right ventricle. In addition, patients who have undergone tetralogy of Fallot repair, particularly those who required a ventriculotomy, may be predisposed to develop late right ventricular failure in the setting of pulmonary insufficiency which leads to right ventricular volume overload. Congenital heart defects associated with increased pulmonary blood flow [e.g., ventricular septal defect (VSD)] must be corrected early to avoid the development of irreversible pulmonary vascular obstructive disease. For unrepaired defects, shunt reversal may occur with patients becoming cyanotic. For these patients with residual defects, right ventricular function is usually preserved for several decades with hypoxemia as the primary problem. Right ventricular function is usually maintained since the defect serves as a "pop-off" valve for the right ventricle under systemic pressure at the expense of developing hypoxemia. In contrast, if the defect is repaired in the setting of pulmonary vascular obstructive disease, the right ventricle is exposed to an acute increase in afterload and will be more likely to fail.

PATHOPHYSIOLOGY

There are inherent differences between the right ventricle (RV) and left ventricle (LV) under normal physiologic conditions. Under normal loading conditions, when the function is not compromised, the right ventricle ejects blood against approximately 25% of the afterload of the left ventricle. This leads to differences in wall thickness due to the La Place relationship, i.e., the left ventricle wall is thicker than the right ventricle wall to minimize wall stress [wall stress = right ventricular systolic pressure (P) × chamber radius $(r)/2$ × wall wall thickness (h)] (3). While the right ventricle can adapt to an increase in volume because it is more compliant than the left ventricle, the right ventricle is less prepared to handle an acute increase in pressure afterload, i.e., thinner wall (4). Therefore, right ventricular systolic performance becomes strongly preload dependent under conditions of acute increases in systolic load, such as a pulmonary embolism. A caveat to this rule is that tricuspid valve regurgitation is very sensitive to changes in ventricular systolic pressure and size (becoming more severe with increases of either) and actually negates the classic Starling effect during alterations in diastolic filling, functioning as a descending limb (5).

For a child who is born with a congenital heart defect with increased right ventricular afterload, e.g., severe pulmonic stenosis or who has had pulmonary hypertension from birth, the right ventricle is better equipped to handle the elevated afterload because it has been exposed to systemic pressure in utero (6) (Fig. 1). For children who develop increased afterload following the normal thinning out of the right ventricle, which occurs within the first decade of life following the normal decrease in the pulmonary vascular resistance, there are certain adaptive changes that occur. If there has been a gradual exposure over time, the right ventricle has the ability to remodel and adapt to the pressure load by recruitment of sarcomeres and hypertrophy of myocytes. The adaptation of the right ventricle to increased afterload such as idiopathic PAH or congenital heart defects with increased right ventricular afterload, e.g., pulmonic stenosis, is a double-edged sword. The right ventricular hypertrophy will assist the right ventricle in pumping against increased afterload; however, this occurs at a cost to left ventricular integrity. Under normal conditions, the right ventricle is crescentic or pancake shaped with the right ventricular free wall and interventricular septum concave around the left ventricle

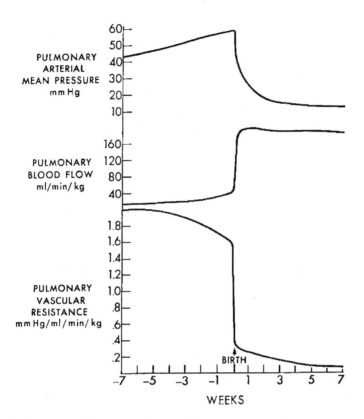

Figure 1   The changes in pulmonary arterial pressure, pulmonary blood flow, and calculated pulmonary vascular resistance during the 7 weeks preceding birth, at birth, and the 7 weeks postnatally. The prenatal data were derived from lambs and the postnatal data from other species. (Reprinted with permission from Ref. 6.)

at both end-diastole and end-systole (Fig. 2). During systole, the left ventricle contracts toward a central axis, while the right ventricular free wall and septum contract in parallel. With right ventricular hypertrophy, the interventricular septal orientation flattens and ultimately commits to the right ventricle in severe cases. This may lead to a vicious cycle of left ventricular diastolic dysfunction and subsequent worsening of right heart failure in severe cases (7,8) (Fig. 2). This has been demonstrated in association with several conditions which include chronic obstructive pulmonary disease (9),

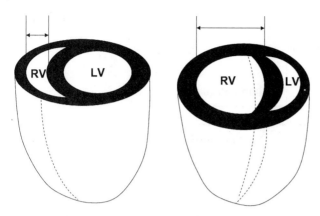

Figure 2 Ventricular geometry of the normal heart (left panel) vs. the hypertensive right ventricle (right panel). The right ventricle is normally crescent shaped, but rounds out and bows toward the left ventricle when there is increased afterload (right panel).

idiopathic PAH (10), ASD (8), and myocardial infarction and is referred to as interventricular dependence. This phenomenon may explain why some patients with severe right ventricular hypertension develop pulmonary vascular congestion in the late stages of their disease. If the pulmonary hypertension becomes severe, there may actually be increased right ventricular volume and size in both systole and diastole due to remodeling of the myocardium (increase in myocyte length) (11). This is likely an attempt to maintain cardiac output by increasing the stroke volume of the failing right ventricle.

There is significant variability between patients in how quickly the right heart fails. Rapid increases in pulmonary arterial pressure are universally not well tolerated unless the right ventricle is already hypertrophied. However, slower alterations in pressure may or may not be accompanied by right ventricular failure, i.e., in some patients, right heart dysfunction develops slowly over decades, while others rapidly develop severe right ventricular dysfunction (12) (Fig. 3). This variability has prompted investigators to study local mechanisms of ventricular adaptation to pressure overload as well as genetic predisposition and biologic variability among patients. For example, in a study by Lowes et al.

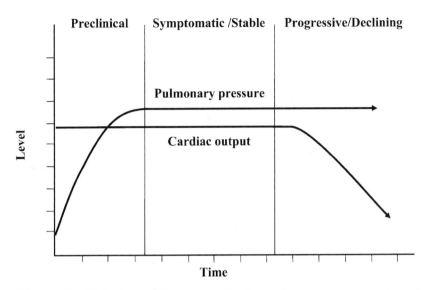

Figure 3 This figure illustrates the hemodynamic progression of untreated idiopathic PAH which ultimately leads to right-sided heart failure with associated decrease in cardiac output and clinical deterioration. (Adapted with permission from Ref. 12.)

(13), investigators compared right ventricular endomyocardial biopsies from intact nonfailing hearts to those with right ventricular failure from idiopathic PAH or idiopathic dilated cardiomyopathy. The investigators used quantitative reverse transcriptase polymerase chain reaction of the RNA obtained from the biopsies to measure expression of genes involved in regulation of contractility and hypertrophy. Measurements were also made in explanted hearts of idiopathic dilated cardiomyopathy and donor nonfailing hearts. They found that in right heart failure from either idiopathic PAH or idiopathic dilated cardiomyopathy, the alpha major histocompatibility complex (α-myosin heavy chain mRNA) was down-regulated and the beta MHC gene expression was up-regulated. This alteration in the major histocompatibility complex isoforms may translate into a decrease in the myosin ATPase enzyme velocity consistent with slowing the speed of contraction. This is just one example of how the ventricle may be subject to local regulation and to changes in genetic expression which may account for the differences in severity between patients with the same degree of afterload. Neurohormonal activation can lead to altered gene expression, changes in myocardial growth and remodeling, and toxicity, ischemia, and energy depletion in left heart failure (Fig. 4) (14). Neurohormonal activation has also been demonstrated in patients with right ventricular failure and normal left ventricular function, which may have implications for the role of this system in the pathophysiology of right-sided heart failure; however, this requires further investigation (15).

There may also be markers of myocardial injury, and thus right ventricular dysfunction for patients with right-sided heart failure. For example, cardiac troponin T has been reported as an independent marker of increased mortality

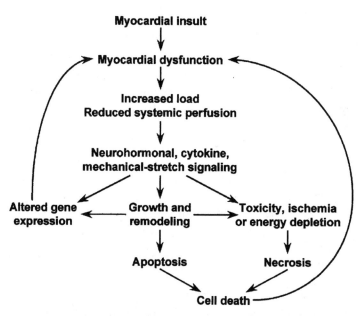

Figure 4 The central role of neurohormonal, cytokine, and mechanical (increased wall stress) signaling pathways in producing adverse biologic effects that lead to progressive myocardial dysfunction and remodeling. A cascade of events leads to altered gene expression and/or cell death, both of which impair myocardial function further. (Reprinted with permission from Ref. 14.)

risk in patients with chronic PAH (16). Similarly, plasma brain natriuretic peptide (BNP) has also been shown to increase in proportion to the extent of right ventricular dysfunction in PAH and may have a strong, independent association with increased mortality rates in patients with idiopathic PAH (17,18). Hyperuricemia may also serve as a prognostic marker for severity of PAH as levels are elevated in severe PAH and correlate with increased mortality (19).

With regard to increased afterload, while one patient may compensate by developing right ventricular hypertrophy in response to increased wall stress based on Laplace's law, another patient may be unable to develop a hypertrophic response by recruiting sarcomeres and thus have "decompensated" heart failure with right heart dilatation and dysfunction. In addition, depending on whether the stimulus is pressure overload or volume overload, the response will lead to different adaptive changes which may or may not compensate for the stimulus (Fig. 5) (3). For the pressure overloaded heart, the expected compensatory effect would be concentric hypertrophy to reduce wall stress. For the volume overloaded/preloaded heart, one develops an increase in end-diastolic wall stress that leads to chamber dilatation as a

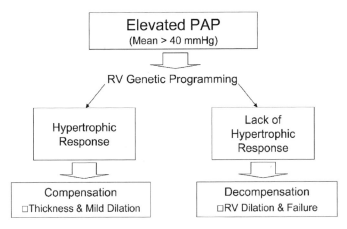

Figure 5 Hypothesis for variable right ventricular response to markedly increased afterload of idiopathic PAH. (Reprinted with permission from Ref. 3.)

compensatory mechanism. Ultimately, the hypertrophied heart will dilate when it begins to fail and the dilated heart will reach a maximum stretch point (Starling's law) before it begins to fail with subsequent hypertrophy. Thus, these mechanisms appear to be somewhat intertwined. For example, in a patient with increased right ventricular afterload from idiopathic PAH or chronic obstructive lung disease, volume overload may occur as a consequence of (1) inadequacy of the right ventricular mass to sustain systolic performance in the presence of increased afterload resulting in increased right ventricular volume at end-diastole as well as end-systole, and (2) tricuspid regurgitation secondary to increased right ventricle afterload (5).

In addition to the physiologic changes that occur within the right heart, there are also structural adaptations of the right heart in response to abnormal loads. Right atrial dilatation occurs when the right atrial pressure increases secondary to increased right ventricular diastolic pressure. In the absence of tricuspid valve abnormalities, the right atrial dilatation is usually secondary to functional tricuspid regurgitation or elevated right ventricular diastolic pressure as seen in right ventricular failure. Right atrial dilatation is one of the known survival parameters for idiopathic PAH patients, with more severe dilatation associated with worse survival (20).

There are certain congenital heart lesions/repairs that warrant separate mention. For patients with hypoplastic left heart syndrome who have undergone a Fontan repair, or patients who have undergone a Mustard or Senning repair for transposition of the great arteries, as well as patients with congenitally corrected transposition of the great vessels, the right ventricle becomes the "systemic ventricle" and pumps to the systemic circulation. The fact that the right heart often fails under these circumstances lends further support to the hypothesis that the right and left ventricle are not only anatomically different, but may have different genetic, neurohormonal, and biochemical programs that influence their function.

DIAGNOSIS

Clinical Findings

Clinical History/Symptoms

The history should explore the duration of symptoms, severity, and possible clues as to the etiology of the right-sided heart failure. The clinical symptoms differ for patients with residual intracardiac or extracardiac defects vs. those without. For patients who do not have intracardiac or extracardiac shunts, i.e., those with underlying pulmonary disease or idiopathic PAH, the symptoms are fairly classic for right-sided heart failure, i.e., manifestations of congestion of the systemic vascular circuit. Some of the features of right heart failure include peripheral edema, ascites, dyspnea on exertion, and syncope. Dyspnea, the most frequent presenting complaint of adults and many children with idiopathic PAH and associated right-sided heart failure, is due to impaired oxygen delivery during physical activity as a result of an inability to increase cardiac output in the presence of increased oxygen demands. Palpitations secondary to arrhythmias may occur if there is significant right atrial dilatation. Infants with large, unrestrictive systemic to pulmonary shunts usually present with signs of congestive heart failure, such as tachypnea, diaphoresis, and failure to thrive. Following years of continued exposure to high shear stress from the left to right shunting, the pulmonary vascular resistance increases, frequently to systemic levels, leading to bidirectional shunting and ultimately to right-to-left shunting. Hypoxemia and cyanosis then ensue, which can be severe. In rare cases, a history of congestive heart failure and/or failure to thrive in infancy is absent. In these patients, reversal of flow may have occurred within the first two years of life. This group may represent a subset of patients who may have never had the normal physiologic fall in the pulmonary vascular resistance after birth or perhaps may represent a subset of patients with an increased susceptibility to pulmonary vascular disease.

Physical Signs

The pediatric cardiologist needs to recognize the physical signs of right-sided heart failure. On physical examination, signs differ for children with and without an intracardiac or extracardiac shunt. In patients who have undergone "corrective" surgery for their congenital heart defects, the physical findings may be identical to patients with idiopathic PAH or other types of PAH. Careful attention should be paid to the cardiac examination, and other signs of systemic venous congestion related to right "pump" failure. The cardiac signs of elevated right ventricular systolic pressure include a loud single P2, murmur of tricuspid insufficiency, and murmur of pulmonary insufficiency. In addition, there may be an S3 or S4 right ventricular gallop. An increase in the pulmonic component of the second heart sound and a right-sided fourth heart sound are early findings. When heard, a right ventricular third heart sound generally reflects advanced disease. A pansystolic murmur of tricuspid regurgitation is very common. The high-pitched diastolic murmur of pulmonary insufficiency may also be heard, and usually relates to the high pulmonary arterial pressures and dilatation of the main pulmonary artery. The P2 intensity may actually become softer as the right ventricle fails. Jugular venous distention may be present with a prominent a wave. Hepatomegaly may also be present. In children, because the liver capsule is more distensible, the size of the liver is a good marker of the degree of right heart failure and response to therapy. Ascites and peripheral edema can also occur in severe cases. Other systemic findings may implicate a systemic cause for the right heart failure or pulmonary hypertension, e.g., rash for systemic lupus erythematosus. Clubbing and cyanosis may be present in children with underlying lung disease or the Eisenmenger syndrome. Clubbing of the digits is very rare following complete surgical repair of a congenital heart defect unless there is underlying pulmonary disease, since these patients are no longer hypoxemic.

The patient with pulmonary hypertension and pulmonary vascular disease with a congenital systemic–pulmonary shunt who has not undergone surgical repair, i.e., Eisenmenger patient, may appear cyanotic at rest. In the early stages of the disease, they may only develop cyanosis with exertion. By definition, all patients with the Eisenmenger syndrome become progressively more cyanotic with exertion. Particular focus on cyanosis should be paid to the oral mucosa and nail beds. In addition, clubbing of the digits may be present. Most patients do not have an increased jugular venous pressure on physical examination, particularly if an interatrial communication is present. On cardiac examination, a right ventricular lift, a loud, palpable, single S2, a high-pitched diastolic murmur of pulmonary insufficiency, and pansystolic murmur of tricuspid insufficiency may also be present. If there is congestive heart failure, peripheral edema, ascites, and hepatosplenomegaly may also be present.

Chest X-Ray

The chest rocntgenogram is an important part of the diagnostic evaluation. The presence of any specific parenchymal disorder should be investigated. In addition, one can rule out significant chest wall deformity by chest x-ray. Furthermore, overall or segmental enlargement of the cardiac silhouette may provide a diagnostic clue. For patients with idiopathic PAH, the classic findings are prominence of the main pulmonary arteries and hilar vessels (Fig. 6). Peripheral pruning is a very late finding. For other defects such as Ebstein's anomaly, there may be additional findings specific for the particular condition, e.g., right atrial enlargement.

ECG

Electrocardiographic findings are seen early in the course of right-sided heart failure. Classic changes may include right axis deviation, right atrial enlargement (P pulmonale), right ventricular hypertrophy, and right ventricular strain patterns (Fig. 7). Right ventricular hypertrophy is reflected in the electrocardiogram by persistent increased voltage over the right precordial leads and a decreased or absent S wave

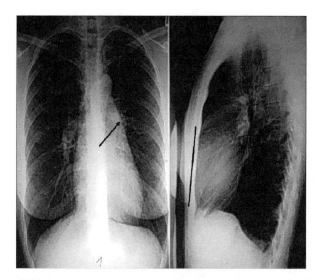

Figure 6 Chest x-ray of a patient with idiopathic PAH demonstrates enlargement of the right ventricle and central pulmonary arteries with pruning of the peripheral pulmonary arteries.

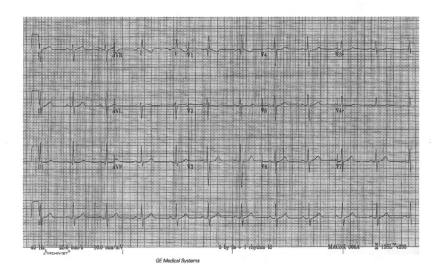

Figure 7 Electrocardiogram demonstrates right axis deviation, right ventricular hypertrophy with a right ventricular strain pattern.

(pure R in V$_3$R and V$_1$). When right ventricular pressure is just below or near systemic levels, upright T waves can be seen over the right precordium with a dominant R wave. When there is suprasystemic right ventricular systolic pressure, a strain pattern may be present over the right chest leads with T wave inversion and J point depression (5). Since prominent right-sided forces are a normal finding in infancy and regress with age, the electrocardiographic interpretation becomes somewhat more difficult in the pediatric population as it must be interpreted in context of the age of the patient and the normal maturational changes that occur. Whereas, the amplitude of the R wave in lead V$_1$ often exceeds the R wave in V$_6$ from birth to six months, the R wave in V$_1$ decreases progressively throughout infancy and childhood, reaching an adult pattern usually by adolescence (5). Therefore, as an example, prominent V$_1$R wave forces in an 8-year old are abnormal, but in a 2-year old may be normal. Additionally, the presence of an associated congenital heart defect may change the axis, e.g., left superior axis in complete atrioventricular canal defect, masking right axis deviation.

Transthoracic Echocardiography

General

Echocardiography for assessment of right heart function has several limitations. In contrast to the left ventricle which is elliptical and easily assessed echocardiographically, the right ventricle is crescent shaped and truncated with separate inflow and outflow portions which are positioned in different planes (21). The right ventricle does not conform to any classic geometric model and volume estimates can be inaccurate (22). This creates a challenge in interpretation of the echocardiogram. Several advances in echocardiographic techniques have been developed in an attempt to overcome these obstacles.

Two-Dimensional (2D) Echocardiography

In normal subjects, 2D echocardiographic imaging provides a good assessment of right ventricular dimensions, shape, and wall thickness (23). By reviewing 2D images one can obtain a qualitative assessment of right ventricular dilatation and/or right ventricular hypertrophy (Fig. 8). In addition, the orientation of the interventricular septum and its commitment to either the right or left ventricle gives a qualitative estimate of right ventricular hypertension, i.e., committed to the left ventricle—less than 50% systemic arterial pressure, flat—approximately 50% systemic arterial pressure, and committed to the right ventricle—suprasystemic arterial pressure. However, in patients with pulmonary disease, assessment of dimensions by 2D imaging is less reliable (24–26). Right ventricle pressure overload is associated with right ventricular free wall hypertrophy, and right ventricle volume overload is associated with right ventricular dilatation and paradoxical interventricular septal motion secondary to elevated right ventricular end-diastolic pressure.

There are several techniques for estimating right ventricular volume and function by 2D echocardiographic imaging. Simpson's method calculates the volume of the right ventricle

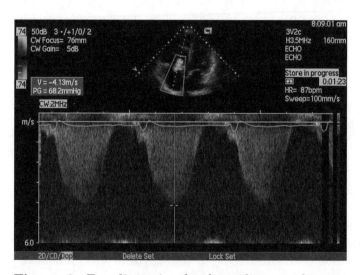

Figure 8 Two-dimensional echocardiogram demonstrates right heart dilatation with tricuspid insufficiency. Doppler technique demonstrates a tricuspid regurgitant pressure gradient of 68 mmHg, consistent with right ventricular systolic hypertension.

based on a summation of the volume of individual slices (21). This can be useful in estimating the right ventricle ejection fraction (EF)%. While there is a good correlation with angiographic RVEF% using Simpson's method, this method is technically challenging in general clinical practice. The eccentricity index can also be helpful in assessing right ventricular volume (degree of septal displacement = ratio of minor axis diameter of left ventricle parallel to septum to that perpendicular to it) (27). The right ventricular area based on single plane subtraction echocardiographic methods has also been shown to correlate with right ventricular ejection fraction (28,29). Tricuspid annular plane systolic excursion (TAPSE) may be another useful measure of right ventricular systolic function. One limitation of this technique is that it only evaluates systolic performance. The use of echocardiographic contrast agents can also be used to assess function, with slow or poor clearance as an indicator of decreased myocardial function.

An assessment of right atrial size may be an important prognostic indicator, with right atrial dilatation being associated with a poor prognosis in patients with idiopathic PAH (20). The presence and size of a pericardial effusion may be another prognostic indicator for patients with right heart failure. It has been demonstrated that effusion size is correlated with right atrial pressure (30). For patients with severe idiopathic PAH, pericardial effusion is common and is associated with right heart failure, impaired exercise tolerance, and a poor 1-year prognosis (20,30).

Doppler Echocardiography

The introduction of Doppler echocardiography was a major advance in echocardiography. This provided a noninvasive technique for estimating systolic pulmonary arterial pressure. To estimate the systolic pulmonary arterial pressure, the peak velocity of the tricuspid regurgitant jet is measured and applied to the Bernouli equation (right ventricle systolic pressure $(mmHg) = 4 \times (tricuspid\ regurgitation\ velocity)^2$ + right atrial pressure (21,31). An estimate of right atrial pressure can be obtained by physical examination, inferior vena cavae measurements, or tricuspid inflow parameters (32,33). One limitation of this technique for measuring systolic pulmonary arterial pressure is that it relies on the presence of tricuspid regurgitation and may be inaccurate if the tricuspid regurgitation is only mild leading to under or overestimation of the systolic pulmonary arterial pressure.

One technique for assessing right ventricular systolic performance is the right ventricular Doppler outflow tract profile including right ventricle pre-ejection time, ejection time, acceleration time, and their ratios (34). These measures are very sensitive to changes in systolic pulmonary arterial pressure, e.g., prolonged pre-ejection time, early systolic peak velocity, and diminished acceleration time.

A Doppler index of myocardial performance (MPI, IMP, or Tei index) has received recent attention (35). It is based on measurements of Doppler derived time intervals during the cardiac cycle, and thus is not limited by the geometry of the right ventricle as some of the other techniques are. By comparing the ratio of the isovolumic contraction and the iso-volumic relaxation periods to the ejection time period, one can calculate the MPI (Fig. 9) (36). The isovolumic contraction time will increase in right ventricular systolic dysfunction as the right ventricular ejection time decreases. Diastolic dys-function is manifested by a prolongation of the isovolumic relaxation time. Therefore, with increasing global right ventricular dysfunction, the MPI will increase. This performance index has been validated in congenital heart disease (36,37), idiopathic PAH (38), right ventricular infarction (39), and chronic lung disease (40). When Eidem et al. (36) investigated the MPI in children and adults with congenital heart disease associated with increased preload (ASD), afterload (pulmon-ary stenosis), or both (L-transposition of the great arteries with severe left atrioventricular valve regurgitation), before and after their surgical repair, no significant change in right ventricular MPI was seen in any postoperative patient group despite relief of the right ventricular volume and/or pressure overload. They concluded that the right ventricular MPI index was relatively independent of the changes in preload or after-load. Yeo et al. (38) also reported a significant correlation

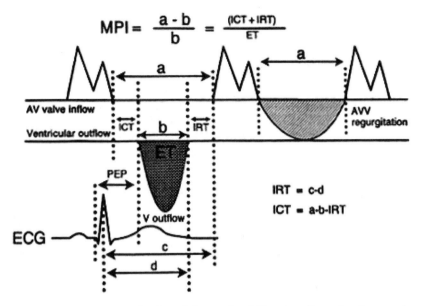

Figure 9 MPI is calculated from the following Doppler intervals: interval "a" represents the interval from cessation to onset of tricuspid valve inflow; interval "b" is RV ejection time (ejection time). The MPI is a ratio of the sum of ICT and IRT divided by ejection time. ICT and IRT can be derived as shown in equations at bottom right. Duration of tricuspid valve regurgitation can be substituted for interval "a". AV, atrioventricular; AVV, atrioventricular valve; ECG, electrocardiogram; V, ventricular. (Reprinted with permission from Ref. 36.)

between the MPI, clinical symptoms, and survival for patients with idiopathic PAH, further supporting its use as a clinical correlate of right heart dysfunction severity. However, there are certain circumstances in which the MPI is not valid, e.g., in the setting of tachyarrhythmias or heart block.

Several echocardiographic techniques can be used to assess right ventricular diastolic function. The measured pulmonary insufficiency pressure gradient (mmHg) can be used as an estimate of right ventricle end-diatolic pressure and pulmonary artery mean pressure (41,42). In addition, the classic technique for assessing diastolic performance is by analyzing the tricuspid inflow pattern. This can be measured as the "E to A ratio" and the deceleration time of early filling (Edt). By evaluating the tricuspid flow velocity profile one can measure the peak velocity of early filling (E velocity), the peak velocity of late filling due to atrial contraction (A velocity), and the Edt. One would expect the E/A ratio to fall and the Edt to be prolonged with right ventricular diastolic dysfunction. Similarly, with left-sided diastolic dysfunction secondary to changes in ventricular geometry with elevated right ventricular systolic function, transmitral flow patterns may be abnormal (Fig. 10) (43). Unfortunately, many variables can affect these measurements so they should be used cautiously. Doppler assessment of the hepatic venous flow or the superior vena caval flow may also help in the assessment of right ventricular diastolic dysfunction. In addition, the right ventricular isovolumic relaxation time is prolonged with diastolic dysfunction (Fig. 9).

Novel echocardiographic techniques including tissue Doppler (44), three-dimensional echocardiography (45), automated

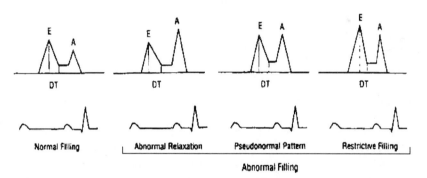

Figure 10 Top: Patterns of transmitral flow with various degrees of ventricular diastolic dysfunction. Bottom: Electrocardiographic tracings corresponding to diagrams. In healthy subjects, the transmitral flow is biphasic, consisting of an initial tall E wave followed by a shorter A wave. The deceleration time (DT) is the interval between the peak early diastolic flow velocity and the onset of diastasis; this parameter measures how rapidly left atrial and left ventricular pressures equalize in early diastole and is related directly to mitral valve area and inversely to ventricular compliance (normal adult 200 ± 40 msec). (Reprinted with permission Ref. 43.)

border detection (46), color kinesis (47), and intracardiac echocardiography (48) may prove useful in assessing right ventricular integrity in the future, however, the current experience in pediatric patients is limited.

Cardiac MRI and MUGA

Magnetic resonance imaging (MRI) can be an excellent tool for imaging the right ventricle, both for anatomic and functional assessments (49). Magnetic resonance imaging provides a direct, noninvasive visualization of the right ventricular chamber as well as the myocardium itself allowing reliable demonstration of morphologic changes in the size and shape of the ventricle, thickness of the myocardium, and presence of abnormal infiltration by fat or edema (Fig. 11) (50). In addition, the MRI does not depend on any geometric assumptions about the right ventricle, and thus calculations of right ventricular mass and volume can be accurately quantified. Multiple-gated equilibrium study (MUGA) can image the entire heart from various angles, assess both systolic and diastolic function, and detect segmental wall-motion abnormalities. This may be a relatively good noninvasive technique for serial assessments of right ventricular function.

Cardiac Catheterization

Right heart catheterization is critical for patients with right heart failure for both diagnostic and therapeutic reasons. There are several important hemodynamic measures during right heart catheterization that assess the severity of right heart dysfunction/failure. These include right atrial pressure, right ventricular systolic and diastolic pressures, pulmonary arterial pressure, pulmonary vascular resistance, pulmonary capillary wedge pressure (as an estimate of left ventricle end-diastolic pressure), cardiac index and gradient across the right ventricular outflow tract and degree of left-to-right or right-to-left shunting (if applicable). If there is significant tricuspid insufficiency, the best method for determining cardiac output is using the Fick technique with

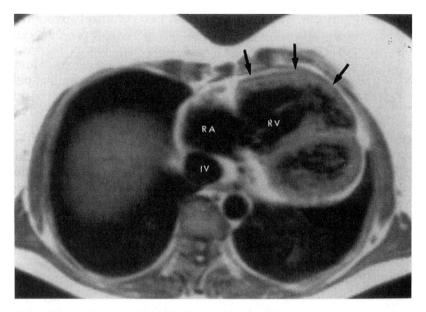

Figure 11 Axial spin echo image of a 24-year old woman with idiopathic PAH. There is rotation of the heart into the left chest and dilatation of both the right ventricle (RV) and right atrium (RA) resulting from the volume load of tricuspid regurgitation. There is increased thickness of the RV free wall (arrows) and flattening of the interventricular septum, resulting from the pressure load caused by increased pulmonary resistance. The inferior vena cava (IV) is moderately dilated. (Reprinted with permission from Ref. 50.)

measured oxygen consumption (51). Angiography may be useful in selected cases to evaluate the degree of right ventricular dysfunction and dilatation, and the degree of tricuspid insufficiency, in addition to other anatomic abnormalities.

MEDICAL MANAGEMENT

General

The medical management of right-sided heart failure is focused on correcting the stimulus if possible (i.e., decreasing the preload or afterload on the right ventricle), alleviating the venous congestion, and improving myocardial performance if possible. Correcting the stimulus may be possible for certain conditions, e.g., ASD closure (increased preload), thrombectomy for pulmonary thrombus (increased afterload), pulmonary valvuloplasty for pulmonary stenosis (increased afterload), and AV valve replacement for congenitally corrected transposition of the great vessels with severe left-sided AV valve regurgitation (increased preload and afterload). The right ventricle has the capacity to remodel even in severe cases of right ventricular failure once the afterload is reduced. For example, in patients with idiopathic PAH and significant right ventricular dysfunction who have undergone lung transplantation alone, the right ventricle almost always recovers following lung transplantation (52,53). Similarly, in adults undergoing ASD repair (surgical or percutaneous), there are rapid improvements in the size of the right ventricle within one month following ASD closure with sustained improvements. However, approximately 23–29% of the adult patients will have residual right heart dilatation (54,55). Among patients who had percutaneous ASD closure, those that had residual right heart dilatation tended to be older (i.e., > 40 years), which suggests that long-standing volume load may have irreversible sequelae (55). This may also explain why the results have not been dramatic for adults following tetralogy of Fallot repair who undergo right ventricular outflow tract reconstruction for severe right heart dilatation secondary to severe pulmonary insufficiency and may have implications about timing of surgery (56).

Pulmonary Vasodilators

Intuitively, one would expect an effective pulmonary vasodilator to reduce the afterload of the right ventricle. Pulmonary vasodilator therapy has been used for the treatment of idiopathic PAH and some forms of secondary pulmonary hypertension based on the premise that pulmonary vasoconstriction plays a role in the development of the pulmonary vascular disease. However, there are important considerations for the use of pulmonary vasodilators for right heart failure depending on the etiology. The pulmonary vasodilators that are currently available in the United States include calcium channel blockers, continuous intravenous epoprostenol (i.e., synthetic prostacyclin), subcutaneous treprostinil (prostacyclin analogue), and the dual endothelin receptor antagonist, bosentan. Drugs currently under investigation include selective endothelin A receptor antagonists, intravenous treprostinil, and sildenafil (phosphodiesterase 5 inhibitor). All of these agents should be used with caution as they often have systemic effects and often may worsen ventilation/perfusion mismatch for patients with underlying lung disease. Therefore, they should only be used after complete hemodynamic evaluation with cardiac catheterization and acute pulmonary vasodilator testing to determine the appropriate therapy.

Systemic Venous Congestion

Although diuretics may be useful for patients with severe right heart failure to relieve hepatic congestion and/or increased intravascular volume, this must be done cautiously to avoid overdiuresis in patients who rely on preload to maintain adequate cardiac output, e.g., following complete repair of tetralogy of Fallot.

Myocardial Performance

For myocardial performance, inotropic agents may be indicated. The efficacy of inotropic agents for right heart failure remains controversial, and its use in patients with right heart dysfunction is adapted from that of patients with left heart dysfunction (57). There have been reports of increased cardiac output with the use of digitalis in patients with PAH with right heart failure (58).

While extracoporeal membrane oxygenation has been used for several years for respiratory failure secondary to persistent pulmonary hypertension of the newborn, its use following cardiac surgery has become more common in the recent past. In postoperative cases of severe right heart failure, mechanical assist devices such as right ventricular assist device (RVAD) or extracoporeal membrane oxygenation may be indicated in an attempt to support the right heart while awaiting recovery of function (59,60). In cases of severe right heart failure which are refractory to medical or surgical therapy and who await transplantation, mechanical assist devices such as RVAD or extracoporeal membrane oxygenation may also serve as a palliative bridge to transplantation. However, for lung transplantation, the estimated waiting time is over 1 year which makes this approach impractical in most circumstances.

Anticoagulation

Patients with significant right-sided heart failure are at risk for thromboembolic events for several reasons: sedentary lifestyle due to self-limitation in the setting of peripheral venous insufficiency, dilation of the right heart, and sluggish pulmonary blood flow. Even a small pulmonary embolus can be life-threatening in patients who cannot vasodilate or recruit additional pulmonary vessels normally; postmortem examinations of patients with pulmonary vascular disease who have died suddenly often demonstrate fresh clot in the pulmonary vascular bed. If warfarin is used, the aim is to maintain the international normalized ratio (INR) at 1.5–2.0 for most patients, with a higher INR for patients who are hypercoagulable, e.g., positive lupus anticoagulant, positive anticardiolipin antibodies, or protein C or protein S deficiency.

Supplemental Oxygen

If lung disease or pulmonary vascular disease is present, supplemental oxygen may be beneficial to decrease alveolar hypoxia which may stimulate pulmonary vasoconstriction. The use of supplemental oxygen may alleviate some of the right ventricular afterload. Thus, patients may also gain clinical benefit. Although recent data demonstrated that supplemental oxygen did not offer a survival benefit for adult patients with Eisenmenger syndrome (61), a previous study demonstrated that the use of supplemental oxygen in children with pulmonary vascular disease during sleep may slow the progression of polycythemia and increase survival (62). There is also evidence that systemic arterial oxygen desaturation may occur in the supine position due to ventilation/perfusion changes within the lung which occur when supine, and that the use of supplemental oxygen attenuates these changes (63). These findings provide further rationale for the use of supplemental oxygen with sleep for selected patients.

In addition, patients who have significant systemic arterial oxygen desaturation with activity due to increased oxygen extraction, in the setting of fixed oxygen delivery, may benefit from supplemental oxygen during exercise. Patients with right-sided heart failure who also have increased oxygen extraction at rest may benefit from supplemental oxygen. During acute respiratory infections, supplemental oxygen may be helpful to prevent worsening hypoxemia. In addition, supplemental oxygen for air travel may be helpful to alleviate alveolar hypoxia related to barometric changes.

INTERVENTIONAL/SURGICAL TREATMENT

At present, interventional/surgical treatment for patients with severe right heart failure is reserved for those patients with advanced disease that is refractory to medical management.

Atrial Septostomy

Patients with idiopathic PAH in whom a foramen ovale is patent live longer than those without a patent foramen ovale (64). Furthermore, patients with Eisenmenger syndrome with an ASD have a better prognosis than idiopathic PAH patients who have an intact atrial septum (65). In postoperative patients with advanced pulmonary vascular disease and right heart failure who have no significant residual communication between the systemic and pulmonary circulation, an atrial septostomy may improve symptoms and survival (66). In particular, for patients with recurrent near-syncope or syncope who have been treated maximally from a medical standpoint, an atrial septostomy may prevent further episodes of syncope by serving as a "pop-off valve" during times of acute pulmonary hypertensive crises. It should be noted that atrial septostomy remains investigational, and should only be performed in an experienced center. In addition, there may be evidence that for a "failing" Fontan with protein losing enteropathy or severe arrhythmias creation of a baffle fenestration may improve the clinical condition (67). Although the patients may appear more cyanotic (particularly with exertion), cardiac output is maintained by right-to-left shunting, and oxygen delivery to the tissues is in fact increased despite the decrease in systemic arterial oxygen saturation (66).

Transplantation

While successful heart–lung transplantation, as well as lung transplantation with repair of congenital heart defect(s) has been available for over 20 years, there are several limitations to these procedures. A limited number of centers can perform the procedures and postoperative care for the patients, and the availability of suitable donors is limited. Furthermore, the high incidence of bronchiolitis obliterans in the transplanted organs of these patients (25–40%) is of great concern (68). Both single and bilateral lung transplantation has been performed in pediatric patients with pulmonary vascular obstructive disease including patients with severe right ventricular failure (69). Thus, lung transplantation with repair of the congenital heart defect appears to be the surgical procedure of choice for virtually all patients in whom left ventricular function is preserved despite severe right ventricular failure. Currently, the overall 1-year, 5-year, and long-term (9-year) survival for lung transplantation, including recipients with all forms of lung disease is 71%, 49%, and 20%, respectively (69). There has not been a significant improvement in survival in the most recent era analyzed (1998–2001 vs. 1992–1998). One must be familiar with the natural history of Eisenmenger syndrome when considering transplantation. For untreated Eisenmenger syndrome, the 5-year and 25-year survival is greater than 80% and 40%, respectively (70). For patients with the Eisenmenger syndrome, the 1-year and 5-year survival following lung transplantation is worse, 52% and 39%, respectively (68). Recent data suggest that for patients with Eisenmenger syndrome secondary to a VSD, heart–lung transplantation may offer a survival benefit over lung transplantation (71). For Eisenmenger patients, we generally reserve transplantation for those patients who are very symptomatic despite optimal medical management, in whom long-term survival is unlikely, i.e., patients in whom the likelihood of 2-year survival is less than 50%. This is in contrast to strategies used in patients with idiopathic PAH, who have a worse long-term prognosis and may require transplantation sooner.

SUMMARY

Right-sided heart failure in children is associated with many conditions which include congenital heart defects, pulmonary disease, and idiopathic PAH. The physiologic impact on the right ventricle can usually be attributed to an increase in preload, afterload, or both. Functional assessment is difficult given the unusual geometry of the right ventricle, however, advances in both echocardiography and MRI have improved the ability to evaluate right heart function. The primary goal in management is to eliminate the stimulus for right ventricular dysfunction if possible. If not, medical management should be tailored to the cause of the right heart dysfunction and may include diuretics, inotropic agents, pulmonary vasodilators, and mechanical support if necessary. We anticipate that with improved longevity for patients with congenital heart disease and for patients with pulmonary hypertension there will be a greater focus on the right heart in the future with continued advances in technology for assessing right ventricular integrity as well as treatment options.

REFERENCES

1. Barst RJ. Recent advances in the treatment of pediatric pulmonary arterial hypertension. Pediatr Clin North Am 1999; 46(2):331–345.
2. Bristow JD, Morris JF, Kloster FE. Hemodynamics of cor pulmonale. Prog Cardiovasc Dis 1966; 9(3):239–258.
3. Bristow MR, Zisman LS, Lowes BD, Abraham WT, Badesch DB, Groves BM, Voelkel NF, Lynch DMB, Quaife RA. The pressure-overloaded right ventricle in pulmonary hypertension. Chest 1998; 114:101S–106S.

4. Konstam MA, Cohen SR, Salem DN, et al. Comparison of left and right ventricular end-systolic pressure–volume relations in congestive heart failure. J Am Coll Cardiol 1985; 5:1326–1334.

5. Konstam MA, Isner JM. The Right Ventricle. Boston: Kluwer Academic Publishers, 1988:21.

6. Rudolph AM. Congenital Diseases of the Heart. Chicago, IL: Year Book Medical Publishers, Inc., 1974.

7. Boxt LM, Katz FJ, Kolb T. Direct quantitation of right and left ventricular volumes with nuclear magnetic resonance imaging in patients with primary pulmonary hypertension. J Am Coll Cardiol 1992; 19:1508–1515.

8. Tanaka H, Tei C, Nakao S, et al. Diastolic bulging of the interventricular septum toward the left ventricle. An echocardiographic manifestation of negative interventricular pressure gradient between left and right ventricles during diastole. Circulation 1980; 62(3):558–563.

9. Mizushige K, Morita H, Senda S, Matsuo H. Influence of right ventricular pressure overload on left and right ventricular filling in cor pulmonale assessed with Doppler echocardiography. Jpn Circ J 1989; 53(10):1287–1296.

10. Louie EK, Rich S, Levitsky S, Brundage BH. Doppler echocardiographic demonstration of the differential effects of right ventricular pressure and volume overload on left ventricular geometry and filling. J Am Coll Cardiol 1992; 19(1):84–90.

11. Werchan PM, Summer WR, Gerdes AM, et al. Right ventricular performance after monocrotaline-induced pulmonary hypertension. Am J Physiol 1989; 256:H1328–H1336.

12. Rich S. Primary pulmonary hypertension. Prog Cardiovasc Dis 1988; 31(3):205–238.

13. Lowes BD, Minobe W, Abraham WT, et al. Changes in gene expression in the intact human heart. Downregulation of alpha-myosin heavy chain in hypertrophied, failing ventricular myocardium. J Clin Invest 1997; 100(9):2315–2324.

14. Bristow MR. Management of heart failure. In: Braunwald E, Zipes D, Libby P, eds. Heart Disease. 6th ed. Philadelphia, PA: WB Saunders.

15. Nootens M, Kaufmann E, Rector T, et al. Neurohormonal activation in patients with right ventricular failure from pulmonary hypertension: relation to hemodynamic variables and endothelin levels. JACC 1995; 26:1581–1585.

16. Torbicki A. Kurzyna M, Kuca P, et al. Detectable serum cardiac troponin T as a marker of poor prognosis among patients with chronic precapillary pulmonary hypertension. Circulation. 2003; 108(7): 844–848.

17. Nagaya N, Nishikimi T, Uematsu M, et al. Plasma brain natriuretic peptide as a prognostic indicator in patients with primary pulmonary hypertension. Circulation 2000; 102:865–870.

18. Nagaya N, Nishikimi T, Okano Y, et al. Plasma brain natriuretic peptide levels increase in proportion to the extent of right ventricular dysfunction in pulmonary hypertension. JACC 1998; 31:202–208.

19. Bendayan D, Shitrit D, Ygla M, et al. Hyperuricemia as a prognostic factor in pulmonary arterial hypertension. Respir Med 2003; 97: 30–33.

20. Raymond RJ, Hinderliter AL, Willis PW, et al. Echocardiographic predictors of adverse outcomes in primary pulmonary hypertension. J Am Coll Cardiol 2002; 39:1214–1219.

21. Burgess MI, Bright-Thomas RJ, Ray SG. Echocardiographic evaluation of right ventricular function. Eur J Echocardiogr 2002; 3(4): 252–262.

22. Jiang L, Handschumacher MD, Hibberd MG, et al. Three-dimensional echocardiographic reconstruction of right ventricular volume: in vitro comparison with two-dimensional methods. J Am Soc Echocardiogr 1994; 7:150–158.

23. Foale F, Nihoyannopoulos P, McKenna W, et al. Echocardiographic measurement of the normal adult right ventricle. Br Heart J 1986; 56(1):33–44.

24. Kaul S, Tei C, Hopkins JM, Shah PM. Assessment of right ventricular function using two-dimensional echocardiography. Am Heart J 1984; 107:526–531.

25. Danchin N, Cornette A, Henriquez A, et al. Two-dimensional echocardiographic assessment of the right ventricle in patients with chronic obstructive lung disease. Chest 1987; 92: 229–233.

26. Vitolo E, Castini D, Colombo A, et al. Two-dimensional echocardiographic evaluation of right ventricular ejection fraction: comparison between three different methods. Acta Cardiol 1988; 43:469–480.

27. Ryan T, Petrovic O, Dillon JC, et al. An echocardiographic index for separation of right ventricular volume and pressure and overload. J Am Coll Cardiol 1985; 5:918–927.

28. Schenk P, Globits S, Koller J, et al. Accuracy of echocardiographic right ventricular parameters in patients with different end-stage lung diseases prior to lung transplantation. J Heart Lung Transplant 2000; 19:145–154.

29. Mongkolsmai D, Williams GA, Goodgold H, Labovitz AJ. Determination of right ventricular ejection fraction by two-dimensional echocardiographic single plane subtraction method. J Am Soc Echocardiogr 1989; 2(2):119–124.

30. Hinderliter AL, Willis PW, Long W, et al. Frequency and prognostic significance of pericardial effusion in primary pulmonary hypertension. Am J Cardiol 1999; 84:481–484.

31. Yock PG, Popp RL. Noninvasive estimation of right ventricular systolic pressure by Doppler ultrasound in patients with tricuspid regurgitation. Circulation 1984; 70:657–662.

32. Simonson JA, Schiller NB. Sonospirometry, a new method for noninvasive estimation of mean right atrial pressure based on two-dimensional echographic measurements of the inferior vena cava during measured inspiration. J Am Coll Cardiol 1988; 11(3):557–564.

33. Naguch SF, Kopelen HA, Zoghbi WA. Relation of mean right atrial pressure to echocardiographic and Doppler parameters of right atrial and right ventricular function. Circulation 1996; 93(6):1160–1169.

34. Weyman AE. Right ventricular outflow tract. Weyman AE, ed. Principles and Practice of Echocardiography. 2nd ed. Philadelphia, PA: Lea & Febiger, 1994:863–900.

35. Tei C. New non-invasive index for combined systolic and diastolic ventricular function. J Cardiol 1995; 26:135–136.

36. Eidem BW, O'Leary PW, Tei C, Seward JB. Usefulness of the myocardial performance index for assessing right ventricular function in congenital heat disease. Am J Cardiol 2000; 86:654–658.

37. Ishii M, Eto G, Tei C, et al. Quantitation of the global right ventricular function in children with normal heart and congenital heart disease: a right ventricular myocardial performance index. Pediatr Cardiol 2000; 21:416–421.

38. Yeo TC, Dujardin KS, Tei C, et al. Value of a Doppler-derived index combining systolic and diastolic time intervals in predicting outcome in primary pulmonary hypertension. Am J Cardiol 1998; 81:1157.

39. Mattioli AV, Vandelli R, Mattioli G. Doppler echocardiographic evaluation of right ventricular function in patients with right ventricular infarction. J Ultrasound Med 2000; 19:831–836.

40. Nishimura E, Ikeda S, Naito T, et al. Evaluation of right-ventricular function by Doppler echocardiography in patients with chronic respiratory failure. J Int Med Res 1999; 27:65–73.

41. Kitabatake A, Inoue M, Asao M. Noninvasive evaluation of pulmonary hypertension by a pulsed Doppler technique. Circulation 1983; 68:302–209.

42. Dabestani A, Mahan G, Gardin JM, et al. Evaluation of pulmonary artery pressure and resistance by pulsed Doppler echocardiography. Am J Cardiol 1987; 59:662–668.

43. Ramachandran SV, Benjamin EJ, Levy D. Congestive heart failure with normal left ventricular systolic function. Clinical approaches to the diagnosis and treatment of diastolic heart failure. Arch Intern Med 1996; 156:146–151.

44. Caso P, Galderisi M, Cicala S, et al. Association between myocardial right ventricular relaxation time and pulmonary arterial pressure in chronic obstructive lung disease: analysis by pulsed Doppler tissue imaging. J Am Soc Echocardiogr 2001; 14:970–977.

45. Papavassiliou DP, Parks WJ, Hopkins KL, Fyfe DA. Three-dimensional echocardiographic measurement of right ventricular volume in children with congenital heart disease validated by magnetic resonance imaging. J Am Soc Echocardiogr 1998; 11:770–777.

46. Geva T, Powell AJ, Crawford EC, et al. Evaluation of regional differences in right ventricular systolic function by acoustic quantification echocardiography and cine magnetic resonance imaging. Circulation 1998; 98:339–345.
47. Vignon P, Weinert L, Mor-Avi V, et al. Quantitative assessment of regional right ventricular function with color kinesis. Am J Respir Crit Care Med 1999; 159:1949–1959.
48. Vazquez de Prada JA, Chen MH, Guerrero JL, et al. Intracardiac echocardiography: in vitro and in vivo validation for right ventricular volume and function. Am Heart J 1996; 131:320–328.
49. Markewicz W, Schtem U, Higgins CB. Evaluation of the right ventricle by magnetic resonance imaging. Am Heart J 1987; 113:8–15.
50. Boxt LM. Magnetic resonance imaging. Clin North Am 1996; 4(2):p. 317 [WB Saunders].
51. Guyton AC, Jones CE, Coleman RG. Circulatory Physiology: Cardiac Output and Its Regulation. 2nd ed. Philadelphia: WB Saunders, 1973.
52. Carere R, Patterson GA, Liu P, et al. The Toronto Lung Transplant Group. Right and left ventricular performance after single and double lung transplantation. J Thorac Cardiovasc Surg 1991; 102(1):115–122 [discussion 122–123].
53. Globits S, Burghuber OC, Koller J, et al. Effect of lung transplantation on right and left ventricular volumes and function measured by magnetic resonance imaging. Am J Respir Crit Care Med 1994; 149(4 Pt 1):1000–1004.
54. Pearlman AS, Borer JS, Clark CE. Abnormal right ventricular septal motion after atrial septal defect closure: etiology and functional significance. Am J Cardiol 1978; 41:295–301.
55. Veldtman GR, Razack V, Siu S, et al. Right ventricular form and function after percutaneous atrial septal defect device closure. J Am Coll Cardiol 2001; 37:2108–2113.
56. Therrien J, Siu SC, McLaughlin PR, Liu PP, Williams WG, Webb GD. Pulmonary valve replacement in adults late after repair of tetralogy of Fallot: are we operating too late? J Am Coll Cardiol 2000; 36: 1670–1675
57. The Digitalis Investigation Group. The effect of digoxin on mortality and morbidity in patients with heart failure. N Engl J Med 1997; 336(8):525–533.
58. Rich S, Seidlitz M, Dodin E, Osimani D, Judd D, Genthner D, McLaughlin V, Francis G. The short-term effects of digoxin in patients with right ventricular dysfunction from pulmonary hypertension. Chest 1998; 114:787–792.
59. Chen JM, Levin HR, Rose EA, et al. Experience with right ventricular assist devices for perioperative right-sided circulatory failure. Ann Thorac Surg 1996; 61:305–310.
60. Rogers AJ, Trento A, Siewers RD, Griffith BP, Hardesty RL, Pahl E, Beerman LB, Fricker FJ, Fischer DR. Extracorporeal membrane

oxygenation for postcardiotomy cardiogenic shock in children. Ann Thorac Surg 1989; 47(6):903–906.

61. Sandoval J, Aguirre JS, Pulido T, Martinez-Guerra ML, Santos E, Alvarado P, Rosas M, Bautista E. Nocturnal oxygen therapy in patients with the Eisenmenger syndrome. Am J Respir Crit Care Med 2001; 164(9):1682–1687.

62. Bowyer JJ, Busst CM, Denison DM, Shinebourne EA. Effect of long-term oxygen treatment at home in children with pulmonary vascular disease. Br Heart J 1985; 55:385–390.

63. Sandoval J, Alvarado P, Martinez-Guerra ML, Gomez A, Palomar A, Meza S, Santos E, Rosas M. Effect of body position changes on pulmonary gas exchange in Eisenmenger's syndrome. Am J Respir Crit Care Med 1999; 159:1070–1073.

64. Rosovec A, Montanes P, Oakley C. Factors that influence the outcome of primary pulmonary hypertension. Br Heart J 1986; 55:449–458.

65. Young DM. Fate of the patient with Eisenmenger's syndrome. Am J Cardiol 1971; 28:658–669.

66. Kerstein D, Levy PS, Hsu DT, et al. Blade balloon atrial septostomy improves survival inpatients with severe primary pulmonary hypertension. Circulation 1995; 91:2028–2035.

67. Rychik J, Rome JJ, Jacobs ML. Late surgical fenestration for complications after the Fontan operation. Circulation 1997; 96(1):33–36.

68. Trulock EP. Lung transplantation for primary pulmonary hypertension. Clin Chest Med 2001; 22:583–593.

69. Boucek MM, Edwards LB, Keck BM, et al. The Registry of the International Society for Heart and Lung Transplantation: sixth official pediatric report—2003. J Heart Lung Transplant 2003; 22(6):636–652.

70. Clarkson PM, Frye RL, DuShane JW, et al. Prognosis for patients with ventricular septal defect and severe pulmonary vascular obstructive disease. Circulation 1968; 38:129.

71. Waddell TK, Bennett L, Kennedy R, et al. Heart–lung or lung transplantation for Eisenmenger syndrome. J Heart Lung Transplant 2002; 21:731–737.

14

Chronic Heart Failure in Congenital Heart Disease

DAPHNE T. HSU

Columbia University Medical Center,
College of Physicians and Surgeons,
Children's Hospital of New York,
New York, New York, U.S.A.

INTRODUCTION

Improved surgical results have decreased the mortality associated with congenital heart defects in the United States from 2.5 to 1.5 per 100,000 population over the past 20 years (1). Despite these advances, chronic heart failure remains an important factor contributing to the long-term morbidity and mortality of patients with congenital heart disease (2–4). Chronic heart failure occurs most commonly in these patients as a result of excessive ventricular volume or pressure load in the setting of normal myocardial function. Primary

567

myocardial dysfunction also occurs in patients with palliated congenital heart disease in the late postoperative period. The presence of a hemodynamically significant congenital heart defect in conjunction with myocardial dysfunction is associated with significant morbidity and mortality (5,6).

The clinical manifestations of chronic heart failure associated with congenital heart disease are a result of the hemodynamic consequences of the specific lesion and the neurohormonal abnormalities that result from the chronic myocardial stress imposed by the lesion. The neurohormonal model of heart failure has gained wide acceptance in the diagnosis and management of adult patients with heart failure (7,8). Although the etiology of heart failure is significantly different in patients with congenital heart disease compared to adult heart failure patients, there is increasing evidence that abnormalities in the neurohormonal axis are similar between the two groups (9–19). Differences in the response of the neurohormonal system to myocardial stress may account for the variable clinical symptomatology seen among patients with the same congenital heart lesion (10,16,20,21). Evaluation of neurohormonal abnormalities in patients with congenital heart disease may prove useful in monitoring disease severity and targeting management strategies.

Medical therapy can be beneficial in patients with congenital heart disease and chronic heart failure, although in most instances, specific surgical or catheter-based therapies are the treatment of choice. This chapter will explore the main causes of chronic heart failure in patients with congenital heart disease and outline management strategies. The focus will be on heart failure in the setting of a biventricular heart, as right-sided heart failure and heart failure associated with single ventricle lesions are discussed in previous chapters.

ETIOLOGIES OF HEART FAILURE IN CONGENITAL HEART DISEASE

The spectrum of hemodynamic abnormalities associated with chronic heart failure in patients with congenital heart disease includes low cardiac output due to increased demand on a normal myocardium, primary systolic myocardial dysfunction, diastolic dysfunction with or without systolic myocardial dysfunction, and, in a situation unique to congenital heart disease, severe cyanosis that limits functional capacity.

Ventricular Volume or Pressure Load and Normal Myocardium

The majority of patients develop evidence of low cardiac output and chronic heart failure as a result of excessive demand on a normal myocardium from either increased ventricular volume or pressure load. The common congenital lesions associated with this type of chronic heart failure are listed in Table 1.

In left-to-right shunt lesions, the left ventricle dilates to maintain cardiac output in the face of a significant shunt from the systemic to the pulmonary circulation. As the ventricle dilates, left ventricular filling pressure increases, and can result in pulmonary edema and pulmonary hypertension. Despite normal myocardial function, cardiac output is diminished if the degree of left ventricular dilatation is unable to compensate for the left-to-right shunt and oxygen delivery to the tissues is impaired. Left ventricular dilatation also occurs in mitral or aortic insufficiency and, similar to a left-to-right shunt, low cardiac output results if the degree of dilatation is unable to compensate for the regurgitant volume.

Table 1 Congenital Heart Lesions with Chronic Heart Failure

Volume overload
  Left-to-right shunt lesions
    Ventricular septal defect
    Atrioventricular septal defect
    Patent ductus arteriosus
    Atrioventricular canal defect
  Valve regurgitation
    Mitral
    Aortic
Pressure overload
  Coarctation of the aorta
  Aortic stenosis (valvar, subvalvar, or supravalvar)
  Multiple levels of ventricular outflow tract obstruction (Shone's complex)

Severe left ventricular outflow tract obstruction can limit ventricular output, especially in the face of increased demand. This can result in symptoms of congestive heart failure, including fatigue and exercise tolerance.

Primary Myocardial Dysfunction

Although less common, primary myocardial dysfunction can occur following surgical repair or palliation of congenital heart disease. Primary myocardial dysfunction has been described in patients with aortic stenosis with longstanding obstruction (22). Primary myocardial dysfunction may also occur as a result of ventricular volume overload from chronic mitral or aortic insufficiency (23–25). In these instances, heart failure can be exacerbated by the presence of an abnormal demand on a diseased myocardium. Rarely, a primary myocardial process that leads to ventricular dysfunction, such as myocarditis, develops unrelated to the presence of a congenital heart defect.

Lesions with a systemic right ventricle such as corrected transposition of the great arteries or transposition of the great arteries following an atrial switch procedure are most prone to the late development of chronic heart failure (5,6,26–28). In patients with corrected transposition of the great arteries and a systemic right ventricle, the development of tricuspid valve insufficiency is a strong predisposing factor to the development of ventricular dysfunction and heart failure (29). The incidence of any symptomatic heart failure (NYHA Class II or higher) following the atrial switch procedure ranges from 22% to 37% within 20 years of surgery (26–28,30,31). The incidence of severe right ventricular failure is 2–8% (26,30,31). Myocardial perfusion defects have been described late following the atrial switch operation and are associated with worse systemic right ventricular function, offering some insight into the mechanism of ventricular failure in this lesion (26).

Diastolic Dysfunction

In addition to abnormalities of ventricular systolic function, abnormalities in diastolic filling have also been described in congenital heart disease, especially with left ventricular outflow tract obstruction. Echocardiographic abnormalities including diminished early peak filling rates and wall thinning have been described in patients with aortic stenosis or coarctation (32–35). Direct catheter measurements of the pressure volume relationship have demonstrated normal passive diastolic relaxation, indicating that the diastolic filling abnormalities are likely due to ventricular hypertrophy and are not a sign of intrinsic abnormalities of the relaxation properties of the myocardium (36–38). Despite the presence of diastolic filling abnormalities, symptoms of pure diastolic dysfunction in the absence of systolic dysfunction are rare in children with congenital heart disease.

Cyanosis

Severe cyanosis can also be a cause of cardiac insufficiency in children with congenital heart disease. These patients will not manifest signs of congestive heart failure; however, exercise limitations can be severe because of low oxygen delivery. In the presence of ventricular dysfunction, cyanosis exacerbates the clinical findings of heart failure.

MANIFESTATIONS OF HEART FAILURE IN CHILDREN WITH CONGENITAL HEART DISEASE

Clinical Features

The clinical manifestations of chronic heart failure in congenital heart disease are a reflection of the hemodynamic stresses placed on the circulatory system by the congenital heart lesion and the neurohormonal abnormalities that result from an inability to compensate for the stresses. The Ross Heart Failure Class, summarized in Table 2, is modeled after the New York Heart Association Heart Failure Class (39), and has been used to grade the degree of heart failure in infants and small children (16). The most common features of heart failure in infants and children are incorporated into the Ross

Table 2   Ross Heart Failure Class

Group I	No limitations or symptoms
Group II	Mild tachypnea or diaphoresis with feedings in infants, dyspnea on exertion in older children, no growth failure
Group III	Marked tachypnea or diaphoresis with feedings or exertion and prolonged feeding times with growth failure from congestive heart failure
Group IV	Symptomatic at rest with tachypnea, retractions, grunting, or diaphoresis

Heart Failure class and include venous congestion, failure to thrive, and, in the older child, exercise intolerance.

Tachypnea

Tachypnea is the most common sign of congestive heart failure in infants. A respiratory rate >50 per min occurs in more than half of infants with a significant left-to-right shunt (10,16,20). The presence of tachypnea has been associated with an increased pulmonary artery pressure and a lower cardiac index, and is a marker for significant hemodynamic compromise (10). The pulmonary abnormalities associated with congenital heart disease and a large left-to-right shunt include lower tidal volume, decreased pulmonary compliance, and higher expiratory airway resistance (40).

Failure to Thrive

Failure to thrive is the most significant complication of chronic heart failure in the child with congenital heart disease. Poor oral intake and failure to thrive were described in association with a large left-to-right shunt over 40 years ago (41). Weight is more severely affected than height, although height can be impaired as well (3,41,42). Failure to thrive in infants with a large left-to-right shunt is in part due to decreased caloric intake (43). In addition, studies of energy expenditure in infants with heart disease have found evidence of increased total energy expenditure (44). Resting energy expenditure is not significantly higher in infants with congenital heart disease compared to normal controls, indicating that the increase in total energy expenditure is due to an increase in the cost of physical activity (4). Despite improvements in medical and surgical management, failure to thrive remains a significant complication in pediatric patients with congestive heart failure and congenital heart disease, and is most common in children less than 3 years of age (3,4). Failure to thrive is the most common indication for intervention in patients with a congenital heart lesion amenable to surgical repair.

Exercise Intolerance

Exercise intolerance is difficult to quantify in infants and small children. The tools developed to grade heart failure in children have included qualitative measures of ability to perform normal age-appropriate activities such as attend school or participate in sports (20,45,46). Exercise testing has been reserved for use in the older child or young adult. The prognostic value of exercise testing in children with heart failure has not been well defined (11,15,47).

Neurohormonal Abnormalities

Neurohormonal Abnormalities in Heart Failure

Neurohormonal abnormalities are widely recognized in the pathogenesis of heart failure in the adult patient (8). There is increasing evidence that abnormalities in the neurohormonal axis contribute to the development of heart failure in patients with congenital heart disease. Activation of the neurohormonal axis has been described in two distinct groups of patients: those with significant ventricular volume overload from a left-to-right shunt and those with primary myocardial dysfunction following reparative or palliative cardiac surgery.

In adult patients, primary myocardial dysfunction or a previous myocardial infarction results in decreased cardiac output and stimulation of the neurohormonal axis, leading to the signs and symptoms of congestive heart failure. The neurohormonal axis is comprised of several components

including the adrenergic and the renin–angiotensin–aldosterone systems (RAAS) along with circulating factors such as
endothelin, vasodilator peptides (atrial natriuretic peptide,
ANP, and B-type natriuretic peptide, BNP), and proinflammatory cytokines including TNF-α and IL-1β. Although
stimulation of these components may be beneficial in the compensatory response to acute heart failure, it has become evident that chronic activation of these systems is maladaptive
and leads to worsening heart failure (7). In patients with congenital heart disease and a significant ventricular volume
overload or primary myocardial dysfunction, decreased
cardiac output occurs and can stimulate a similar cascade of
events leading to activation of the neurohormonal axis (11).

Neurohormonal Abnormalities in Ventricular Volume Overload

Several studies have confirmed the presence of abnormalities
in the adrenergic and RAAS systems in infants with a left-to-
right shunt, supporting the concept of neurohormonal activation in heart failure secondary to congenital heart disease
(9,10,16,17,19,48). The Ross Heart Failure Classification
was originally developed to evaluate the relationship between
plasma catecholamine levels and the degree of clinical heart
failure (48). A significant positive association was demonstrated between plasma norepinephrine levels and the Ross
Heart Failure Class in 61 children with a left-to-right shunt.
Wu et al. (19) similarly found a positive correlation between
elevations in the plasma norepinephrine levels and the degree
of left-to-right shunt flow and pulmonary artery systolic pressure. This study also measured β-adrenergic receptor density
and found that receptor density was significantly lower in
patients with heart failure, indicating a downregulation of
the adrenergic system in the face of elevated levels of circulating catecholamines. Following surgical repair, serum plasma
norepinephrine levels return to normal, heart failure class
improves and β-adrenergic receptor density increases (19,48).
    Activation of the RAAS in infants with a left-to-right
shunt and congestive heart failure was demonstrated in a

study that measured plasma renin activity and aldosterone and norepinephrine levels in 47 infants undergoing cardiac catheterization (9). Neurohormone levels were compared to the hemodynamic measurements obtained during catheterization and to a modified heart failure score that included respiratory rate, weight gain, diaphoresis, and the need for diuretic therapy. Higher plasma renin activity was associated with a higher heart failure score and lower mean arterial pressure, suggesting that relative hypotension is one of the factors stimulating the RAAS system in these infants.

Further evidence of neurohormonal activation in infants with congestive heart failure is found in the study by Buchhorn et al. that compared the clinical symptoms of heart failure, including respiratory rate and weight gain, with evidence of neurohormonal activation in infants with a left-to-right shunt. Norepinephrine and epinephrine levels and plasma renin activity were measured and compared with symptoms, hemodynamic findings at catheterization, and heart rate variability on a 24-hour Holter monitor recording. Infants with tachypnea had a 5.1-fold higher plasma renin activity and 2.3-fold higher norepinephrine levels compared to patients with congenital heart disease without significant tachypnea. Elevations in norepinephrine levels, plasma renin activity, and heart rate were inversely correlated with weight gain. This study demonstrates the interrelationships between neurohormonal abnormalities and the clinical signs of heart failure (10).

Other abnormalities of the neurohormonal axis have been reported in children with congenital heart disease and include alterations in autonomic tone and elevations in circulating BNP levels. In a study of heart rate variability in 258 children with various forms of congenital heart disease, including volume load, pressure load, and single ventricle lesions, a decrease in the time- and frequency-domain measures of heart rate variability was correlated with the presence of Class II–IV heart failure (21). The degree of impairment in heart rate variability could not be correlated with the underlying cardiac disease or hemodynamic data from cardiac catheterization. These data suggest the presence of autonomic dysfunction in the setting of heart failure in children. A recent cross-sectional study measured BNP levels in a heterogeneous group of 107 patients with congenital heart disease undergoing catheterization (13). The levels of BNP were elevated in children with left ventricular outflow tract obstruction; however, no correlation was made between BNP levels and the presence of heart failure. The latter finding may be due to the small number of patients with a significant left-to-right shunt in this series.

Neurohomonal Abnormalities with Primary Myocardial Dysfunction

As the population of survivors with congenital heart disease ages, the incidence of heart failure may increase overtime due to the chronic myocardial stress that occurs from intrinsic abnormalities of the myocardium. An increasing number of studies report neurohormonal activation following repair of congenital heart disease, especially in the adolescent and young adult populations.

A large study correlated heart failure class with hemodynamic findings at cardiac catheterization, exercise test results, ejection fraction determinations, heart rate variability, and neurohormonal activity in patients following repair of congenital heart disease lesions that ranged from closure of an atrial or ventricular septal defect to repair of left or right ventricular outflow tract obstruction (15). Elevations in plasma renin activity and norepinephrine were associated with worse heart failure class, although the relationship was not step-wise, with norepinephrine level elevation occurring only with Class II–IV heart failure. The levels of vasoactive peptides (ANP and BNP) significantly increased in a stepwise fashion with increasing heart failure class. Cardiac autonomic nervous activity was reduced in all patients with congenital heart disease compared to a control population, but did not correlate with the severity of heart failure. Similar results correlating neurohormonal activation and heart failure class were found in a study of patients with single ventricle physiology, tetralogy of Fallot or complex heart disease (12). Levels of ANP, BNP, endothelin-1, and norepinephrine were significantly higher than control patients, even in patients with asymptomatic congenital heart disease, and increased in a stepwise fashion with increasing heart failure severity. Activation of the RAAS also occurred in symptomatic patients. Evidence of neurohormonal activation was not associated with a particular congenital heart lesion, suggesting that neurohormonal abnormalities may be the final common pathway in patients with repaired congenital heart disease who develop heart failure.

EVALUATION OF HEART FAILURE

Grading Heart Failure Severity in Children

Several different methods have been suggested to grade the severity of heart failure in children with congenital heart disease (9,16,20,45). Functional limitations are difficult to assess in infants and small children, thus symptoms often serve as a surrogate for exercise tolerance. Careful assessment of respiratory status, weight gain, and evidence of venous congestion are the cornerstones of all proposed grading systems for heart failure in children. The New York University grading system also includes laboratory findings, such as chest x-ray and echocardiographic indices, and the need for medical therapy; this system has not been extensively validated (45). The Ross Heart Failure Class has gained wider acceptance amongst heart failure specialists and was adopted as the rating scale for heart failure in children by the 1994 Canadian Consensus on Heart Failure (16,49).

Laboratory Assessment of Heart Failure

Echocardiography

Echocardiography remains the cornerstone in the evaluation of the anatomy and hemodynamic consequences of congenital heart lesions. In patients with volume overload heart failure, the degree of volume overload can be assessed by qualitative and quantitative two-dimensional echocardiography and Doppler echocardiography can be used to detect evidence of diastolic filling abnormalities (32–35). In patients with repaired congenital heart disease, echocardiography is a useful screening tool for the presence of ventricular dysfunction, although quantitative assessment of right ventricular function is limited (50).

Cardiac Catheterization

Cardiac catheterization is rarely indicated in the assessment of heart failure in congenital heart disease with volume overload from a left-to-right shunt. Management decisions are made by evaluating the clinical and hemodynamic consequences of the cardiac lesion. The clinical severity of the heart failure and information available from echocardiographic measurements of ventricular volume and intracardiac hemodynamics are sufficient to determine the need for surgery in the vast majority of cases. In the patient with heart failure following repair or palliation of congenital heart disease, the indications for catheterization include the evaluation and treatment of residual heart lesions and assessment of ventricular filling pressures and cardiac output (15).

Exercise Testing

Exercise testing has been shown to be useful in the evaluation of adult patients with heart failure (51,52). The clinical significance of exercise testing in the patient with congenital heart disease is not well defined. Abnormalities in peak VO2 are found in asymptomatic patients with congenital heart disease and in a study by Ohuchi et al. (15,47), a stepwise decrease in peak VO2 was seen with increasing heart failure class (12).

Neurohormonal Levels

As detailed in the above sections, evidence of activation of the adrenergic and RAAS systems and elevations of BNP and ANP levels are found in patients with congenital heart disease and heart failure. The clinical utility of measurements of neurohormonal markers in predicting outcomes of heart failure has not been proven. Further study regarding the prognostic significance of elevated vasoactive peptides levels in the setting of congenital heart disease is needed prior to the incorporation of routine measurement of ANP and BNP levels into clinical practice.

THERAPY

The choice between medical and surgical or catheter-based management of chronic heart failure in patients with congenital heart disease depends on the type of lesion, the degree of heart failure, and the surgical options available. The following sections outline disease-specific management issues.

Volume Overload Lesions

In infants who present with significant congenital heart disease and severe heart failure, urgent surgical intervention is indicated and medical management is indicated only to stabilize the patient prior to operation. In patients with less severe heart failure, medical management is often indicated, especially when surgical outcome would be improved by somatic growth, or in patients with a lesion that may become less hemodynamically significant over time, such as a ventricular septal defect, where medical management may eliminate the need for surgery.

Medical Management

The initial management of infants with volume overload lesions includes diuretic therapy to decrease pulmonary edema and improve respiratory status. The use of digoxin in this setting is controversial, as the ventricular systolic function is often normal to hyperdynamic. Few studies have been performed to evaluate digoxin in volume overload lesions (53,54). A catheter-based study of the effects of a single dose of digoxin in infants with a large ventricular septal defect demonstrated favorable effects in infants with relatively low systemic and pulmonary resistance, however, in patients with a high systemic or pulmonary vascular resistance, the dose increased left atrial pressure (55). Despite this ongoing controversy, the use of digoxin is common in infants and children with ventricular volume overload heart failure.

Optimizing nutritional status is an important intervention in the treatment of the infant with a volume overload lesion. Increasing the caloric density of the formula and/or providing continuous enteral feeds may be necessary to meet metabolic demands and increase weight gain (43,56). Recent reports document low morbidity and increased weight gain with the use of a percutaneous endoscopic gastrostomy and continuous enteral feeding (57,58).

Abnormalities in the adrenergic and RAAS system have been documented in infants with left-to-right shunt lesions. The use of angiotensin-converting enzyme inhibitors or β-adrenergic receptor blockers is controversial in patients with volume overload heart failure. There have been many small series reporting the use of angiotensin-converting enzyme inhibition in the setting of heart failure in infants, with variable results (59–63). A comparison of low dose captopril vs. propranolol therapy in 22 infants with predominantly single ventricle lesions was reported by Buchhorn et al. (46). In this retrospective analysis, 11 infants who received low dose captopril between the years 1993 and 1995 were compared to 11 infants who received propranolol between the years 1996 and 1998. The propranolol group had a lower heart failure score and better weight gain compared to the captopril treated group after 3 months of therapy. A small, open label, randomized monocenter study compared the addition of β-adrenergic receptor blockers to digoxin and diuretics in infants with a significant left-to-right shunt. After two and a half weeks, the infants who received β-adrenergic receptor blockers had an improved heart failure score, lower renin levels, and lower mean heart rates compared to baseline and to the control group (64).

Surgical Management

With advances in the surgical management of neonates and infants with congenital heart disease, mortality following open heart repair of left-to-right shunt lesions has decreased significantly over the past 20 years (1). Surgical repair for simple cardiac lesions can safely be performed in even premature infants (65). The ability to perform surgical intervention at an earlier age has decreased the role of medical therapy in these infants. Currently, surgery is recommended for a simple left-to-right shunt lesion at any age if the patient has manifestations of heart failure, especially failure to thrive, and is not responsive to medical therapy.

Pressure Overload Lesions

Evidence of inadequate cardiac output in patients with left ventricular outflow obstruction is an indication for surgical or catheter-based intervention. Medical management does not have a role in the management of heart failure in these lesions if systolic ventricular function is preserved. In the setting of impaired systolic function and left ventricular outflow obstruction, ventricular dysfunction may persist following intervention for the primary lesion or intervention may be precluded because of the high procedural risk associated with depressed ventricular function. In these cases, medical therapy of chronic left ventricular systolic dysfunction as outlined in the following chapter is indicated.

Primary Myocardial Dysfunction in the Postoperative Patient

Heart failure can occur due to primary myocardial dysfunction in the postoperative patient (11,12,15,27,30,31,37,38,47,66). Abnormal activation of the neurohormonal axis has been demonstrated in this setting. Although no randomized studies have been performed to evaluate the effect of angiotensin-converting enzyme inhibition or β-adrenergic receptor blockers in the treatment of ventricular dysfunction in the setting of congenital heart disease, evidence of neurohormonal activation suggests that these therapies may be effective. The approach to medical therapy in patients with congenital heart disease and symptomatic right or left ventricular systolic dysfunction may include the use of diuretics, angiotensin-converting enzyme inhibitors, and potentially β-adrenergic receptor blockers. Further studies of the effectiveness of specific medical therapies in these lesions will help clarify these recommendations. The role of prophylactic medical therapy in the patient with asymptomatic ventricular dysfunction is not defined at present.

Surgical or catheter-based therapeutic interventions play an important role in the management of patients with ventricular dysfunction and associated defects, such as ventricular outflow tract obstruction, residual left-to-right shunt lesions or valvar insufficiency. Careful evaluation and treatment of residual defects are essential to optimizing cardiac performance in the patient with primary ventricular dysfunction. Aggressive diagnostic approaches should be used to identify the presence of a residual lesion amenable to correction.

A unique two-step surgical approach has been proposed to treat significant systemic right ventricular dysfunction in patients with transposition of the great arteries following a Mustard or Senning atrial switch procedure. Initially a pulmonary artery banding procedure is performed to prepare the subpulmonary left ventricle. Once the left ventricle has hypertrophied, an arterial switch procedure is performed and the left ventricle becomes the systemic ventricle. The success of this procedure has been mixed, with a reported operative mortality rate of 16%; however, left ventricular function was normal in 91% of the operative survivors (67).

Heart Transplantation

Heart transplantation has become an accepted therapy for the patient with congenital heart disease and end-stage heart failure unresponsive to medical or surgical intervention. In a series of patients listed for heart transplantation with congenital heart disease, biventricular lesions comprised 33% of the population (5). The most common lesions were transposition complex and left-sided obstructive lesions. Congenital heart disease poses special management challenges for the transplant surgeon and cardiologist. Associated anatomic or hemodynamic abnormalities often require surgical attention at the time of transplantation or can complicate the post-transplant course. Congenital heart disease is a risk factor for mortality in the first year (2). Despite this early mortality risk, the reported 65% 5-year survival after heart transplantation in patients with congenital heart disease is not significantly different from survival reported in patients with cardiomyopathy who undergo transplantation (68). Heart transplantation should be considered in any patient with congenital heart disease who is refractory to therapy.

REFERENCES

1. Boneva R, Botto L, Moore C, Yang Q, Correa A, Erickson J. Mortality associated with congenital heart defects in the United States: trends and racial disparities, 1979–1997. Circulation 2001; 103:2376–2381.
2. Boucek M, Edwards L, Keck B, Trulock E, Taylor D, Mohacsi P, Hertz J. The registry of the International Society for Heart and Lung Transplantation: sixth official pediatric report—2003. J Heart Lung Transplant 2003; 22:636–652.
3. Cameron J, Rosenthal A, Olson A. Malnutrition in hospitalized children with congenital heart disease. Arch Pediatr Adolesc Med 1995; 149:1098–1102.
4. Leitch C. Growth, nutrition and energy expenditure in pediatric heart failure. Prog Ped Card 2000; 11:195–202.
5. Mital S, Addonizio LJ, Lamour JM, Hsu DT. Outcome of children with end-stage congenital heart disease waiting for cardiac transplantation. J Heart Lung Transplant 2003; 22:147–153.
6. Rosenthal D, Dubin A, Chin C, Faco D, Gamber P, Bernstein P. Outcome while awaiting heart transplantation in children: a comparison of congenital heart disease and cardiomyopathy. J Heart Lung Transplant 2000; 18:751–755.
7. Braunwald E, Bristow M. Congestive heart failure: fifty years of progress. Circulation 2000; 102:IV-14–IV-23.
8. McMurray J, Pfeffer M. New therapeutic options in congestive heart failure: Part I. Circulation 2002; 105:2099–2106.
9. Buchhorn R, Ross R, Bartmus D, Wessel A, Hulpke-Wette M, Bursch J. Activity of the renin–angiotensin–aldosterone and sympathetic nervous system and their relation to hemodynamic and clinical abnormalities in infants with left-to-right shunts. Int J Cardiol 2001; 70:225–230.
10. Buchhorn R, Hammersen A, Bartmus D, Bursch J. The pathogenesis of heart failure in infants with congenital heart disease. Cardiol Young 2001; 11:498–504.
11. Bolger A, Coats A, Gatzoulis M. Congenital heart disease: the original heart failure syndrome. Eur Heart J 2002; 24:970–976.

12. Bolger A, Sharma R, Li W, Leenarts M, Kalra P, Kemp M, Coats A, Anker S, Gatzoulis M. Neurohormonal activation and the chronic heart failure syndrome in adults with congential heart disease. 2002; 106:92–99.

13. Cowley C, Bradley J, Shaddy R. B-type natriuretic peptide levels in congenital heart disease. Pediatr Cardiol. Epub ahead of Print, 2004; 25:336–340.

14. Kunii Y, Kamada M, Ohtsuki S, Araki T, Kataoka K, Kageyama M, Nakagawa N, Seino Y. Plasma brain natriuretic peptide and the evaluation of volume overload in infants and children with congenital heart disease. Acta Med Okayama 2003; 57:191–197.

15. Ohuchi H, Takasugi H, Ohashi H, Okada Y, Yamada O, Ono Y, Yagihara T, Echigo S. Stratification of pediatric heart failure on the basis of neurohormonal and cardiac autonomic nervous activities in patients with congenital heart disease. Circulation 2003; 108:2368–2376.

16. Ross R, Daniels S, Schwartz D, Hannon D, Shukla R, Kaplan S. Plasma norepinephrine levels in infants and children with congestive heart failure. Am J Cardiol 1987; 59:911–914.

17. Scammell A, Diver M. Plasma renin activity in infants with congenital heart disease. Arch Dis Child 1987; 62:1136–1138.

18. Suda K, Matsumura M, Matsumoto M. Clinical implication of plasma natriuretic peptides in children with ventricular septal defect. Pediatr Int 2003; 45:249–254.

19. Wu J, Chang H, Huang T, Chiang C, Chen S. Reduction in lymphocyte β adrenergic receptor density in infants and children with heart failure secondary to congenital heart disease. Am J Cardiol 1996; 77:170–174.

20. Ross R, Bollinger R, Pinsky W. Grading the severity of congestive heart failure in infants. Pediatr Cardiol 1992; 13:72–75.

21. Massin M, von Bernuth G. Clinical and haemodynamic correlates of heart rate variability in children with congenital heart disease. Eur J Pediatr 1998; 157:967–971.

22. Jindal R, Saxena A, Kothari S, Juneja R, Shrivastava S. Congenital severe aortic stenosis with congestive heart failure in late childhood and adolescence: effect on left ventricular function after balloon valvuloplasty. Cathet Cardiovasc Interv 2000; 51:168–172.

23. Krishnan U, Gersony W, Berman-Rosenzweig E, Apfel H. Late left ventricular function after surgery for children with chronic symptomatic mitral regurgitation. Circulation 1997; 96:4280–4285.

24. Murakami T, Nakazawa MTN, Momma K. Prediction of postoperative left ventricular pump function in congenital mitral regurgitation. Pediatr Cardiol 1999; 20:418–421.

25. Borer J, Bonow R. Contemporary approach to aortic and mitral regurgitation. Circulation 2003; 108:2432–2438.

26. Lubiszewska B, Gosiewska E, Hoffman P, Teresinska A, Rozanski J, Piotrowski W, Rydlewska-Sadowska W, Kubicka K, Ruzyllo W. Myo-

cardial perfusion and function of the systemic right ventricle in patients after atrial switch procedure for complete transposition: long-term follow-up. J Am Coll Cardiol 2000; 36:1365–1370.

27. Piran S, Veldtman G, Siu S, Webb G, Liu P. Heart failure and ventricular dysfunction in patients with single or systemic right ventricles. Circulation 2002; 105:1189–1194.

28. Sarkar D, Bull C, Yates R, Wright D, Scullin S, Gewillig M, Claryton R, Tunstill A, Deanfield J. Comparison of long-term outcomes of atrial repair of simple transposition with implications for a late arterial switch strategy. Circulation 1999; 100:II176–II181.

29. Beauchesne L, Warnes C, Connolly H, Ammash N, Tajik A, Danielson G. Outcome of the unoperated adult who presents with congenially corrected transposition of the great arteries. J Am Coll Cardiol 2002; 40:285–290.

30. Trusier G, Williams W, Duncan F, Hesslein P, Benson L, Freedom R, Isukawa T, Qlley P. Results with the Mustard operation in simple transposition of the great arteries 1963–1985. Ann Surg 1987; 206: 251–260.

31. Wilson N, Clarkson P, Barratt-Boyes B, Calder A, Whitlock R, Easthope R, Neutze J. Long-term outcome after the Mustard repair for simple transposition of the great arteries, 28-year follow-up. J Am Coll Cardiol 1998; 32:758–765.

32. Fifer M, Bonrow K, Colan S, Lorell B. Early diastolic left ventricular function in children and adults with aortic stenosis. J Am Coll Cardiol 1985; 5:1147–1154.

33. Meliones J, Snider A, Server G, Shaffer E. Rocchini A, Beekman R, Rosenthal A, Dick M, Peters J, Reynolds P. Pulsed Doppler assessment of left ventricular diastolic filling in children with left ventricular outflow obstruction before and after balloon angioplasty. Am J Cardiol 1989; 63:231–236.

34. Villari B, Hess O, Kaufmann P, Krogmann O, Grimm J, Karyenbuehl H. Effect of aortic valve stenosis (pressure overload) and regurgitation (volume overload) on left ventricular systolic and diastolic function. Am J Cardiol 1992; 69:923–934.

35. Tede N, Child J. Diastolic dysfunction in patients with congenital heart disease. Cardiol Clin 2000; 18:491–499.

36. Banerjee A, Mendelsohn A, Knilans T, Meyer R, Schwartz P. Effect of myocardial hypertrophy on systolic and diastolic function in children: insights from the force–frequency and relaxation–frequency relationships. J Am Coll Cardiol 1998; 32:1088–1095.

37. Sandor G, Oiley P. Determination of left ventricular diastolic chamber stiffness and myocardial stiffness in patients with congenital heart disease. Am J Cardiol 1982; 49:771–779.

38. Sandor G, Puterman M, Patterson M, Tipple M, Vince E. Effect of pressure loading, volume loading and surgery on left ventricular chamber and myocardial stiffness in congenital heart disease, with a

reevaluation of normal pediatric values. J Am Coll Cardiol 1986; 8: 371–378.

39. The Criteria Committee of the New York Heart Association. Diseases of the Heart and Blood Vessels: Nomenclature and Criteria for Diagnosis. Boston: Little, Brown and Co., 1964; 112.

40. Yau K, Fang L, Wu M. Lung mechanics in infants with left-to-right shunt congenital heart disease. Pediatr Pulmonol 1996; 21:42–47.

41. Mehrizi A, Drash A. Growth disturbance in congenital heart disease. J Pediatr 1962; 61:418–429.

42. Thommessen M, Heiberg A, Kase B. Feeding problems in children with congenital heart disease: the impact on energy intake and growth outcome. Eur J Clin Nutr 1992; 46:457–464.

43. Yahav J, Avigad S, Frand M, Shem-Tov A, Barzilay Z, Linn S, Jonas A. Assessment of intestinal and cardiorespiratory function in children with congenital heart disease on high-caloric formulas. J Pediatr Gastroenterol Nutr 1985; 4:778–785.

44. Menon G, Poskill E. Why does congential heart disease cause failure to thrive? Arch Dis Child 1985; 60:1134–1139.

45. Connelly P, Rutkowski M, Auslender M, Artment M. The New York University Pediatric Heart Failure Index: a new method of quantifying chronic heart failure severity in children. J Pediatr 2001; 138: 64–648.

46. Buchhorn R, Ross R, Huipke-Wette M, Bartmus D, Wessel A, Schulz R, Bursch J. Effectiveness of low dose captopril versus propranolol therapy in infants with severe congestive failure due to left-to-right shunts. Int J Cardiol 2000; 76:227–233.

47. Ohuchi H, Suzuki H, Toyohara K, Tatsumi K, Ono Y, Arakaki Y, Echigo S. Abnormal cardiac autonomic nervous activity after right ventricular outflow tract reconstruction. Circulation 2000; 102:2732–2738.

48. Ross R, Daniels S, Schwartz D, Hannon D, Kaplan S. Return of plasma norepinephrine to normal after resolution of congestive heart failure in congenital heart disease. Am J Cardiol 1987; 60:1411–1413.

49. Johnstone D, Abdulla A, Arnold J, Bernstein V, Bourass M, Brophy J, Davies R, Gardner M, Hoeschen R, Mickleborough L, Moe G, Montague T, Paguet M, Rouleau J-L, Yusuf S. Diagnosis and management of heart failure. Canadian Cardiovascular Society. Can J Cardiol 1994; 10:613–631.

50. Helbing W, Bosch H, Maliepaard C, Rebergen S, van der Geest R, Hansen B, Ottenkamp J, Reiber J, de Roos A. Comparison of echocardiographic methods with magnetic resonance imaging for assessment of right ventricular function in children. Am J Cardiol 1995; 76: 589–594.

51. Arena R, Myers J, Aslam S, Varughese E, Peberdy M. Peak VO2 and VEA/CQ2 slope in patients with heart failure: a prognostic comparison. Am Heart J 2004; 147:354–360.

52. Hunt SA, Baker DW, Chin MH, Cinguegrani MP, Feldmanmd AM, Francis GS, Ganiats TG, Goldstein S, Gregoratos G, Jessup ML, Noble RJ, Packer M, Silver MA, Stevenson LW, Gibbons RJ, Antman EM, Alpert JS, Faxon DP, Fuster V, Jacobs AK, Hiratzka LF, Russell RQ, Smith SC Jr. ACC/AHA Guidelines for the Evaluation and Management of Chronic Heart Failure in the Adult: Executive Summary. A Report of the American College of Cardiology/American Heart Association Task Force on Practice Guidelines (Committee to Revise the 1995 Guidelines for the Evaluation and Management of Heart Failure). Circulation 2001; 104:2296–3007.

53. Berman WJ, Yabek S, Dillon T, Niland C, Corlew S, Christensen P. Effects of digoxin in infants with congested circulatory state due to a ventricular septal defect. N Engl J Med 1983; 308:363–366.

54. Redington A, Carvalho J, Shinebourne E. Does digoxin have a place in the treatment of the child with congentil heart diseace? cardiovasc Drugs ther. 1989;1;21-22.

55. Seguchi M, Nakazawa M, Momma K. Further evidence suggesting a limited role of digitalis in infants with circulatory congestion secondary to large ventricular septal defect. Am J Cardiol 1999; 83:1408–1411.

56. Schwarz S, Gewitz M, See C, Berezin S, Glassman M, Medow C, Fish B, Newman L. Enteral nutrition in infants with congenital heart disease and growth failure. Pediatrics 1990; 86:368–373.

57. Hofner G, Behrens R, Koch A, Singer H, Hofbeck M. Enteral nutritional support by percutaneous endoscopic gastrostomy in children with congenital heart disease. Pediatr Cardiol 2000; 21:341–346.

58. Ciotti G, Holzer R, Pozzi M, Dalzell M. Nutritional support via percutaneous endoscopic gastrostomy in children with cardiac disease experiencing difficulties with feeding. Cardiol Young 2002; 12:537–541.

59. Frenneaux M, Stewart R, Newman C, Hallidie-Smith K. Enalapril for severe heart failure in infancy. Arch Dis Child 1989; 64:219–223.

60. Dutertre J, Billaud E, Autret E, Chantepie A, Oliver I, Laugier J. Inhibition of angiotensin converting enzyme with enalapril maleate in infants with congestive heart failure. Br J Clin Pharmac 1993; 35: 528–530.

61. Scammell A, Arnold R, Wilkinson J. Captopril in treatment of infant heart failure: a preliminary report. Int J Cardiol 1987; 16:295–301.

62. Shaw N, Wilson N, Dickinson D. Captopril in heart failure secondary to a left to right shunt. Arch Dis Child 1988; 63:360–363.

63. Rheuban K, Carpenter M, Ayers C, Gutgesell H. Acute hemodynamic effects of converting enzyme inhibition in infants with congestive heart failure. J Pediatr 1990; 117:668–670.

64. Buchhorn R, Hulpke-Wette M, Hilgers R, Bartmus P, Wessel A, Bursch J. Propranolol treatment of congestive heart failure in infants with congenital heart disease: the CHF-PRO-INFANT trial. Int J Cardiol 2001; 79:167–173.

65. Reddy V, McElhinney D, Sagrado T, Parry A, Teitel D, Hanley F. Results of 102 cases of complete repair of congenital heart defects in patients weighing 700 to 2500 grams. J Thorac Cardiovasc Surg 1999; 117:324–331.
66. Sandor G, Freedom R, Williams W, LeBland J, Trusier G, sPatterson M. Left ventricular systolic and diastolic function after two-stage anatomic correction of transposition of the great arteries. Am Heart J 1988; 115:1257–1262.
67. Poirier N, Mee R. Left ventricular reconditioning and anatomical correction for systemic right ventricular dysfunction. Semin Thorac Cardiovasc Surg Pediatr Card Surg Annu 2003; 3:198–215.
68. Hsu DT, Quaegebeur J, Michler R, Smith C, Rose E, Kichuk M, Gersony W, Douglas J, Addonizio LJ. Heart transplantation in children with congenital heart disease. J Am Coll Cardiol 1995; 26:743–749.

15

Medical Management of Chronic Systolic Left Ventricular Dysfunction in Children

ROBERT E. SHADDY

Division of Pediatric Cardiology,
University of Utah,
School of Medicine,
Salt Lake City, Utah, U.S.A.

Chronic left ventricular (LV) systolic dysfunction in children is much less common than in adults. This chapter will primarily focus on the diagnosis and treatment options for LV systolic dysfunction in children, since many other related topics such as etiologies and clinical consequences will be covered in detail in other chapters in this book.

ETIOLOGIES

In adults, the etiology of LV dysfunction is most commonly secondary to coronary artery disease. In contrast, LV dysfunction in children occurs due to intrinsic abnormalities of the LV myocardium (cardiomyopathies), postoperative abnormalities of ventricular function, congenital or acquired coronary artery abnormalities, and inflammatory or toxic insults to the LV. The pathophysiologies of these disorders are at least partially dependent on the etiologies and the extent of the disturbances to LV function. The final common pathophysiologic pathway of this LV dysfunction is the neurohormonal and cytokine activation with its resultant constellation of signs and symptoms of heart failure. Many of these topics are covered in detail in other chapters of this book, and the reader is directed to these chapters for a complete discussion of these etiologies. This chapter will highlight similarities and any differences between groups with regard to treatment modalities.

Diagnosis

In an asymptomatic child, the diagnosis of LV dysfunction requires a strong index of suspicion. Most children and adults can tolerate a moderate decrease in their systolic LV function before symptoms become manifest. Most patients with systolic LV dysfunction will have some degree of diastolic LV dysfunction. Systolic dysfunction is generally easier to recognize and quantitate than diastolic dysfunction. However, noninvasive diagnosis of both abnormalities can be achieved with the use of echocardiography and newer modalities such as magnetic resonance imaging.

Clinical Consequences

Left ventricular dysfunction in children can cause a large variety of symptoms. These include tachypnea, tachycardia, and poor weight gain, particularly in infants and small children. Older children also demonstrate symptoms of exercise intolerance, and often present with symptoms of gastrointestinal upset due to the concomitant right-sided heart failure that can accompany left-sided heart failure. Cardiovascular collapse and even sudden death are seen in the setting of severe heart failure due to LV systolic dysfunction.

Medical Management

At the current time, there is a very limited evidence base for the treatment of chronic systolic LV dysfunction in children. In fact, most of the treatment strategies used in children are extrapolated from trials in adults with chronic heart failure. Although there is good rationale for doing this, there are significant differences between children and adults that should be taken into account when extrapolating trials in adults to therapies in children without appropriate study. For example, there are possible age-related differences between children and adults (and between younger and older children) with regard to multiple areas including myocardial receptors, myocardial performance, and response to drug treatment; there are probable differences between children and adults with regard to pharmacokinetics; and definite differences between the substrate for LV dysfunction between children and adults, since the majority of the adults in heart failure trials have had a myocardial infarction, whereas this represents a small minority of children. Thus, there are limitations and possible even dangers in extrapolating the treatment of systolic LV dysfunction in adults to children. More prospective, randomized trials are needed to define the best therapies.

The best therapies for heart failure in adults are still being elucidated, but can best be defined through understanding the failing myocardium (1,2). In the failing adult myocardium, the β_1/β_2-adrenergic receptor ratio changes from about 80/20 to about 50/50. β_1-Adrenergic receptors are downregulated and uncoupled, and the β_2-adrenergic receptors are uncoupled. There is upregulation of β-adrenergic receptor kinase and inhibitory G protein, both of which contribute to the receptor uncoupling. Finally, there is downregulation of adenylyl cyclase. Some consider the cumulative effect of these actions to provide a partial "shield" for the myocardium

against the harmful stimuli of chronic adrenergic stimulation
(1). In heart failure, chronic adrenergic stimulation of myocytes causes alterations in gene expression leading to myocyte
dysfunction (3). There are reexpression of fetal genes for
myocyte hypertrophy, in addition to increased sarcoplasmic
reticulum Ca^{++} ATPase (SERCA2) and adult forms of myosin
heavy chain and troponin. These changes result in cell loss
and apoptosis, cell and chamber remodeling, and altered
interstitial matrix, including depletion of fibrillar collagen
and activation of matrix metalloproteinases (1,3). In the failing pediatric myocardium, there is downregulation of β-adre-
nergic receptor density in infants with left-to-right shunts
and children with severe cyanotic or acyanotic congenital
heart disease (4). A higher degree of downregulation has been
found to correlate with a worse postoperative course (5). These
and other molecular, cellular, and physiologic changes associated with heart failure provide a rationale for the efficacy
of β-adrenergic receptor blockade and other treatments directed toward the neurohormonal changes seen in heart failure.

Diuretics

Diuretics are thought to be a necessary, but not sufficient part
of the treatment of patients with heart failure and fluid overload. There are no long-term studies of diuretics in heart failure, so the effects of diuretics on morbidity and mortality are
unknown. With the exception of spironolactone (a steroid that
blocks aldosterone), conventional diuretics used in the treatment of heart failure block specific ion-transport proteins in
renal tubular cells and therefore inhibit the reabsorption of
solutes (6). These are very effective in relieving volume overload and congestive symptoms in heart failure, but can activate the renin–angiotensin–aldosterone and sympathetic
nervous systems. Thus, conventional diuretics are indicated
for patients with fluid overload due to chronic LV systolic
dysfunction.

The aldosterone antagonists, spironolactone and eplerenone, have been shown to reduce mortality in adults with
heart failure (Table 1) (7,8). Plasma aldosterone levels are

Table 1 Summary of Selected Drug Trials in Heart Failure in Adults

Trial (Year of publication)	Entry criteria	n	Therapy	Outcome
RALES (1999)	NYHA III–IV LVEF ≤ 35%	1,663	Spironolactone vs. placebo	Decreased mortality and heart failure hospitalizations
EPHESUS (2003)	Recent MI LVEF < 40%	6,642	Eplerenone vs. placebo	Decreased mortality and cardiovascular hospitalizations
RADIANCE (1993)	NYHA II–III LVEF ≤ 35%	178	Continued digoxin or switched to placebo	Increased heart failure in those switched to placebo
DIG (1997)	NYHA II–III LVEF < 45%	6,800	Digoxin vs. placebo	Decreased hospitalization
CONSENSUS (1987)	NYHA IV	253	Enalapril vs. placebo	Decreased mortality
SOLVD (1991)	NYHA I–IV LVEF < 35%	2,569	Enalapril vs. placebo	Decreased mortality and heart failure hospitalizations
ELITE (1997)	NYHA II–IV LVEF < 40%	722	Captopril vs. losartan	Decreased mortality with losartan
ValHeFT (2001)	NYHA II–IV LVEF < 40%	5,010	Valsartan vs. placebo	Improved combined endpoint of mortality and morbidity
MOCHA (1995)	NYHA II–IV LVEF < 35%	345	Carvedilol vs. placebo	Dose-dependent decrease in mortality
PRECISE (1995)	NYHA II–IV LVEF < 35%	278	Carvedilol vs. placebo	Decrease in combined risk of mortality and morbidity
MERIT-HF (1999)	NYHA II–IV LVEF < 40%	3,991	Metoprolol vs. placebo	Decreased mortality
CIBIS-II (1999)	NYHA III–IV LVEF < 40%	2,647	Bisoprolol vs. placebo	Decreased mortality and

(Continued)

Table 1 Summary of Selected Drug Trials in Heart Failure in Adults (*Continued*)

Trial (Year of publication)	Entry criteria	n	Therapy	Outcome
				hospitalizations
COPERNICUS (2002)	LVEF < 35% NYHA III–IV	2,289	Carvedilol vs. placebo	Decreased mortality and hospitalizations
COMET (2003)	LVEF < 25% NYHA II–IV	3029	Carvedilol vs. metoprolol	Decreased mortality with carvedilol
InSYNC (2002)	LVEF < 35% NYHA II–IV QRS > 130 msec	453	Cardiac resynchronization or no resynchronization	Decreased symptoms and hospitalizations
GESICA	LVEF < 35% NYHA II–IV	516	Amiodarone vs. placebo	Decreased mortality and hospitalizations
AVID (1997)	LVEF < 40% Resuscitated VF, or VT with symptoms or	1016	ICD vs. drug therapy	Decreased mortality with ICD
MUSTT (1996)	CAD and induced sustained VT	704	Antiarrhythmic therapy vs. no antiarrhythmic therapy	Decreased mortality with antiarrhythmic therapy
MADIT I (1996)	LVEF < 35% NYHA I–IV, VT	196	ICD vs. conventional therapy	Decreased mortality with ICD

Abbreviations: CAD = coronary artery disease; ICD = implantable cardioverter/defibrillator; LVEF = left ventricular ejection fraction; MI = myocardial infarction; NYHA = New York Heart Association; VF = ventricular fibrillation; VT = ventricular tachycardia.

elevated in heart failure, both because of increased production and reduced hepatic clearance. The mechanisms of aldosterone-mediated potentiation of heart failure are still being defined, but include increased myocardial fibrosis, increased angiotensin-converting enzyme (ACE) and endothelin activity, increased free radical production, and decreased adrenal nitric oxide. The use of aldosterone antagonists is currently recommended in adults with heart failure, but these patients must be carefully selected and monitored for evidence of hyperkalemia and/or renal dysfunction.

Digoxin

Digoxin is a cardiac glycoside, a class of drugs that have been used in the treatment of heart failure for at least three centuries. Its primary mechanism of action is through inhibition of the sarcolemmal Na^+/K^+-ATPase sodium pump. Inhibition of the sarcolemmal Na^+/K^+-ATPase sodium pump results in increased intracellular sodium and the subsequent increase in intracellular calcium through inhibition of the Na^+/Ca^+ exchanger. This increase in intracellular calcium results in increased contractility. Digoxin also has beneficial effects in heart failure beyond the myocyte. It decreases circulating plasma norepinephrine levels, and reduces sympathetic tone (9–11). Digoxin has acute beneficial hemodynamic effects in adults with heart failure, manifested as an increase in cardiac output and LV ejection fraction, as well as a decrease in LV filling pressure, pulmonary capillary wedge pressure, and systemic vascular resistance (12,13).

There is good evidence that digoxin improves symptoms in adults with heart failure, although there is no evidence that it improves survival. The randomized assessment of digoxin on inhibitors of angiotensin-converting enzyme (RADIANCE) trial demonstrated that patients withdrawn from digoxin had significantly worsened heart failure symptoms and exercise tolerance (Fig. 1) (14). The digitalis investigators group (DIG) trial showed no differences in mortality in those treated with digoxin and those treated with placebo over a 3-year period, although there were significantly fewer

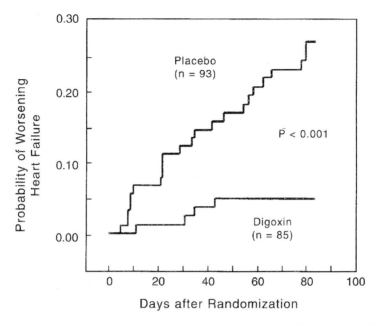

Figure 1 Kaplan–Meier analysis of the cumulative probability of worsening heart failure in the patients continuing to receive digoxin and those switched to placebo. (Reprinted with permission from Ref. 14.)

cardiovascular hospitalizations in the digoxin-treated group (15). These data and others suggest that digoxin improves symptoms but not survival in adults with heart failure.

Toxicity of digoxin has been correlated with higher serum digoxin concentrations, particularly >2.0 ng/mL in adults. Hypokalemia and hypomagnesemia are commonly associated with diuretic use in heart failure and increase toxicity. Major signs of digoxin toxicity are cardiac arrhythmias, gastrointestinal disturbances, and neurologic changes. Increased automaticity (premature ventricular beats) or impaired conduction (sinus bradycardia or atrioventricular block) are seen with digoxin toxicity and often require withdrawal of the drug. Amiodarone, verapamil, spironolactone, flecainide, Pediatrics/ropafenone, and carvedilol have all been associated with increased serum digoxin concentrations, requiring monitoring

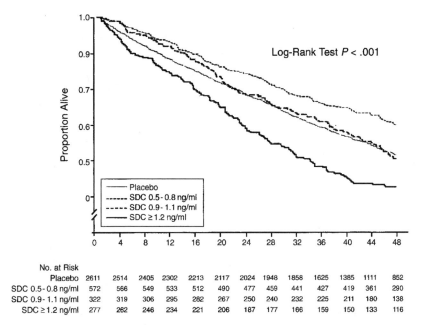

No. at Risk

Placebo	2611	2514	2405	2302	2213	2117	2024	1948	1858	1625	1385	1111	852
SDC 0.5-0.8 ng/ml	572	566	549	533	512	490	477	459	441	427	419	361	290
SDC 0.9-1.1 ng/ml	322	319	306	295	282	267	250	240	232	225	211	180	138
SDC ≥1.2 ng/ml	277	262	246	234	221	206	187	177	166	159	150	133	116

Figure 2 Kaplan–Meier survival analysis for all-cause mortality. SDC indicates serum digoxin concentration. The figure presents the cumulative survival rates for patients assigned to placebo and patients assigned to digoxin in three SDC groups over a mean follow-up of 37 months. (Reprinted with permission from Ref. 17.)

of serum digoxin concentrations when given to a patient receiving digoxin, with concomitant reduction in digoxin dosing in many cases (16). Serial serum digoxin concentration monitoring has often not been routinely recommended unless toxicity is suspected or changes in renal function occur. However, recent evidence from studies in adults suggest that higher serum digoxin concentrations (>1.2 ng/mL) are associated with higher mortality, higher rates of hospitalization, and greater toxicity (17) (Fig. 2). Thus, lower serum digoxin concentrations may be preferable in order to attain the benefit of the drug without increasing adverse effects.

The efficacy of digoxin in the treatment of heart failure in children is unknown. Small, uncontrolled, studies examining the acute hemodynamic effects of digoxin in children with heart failure due to large left-to-right shunts are conflicting, some showing benefit and others showing no benefit (18–20). There are no data on the efficacy of digoxin in heart failure in children with LV systolic dysfunction. Thus, the effects of digoxin on symptoms and/or survival are unknown.

Angiotensin-Converting Enzyme Inhibitors

Multiple prospective, randomized trials studying thousands of adults have definitively shown that ACE inhibitors improve LV ejection fraction, symptoms, and survival in heart failure (21–23). These benefits are seen not only with symptomatic heart failure, but also asymptomatic systolic LV dysfunction (24). The mechanisms of action through which ACE inhibitors benefit patients with heart failure are still a matter of debate. ACE is the enzyme responsible for the conversion of angiotensin I to angiotensin II. Angiotensin II stimulates vasoconstriction, aldosterone release, and cardiac hypertrophy. ACE is identical to kinase II, the inhibition of which results in increased bradykinin and is thus thought to be responsible for the common adverse effect of cough seen with ACE inhibitors. ACE inhibitors reduce afterload, preload, and systolic wall stress. Many of their properties may be beneficial in heart failure, including vasodilation, increase in bradykinin, ventricular remodeling, improved renal function, and blunting the hypertrophic and apoptotic effects of angiotensin II within the myocardium. Although aspirin may abrogate the effects of ACE inhibitors through its inhibition of the production of vasodilating prostaglandins, recent reviews suggest that there is only weak evidence that aspirin actually clinically lessens the benefit of ACE inhibitors in heart failure (25).

Definitive evidence that ACE inhibitors improve LV function, symptoms or survival in children with heart failure is lacking. Many small open-label studies with ACE inhibitors suggest that ACE inhibitors may acutely benefit children with large left-to-right intracardiac shunts (26–30). There also may be benefit in children with dilated (but not restrictive) cardiomyopathy (31,32). However, the only prospective, randomized trial of ACE inhibitors in children with heart disease failed to show any improvement in exercise capacity in children with single ventricle after the Fontan operation (33). This study was limited by the fact that these children were not in heart failure, and the possibility that exercise capacity is not a good endpoint in heart failure trials. Another study prospectively comparing two groups at two different hospitals showed a shorter duration and lesser amount of pleural drainage after bi-directional cavopulmonary shunt in patients treated with enalapril compared to those not treated with enalapril (34).

A large number of ACE inhibitors are currently used in adults with heart failure. ACE inhibitors differ in the chemical structure of their active moieties, in potency, in bioavailability, in plasma half-life, in route of elimination, in their distribution affinity for tissue-bound ACE, and whether they are administered as prodrugs (35). Regardless of which ACE inhibitor is being used, it should be started at a low-dose and then gradually increased as tolerated, watching for signs of hypotension and/or renal dysfunction. There is conflicting evidence whether or not higher doses of ACE inhibitors are beneficial to lower doses (36,37). Particularly, if one is considering adding β-blocker therapy, it can be argued that lower doses of ACE inhibitors may be preferable.

Angiotensin Receptor Blockers

Angiotensin II receptor blockers (ARBs) directly block the effects of angiotensin II at the receptor level. There are theoretical advantages of ARBs over ACE inhibitors. For instance, ARBs do not increase bradykinin levels as ACE inhibitors do, an effect that is responsible for the common adverse effect of cough seen with ACE inhibitors. The first study comparing an ACE inhibitor (captopril) to an ARB (losartan), the Evaluation of Losartan in the Elderly (ELITE) trial, showed no difference in the primary endpoint (heart failure hospitalizations) in elderly patients with heart failure, but an unexpected statistically significant improvement in survival with losartan (38). However, the follow-up study, ELITE II, failed to show a significant survival benefit from ARBs over ACE inhibitors (39). In the Valsartan in Heart Failure Trial (Val-HeFT), the ARB valsartan or placebo was added to therapy including digoxin, diuretics, ACE inhibitors, and β-blockers. The addition of valsartan had no effect on all-cause mortality, but provided a 13% reduction in combined morbidity and mortality (40). On the basis of these and other studies, the use of ARBs is currently only recommended for patients with heart failure who are unable to tolerate ACE inhibitors. The little data available on the use of ARBs in children are primarily limited to its use in pediatric hypertension (41,42).

β-Adrenergic Receptor Blockers

β-Adrenergic receptor blockers (β-blockers) were long considered to be contraindicated in patients with heart failure because of the theoretical concerns of the deleterious effects of blocking sympathetic stimulation to the failing heart. After Waagstein's initial report of improvement in a small group of adults with heart failure treated with β-blockers (43), a large number of small open-label studies were published in the 1980s and early 1990s suggesting that β-blockers may benefit patients with heart failure (44–47). Although the first prospective, randomized, placebo-controlled trials of β-blockers in heart failure suggested a possible benefit on both symptoms and mortality in patients with heart failure due to ischemic or nonischemic LV dysfunction, these studies were statistically underpowered to conclusively prove any significant benefits of β-blockers over placebo (47–49). However, in 1996, two placebo-controlled, prospective, randomized, double-blind trials demonstrated a significant mortality benefit from carvedilol in adults with mild-to-moderate heart failure. The Multicenter Oral Carvedilol Heart Failure Assessment (MOCHA) trial compared placebo to low (6.25 mg twice daily), medium (12.5 mg twice daily), or high (25 mg twice daily), dose carvedilol in adults with ischemic or nonischemic LV dysfunction and heart failure (50). There was a significant dose-dependent reduction in mortality and heart failure hospitalizations, in addition to a dose-dependent increase in LV ejection fraction in patients receiving carvedilol. Interestingly, this dose-dependent improvement was most evident in patients with dilated cardiomyopathy, suggesting a continued benefit of higher dose carvedilol in this group of patients not seen after myocardial infarction. The US Carvedilol study showed a remarkable 67% reduction in mortality in patients with mild-to-moderate heart failure treated with carvedilol when compared to placebo (51). These two studies, for the first time, demonstrated a significant benefit of β-blockers in adults with heart failure with regard to symptoms, LV systolic function and survival. Soon after this, the Metoprolol CR/XL Randomized Intervention Trial (MERIT) reported a study in which 3991 adults with ischemic or nonischemic cardiomyopathy and mild-to-moderate heart failure were randomized to either placebo or metoprolol (up to 200 mg/day) (52). In this study, the primary endpoint was all-cause mortality, and patients receiving metoprolol had a significant (52) reduction in mortality compared to placebo ($p = 0.0001$). In 1999, the follow-up study to the Cardiac Insufficiency Bisoprolol (CIBIS) trial, CIBIS-II, randomized 2647 adults with ischemic or nonischemic cardiomyopathy and mild-to-moderate heart failure to either placebo or bisoprolol. In contrast, to the first CIBIS trial where the maximal dose of bisoprolol was 5 mg/day, in CIBIS-II the maximal dose was 10 mg/day (53). The primary endpoint was all-cause mortality, and bisoprolol treatment was associated with a significant 29% reduction in mortality ($p = 0.0001$) in addition to a significant 33% reduction in sudden death ($p = 0.0001$). The reduction in sudden death mortality seen in this and other β-blocker studies suggests that β-blockers reduce mortality not only by decreasing the progression of heart failure, but also by reducing the fatal arrhythmias associates with it as well. Up to this time, these trials had focused on adults with mild-to-moderate heart failure. In 2001, the Carvedilol Prospective Randomized Cumulative Survival (COPERNICUS) trial randomized 2389 adults in 334 centers with ischemic or nonischemic cardiomyopathy and severe heart failure to placebo or carvedilol (25 mg twice dialy) (54) (Fig. 3). There was a significant 35% reduction in all-cause mortality in the carvedilol group ($p = 0.001$) compared to placebo. On the basis of these studies, carvedilol has now been recommended for all adults with stable heart failure, mild, moderate, or severe.

Since all three of these β-blockers have been shown to improve LV function, symptoms and survival in adults with heart failure, the next question was whether one β-blocker is better than another. Sanderson et al. (55) compared metoprolol to carvedilol in 51 adults with heart failure and found similar improvements in both groups with regard to LV ejection fraction, symptoms, and exercise capacity. However, carvedilol had greater effects than metoprolol on blood pressure, LV end-diastolic dimension, and mitral valve inflow.

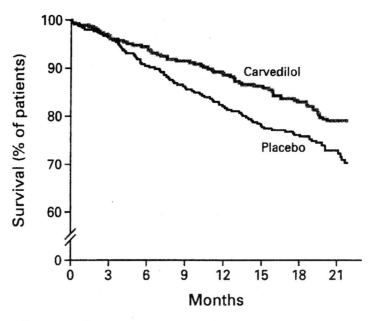

NO. OF PATIENTS AT RISK

Placebo	1133	937	703	580	446	286	183	114
Carvedilol	1156	947	733	620	479	321	208	142

Figure 3 Kaplan–Meier analysis of time to death in the placebo group and the carvedilol group. (Reprinted with permission from Ref. 54.)

Metra et al. (56) also found differences between metoprolol and carvedilol in a study in which they randomized 150 adults with heart failure to either metoprolol or carvedilol. They found that patients receiving carvedilol, when compared to metoprolol, had larger increases in LV ejection fraction at rest and LV stroke work and stroke volume with exercise, and greater decreases in pulmonary artery and pulmonary capillary wedge pressures, although they had less improvement in maximal exercise tolerance. Packer et al. (57), subsequently, performed a meta-analysis of 19 trials of either metoprolol or carvedilol, and showed that there are larger increases in LV ejection fraction with carvedilol than seen with metoprolol. In the Carvedilol or Metoprolol European Trial (COMET), 3029 adults with New York Heart Association Class II–IV symptoms, to treatment with wither metoprolol (target dose 50 mg twice daily) or carvedilol (target dose 25 mg twice daily). Over a 58-month period, carvedilol treatment had a lower all-cause mortality (34%) than metoprolol (40%) ($p = 0.0017$), demonstrating a mortality benefit of carvedilol over metoprolol (Fig. 4).

The current experience with β-blockade in pediatric heart failure is generally anecdotal, although prospective randomized trials are underway. Initial experience with metoprolol in a handful of patients with heart failure due to systemic ventricular systolic dysfunction suggested potential benefit (59,60). A subsequent multicenter retrospective analysis of 15 children (2.5–15 years of age) who received metoprolol due to systemic ventricular systolic dysfunction demonstrated improvement in LV systolic echocardiographic indices and symptoms (61). However, not all patients showed improvement during treatment with metoprolol (Fig. 5), and it was not possible to discern from this retrospective analysis whether the improvement seen in some patients was due to the metoprolol or the natural history of their disease (62). The first report of the use of carvedilol in children with heart failure was again a retrospective analysis of the use of this drug in 46 patients at six institutions (63). In this study, there was a small but statistically significant increase in LV echocardiographic fractional shortening (16–19%) and

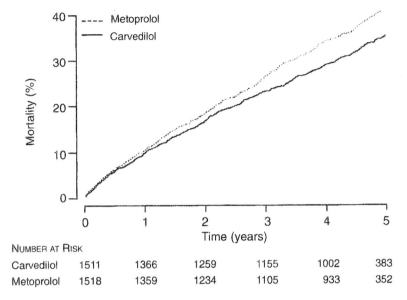

Figure 4 Kaplan–Meier estimates of all-cause mortality for each treatment, carvedilol or metoprolol. (Reprinted with permission from Ref. 58.)

ejection fraction (32–41%). Although there was no actual endpoint since it was a retrospective analysis, most patients improved symptoms at some point in time during the study. However, there were frequent (54%) concomitant medication adjustments, and 30% of patients had an adverse outcome defined as death, transplantation, or placement of a ventricular assist device. Gachara et al. (64) have reported their experience with the use of carvedilol in eight infants with dilated cardiomyopathy and ejection fraction <30%. At 4.5 months after initiation of treatment, these patients showed improvement in both echocardiographic LV ejection fraction and symptoms, and the authors reported no significant adverse events or deaths in this small group. Azeka et al. (65) reported a small prospective, randomized, double-blind, placebo-controlled trial of carvedilol in children with heart failure and dilated cardiomyopathy. In the group treated with carvedilol, there were four deaths and one patient underwent

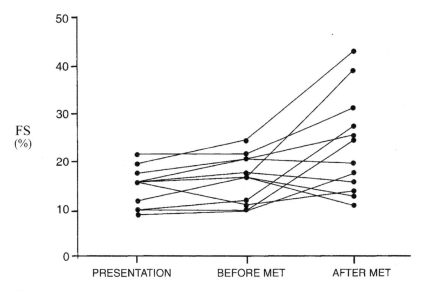

Figure 5 Fractional shortening (FS) in patients treated with metoprolol at three points in time: (1) presentation, which was the time the patient was first diagnosed with cardiomyopathy and after stabilization on conventional medications; (2) before metoprolol, just before starting metoprolol and after having been maintained on conventional medications for a mean period of 22.5 ± 9 months (range 0.5–119 months); and (3) after metoprolol, after receiving metoprolol for a mean period of 23.2 ± 7 months (range 1.2–102 months). (Reproduced with permission from Ref. 61.)

heart transplantation. In the placebo group, there were two deaths and two patients underwent heart transplantation. In those who survived and were not transplanted, there were significantly improved LV ejection fraction and symptoms in the carvedilol group compared with the placebo group. Although the mortality was actually higher in the carvedilol group, the numbers of patients enrolled in this study preclude meaningful interpretation of this finding. Pharmacokinetic analysis of carvedilol in children has shown that the elimination half-life of carvedilol in children is less than in adults, suggesting that optimal dosing strategies of carvedilol in children are different than in adults (66). There have also been case reports of carvedilol improving pulmonary hypertension in a child with dilated cardiomyopathy and pulmonary hypertension (67). Carvedilol increases serum levels of digoxin in children and thus one needs to exercise caution and check serum digoxin levels in children if one adds carvedilol to a regimen of anticongestive heart failure medication including digoxin (16). There are no definitive studies in pediatrics comparing one β-blocker to another. Williams et al. (68) were unable to demonstrate any demonstrable difference between metoprolol and carvedilol in a small retrospective study of these drugs use in children with heart failure at a single institution.

Buchhorn et al. (5,69–73) have published a large body of work on the use of β-blockers (primarily propranolol) in children with heart failure due to left-to-right shunts pre- and postoperatively. Their data suggest that β-blockers in these patients improve symptoms and decrease plasma renin levels, and are superior to low-dose ACE inhibitors. Furthermore, these authors have shown that β-blockers in children with heart failure partially prevent downregulation of β_2 receptor and angiotensin-2 receptor genes and upregulation of endothelin A receptor and connective tissue growth factor genes. In addition, there is also evidence for β-blockade to reverse depressed heart rate variability in infants with heart failure.

New Treatment Strategies

Resynchronization therapy has been studied in adults with symptomatic heart failure due to systolic dysfunction (LV ejection fraction <35%, New York Heart Association functional class III–IV) and prolonged QRS duration >120 msec who were receiving appropriate medical therapy for heart failure. These trials were randomized and included a control group who received the device but did not receive resynchronization therapy for 6 months. The MIRACLE trial and InSYNC trial both reported significant improvements in symptoms and exercise capacity with resynchronization therapy (74,75). On the basis of this, biventricular pacing is now recommended in adults with heart failure and prolonged QRS interval on

ECG. Electrical resynchronization may also be beneficial in patients with heart failure from a failing right ventricle with a prolonged QRS duration, although more study is needed in this area before making recommendations (76).

Since a significant portion of the mortality seen in chronic heart failure is due to sudden arrhythmic death, methods aimed at reducing arrhythmias may help decrease mortality in heart failure. Generally, antiarrhythmic medications have not been shown to decrease mortality in adults with heart failure, and in some instances have actually had a harmful effect (77). In the GESICA trial, amiodarone conferred a 28% reduction in overall mortality compared to placebo in adults with heart failure symptoms and systolic LV dysfunction (78). The role of implantable cardioverters/defibrillators (ICDs) is still being defined in heart failure in adults. Three large randomized trials comparing antiarrhythmic therapy vs. ICD implantation in the secondary prevention (i.e., previous resuscitation from of life-threatening arrhythmia) of sudden death have been published: The Antiarrhythmics Versus Implantable Defibrillator (AVID) trial (79), the Canadian Implantable Defibrillator Study (CIDS) (80), and the Cardiac Arrest Study Hamburg (CASH) (81). In each of these studies, mortality in the ICD group was either statistically significantly lower in the ICD group than the antiarrhythmic group, or there was a nonsignificant trend (82). Similarly, three large randomized trials comparing ICDs to conventional medical therapy in the primary prevention of sudden death have also shown a mortality benefit in patients after myocardial infarction: the Multicenter Automatic Defibrillator Implantation Trial (MADIT), the Multicenter Unsustained Tachycardia Trial (MUSTT), and MADIT II (83–85). Further trials are underway looking at the role of ICDs in nonischemic cardiomyopathy in adults with heart failure. The role of ICDs in children with heart failure is unknown. However, in patients who are thought to be at risk for life-threatening arrhythmias, one should strongly consider placement of an ICD to prevent sudden death. Since the incidence of sudden death in children with heart failure is so low, it is unlikely that an adequately powered trial could

ever be done in this patient population in order to definitively define the role of ICDs in this group of patients with
heart failure.

In addition to digoxin, diuretics (including aldosterone
antagonists), ACE inhibitors, and β-blockers, other treatments have also been found to be beneficial in selected adults
with heart failure. Omapatrilat is a dual inhibitor of both
ACE and neutral endopeptidase. This drug has been shown
to reduce the risk of death and hospitalization in adults with
chronic heart failure, but not necessarily better than ACE
inhibition alone (86). Not all new therapeutic strategies have
proven to be effective in the treatment of heart failure. For
example, new mechanisms of blocking adrenergic effects on
the failing heart have been studied. Moxonidine is a selective
imidazoline ligand that acts specifically on central nervous
system receptors to decrease sympathetic outflow. Two studies examined moxonidine in adults with heart failure: the
Moxonidine Safety and Efficacy (MOXSE) study, and the
Moxonidine Congestive Heart Failure (MOXCON) trial.
There was a dose-related increase in serious adverse effect
in the moxonidine-treated group in the MOXSE trial and an
increase in mortality in the moxonidine-treated group in the
MOXCON trial (87). These studies suggest that the trend
toward an increase in serious adverse events in patients treated with moxonidine may represent the fundamental differences between antiadrenergic treatment via sympatholysis
as seen with moxonidine vs. β-adrenergic receptor blockade.
Tumor necrosis factor (TNF) α blockade was thought to have
theoretical advantages in the treatment of heart failure
because of the observations that TNF exerts negative inotropic effects on the heart and is capable of promoting fibrosis,
hypertrophy, and cardiomyopathy in animal models (88). Circulating TNF levels have also been shown to be elevated in
adults with heart failure and cachexia (89). Because of the
potential benefits of anticytokine therapy in mice with heart
failure, clinical investigators began to explore the effects of
anticytokine therapy in humans with heart failure. A Phase
I trial with etanercept, a soluble recombinantly produced chimeric TNF antagonist, showed benefit in a small number of

patients with heart failure (90). However, two large-scale clinical trials of etanercept in adults with New York Heart Association class II–IV heart failure symptoms (RENAISSANCE and RECOVER) were stopped because of lack of efficacy (91). Finally, endothelin-1 (ET-1) antagonists have not been found yet to be efficacious in heart failure treatment, despite theoretical advantages. ET-1 is a vasoconstrictor peptide that is partially responsible for the increased peripheral vascular resistance seen in heart failure. ET-1 is elevated in patients with heart failure and correlates with hemodynamic severity and symptoms (92). However, in the Endothelin Antagonist Bosentan for Lowering Cardiac Events in Heart Failure (ENABLE) trial, the nonselective ET receptor antagonist bosentan, actually conferred an early risk of worsening heart failure compared to placebo (93). Thus, ET-1 antagonists are not currently recommended for the treatment of heart failure.

Recommendations

Based on the available evidence, including the trials described above, a joint task force of the American College of Cardiology and the American Heart Association published practice guidelines for the evaluation and management of chronic heart failure in adults in 2001 (94). All recommendations in this document followed the format of previous American College of Cardiology and the American Heart Association guidelines:

Class I: Conditions for which there is evidence and/or general agreement that a procedure/therapy is useful and effective.

Class II: Conditions for which there is conflicting evidence and/or a divergence of opinion about the usefulness/efficacy of performing the procedure/therapy.

Class (IIa): Weight of evidence/opinion in favor of usefulness/efficacy.

Class (IIb): Usefulness/efficacy less well established by evidence/opinion.

Class III: Conditions for which there is evidence and/or general agreement that a procedure/therapy is not useful/effective and in some cases may be harmful.

The level of evidence on which these recommendations were based was ranked as level A when the data were derived from multiple randomized clinical trials, level B when the data were derived from a single randomized trial or nonrandomized studies, and level C when the consensus opinion of experts was the primary source of recommendation.

Although these guidelines were developed for adults with heart failure, many of these guidelines are potentially applicable to pediatrics, particularly older children with LV dysfunction. The committee made the following recommendations.

For patients with asymptomatic LV systolic dysfunction:

Class I

ACE inhibition in patients with reduced LV ejection fraction (level of evidence: B).
β-Adrenergic blockade in patients with reduced LV ejection fraction (level of evidence: B).

Class III

Treatment with digoxin in patients with left ventricular dysfunction who are in sinus rhythm (level of evidence: C).
Routine use of nutritional supplements to treat structural heart disease or prevent the development of symptoms (level of evidence: C).

For patients with symptomatic LV systolic dysfunction:

Class I

Diuretics in patients with evidence of fluid retention (level of evidence: A).
ACE inhibition in all patients unless contraindicated (level of evidence: A).

β-Adrenergic blockade in all stable patients unless contraindicated (level of evidence: A).

Digitalis for treatment of symptoms unless contraindicated (level of evidence: A).

Class IIa

Spironolactone in patients with recent or current Class IV symptoms, preserved renal function, and normal potassium concentration (level of evidence: B).

Exercise training as an adjunctive approach to improve clinical status in ambulatory patients (level of evidence: A).

Angiotensin receptor blockade in patients who are being treated with digitalis, diuretics, and a β-blocker and who cannot be given ACE inhibitors because of cough or angioedema (level of evidence: A).

Class IIb

Anticoagulation in patients with heart failure who do not have atrial fibrillation or a previous thromboembolic event (level of evidence: B or C).

Class III

Long-term intermittent use of an infusion of positive inotropic drug (level of evidence: C).

Use of angiotensin receptor blockade instead of an ACE inhibitor in patients (a) who have not been given or who can tolerate ACE inhibitors or (b) have not been tried on β-blockers (level of evidence: B).

Use of a calcium-channel blocking drug as treatment for heart failure (level of evidence: B).

Routine use of nutritional supplements (coenzyme Q10, carnitine, taurine, and antioxidants) or hormones (growth hormone or thyroid hormone) for the treatment of heart failure (level of evidence: C).

The evidence base for deriving recommendations for the treatment of chronic heart failure in children is lacking. In older children, particularly those with systolic LV dysfunction, it is reasonable to consider the use of the guidelines described above. However, unknown dosing strategies and/or age-related differences in response to therapy require that clinicians exercise caution in using these adult heart failure guidelines in children until better data are available to guide therapy. Multicenter trials are underway to help provide the evidence base that will be necessary to allow optimizing medical therapy of chronic LV systolic dysfunction in children.

REFERENCES

1. Bristow MR. Mechanism of action of beta-blocking agents in heart failure. Am J Cardiol 1997; 80(11A):26L–40L.
2. Port JD, Bristow MR. Altered beta-adrenergic receptor gene regulation and signaling in chronic heart failure. J Mol Cell Cardiol 2001; 33(5):887–905.
3. Colucci WS, Sawyer DB, Singh K, Communal C. Adrenergic overload and apoptosis in heart failure: implications for therapy. J Card Fail 2000; 6(2 suppl 1):1–7.
4. Kozlik-Feldmann R, Kramer HH, Wicht H, Feldmann R, Netz II, Reinhardt D. Distribution of myocardial beta-adrenoceptor subtypes and coupling to the adenylate cyclase in children with congenital heart disease and implications for treatment. J Clin Pharmacol 1993; 33(7):588–595.
5. Buchhorn R, Hulpke-Wette M, Ruschewski W, et al. Beta-receptor downregulation in congenital heart disease: a risk factor for complications after surgical repair? Ann Thorac Surg 2002; 73(2):610–613.
6. Costello-Boerrigter LC, Boerrigter G, Burnett JC Jr. Revisiting salt and water retention: new diuretics, aquaretics, and natriuretics. Med Clin North Am 2003; 87(2):475–491.
7. Pitt B, Zannad F, Remme WJ, et al. The effect of spironolactone on morbidity and mortality in patients with severe heart failure. Randomized Aldactone Evaluation Study Investigators. N Engl J Med 1999; 341(10):709–717.
8. Pitt B, Remme W, Zannad F, et al. Eplerenone, a selective aldosterone blocker, in patients with left ventricular dysfunction after myocardial infarction. N Engl J Med 2003; 348(14):1309–1321.
9. Alicandri C, Fariello R, Boni E, et al. Captopril versus digoxin in mild-moderate chronic heart failure: a crossover study. J Cardiovasc Pharmacol 1987; 9(suppl 2):S61–S67.

10. Krum H, Bigger JT Jr, Goldsmith RL, Packer M. Effect of long-term digoxin therapy on autonomic function in patients with chronic heart failure. J Am Coll Cardiol 1995; 25(2):289–294.

11. Gheorghiade M, Ferguson D. Digoxin. A neurohormonal modulator in heart failure? Circulation 1991; 84(5):2181–2186.

12. Ribner HS, Plucinski DA, Hsieh AM, et al. Acute effects of digoxin on total systemic vascular resistance in congestive heart failure due to dilated cardiomyopathy: a hemodynamic-hormonal study. Am J Cardiol 1985; 56(13):896–904.

13. Gheorghiade M, St Clair J, St Clair C, Beller GA. Hemodynamic effects of intravenous digoxin in patients with severe heart failure initially treated with diuretics and vasodilators. J Am Coll Cardiol 1987; 9(4):849–857.

14. Packer M, Gheorghiade M, Young JB, et al. Withdrawal of digoxin from patients with chronic heart failure treated with angiotensin-converting-enzyme inhibitors. RADIANCE Study. N Engl J Med 1993; 329(1):1–7.

15. The Digitalis Investigation Group. The effect of digoxin on mortality and morbidity in patients with heart failure. N Engl J Med 1997; 336(8):525–533.

16. Ratnapalan S, Griffiths K, Costei AM, Benson L, Koren G. Digoxin–carvedilol interactions in children. J Pediatr 2003; 142(5):572–574.

17. Rathore SS, Curtis JP, Wang Y, Bristow MR, Krumholz HM. Association of serum digoxin concentration and outcomes in patients with heart failure. JAMA 2003; 289(7):871–878.

18. Berman W Jr, Yabek SM, Dillon T, Niland C, Corlew S, Christensen D. Effects of digoxin in infants with congested circulatory state due to a ventricular septal defect. N Engl J Med 1983; 308(7):363–366.

19. Kimball TR, Daniels SR, Meyer RA, et al. Effect of digoxin on contractility and symptoms in infants with a large ventricular septal defect. Am J Cardiol 1991; 68(13):1377–1382.

20. Seguchi M, Nakazawa M, Momma K. Further evidence suggesting a limited role of digitalis in infants with circulatory congestion secondary to large ventricular septal defect. Am J Cardiol 1999; 83(9): 1408–1411, A8.

21. The CONSENSUS Trial Study Group. Effects of enalapril on mortality in severe congestive heart failure. Results of the Cooperative North Scandinavian Enalapril Survival Study (CONSENSUS). N Engl J Med 1987; 316(23):1429–1435.

22. Cohn JN, Johnson G, Ziesche S, et al. A comparison of enalapril with hydralazine-isosorbide dinitrate in the treatment of chronic congestive heart failure. N Engl J Med 1991; 325(5):303–310.

23. The SOLVD Investigators. Effect of enalapril on survival in patients with reduced left ventricular ejection fractions and congestive heart failure. N Engl J Med 1991; 325(5):293–302.

24. Yusuf S, Pepine CJ, Garces C, et al. Effect of enalapril on myocardial infarction and unstable angina in patients with low ejection fractions. Lancet 1992; 340(8829):1173–1178.

25. Teo KK, Yusuf S, Pfeffer M, et al. Effects of long-term treatment with angiotensin-converting-enzyme inhibitors in the presence or absence of aspirin: a systematic review. Lancet 2002; 360(9339):1037–1043.

26. Shaddy RE, Teitel DF, Brett C. Short-term hemodynamic effects of captopril in infants with congestive heart failure. Am J Dis Child 1988; 142(1):100–105.

27. Montigny M, Davignon A, Fouron JC, Biron P, Fournier A, Elie R. Captopril in infants for congestive heart failure secondary to a large ventricular left-to-right shunt. Am J Cardiol 1989; 63(9):631–633.

28. Lloyd TR, Mahoney LT, Knoedel D, Marvin WJ Jr, Robillard JE, Lauer RM. Orally administered enalapril for infants with congestive heart failure: a dose-finding study. J Pediatr 1989; 114(4 Pt 1): 650–654.

29. Rheuban KS, Carpenter MA, Ayers CA, Gutgesell HP. Acute hemodynamic effects of converting enzyme inhibition in infants with congestive heart failure. J Pediatr 1990; 117(4):668–670.

30. Boucek MM, Chang RL. Effects of captopril on the distribution of left ventricular output with ventricular septal defect. Pediatr Res 1988; 24(4):499–503.

31. Bengur AR, Beekman RH, Rocchini AP, Crowley DC, Schork MA, Rosenthal A. Acute hemodynamic effects of captopril in children with a congestive or restrictive cardiomyopathy. Circulation 1991; 83(2): 523–527.

32. Lewis AB, Chabot M. The effect of treatment with angiotensin-converting enzyme inhibitors on survival of pediatric patients with dilated cardiomyopathy. Pediatr Cardiol 1993; 14(1):9–12.

33. Kouatli AA, Garcia JA, Zellers TM, Weinstein EM, Mahony L. Enalapril does not enhance exercise capacity in patients after Fontan procedure. Circulation 1997; 96(5):1507–1512.

34. Thompson LD, McElhinney DB, Culbertson CB, et al. Perioperative administration of angiotensin converting enzyme inhibitors decreases the severity and duration of pleural effusions following bidirectional cavopulmonary anastomosis. Cardiol Young 2001; 11(2):195–200.

35. Brown NJ, Vaughan DE. Angiotensin-converting enzyme inhibitors. Circulation 1998; 97(14):1411–1420.

36. Packer M, Poole-Wilson PA, Armstrong PW, et al. Comparative effects of low and high doses of the angiotensin-converting enzyme inhibitor, lisinopril, on morbidity and mortality in chronic heart failure. ATLAS Study Group. Circulation 1999; 100(23):2312–2318.

37. van Veldhuisen DJ, Genth-Zotz S, Brouwer J, et al. High-versus low-dose ACE inhibition in chronic heart failure: a double-blind, placebo-controlled study of imidapril. J Am Coll Cardiol 1998; 32(7): 1811–1818.

38. Pitt B, Segal R, Martinez FA, et al. Randomised trial of losartan versus captopril in patients over 65 with heart failure (Evaluation of Losartan in the Elderly Study, ELITE). Lancet 1997; 349(9054): 747–752.

39. Pitt B, Poole-Wilson PA, Segal R, et al. Effect of losartan compared with captopril on mortality in patients with symptomatic heart failure: randomised trial—the Losartan Heart Failure Survival Study ELITE II. Lancet 2000; 355(9215):1582–1587.

40. Cohn JN, Tognoni G. A randomized trial of the angiotensin-receptor blocker valsartan in chronic heart failure. N Engl J Med 2001; 345(23):1667–1675.

41. Friedman AL. Approach to the treatment of hypertension in children. Heart Dis 2002; 4(1):47–50.

42. Marino MR, Vachharajani NN. Pharmacokinetics of irbesartan are not altered in special populations. J Cardiovasc Pharmacol 2002; 40(1):112–122.

43. Waagstein F, Hjalmarson A, Varnauskas E, Wallentin I. Effect of chronic beta-adrenergic receptor blockade in congestive cardiomyopathy. Br Heart J 1975; 37(10):1022–1036.

44. Waagstein F, Hjalmarson A, Swedeberg K, Wallentin I. Beta-blockers in dilated cardiomyopathies: they work. Eur Heart J 1983; 4(suppl A):173–178.

45. Eichhorn EJ, Bedotto JB, Malloy CR, et al. Effect of beta-adrenergic blockade on myocardial function and energetics in congestive heart failure. Improvements in hemodynamic, contractile, and diastolic performance with bucindolol [see comments]. Circulation 1990; 82(2):473–483.

46. Olsen SL, Gilbert EM, Renlund DG, Taylor DO, Yanowitz FD, Bristow MR. Carvedilol improves left ventricular function and symptoms in chronic heart failure: a double-blind randomized study. J Am Coll Cardiol 1995; 25(6):1225–1231.

47. Gilbert EM, Anderson JL, Deitchman D, et al. Long-term beta-blocker vasodilator therapy improves cardiac function in idiopathic dilated cardiomyopathy: a double-blind, randomized study of bucindolol versus placebo. Am J Med 1990; 88(3):223–229.

48. CIBIS Investigators and Committees. A randomized trial of beta-blockade in heart failure. The Cardiac Insufficiency Bisoprolol Study (CIBIS). Circulation 1994; 90(4):1765–1773.

49. Waagstein F, Bristow MR, Swedberg K, et al. Beneficial effects of metoprolol in idiopathic dilated cardiomyopathy. Metoprolol in Dilated Cardiomyopathy (MDC) Trial Study Group. Lancet 1993; 342(8885):1441–1446.

50. Bristow MR, Gilbert EM, Abraham WT, et al. Carvedilol produces dose-related improvements in left ventricular function and survival in subjects with chronic heart failure. MOCHA Investigators. Circulation 1996; 94(11):2807–2816.

51. Packer M, Colucci WS, Sackner-Bernstein JD, et al. Double-blind, placebo-controlled study of the effects of carvedilol in patients with moderate to severe heart failure. The PRECISE Trial. Prospective Randomized Evaluation of Carvedilol on Symptoms and Exercise [see comments]. Circulation 1996; 94(11):2793–2799.

52. Effect of metoprolol CR/XL in chronic heart failure: Metoprolol CR/XL Randomised Intervention Trial in Congestive Heart Failure (MERIT-HF). Lancet 1999; 353(9169):2001–2007.

53. The Cardiac Insufficiency Bisoprolol Study II (CIBIS-II): a randomised trial. Lancet 1999; 353(9146):9–13.

54. Packer M, Fowler MB, Roecker EB, et al. Effect of carvedilol on the morbidity of patients with severe chronic heart failure: results of the carvedilol prospective randomized cumulative survival (COPERNICUS) study. Circulation 2002; 106(17):2194–2199.

55. Sanderson JE, Chan SK, Yip G, et al. Beta-blockade in heart failure: a comparison of carvedilol with metoprolol. J Am Coll Cardiol 1999; 34(5):1522–1528.

56. Metra M, Giubbini R, Nodari S, Boldi E, Modena MG, Dei Cas L. Differential effects of beta-blockers in patients with heart failure: a prospective, randomized, double-blind comparison of the long-term effects of metoprolol versus carvedilol. Circulation 2000; 102(5): 546–551.

57. Packer M, Antonopoulos GV, Berlin JA, Chittams J, Konstam MA, Udelson JE. Comparative effects of carvedilol and metoprolol on left ventricular ejection fraction in heart failure: results of a meta-analysis. Am Heart J 2001; 141(6):899–907.

58. Poole-Wilson PA, Swedberg K, Cleland JG, et al. Comparison of carvedilol and metoprolol on clinical outcomes in patients with chronic heart failure in the Carvedilol Or Metoprolol European Trial (COMET): randomised controlled trial. Lancet 2003; 362(9377):7–13.

59. Shaddy RE, Olsen SL, Bristow MR, et al. Efficacy and safety of metoprolol in the treatment of doxorubicin-induced cardiomyopathy in pediatric patients. Am Heart J 1995; 129(1):197–199.

60. Shaddy RE. Beta-blocker therapy in young children with congestive heart failure under consideration for heart transplantation. Am Heart J 1998; 136(1):19–21.

61. Shaddy RE, Tani LY, Gidding SS, et al. Beta-blocker treatment of dilated cardiomyopathy with congestive heart failure in children: a multi-institutional experience. J Heart Lung Transplant 1999; 18(3):269–274.

62. Lewis AB. Late recovery of ventricular function in children with idiopathic dilated cardiomyopathy. Am Heart J 1999; 138(2 Pt 1):334–338.

63. Bruns LA, Chrisant MK, Lamour JM, et al. Carvedilol as therapy in pediatric heart failure: an initial multicenter experience. J Pediatr 2001; 138(4):505–511.

64. Gachara N, Prabhakaran S, Srinivas S, Farzana F, Krishnan U, Shah MJ. Efficacy and safety of carvedilol in infants with dilated cardiomyopathy: a preliminary report. Indian Heart J 2001; 53(1):74–78.
65. Azeka E, Franchini Ramires JA, Valler C, Alcides Bocchi E. Delisting of infants and children from the heart transplantation waiting list after carvedilol treatment. J Am Coll Cardiol 2002; 40(11):2034–2038.
66. Laer S, Mir TS, Behn F, et al. Carvedilol therapy in pediatric patients with congestive heart failure: a study investigating clinical and pharmacokinetic parameters. Am Heart J 2002; 143(5):916–922.
67. Horenstein MS, Ross RD, Singh TP, Epstein ML. Carvedilol reverses elevated pulmonary vascular resistance in a child with dilated cardiomyopathy. Pediatr Cardiol 2002; 23(1):100–102.
68. Williams RV, Tani LY, Shaddy RE. Intermediate effects of treatment with metoprolol or carvedilol in children with left ventricular systolic dysfunction. J Heart Lung Transplant 2002; 21(8):906–909.
69. Buchhorn R, Bartmus D, Siekmeyer W, Hulpke-Wette M, Schulz R, Bursch J. Beta-blocker therapy of severe congestive heart failure in infants with left to right shunts. Am J Cardiol 1998; 81(11): 1366–1368.
70. Buchhorn R, Hulpke-Wette M, Wessel A, Bursch J. Beta-blocker therapy in an infant with pulmonary hypertension. Eur J Pediatr 1999; 158(12):1007–1008.
71. Buchhorn R, Ross RD, Hulpke-Wette M, et al. Effectiveness of low dose captopril versus propranolol therapy in infants with severe congestive failure due to left-to-right shunts. Int J Cardiol 2000; 76(2–3):227–233.
72. Buchhorn R, Hulpke-Wette M, Hilgers R, Bartmus D, Wessel A, Bursch J. Propranolol treatment of congestive heart failure in infants with congenital heart disease: the CHF-PRO-INFANT Trial. Congestive heart failure in infants treated with propanol. Int J Cardiol 2001; 79(2–3):167–173.
73. Buchhorn R, Hulpke-Wette M, Ruschewski W, et al. Effects of therapeutic beta blockade on myocardial function and cardiac remodelling in congenital cardiac disease. Cardiol Young 2003; 13(1):36–43.
74. Abraham WT, Fisher WG, Smith AL, et al. Cardiac resynchronization in chronic heart failure. N Engl J Med 2002; 346(24):1845–1853.
75. Young JB, Abraham WT, Smith AL, et al. Combined cardiac resynchronization and implantable cardioversion defibrillation in advanced chronic heart failure: the MIRACLE ICD Trial. JAMA 2003; 289(20):2685–2694.
76. Dubin AM, Feinstein JA, Reddy VM, Hanley FL, Van Hare GF, Rosenthal DN. Electrical resynchronization: a novel therapy for the failing right ventricle. Circulation 2003; 107(18):2287–2289.
77. Echt DS, Liebson PR, Mitchell LB, et al. Mortality and morbidity in patients receiving encainide, flecainide, or placebo. The Cardiac Arrhythmia Suppression Trial. N Engl J Med 1991; 324(12):781–788.

78. Singh SN, Fletcher RD, Fisher SG, et al. Amiodarone in patients with congestive heart failure and asymptomatic ventricular arrhythmia. Survival Trial of Antiarrhythmic Therapy in Congestive Heart Failure. N Engl J Med 1995; 333(2):77–82.

79. The Antiarrhythmics versus Implantable Defibrillators (AVID) Investigators. A comparison of antiarrhythmic-drug therapy with implantable defibrillators in patients resuscitated from near-fatal ventricular arrhythmias. N Engl J Med 1997; 337(22):1576–1583.

80. Connolly SJ, Gent M, Roberts RS, et al. Canadian implantable defibrillator study (CIDS): a randomized trial of the implantable cardioverter defibrillator against amiodarone. Circulation 2000; 101(11): 1297–1302.

81. Kuck KH, Cappato R, Siebels J, Ruppel R. Randomized comparison of antiarrhythmic drug therapy with implantable defibrillators in patients resuscitated from cardiac arrest: the Cardiac Arrest Study Hamburg (CASH). Circulation 2000; 102(7):748–754.

82. Estes NA III, Weinstock J, Wang PJ, Homoud MK, Link MS. Use of antiarrhythmics and implantable cardioverter-defibrillators in congestive heart failure. Am J Cardiol 2003; 91(6A):45D–52D.

83. Moss AJ, Hall WJ, Cannom DS, et al. Improved survival with an implanted defibrillator in patients with coronary disease at high risk for ventricular arrhythmia. Multicenter Automatic Defibrillator Implantation Trial Investigators. N Engl J Med 1996; 335(26): 1933–1940.

84. Buxton AE, Lee KL, Fisher JD, Josephson ME, Prystowsky EN, Hafley G. A randomized study of the prevention of sudden death in patients with coronary artery disease. Multicenter Unsustained Tachycardia Trial Investigators. N Engl J Med 1999; 341(25): 1882–1890.

85. Moss AJ, Zareba W, Hall WJ, et al. Prophylactic implantation of a defibrillator in patients with myocardial infarction and reduced ejection fraction. N Engl J Med 2002; 346(12):877–883.

86. Packer M, Califf RM, Konstam MA, et al. Comparison of omapatrilat and enalapril in patients with chronic heart failure: the Omapatrilat Versus Enalapril Randomized Trial of Utility in Reducing Events (OVERTURE). Circulation 2002; 106(8):920–926.

87. Swedberg K, Bristow MR, Cohn JN, et al. Effects of sustained-release moxonidine, an imidazoline agonist, on plasma norepinephrine in patients with chronic heart failure. Circulation 2002; 105(15): 1797–1803.

88. Lisman KA, Stetson SJ, Koerner MM, Farmer JA, Torre-Amione G. The role of tumor necrosis factor alpha blockade in the treatment of congestive heart failure. Congest Heart Fail 2002; 8(5):275–279.

89. Levine B, Kalman J, Mayer L, Fillit HM, Packer M. Elevated circulating levels of tumor necrosis factor in severe chronic heart failure. N Engl J Med 1990; 323(4):236–241.

90. Deswal A, Bozkurt B, Seta Y, et al. Safety and efficacy of a soluble P75 tumor necrosis factor receptor (Enbrel, etanercept) in patients with advanced heart failure. Circulation 1999; 99(25):3224–3226.

91. Mann DL, Deswal A, Bozkurt B, Torre-Amione G. New therapeutics for chronic heart failure. Annu Rev Med 2002; 53:59–74.

92. McMurray JJ, Ray SG, Abdullah I, Dargie HJ, Morton JJ. Plasma endothelin in chronic heart failure. Circulation 1992; 85(4): 1374–1379.

93. Kalra PR, Moon JC, Coats AJ. Do results of the ENABLE (Endothelin Antagonist Bosentan for Lowering Cardiac Events in Heart Failure) study spell the end for non-selective endothelin antagonism in heart failure? Int J Cardiol 2002; 85(2–3):195–197.

94. Hunt SA, Baker DW, Chin MH, et al. ACC/AHA Guidelines for the Evaluation and Management of Chronic Heart Failure in the Adult: Executive Summary A Report of the American College of Cardiology/American Heart Association Task Force on Practice Guidelines (Committee to Revise the 1995 Guidelines for the Evaluation and Management of Heart Failure): Developed in Collaboration With the International Society for Heart and Lung Transplantation; Endorsed by the Heart Failure Society of America. Circulation 2001; 104(24): 2996–3007.

16

Nutritional Aspects of Pediatric Heart Failure

CATHERINE A. LEITCH

Section of Neonatal–Perinatal Medicine,
Department of Pediatrics, Indiana University
Medical Center, Indianapolis, Indiana, U.S.A.

Growth impairment in infants and children with congenital heart disease (CHD) is well documented. The greatest severity of growth retardation is usually found in infants with congestive heart failure (CHF) associated with ventricular septal defect (1), patent ductus arteriosus (2), transposition of the great arteries, or coarctation of the aorta (3). Although the etiology for this growth impairment remains unknown, CHD and/or CHF can affect growth by causing insufficient caloric intake due to an actual decrease in the number of calories consumed or to malabsorption of the ingested calories (4,5), or by causing an increase in energy expenditure of patients with the disease (6–10). Chronic hypoxia has also been implicated as a cause of growth impairment in infants with cyanotic CHD (11–13). Whatever the cause of growth impairment in these infants, it is clear that adequate nutrition is crucial to allow for proper growth and neurodevelopment and to decrease surgical risk (14).

More than 35 years ago, Mehrizi and Drash (11) reported that 55% of children with CHD were below the 16th percentile for weight, 52% were below the 16th percentile for height, and 27% were below the 3rd percentile for both. In the intervening years, considerable progress has been made in both surgical management and nutritional intervention for these patients, so it might be expected that the number of malnourished infants and children with CHD would have decreased. A study by Cameron et al. (15) examined 150 hospitalized patients ranging in age from newborn to 24 years. Despite improvements in the care of the pediatric patient with CHD, up to 70% of patients with either cyanosis and/or CHF, and up to 60% of patients with left-to-right shunts remain malnourished.

At birth, infants with CHD usually have weights appropriate for gestational age. However, growth problems usually become evident early in life (2,4,7,9,16–19). Weight is often more affected than height and boys tend to be more malnourished than girls (1,18,20). The severity and pattern of growth restriction are related to the type of cardiac lesion and their hemodynamic effects (11), although weight and height are not always directly related to the severity of CHD or CHF (21,22). In patients with cyanotic CHD (e.g., transposition of the great arteries, tetralogy of Fallot), both weight and height tend to be equally reduced (11), whereas in patients with acyanotic lesions (e.g., secundum atrial septal defect, ventricular septal defect, or patent ductus arteriosus) weight is affected more than height (11,23). Patients with pulmonary stenosis or coarctation of the aorta generally have normal growth patterns, although impairment in linear growth relative to weight has been observed (11,24,25).

The discrepancy between weight gain and linear growth is most striking in infants with CHF and/or large left-to-right shunting. These infants tend to weigh less than cyanotic children. Indeed, the incidence of growth failure is highest in infants with ventricular septal defects (26). It has been suggested that this may be due in part to the greater occurrence of pulmonary hypertension and CHF in children with left-to-right shunts (27). When bone age (skeletal maturity) has been measured, skeletal retardation was associated with retardation in both height and weight, but was not necessarily parallel to it (1,17,28). Delay in skeletal maturation has been shown to be related to the severity of hypoxemia in patients with cyanotic CHD and can also be demonstrated in infants with CHF (28).

The role of hypoxemia as a primary cause for growth retardation is unclear. Some studies have shown significant differences in growth between cyanotic and acyanotic children with CHD (11–13) while others have not (18,29). Patients with CHD without associated CHF (e.g., tetralogy of Fallot) are only moderately underdeveloped, whereas those with associated CHF (e.g., D-transposition of the great arteries) are usually more severely affected. Significant differences have been observed in both mental and motor skills between infants in CHF and infants not in CHF, with the infants in CHD achieving lower scores (30). Of the infants in CHF, 49% were also hypoxemic.

Delayed skeletal maturation (28) and growth in adolescents with CHD (31) have been related directly to the severity of the hypoxemia. The delay in adolescence in patients with CHD (11–13) suggests possible endocrine involvement. Pubescence in very cyanotic children may be delayed and not begin until a height age of 12–13 years is reached.

The timing of surgical repair may also influence growth in these children. Recent surgical advances have led to correction of many congenital heart defects in the first year of life. This is due to improvements in both of pre- and postoperative care (32) as well as developments in enteral nutrition (33–37). Early surgical repair resulting in the elimination of CHF and hypoxemia often alleviates malnutrition and may lead to catch-up growth in these infants (38,39). However, in older children, the effects of surgery on growth are not as clear, with some children displaying catch-up growth and others continuing to lag (18,40–42).

ENERGY EXPENDITURE

Total energy expenditure (TEE) is the sum of three components: resting energy expenditure (REE), energy expended in physical activity, and dietary-induced thermogenesis. The relative contribution of each component to the total varies with age, gender, body composition, and health. The REE is the minimum amount of energy required to sustain life in a resting state in a neutral thermal environment several hours after food or physical activity. It includes the work of breathing, heart function, thermal regulation, and other essential tissue and cellular functions and is the largest component of TEE, comprising approximately 60% of the TEE in healthy adults and 80% in the newborn. Measurement of REE is thus useful in estimating total energy needs of healthy subjects under ideal conditions and in detecting differences in basal metabolic processes in different populations. The magnitude of the physical activity component is subject to voluntary control, and ranges from around 10% in newborn infants to approximately 30% of TEE in normal adults. Diet-induced thermogenesis constitutes the remainder of TEE and is the amount of energy expenditure above REE after a meal and includes the cost of absorption, metabolism, and storage of food. Positive energy balance is achieved when metabolizable energy intake is greater than energy expenditure. Only then is growth possible, with excess energy stored as new tissue. If exogenous metabolizable energy intake is less than expenditure, energy balance is negative and body energy stores must be mobilized to meet ongoing energy needs.

The REE is typically measured using open circuit indirect calorimetry. This is performed with a patient under a plastic hood, while air is pulled through the hood by a suction pump. By measuring the flow rate, and the change in concentration of both O_2 and CO_2, oxygen consumption and carbon dioxide production can be measured. This method is noninvasive and measurements are taken over a period of minutes to hours. It must be emphasized that, while REE is a useful starting point in assessing the energy requirements of an individual, it is only one component of the total energy requirement of that individual. As such, it is not the parameter on which dietary recommendations should be made. The TEE includes contributions of all components and is a determination of the *actual* amount of energy used by that individual.

The TEE can be measured independently, or it can be estimated from the sum of measurements of individual components extrapolated over long time periods. In addition to errors associated with extrapolation, measurements of individual components are disruptive to the subject's normal lifestyle and thus may produce atypical results. Measurements of TEE using the doubly labeled water method are being performed in more and more laboratories. These measurements are not invasive, do not interfere with the patient's lifestyle, do not require extrapolation, and provide data on the amount of energy actually used by the patient over a long period of time. This technique utilizes water labeled with tracer amounts of the stable isotopes deuterium (^2H) and ^{18}O. A tracer dose of deuterium-labeled water (^2H_2O) and ^{18}O-labeled water ($H_2{}^{18}O$) is administered. The tracers distribute throughout the entire body water pool over a short period (approximately 4–12 hr); the concentrations (or enrichment) of the deuterium and ^{18}O labels in water are then measured in urine, saliva, or blood. Over a period of time ranging from 3 to 10 days for neonates and from 1 to 3 weeks for adults, both labels are lost from the body. However, they are lost at different rates. The deuterium label is lost as water (from urinary and evaporative losses) while the ^{18}O label is lost as both water and CO_2. The difference between the elimination rates of the two isotopes reflects CO_2 production. From this CO_2 production rate and an assumed respiratory quotient, total daily energy expenditure can be determined. The significant advantage of this method is that the TEE can be estimated noninvasively in free-living individuals over fairly long periods of time.

Elevated metabolic rate has been proposed as a cause of failure to thrive in infants with CHD (4,6,20,43). Several studies using respiratory calorimetry have shown that infants with CHD have high REE as well as low energy intakes compared to age-matched controls (6,20,35,43). However, these study populations all included patients with a variety of cyanotic and acyanotic defects. Krauss and Auld (44) used respiratory calorimetry to compare the REE of infants <1 month old with CHF and age-matched infants without CHF and found that the REE of infants with CHF were significantly greater than those of infants without CHF. However, their study groups were heterogeneous with respect to the type of lesion, severity of CHD, degree of cyanosis, and presence of respiratory distress. Lees et al. (43) and Stocker et al. (6) showed that increased oxygen consumption correlates with increasing severity of CHF. Leitch et al. (7) studied a group of infants with cyanotic CHD and a group of age-matched healthy infants in 2 weeks of age and again in 3 months of age. No significant differences were found between groups in REE at either study time. Ackerman et al. (9) studied a group of 4-month-old infants with ventricular septal defects and a group of age-matched infants and found no differences in REE between the two groups.

The REE results for infants ranging in age from 9 hr to 4 months are summarized in Fig. 1 (7,9,10,19,35,44). From these limited data, it appears that infants with CHD have very similar REE to those of healthy, age-matched infants (58.4 ± 16.8 kcal/kg/day for infants with CHD vs. 54.7 ± 14.7 kcal/kg/day for healthy infants). Infants with CHF had a trend toward the highest REE (70.7 ± 16.3 kcal/kg/day). No differences between groups were statistically significant. Farrell et al. (10) examined the REE of 4-month-old infants with VSD and healthy age-matched control (CTL) infants. The VSD group was subdivided in infants without CHF (*n*-CHF group) and those with CHF (CHF group). As shown in Fig. 2, no significant differences were found among the groups. The *n*-CHF and CTL groups were nearly identical with REE of 44.3 ± 8.2 kcal/kg/day and 44.0 ± 12.4 kcal/kg/day,

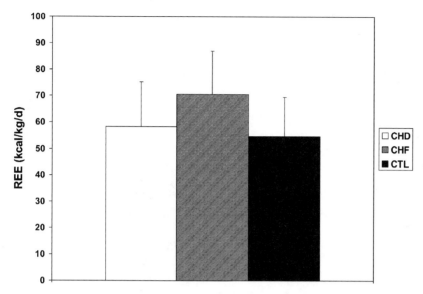

Figure 1 Comparison of REEs of infants ranging in age from 9 hr to 4 months. No significant differences are found between infants with CHD or CHF and healthy control (CTL) infants.

respectively. The CHF infants had an REE of 52.3 ± 14.1 kcal/kg/day.

There have only been a limited number of studies using the doubly labeled water method to measure TEE in infants with CHD. Barton et al. (45) studied 3–6-month-old infants with severe CHD and found that these infants had significantly increased TEE relative to healthy infants before surgery (101.6 ± 9.6 kcal/kg/day vs. a literature value of 66.9 ± 14.3 kcal/kg/day for healthy infants). Intake in CHD patients was only 82% of the estimated average requirement recommended for age. Four patients were studied immediately after surgery; no consistent pattern of change in energy expenditure was observed in this small group. While the results of that investigation suggest an increase in TEE associated with CHD, the infants had a variety of cyanotic and acyanotic defects and four of eight infants were in CHF. In addition, the investigators did not study healthy infants themselves, relying instead on literature values obtained by

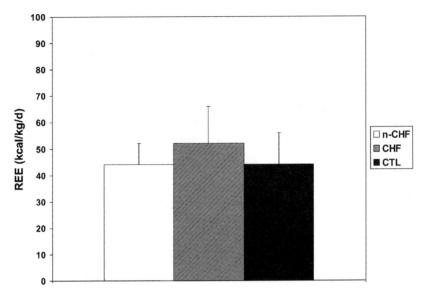

Figure 2 Comparison of REEs of 4-month-old infants with VSD and healthy control (CTL) infants. The VSD infants were subdivided into a group not being treated for CHF (*n*-CHF) and infants with CHF. No significant differences were found between the VSD infants and the CTL infants.

other investigators in separate laboratories at different times. Mitchell et al. (46) studied 4–33-month-old children before and immediately after cardiac surgery. They found increased TEE in some children before surgery and a significant postoperative reduction in TEE in most children, with values falling below those of healthy children not undergoing surgery. They attributed this reduction to a decrease in physical activity. Once again, the study population was extremely heterogeneous: a wide age range was included, the children had a variety of cyanotic and acyanotic defects, and surgical procedures ranged from palliative procedures to complete repair. Leitch et al. (7) examined the TEE in infants with cyanotic CHD and healthy infants and found a 21% increase in TEE in the infants with cyanotic CHD in 2 weeks of age and a 30% increase in 3 months of age, compared with the healthy, age-matched infants. Ackerman et al. (9) compared the TEE of a group of 4-month-old infants with ventricular septal defects and age-matched healthy infants and found a 40% increase in TEE in the infants with ventricular septal defects. Since no differences were found in REE between groups in either of these studies, the increased TEE was attributed to an elevated cost of physical activity in the infants with CHD. The same group has shown (10) that TEE is significantly higher in infants with VSD and CHF (CHF group) than in infants with VSD who are not being treated for CHF (n-CHF group); 92.3 ± 20.4 kcal/kg/day vs. 77.0 ± 17.2 kcal/kg/day. In addition, the TEE of the infants in the n-CHF group is significantly greater than that of healthy controls (61.3 ± 9.2 kcal/kg/day). Figure 3 shows the relationship between TEE and the severity of the VSD as indicated by the pulmonary-to-systemic blood flow ($Q_p:Q_s$) ratio. A strong positive relationship was found between these parameters ($p \leq 0.0001$).

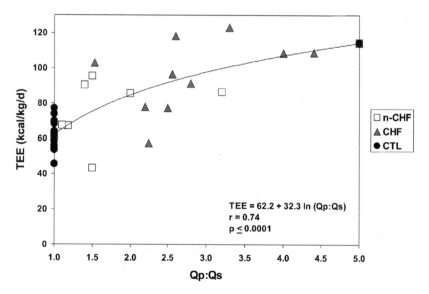

Figure 3 Plot of $Q_p:Q_s$ ratio vs. TEE of 3–4-month-old infants. The solid line represents the logarithmic regression line. The TEE is strongly and positively correlated with the $Q_p:Q_s$ ratio ($p \leq 0.0001$).

Figure 4 summarizes the existing results for total daily energy expenditure in infants with CHD and CHF ranging in age from 3 to 5 months (7–9,45). These results show a significant (~50%) increase in TEE of infants with CHD or CHF compared to healthy age-matched infants; 89.9 ± 6.9 kcal/kg/day, 91.5 ± 20.0 kcal/kg/day and 65.0 ± 6.2 kcal/kg/day, respectively ($p \leq 0.01$).

Studies carried out in neonates (47), infants (48,49), and children (50) several days postoperatively have shown that cardiovascular surgery does not significantly alter REE. Jones et al. (48) found that heart rate, respiratory rate, and REE in stable infants < 4 months of age increase immediately after the operation, but return to baseline values within 12–24 hr. Puhakka et al. (51) reported similar results in infants up to 1 year of age. There are presently no data on the long-term changes in REE, if any, that occur in infants after cardiac surgery. However, infants with ventricular

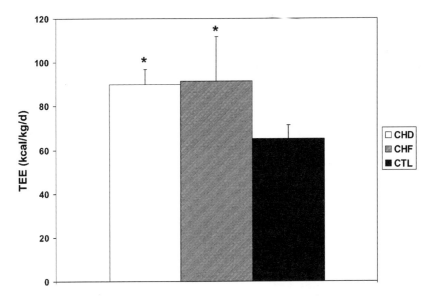

Figure 4 Comparison of literature data for TEEs of infants with CHD and CHF ranging in age from 3 to 5 months. The TEE of infants with CHD and CHF are significantly increased relative to that of healthy age-matched control (CTL) infants ($p \leq 0.01$).

septal defects have been shown to have accelerated weight gain after surgery as compared to infants undergoing repair of tetralogy of Fallot (38,52) or transposition of the great arteries (38). One possible explanation of these results is a gradual decrease in energy expenditure in infants after surgical repair, thus effectively making additional energy available for growth.

ENERGY INTAKE

Poor nutrition may play a major role in growth retardation in patients with CHD, and may be especially important in patients with CHF (4,17,18,20,27,35,37,39,53–56). Some investigators have reported caloric intakes in these patients that are lower than expected for chronological age or body weight (4,20,35,37,56), while others have reported adequate caloric intake for age and weight (7,9,10). Several authors (6,19,20,22,33) have shown a correlation between inadequate caloric intake and malnutrition in infants with CHD. Although no definitive explanation for malnutrition in these patients exists at the present time, several possibilities for decreased caloric intake in these infants have been proposed, including fatigue upon feeding, anorexia, vomiting, and fluid restriction (4,37,43,57).

Malabsorption of available nutrients has also been suggested as a cause of growth failure in infants with CHD. Sondheimer and Hamilton (5) speculated that gastrointestinal maturation and function were delayed in children with severe CHD. No consistent pattern of gastrointestinal abnormality was seen in the infants studied; protein-losing enteropathy and steatorrhea were the most common problems noted. Excessive protein losses were reported in 4 out of 8 children with cyanotic CHD and in 4 out of 12 children with CHF. All patients remained in positive nitrogen balance during the study period. Major gastrointestinal malformations are found in approximately 8% of infants with CHD (58). Nutrient intake in patients with CHF may also be decreased due to hepatomegaly causing reduced gastric volume and increased discomfort.

It has also been proposed that CHF may cause edema of the gut leading to dysmotility and malabsorption (5,56).

Additional evidence for insufficient caloric intake in these patients can be found from studies demonstrating short-term gains in weight and/or length in response to enteral feedings (37,53,54,56). In each of these studies, a caloric intake of 140–200 kcal/kg/day was required to cause catch-up growth. These caloric intakes were only achieved through the use of 24-hr nasogastric or duodenal feedings. Only 50% of the infants studied gained weight on a caloric intake of 149 kcal/kg/day, with consistent weight gain occurring only in patients receiving over 170 kcal/kg/day. However, all these studies clearly demonstrated that infants with CHD do grow when given a large caloric intake, regardless of the type of lesion or presence of CHF.

Table 1 summarizes the results of several studies in which caloric intakes were measured in infants with CHD and/or

Table 1 Energy Intake in Infants with CHD and CHF and Age-Matched Healthy Infants

Group	Age (months)	Energy intake (kcal/kg/day)	Typical energy intake (59) (kcal/kg/day)	Reference
CHD	2.5	107	100	19
CHD	2.6	76	96	35
CHD	5.0	103	94	45
CHD	0.5	97	120	7
CHD	3.0	102	95	7
CHD	4.1	91	95	9
CHD	4.1	88	95	10
CHF	3.2	108	95	19
CHF	4.2	95	95	37
CHF	2.9	105	95	35
CHF	4.0	132	96	45
CHF	4.3	103	95	8
CHF	4.2	102	95	10
Mean ± SD				
CHD	3.1 ± 1.5	94.9 ± 10.7	99.3 ± 9.3	
CHF	3.8 ± 0.6	107.5 ± 12.8	95.2 ± 0.4	
All	3.4 ± 1.2	100.7 ± 13.0	97.4 ± 6.9	

CHF. Several different methods were used in these studies to assess caloric intake: dietary records (37,45), energy balance techniques (35), and isotope dilution (7–9). These results are compared with values for typical daily caloric intakes of healthy age-matched infants (59). All daily caloric intakes are expressed in units of kcal/kg/day to facilitate comparison among the different studies. The results of these studies show that infants with CHD do have a slightly lower daily caloric intake than typical age-matched infants (94.9 ± 10.7 kcal/ kg/day for infants with CHD vs. 99.3 ± 9.3 kcal/kg/day for healthy infants). However, infants with CHF appear to have higher daily caloric intakes than those of typical age-matched infants (107.5 ± 12.8 kcal/kg/ day for infants with CHF vs. 95.2 ± 0.4 kcal/kg/day for age-matched healthy infants). Since the infants with CHD and/or CHF were noted to be smaller than normal for age, this would indicate that the daily caloric intakes in these infants are appropriate for age, but are not adequate to meet daily energy requirements for normal growth and certainly inadequate for catch-up growth.

Malnutrition and growth disturbances related to CHD or CHF in this population might ultimately result in increased surgical risk at the time of palliation or repair (4,60). These infants and children are also at risk for the consequences of long-term malnutrition including continued growth failure even after surgical repair, and delayed motor and cognitive development (61).

NUTRITIONAL SUPPORT

The major goals of nutritional support for these patients are to provide sufficient calories and protein to allow for normal growth and to prevent the breakdown of lean body mass. In addition, it is necessary to provide sufficient calories to make up for past deficiencies and to allow for catch-up growth. It has been estimated that energy intakes of ~150 kcal/kg/day or greater would be required in order to achieve normal weight gain during the early life (37,45,53,54,56). Due to restricted fluid intake and the use of diuretic therapy, the caloric density of infant formula or breast milk may have to be increased to 30 kcal/oz or greater (37). Achieving sufficient energy intake while limiting fluid intake may require the use of a nasogastric tube or gastrostomy.

There is little known about the protein metabolism or protein requirements of infants with CHD. Breast milk and most commercially available infant formulas typically contain between 5% and 12% of total calories as protein. Fomon and Ziegler (62) have suggested a formula of 9% protein, 60% carbohydrate, and 31% fat for infants with CHD. Once the protein needs are met, the caloric value of the formula or breast milk may be increased by addition of glucose polymer or fat (35).

Patients undergoing diuretic treatment may also have electrolyte imbalances and may require supplementation. Potassium and chloride depletions are common and calcium, magnesium, and zinc may also be depleted (63).

SUMMARY

Growth retardation occurs frequently in infants and children with CHD, and the severity of growth retardation appears to be greatest in patients with CHF. Energy intake less than energy expenditure is undoubtedly a significant factor in these patients. Some patients with CHD simply consume too few calories to permit adequate growth. However, it appears that many of these patients are in fact consuming adequate caloric intake for age, yet still experience growth delay. This would indicate that either substantial malabsorption of nutrient intake occurs in these infants and children or that their energy expenditures are higher than those of age-matched healthy children. The data currently available do not indicate that malabsorption is a significant problem in this population as a whole.

Numerous studies have demonstrated increased metabolic rates in infants and children with CHD. The bulk of the evidence indicates that these infants have significantly elevated metabolic rates compared to healthy age-matched infants. Although caloric intake of infants with CHD or CHF may be adequate for age, it is inadequate to meet these substantially increased energy expenditures and still allows normal growth or catch-up growth to occur. High caloric intakes are required to make up nutritional deficits in order to allow for growth and normal neurodevelopment and to decrease surgical risk.

Additional studies are needed of the energy expenditures of patients with specific cardiac defects, and especially of patients with CHF, in order to accurately assess their caloric requirements. Dietary intervention studies can then be designed to supply sufficient caloric intake to exceed energy expenditure and permitting normal growth in these patients.

REFERENCES

1. Menahem S, Venables AW. Pulmonary artery banding in isolated or complicated ventricular septal defects. Brit Heart J 1972; 34:87–94.
2. Krovetz L. Weight gain in children with patent ductus arteriosus. Dis Chest 1963; 44:273.
3. Suoninen P. Physical growth of children with congenital heart disease. Acta Paediatr Scand 1971; 225(suppl):1–50.
4. Krieger I. Growth failure and congenital heart disease. Energy balance in infants. Am J Dis Child 1970; 120:497–502.
5. Sondheimer J, Hamilton J. Intestinal function in infants with severe congenital heart disease. J Pediatr 1978; 92:572–578.
6. Stocker F, Wilkoff W, Miettinen O, Nadas A. Oxygen consumption in infants with heart disease: relationship to severity of congestive heart failure, relative weight, and caloric intake. J Pediatr 1972; 80:43–51.
7. Leitch CA, Karn CA, Peppard RJ, et al. Increased energy expenditure in infants with cyanotic congenital heart disease. J Pediatr 1998; 133:755–760.
8. Leitch C, Wright-Coltart S, Schamberger M, Farrell A. Energy expenditure in infants with hypoplastic left heart syndrome. Pediatr Res 2002; 51:39A.
9. Ackerman IL, Karn CA, Denne SC, Ensing GJ, Leitch CA. Total but not resting energy expenditure is increased in infants with ventricular septal defects. Pediatrics 1998; 102:1172–1177.
10. Farrell A, Schamberger M, Olson I, Leitch C. Large left to right shunts and congestive heart failure increase total energy expenditure in infants with ventricular septal defect. Am J Cardiol 2001; 87:1128–1131.

11. Mehrizi A, Drash A. Growth disturbance in congenital heart disease. J Pediatr 1962; 61:418–429.

12. Linde L, Rasof B, Dunn J. Longitudinal studies of intellectual and behavioral development in children with congenital heart disease. Acta Paediat Scand 1970; 59:169–176.

13. Campbell M, Reynolds G. The physical and mental development of children with congenital heart disease. Arch Dis Child 1949; 24:294.

14. Stoch MB, Smythe PM, Moodie AD, Bradshaw D. Psychosocial outcome and CT findings after gross undernourishment during infancy: a 20-year developmental study. Dev Med Child Neurol 1982; 24:419–436.

15. Cameron JW, Rosenthal A, Olson AD. Malnutrition in hospitalized children with congenital heart disease. Arch Pediatr Adolesc Med 1995; 149:1098–1102.

16. Naeye R. Anatomic features of growth failure in congenital heart disease. Pediatrics 1967; 29:433–440.

17. Bayer L, Robinson S. Growth history of children with congenital heart diseases. Am J Dis Child 1969; 117:564–572.

18. Feldt R, Strickler G, Weidman W. Growth of children with congenital heart disease. Am J Dis Child 1969; 117:573–579.

19. Huse D, Feldt R, Nelson R, Novak L. Infants with congenital heart disease. Am J Dis Child 1975; 129:65–69.

20. Menon G, Poskitt E. Why does congenital heart disease cause failure to thrive?. Arch Dis Child 1985; 60:1134–1139.

21. Thommessen M, Heiberg A, Kase B, Larsen S, Riis G. Feeding problems, height and weight in different groups of disabled children. Acta Paediatr Scand 1991; 80:527–533.

22. Thommessen M, Heiberg A, Kase B. Feeding problems in children with congenital heart disease: the impact on energy intake and growth outcome. Eur J Clin Nutr 1992; 46:457–464.

23. Umansky R, Hauck A. Factors in the growth of children with patent ductus arteriosus. Pediatrics 1962; 30:540–550.

24. Robinson S, Bayer L. Growth history of children with congenital heart defects. I. Effects of operative intervention. Child Dev 1969; 40:315–346.

25. Strangeway A, Fowler R, Cunningham K, Hamilton J. Diet and growth in congenital heart disease. J Pediatr 1976; 57:57–86.

26. Greecher C. Congenital heart disease: a nutritional challenge. Nutr Focus 1990; 5:1–6.

27. Salzer H, Haschke F, Wimmer M, Heil M, Schilling R. Growth and nutritional intake of infants with congenital heart disease. J Pediatr Cardiol 1989; 10:17–23.

28. Danilowicz D, Presti S, Colvin S, Galloway A, Langsner A, Doyle E. Results of urgent or emergency repair for symptomatic infants under one year of age with single or multiple ventricular septal defect. Am J Cardiol 1992; 69:699–701.

29. Adams F, Lund G, Disenhouse R. Observations on the physique and growth of children with congenital heart disease. J Pediatr 1954; 44:674–680.
30. Aisenberg R, Rosenthal A, Nadas A, Wolff P. Developmental delay in infants with congenital heart disease: correlation with hypoxemia and congestive heart failure. Ped Cardiol 1982; 3:133–137.
31. White R Jr, Jordan C, Fischer K, et al. Delayed skeletal growth and maturation in adolescent congenital heart disease. Invest Radiol 1971; 6:326–332.
32. Castenada A, Meyer J, Jonas R, Lock J, Wessel D, Hickey P. The neonate with critical congenital heart disease: repair—a surgical challenge. J Thorac Cardiovasc Surg 1989; 98:869–875.
33. Unger R, DeKleermaeker M, Gidding S. Improved weight gain with dietary intervention in congenital heart disease. AJDC 1992; 146:1078–1084.
34. Forchielli M, McColl R, Walker W, Lo C. Children with congenital heart disease: a nutrition challenge. Nutr Rev 1994; 52:348–353.
35. Jackson M, Poskitt E. The effects of high-energy feeding on energy balance and growth in infants with congenital heart disease and failure to thrive. Br J Nutr 1991; 65:131–143.
36. Hansen S, Dorup I. Energy and nutrient intakes in congenital heart disease. Acta Paediatr 1993; 82:166–172.
37. Schwarz S, Gewitz M, See C, et al. Enteral nutrition in infants with congenital heart disease and growth failure. Pediatrics 1990; 86:368–373.
38. Sholler G, Celermajer J. Cardiac surgery in the first year of life: the effect on weight gain of infants with congenital heart disease. Acta Paediatr J 1986; 22:305–308.
39. Levy RJ, Rosenthal A, Castaneda AR, Nadas AS. Growth after surgical repair of simple D-transposition of the great arteries. Ann Thoracic Surg 1978; 25:225–230.
40. Levy R, Rosenthal A, Miettinen O, Nadas A. Determinants of growth in patients with ventricular septal defect. Circulation 1978; 57: 793–797.
41. Weintraub RG, Menahem S. Early surgical closure of a large ventricular septal defect: influence on long-term growth. J Am Coll Cardiol 1991; 18:552–558.
42. Schuurmans F, Pulles-Heintzberger C, Gerver W, Kester A, P-Ph Forget. Long-term growth of children with congenital heart disease: a retrospective study. Acta Paediatr 1998; 87:1250–1255.
43. Lees M, Bristow J, Griswold H, Olmsted R. Relative hypermetabolism in infants with congenital heart disease and undernutrition. Pediatrics 1965; 36:183–191.
44. Krauss A, Auld A. Metabolic rate of neonates with congenital heart disease. Arch Disease Child 1975; 50:539–541.

45. Barton J, Hindmarsh P, Scrimgeour C, Rennie M, Preece M. Energy expenditure in congenital heart disease. Arch Dis Child 1994; 70: 5–9.

46. Mitchell I, Davies P, Day J, Pollock J, Jamieson M, Wheatley D. Energy expenditure in children with congenital heart disease, before and after cardiac surgery. J Thorac Cardiovasc Surg 1994; 107:374–380.

47. Shanbhogue R, Lloyd D. Absence of hypermetabolism after operation in the newborn infant. JPEN 1992; 16:333–336.

48. Jones M, Pierro A, Hammond P, Lloyd D. The effect of major operations on heart rate, respiratory rate, physical activity, temperature and respiratory gas exchange in infants. Eur J Pediatr Surg 1995; 5:9–12.

49. Jones M, Pierro A, Hammond P, Lloyd D. The metabolic response to operative stress in infants. J Pediatr Surg 1993; 128:1258–1263.

50. Gebara B, Gelmini M, Sarnaik A. Oxygen consumption, energy expenditure, and substrate utilization after cardiac surgery in children. Crit Care Med 1992; 20:1550–1554.

51. Puhakka K, Rasanen J, Leijala M, Peltola K. Oxygen consumption following pediatric cardiac surgery. J Cardiothorac Vasc Anesthesia 1994; 8:642–648.

52. Gingell R, Pieroni D, Hornung M. Growth problems associated with congenital heart disease in infancy. Lebenthal E, ed. Textbook of Gastroenterology and Nutrition in Infancy. New York: Raven, 1981: 853–860.

53. Bougle D, Iselin M, Kahyat A, Duhamel J-F. Nutritional treatment of congenital heart disease. Arch Dis Child 1986; 61:799–801.

54. Vanderhoof J, Hofschire P, Baluff M, et al. Continuous enteral feedings. An important adjunct to the management of complex congenital heart disease. Am J Dis Child 1982; 136:825–827.

55. Baum D, Beck R, Kodama A, Brown B. Early heart failure as a cause of growth and tissue disorders in children with congenital heart disease. Circulation 1980; 62:1145–1151.

56. Yahav J, Avigad S, Frand M, et al. Assessment of intestinal and cardiorespiratory function in children with congenital heart disease on high-caloric formulas. J Pediatr Gastroenterol Nutr 1985; 4: 778–785.

57. Weintraub R, Menahem S. Growth and congenital heart disease. J Paediatr Child Health 1993; 29:95–98.

58. Rosenthal A. Congenital cardiac anomalies and gastrointestinal malformations. In: Pierpont M, Moller J, eds. Genetics of Cardiovascular Disease. Boston: Martinus Nijhoff, 1987:113–126.

59. Fomon S, Bell E. Energy. In: Fomon S, ed. Nutrition of Normal Infants. St. Louis: Mosby Yearbook Inc., 1993:103–120.

60. Balaguru D, Artman M, Auslender M. Management of heart failure in children. Curr Problems Pediatr 2000; 30:1–35.

61. Loeffel F. Developmental considerations of infants and children with congenital heart disease. Heart Lung 1985; 14:214–217.
62. Fomon SJ, Ziegler EE. Nutritional management of infants with congenital heart disease. Am Heart J 1972; 83:581–588.
63. Kleinman R.E. ed. Pediatric Nutrition Handbook. Elk Grove Village: American Academy of Pediatrics, 2004.

17

Heart Failure Postpediatric Heart Transplantation

MARK BOUCEK

Department of Pediatric Cardiology,
The Children's Hospital/UCHSC,
Denver, Colorado, U.S.A.

BACKGROUND

Cardiomyopathic disease is the most common diagnosis leading to heart transplantation in pediatric recipients. In transplanted infants less than 1 year of age about 30% had the diagnosis of myopathy. For the childhood age years, the percentage increases to 52% and for the adolescent population about 62% (1). The current pediatric transplant survival curves suggest a graft half-life of approximately 15 years and probably longer for infant and childhood recipients (1). These results are encouraging for patients who have undergone orthotopic cardiac transplantation.

One does not normally think of heart failure occurring post-transplant. However, the survival data also imply that there are a significant number of patients (approximately 35% by 15 years) that are at risk for heart failure and either death or the need for retransplantation. Of patients with late death following transplantation 30% have coronary vasculopathy potentially leading to ischemic myopathy, another 12% have acute rejection, and 20% are coded as having graft failure (1). Thus, heart failure remains a threat even following orthotopic cardiac transplantation.

In nontransplanted pediatric patients, myopathic disease is frequently due to metabolic or genetic causes in about one-third of patients and approximately 50% have underlying congenital heart disease (2). Classic myocarditis or inflammatory myopathy is felt to occur infrequently, in perhaps 5–10% of pediatric patients with heart failure. The transplant recipient has a different spectrum of etiologies leading to heart failure than their pediatric myopathic counterparts. In fact, the heart transplant recipient is more imitative of the etiologies leading to heart failure in adults where ischemic etiologies play a greater role in the development of late heart failure (3).

Although there are both immune and nonimmune factors that could lead to heart failure following transplantation, orthotopic cardiac replacement is fundamentally an immunologic event. These factors are listed in Table 1. Post-transplant the rate of myopathic disease progression due to immune factors

Table 1 Heart Failure Following Cardiac Transplantation

Immune factors	Nonimmune factors
1. Cytokine induced depressed myocyte function	Donor ischemic injury
2. Direct myocyte injury and death	Hypertension
3. Vasculopathy and ischemia	Hyperlipidemia
4. Inflammatory induced fibrosus	Atrial ventricular dys-synchrony
5. Conduction system rejection	Tricuspid valve insufficiency from mechanical injury
6. Apoptosis/failure to repair	Neurogenic uncoupling
7. Immunosuppressant drug toxicity	

is often so rapid that nonimmune factors such as donor injury, hypertension, hyperlipidemia, atrial dys-synchrony, and neurogenic uncoupling do not have an opportunity to significantly impair cardiac function before immunologic events intercede. As long-term survival improves due to improved regulation of the immune factors following heart transplantation, it is possible that late heart failure due to nonimmune factors may become more of an issue. Fundamental to both immune and nonimmune mechanisms may be the impaired ability of the transplanted organ to regenerate and recover from insults from any etiology. The role of ongoing programed cell death or apoptosis (4), and the ability of cardiac cellular components to regenerate presumably from local tissue or trafficked stem cells is an unknown area. Regenerative potential could be a significant target of immune mechanisms and a late contributor to heart failure. Thus, even with nonimmune insults to cardiac function immune mechanisms may affect the rate of disease progression.

MECHANISMS

Immunologic mechanisms predominate in situations of heart failure following orthotopic cardiac transplantation in pediatric recipients (Fig. 1). The cardiac allograft presents a number of immunologic targets. Host immune effector mechanisms which attack these diverse targets can present with the final common pathway of heart failure. The allograft presents disparate major HLA antigens to the host. In addition, there are other common disparate antigens on the cellular components of the allograft. Host cellular cytotoxic or humoral (antibody) recognition of these common antigenic differences from the host can result in acute diffuse graft failure. Usually CD8 positive T-lymphocytes recognize class I MHC antigen presentation *directly* from the graft and can function as effector CD8 positive T-cells. CD4 positive T-cells and B-cells can process donor antigen *indirectly* via HLA class II and result in cytokine or antibody mediated direct graft injury and dysfunction (5). Alternatively, CD4 T-cells can provide necessary "help" to CD8 T-cells or cells of the innate immune system to cause graft dysfunction/destruction (6). Antigen

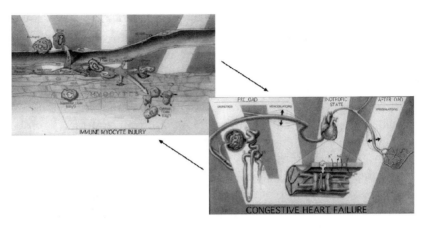

Figure 1 Schematic representation of the interaction between inflammation and immunity, myocyte dysfunction, and the development of congestive heart failure. Conversely, the hemodynamic and neurohumoral derangements with congestive heart failure may lead to altered immune recognition of the myocyte.

presentation through the *direct* pathway does not necessarily require host professional antigen presenting cells (APC) which typically present both MHC class I and class II antigens. Donor professional APCs such as dendritic cells, macrophages, donor T-cells and even endothelial cells on the graft vasculature can also present class II MHC antigens from the graft *directly* to the host T-cell population.

The *direct* pathway and/or *indirect* pathway can lead to injury to the graft at multiple sites including myocytes, often directly through cytokine release such as tumor necrosis factor, IL-6, etc., or through the vascular bed by interrupting microvascular and tissue perfusion (7). This latter effect on the vasculature can add an ischemic component to the inflammatory injury which impairs myocyte function (8). With time, B-lymphocyte contribution can become evident with circulating antibodies which are localized to the myocardium and vasculature triggering complement involvement and widespread inflammatory impairment to graft function.

In addition to the *direct* pathway, antigen from various cellular components of the graft can be processed by host tissue histiocytes and dendritic cells (APCs) which then present the antigen through the MHC class II receptor to host T-cells via the T-cell receptor complex. This activates a population of effector and memory T-cells which can cause acute and recurring injury to the graft directed at any of the cellular components. This *indirect* pathway is felt to be an important mechanism of chronic graft vasculopathy (9). We have already mentioned the myocyte and vascular endothelium but other graft cellular components can become specific targets for immune reactivity. These would include smooth muscle cells, fibroblasts in the interstitium, ganglion cells (Fig. 2), specialized conducting tissue such as the Purkinje fibers and graft based stem cells. The immune system may even differentiate between right and left ventricular myocytes, atrial myocytes, the supporting connective tissue framework, and the epicardial lining of the pericardial sack. Evidence that the immune system has the ability to differentiate cellular components of the donor graft is demonstrated by the specific, yet multiple

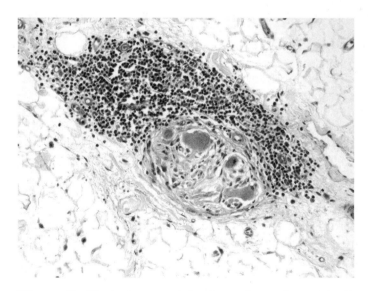

Figure 2 Pentachrome stained specimen demonstrating massive lymphocyte infiltration of a cardiac ganglion and neural vascular bundle (×20).

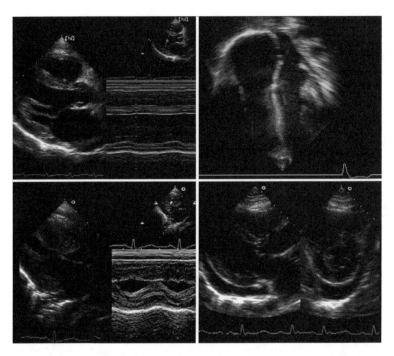

Figure 3 Typical echocardiographic appearances of the four classic patterns of rejection are shown. The upper left panel demonstrates depressed systolic function, ventricular dilatation, and eccentric hypertrophy. The upper right hand panel demonstrates relatively selective right ventricular dilation and dysfunction, a pattern that is frequently associated with severe tricuspid regurgitation. The lower left panel demonstrates a form of rejection relatively unique to pediatric patients associated with marked hypertrophy and left ventricular outflow tract obstruction. The lower right echocardiogram demonstrated a pericardial effusion with preserved ventricular function.

echocardiographic changes associated with acute rejection as shown in Fig. 3. Rejection can cause unique patterns of cardiac dysfunction including ventricular hypertrophy, dilation, valvar insufficiency, and pericardial effusion.

A less well-recognized population of cellular targets is the pluripotent and committed stem cell lineage present throughout the myocardium which may be necessary for myocardial repair (10). If this cell line is immunologically identified by the host, the ability of the graft to repair injury from either immune or nonimmune causes may be compromised. Failure to repair injury may encourage early senescence of a graft even in a pediatric recipient. Whether stem cells of host lineage can replace donor stem cells to repair graft injury is unknown. Reports of host cells populating graft locations have appeared (11). It is uncertain at which stage of cell maturation that graft repopulation occurs. The specific immune mechanisms used in injuring the graft have been described in detail elsewhere (12).

The recognition that immune mechanisms figure prominently in subsequent graft failure and graft loss following heart transplantation has led to expanded pharmacologic approaches to regulating the immune response. Although the pharmaco–immuno therapy that is currently available is much more specific than in the early days of transplantation, many of these drugs affect common cellular pathways of activation (13). These myocellular activation pathways are involved in regeneration, hypertrophy, and function (14). The best understood pharmacologic mechanisms which can interact with cardiac function are the pathways of calcineurin-dependent activation and tacrolimus binding (15). Cyclosporin was the prototypical calcineurin antagonist. Tacrolimus has seen increasing usage at the expense of cyclosporin over the last 10 years. Both of these agents can interfere with important pathways for the development of physiologic and pathologic hypertrophy of the normal heart. Without the coexisting stimulus of inflammation and regeneration, it is uncommon to see a direct effect of these immunomodulators on cardiac function. Patients with renal or hepatic transplantation usually do not show significant cardiac effects from calcineurin inhibitors (15). However, following cardiac transplantation, there are multiple stimuli to the myocyte for hypertrophy, remodeling, and regeneration which may involve the calcineurin pathway. There has been little clinical data which explores the interaction of these immunosuppressive drugs and their therapeutic levels on intrinsic cardiac functional pathways.

In infants and childhood cardiac transplant recipients, a unique scenario of obliterative hypertrophy has been described. This hypertrophic process appears to require the stimuli of rejection but may be an example of disturbed calcineurin pathways (16). Steroids are also widely used in acute and chronic immunosuppressive regimens. Of course, there are direct myocellular effects of chronic steroid administration which can result in hypertrophy and pathologic remodeling leading to impairment in cardiac function. Most immunosuppressive regimens today strive to achieve minimization of the steroid dose and duration of exposure which may abrogate the myotoxic effects of steroids. There are other systemic effects of chronic steroid administration such as hyperlipidemia and hypertension which may interplay with vascular inflammation due to rejection and myocyte remodeling in response to increased afterload. The end result of systemic steroid use creates a hostile environment for the cardiac allograft which enhances graft injury and may have the ultimate deleterious effect of increasing graft antigen presentation to the host with subsequent immunologic injury.

The remainder of this chapter will focus on the timing of heart failure postheart transplantation with an evaluation of acute graft dysfunction occurring within the first six months after transplantation and late graft dysfunction which occurs between six months to years following the transplant event. Finally, a brief discussion of treatment mechanisms that are unique to the post-transplant recipient who develops heart failure will be discussed.

EARLY GRAFT FAILURE

Heart failure which occurs in the first six months after transplant is most likely due to graft injury occurring at the time of organ donation/at transplant or acute allograft rejection (1). Early graft dysfunction can have multiple etiologies including injury associated with the cause of brain death in the donor, brain death itself and ischemia from donor organ procurement, transport and implantation (17). Graft injury at the time of transplant is usually but not always reversible.

The repair mechanisms needed to recover graft function may also be injured. The process of injury and repair is associated with inflammatory signals (18) which may interact with the other main mechanism of dysfunction, early acute rejection. Cell death due to ischemia or injury, unlike programed cell death, causes a local inflammatory reaction. The inflammatory reaction presents markers of injury recognized as danger by the immune effector cells. The immune cells are then activated to eliminate inflammatory and cellular debris.

In the case of organ transplantation, antigens unique to the graft are presented in this environment of injury and inflammation to a sensitized host immune system. This early sequence of events can lead to the development of memory T-cells which have become sensitized to graft antigens (19). These memory T-cells are a legacy which represent a future threat of graft rejection/injury which extends beyond the leading cause of early graft failure, early acute allograft rejection.

Graft dysfunction due to donor or transplant related issues is usually reversible over days to months. Systolic dysfunction returns to normal within days but diastolic parameters may take weeks to recover (20). Fibrosis occurring in response to severe graft injury may cause diastolic dysfunction that can persist indefinitely. In fact, restrictive filling patterns have been described in heart transplant recipients even years post-transplant (21). Early graft systolic dysfunction responds to the usual combination of inotropic and vasodilating agents. Milrinone is most frequently used and has the additional benefit of pulmonary vasodilation which can improve right ventricular dysfunction. When the ischemic injury to the graft is severe, thinning of the myocardial wall occurs with dilation of the ventricle. The resulting eccentric hypertrophy and systolic dysfunction may persist and appears in many respects like a typical dilated cardiomyopathy. Our experience suggests that these dilated dysfunctional allografts may slowly demonstrate remodeling over years but do not fully recover the appropriate wall stress relationship and remain at risk for late progression to heart failure with or without graft rejection (Fig. 4). The presence of heart block in the graft is associated with ventricular dysfunction that is due to severe graft injury and is a marker for dysfunction that likely will persist for years.

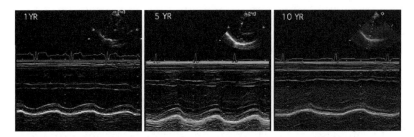

Figure 4 Serial M mode echocardiographic studies performed at 1, 5, and 10 years post-transplant in a patient with ischemic donor injury at the time of transplant. There has been little change or remodeling present in the graft which continues with adequate cardiac function up to 10 years post-transplant.

Acute allograft rejection is the leading cause of early graft failure. Mature memory T-cells with pre-existing receptors for graft antigens can differentiate and mount an immunologic attack against the graft within days. Sensitized hosts are at greatest risk of acute graft injury. Even without prior sensitization, the host immune system may become activated by graft antigens within days to weeks. The greatest risk for acute rejection and graft failure occurs within 2–6 weeks after transplant (22). As mentioned earlier, there is likely an interaction between graft injury at transplant, inflammation and later acute allograft rejection. Thus, at the time of transplant, nonimmune graft insults magnify the potential for immunologic recognition of the graft as danger and subsequent acute rejection and development of memory T-cells. These memory T-cells remain a risk for activation and rejection years into the future.

DIAGNOSIS OF ACUTE REJECTION

Acute graft rejection can occur at anytime post-transplant with a peak incidence at 6 weeks and then decreasing to basal levels by six months post-transplant. Much ado has been made concerning the diagnosis of acute rejection (23). Still the criteria for rejection are largely institution specific (24).

When heart failure occurs in the early weeks to months posttransplant, the diagnosis of acute graft rejection is always primary. Confirmation with histology on endomyocardial biopsy (EMB) may or may not be helpful. In fact, patients with heart failure frequently lack the typical findings on EMB of lymphocyte infiltration (25). Pediatric patients with clinical evidence of heart failure and echocardiographic evidence of ventricular dysfunction have the greatest risk of dying from acute rejection regardless of the findings on biopsy (26). The EMB may be most helpful in excluding other causes of heart failure such as infection with cytomegaloviruses or infiltration such as a lymphoproliferative process.

The diagnosis of acute graft rejection causing heart failure is presumptive and is confirmed by clinical and echocardiographic response to rejection therapy. Rejection may be recalcitrant to conventional treatment with corticosteroids and or anti-T-cell antibodies. The diagnosis of rejection remains foremost particularly if other rare forms of myopathy are excluded on biopsy or serologic testing. Persistence with antirejection therapy is required and may respond to an escalation in treatment such as the use of plasmapheresis (27).

CLINICAL PRESENTATION OF ACUTE REJECTION

Acute allograft rejection is an immune initiated event that may have multiple mechanisms. Immune cytokine mediators such as TNF or IL_{2-6} can have a direct myocardial depressant effect (28). Direct cytotoxicity can also occur with myocyte death or triggered apoptosis (29). Vascular compromise can occur following direct endothelial injury and disturbed permeability or microvascular function. Antibody deposition and complement activation can amplify the immune response causing loss of vascular integrity, thrombosis, and ischemia (30). This particular scenario has been termed vascular rejection, a clinically severe form of rejection which may be difficult to treat with usual therapies (31).

The earliest clinical presentation of acute rejection reflects the early hemodynamic effects of rejection. Diastolic function is usually impaired first resulting in elevated filling pressures, congestion, and edema. This early phase may be seen with relatively preserved systolic function on echo and only mild changes in cardiac output. With time, the diastolic dysfunction may progress to ventricular dilation. However, in the setting of acute rejection early post-transplant, the immune response is usually vigorous and systolic dysfunction rapidly ensues. Cardiac output then becomes markedly impaired with subsequent renal insufficiency and end organ ischemia. Heart failure in this scenario may still be (usually is) reversible but requires emergent therapy and cardiovascular support possibly including ventricular assist or ECMO.

Heart failure from rejection may have an insidious onset but once present, clinical deterioration is rapid and, there is little myocardial reserve since the myocardium is acutely inflamed. Thus, the goal of most immunosuppressive regimens is to suppress early graft rejection while the inflammation from the surgery subsides and immune regulation can develop. As the environment "cools" late after transplant, the immune response usually is less vigorous and rejection develops more slowly allowing clinical presentation, diagnosis, and treatment. Most rejection surveillance protocols also aim to detect rejection before clinical symptoms of heart failure develop. Like rejection diagnosis, rejection surveillance protocols are largely institution specific and none are perfect. Thus, the goal of transplant programs is to eliminate the substrate for allograft rejection and prevention of the immunologic cascade leading to graft injury. Since, immunosuppression alone is either ineffective or toxic, strategies to encourage immune tolerance have been forefront in clinical transplantation. To date, the goal is still elusive.

LATE HEART FAILURE POST TRANSPLANTATION

Heart failure presenting after the first six months post-transplant can be subdivided into acute and chronic heart failure. Acute presentation of the clinical symptoms of heart failure along with measures of myocardial dysfunction indicates allograft rejection. There is a low but constant hazard for late acute rejection months or years post-transplant. The reasons why a previously quiescent immune system becomes activated and results in acute graft dysfunction are largely unknown. Antecedent infections with activation of the immune system which results in a spillover leading to allograft rejection has been implicated but there are little hard data to make a definite cause and effect. Injury to the allograft such as with viral myocarditis could present graft antigens again in an inflamed environment (32) prompting the immune system to react to antigens it had previously tolerated. The late surviving cardiac allograft acts as a chimeric state since foreign antigens are coexisting with the host. In a truly tolerant situation, the cardiac allograft would help to maintain tolerance toward its own antigens within the host. However, following transplantation, true tolerance and true chimerism are rarely achieved. Rather a state of peripheral regulation of the immune system by regulatory T-cells allows the graft to continue to survive despite its antigenic differences and recognition of those differences by the immune system (33). These regulatory T-cells populations are being increasingly recognized as the critical step necessary for long-term graft function (34). Another possible scenario to explain late acute rejection could be that an antecedent infection has a suppressive affect on these regulatory T-cells allowing the immune system to mount an alloimmune response toward the graft.

Early events at the time of transplantation likely leave a legacy well into the future. Rejection occurring within the first year post-transplant has been related to an increased risk for late rejection and death years post-transplant (1). Perhaps both the strength of the immune response to the graft antigens at the time of transplantation and the strength of the regulatory cell population that developed post-transplantation dictate a balance leading to graft survival. Factors that would encourage an immune response to graft antigens in a hostile fashion at the time of transplant would tilt the balance toward rejection occurring at any time. On the other hand, stimulation of regulatory pathways at the time of transplant probably protects against rejection throughout the life of the graft. Unfortunately, these same regulatory cell lines can be immunosuppressed by the drugs used to control the native immune response to the allograft. Thus, there may be a complex interaction between sensitization, regulation and immunosuppression. The immunosuppressive protocol may be the wild card that has the potential both to suppress rejection and suppress tolerizing or regulatory T-cell pathways.

ADOLESCENT RECIPIENTS

In adolescent heart transplant recipients, there appears to be a greater risk of late rejection and death as compared to childhood or infant recipients. The decrement in survival with time for adolescents appears steeper than younger recipients throughout 15 years of followup (1). There is uncertainty as to whether this "adolescent risk" is a biologic phenomenon associated with pubertal changes, etc., or a behavioral phenomenon. In adolescents, with many forms of chronic disease, noncompliance with medical regimen is part and parcel of the drive for independence and autonomy critical to adolescent development. Reports in heart transplantation have also indicated a real problem with noncompliance and subsequent acute rejection and death (35). The issue of adolescent noncompliance has been a subject of intense interest but therapeutic futility. It would seem that the adolescent is destined to challenge the vulnerability associated with stopping immunosuppressive medications.

If this were the only explanation for the "adolescent risk," then we should see an increase in mortality in childhood and infant recipients as they reach adolescent years. However, if there are developmental changes in the immune system at the time of transplant with adolescence that affect the balance between regulation and rejection, then they may be at increased risk of acute rejection regardless of compliance. If there are immunologic differences at the time of transplant, perhaps the infant and childhood recipient would be somewhat more protected when they reach adolescence and become noncompliant since they would have years of graft survival in the host and presumably well-developed regulatory T-cell populations. In either case, the dilemma of adolescents and medical noncompliance gives urgency to protocols which would enhance the development of tolerance to the allograft.

LATE ALLOGRAFT REJECTION

The presentation and diagnosis of acute allograft rejection resulting in heart failure late post-transplant is a little different than what is seen with the patient in the early post-transplant period. Patients who are years out from transplant generally are not undergoing the same degree of immune/rejection surveillance by the health care team. Also, the patient and the family tend to be less acutely tuned to changes which might suggest graft rejection. Thus, patients presenting with late rejection often have been ill for days and perhaps weeks and characteristically will show the echocardiographic changes of acute ventricular dilatation and abnormal left ventricular systolic function. The filling pressures are usually markedly elevated and the patients present with the symptoms of congestive failure and low cardiac output. As mentioned earlier, the EMB may or may not be diagnostic in such a setting. The identification of a relatively acute change certainly points toward the diagnosis of acute rejection. Treatment with antirejection therapy is similar to what is used in the early post-transplant period. The response to treatment in patients who have late rejection is usually quite slow and the patients may be critically ill for several days before significant improvement is detected. If the treatment is initiated and the patient responds, one would expect slow but near complete recovery. The slow rate of recovery in patients with late presenting rejection may be in part due to the fact that the rejection has been present for some time before medical attention was sought.

Heart failure that occurs late after the transplant procedure that has a more insidious onset is usually not due to acute allograft rejection. In the registry of the International Society of Heart and Lung Transplantation, approximately 20% of patients with late mortality are coded as having graft failure rather than acute rejection. This late graft failure can have both immune and nonimmune contributors. Allograft vasculopathy and subsequent myocardial ischemia can develop over months with a progressive deterioration in cardiac function. This ischemic form of heart failure is more akin to what would be seen in adult patients with advanced atherosclerotic disease. However, the rate of progression in the transplant recipient is accelerated. Post-transplant graft vasculopathy is an immune related event felt to be due to indirect antigen presentation and CD4 T-cell activation and assault toward both the endothelium and vessel wall (9,36). This immunologic process leads to intimal proliferation, loss of endothelial responses and regulation, and ultimately vessel occlusion. Antirejection therapy can slow or even halt the progress of graft vasculopathy (9,37). We have noted regression in graft vasculopathy with rejection therapy (Fig. 5). If the rate of progression is retarded with therapeutic maneuvers, then this form of graft vasculopathy can take on many of the features more typical of atherosclerotic disease in the normal adult host. In its aggressive form, the disease is diffuse throughout the vascular bed although there may be focal areas of accentuation. With loss of microvascular function, there can be subendocardial ischemia and subsequent fibrosis with a slow progression

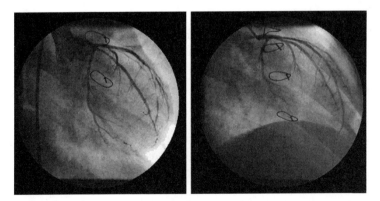

Figure 5 Left coronary artery angiography demonstrating severe post-transplant coronary artery disease in the left coronary artery system, particularly the left anterior descending. In the right hand panel, a followup study approximately 1 year later demonstrates improvement in the severe luminal irregularities, stenosis, and beading noted in the initial study shown in the left hand panel.

toward ventricular dysfunction. Once ventricular dysfunction and heart failure have developed in response to graft vasculopathy, there are few, if any, therapeutic options other than proceeding with retransplantation. Appropriate surveillance and early detection of graft vasculopathy and institution of therapeutic regimens may prevent progression and the development of ischemic myopathy and late heart failure.

Heart failure may also occur without graft vasculopathy. In these patients, the mechanisms are less clear. As discussed at the beginning of this chapter, it is possible that the repair mechanisms intrinsic to myocardial homeostasis and function could be targets of an immune response otherwise unrecognized. The ability of stem cells to replenish and repair the intact myocardium is an area of active research and the transplant patient may in fact be a model of failure to repair. These patients with late graft failure and a normal vascular supply often have an EMB that is unremarkable in terms of the inflammatory reaction. The typical findings on EMB are that of extensive fibrosis (Fig. 6). As mentioned earlier, pediatric

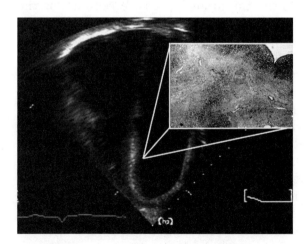

Figure 6 Apical echocardiographic image and histologic insert of a patient with late restrictive physiology and normal coronary arteries. The insert demonstrates the pale area consisting of fibrotic tissue that was extensive throughout the myocardium despite a minimal history of rejection.

patients frequently show restrictive physiology with invasive evaluation performed late post-transplant (21). This observation provides further credence for failure to repair either a previous injury or an ongoing remodeling of the ventricular mass. Diagnostically, the presentation of late congestive failure with ventricular dilatation and dysfunction and an unremarkable EMB and coronary angiography leads to the diagnosis of the syndrome of late graft failure. These patients clinically have a slow progression of disease and may be candidates for the usual therapeutic regimen employed for heart failure although data on therapeutic regimens in transplant recipients are lacking. These treatments are discussed elsewhere throughout this book and will not be repeated at this point.

NONIMMUNE CAUSES OF LATE HEART FAILURE

The nonimmune causes of late graft dysfunction and heart failure can be due to the immunosuppressive regimen or the rejection surveillance regimen. Hypertension is a frequent morbidity following heart transplantation occurring in as many as 60% by 5 years and has been associated with steroid immunosuppressive use (1). The calcineurin antagonist, cyclosporin and tacrolimus, may also cause chronic long-term renal dysfunction leading to hypertension (38). The class of immunosuppressive agents that operate through the target of rapamycin (TOR) also can have nephrotoxic and hyperlipidemic effects (39). The TOR class of immunosuppressive agents has become an area of great interest since they are known to inhibit smooth muscle proliferation and may interfere with growth factors necessary for the development of graft vasculopathy. This may be a therapeutic line that will see increasing use in an attempt to limit the development or progressive graft vasculopathy (37). However, the TOR class of immunosuppressive agents may have toxicity beyond the renal system which could affect graft remodeling and late graft function and long-term followup with rapamycin is lacking.

Rejection surveillance is frequently done with the use of EMB. Generally, the biopsy procedure is a low risk and low morbidity procedure, but, at least in adult heart transplant recipients, there is a troubling late occurrence of severe tricuspid insufficiency possibly related to biopsy injury (40). Patients with severe tricuspid insufficiency can present with late heart failure and impairment of left ventricular function due to severe right ventricular volume overload. Repair or replacement of the tricuspid valve may relieve the symptoms of heart failure in this group of patients. Tricuspid repair may be required in up to 5% of transplant recipients at some point (41).

The cardiac allograft is denervated at the time of transplant and depends on circulating hormones to respond to physiologic demand. There is probably some degree of reinnervation in most transplant recipients but often it is incomplete (42). The lack of neurohumoral coupling between the graft and the circulatory system can impair the response to exercise need and result in symptoms of exercise induced cardiac insufficiency. However, in most patients, this uncoupling is clinically silent or can be corrected for with conscious anticipation and preparation for exercise. Occasionally, pacemaker therapy has been required (43). The role of the neuroendocrine system in maintenance of cardiac homeostasis has not been worked out in light of the denervation or incomplete reinnervation of the cardiac transplant recipient and may contribute to the risk of late heart failure.

Rarely, a reoccurrence of the primary disease process that resulted in the need for transplantation can occur in the cardiac allograft as well. Patients with hemochromatosis secondary to repeated transfusions could be an example of recurrence of native disease.

The therapeutic responses to the nonimmune causes for late heart failure post-transplantation are dependent on an appropriate diagnosis. In some cases, this may lead to a specific treatment such as tricuspid valve repair; in others, nonspecific heart failure therapy may be all that can be offered. As yet, there are not enough late survivors who have developed nonspecific heart failure post-transplantation to make any prognostic certainties. However, in some patients, it is clear that they may progress to the need for retransplantation. Yet, despite almost 20 years of pediatric heart transplantation, less than 5% of patients undergoing transplantation in the current period are doing so for the purpose of retransplantation. Thus late graft failure fortunately seems to remain a low frequency event at least through 15–20 years post-transplantation. Ongoing vigilance for early heart failure is required since there are multiple immune and nonimmune mechanisms that could lead to progressive heart failure as we proceed further out from the date of transplantation.

REFERENCES

1. Boucek MM, Edward LB, Keck BM, Trulock EP, Taylor DO, Mohacsi PJ, Hertz MI. The Registry of the International Society for Heart and Lung Transplantation: Sixth Official Pediatric Report—2003. J Heart Lung Transplant 2003; 22(6):636–652.
2. Lipshultz SE, Sleeper LA, Towbin JA, Lowe AM, Orav EJ, Cox GF, et al. The incidence of pediatric cardiomyopathy in two regions of the United States. N Engl J Med 2003; 348(17):1647-1655.
3. Taylor DO, Edwards LB, Mohacsi PJ, Boucek MM, Trulock EP, Keck BM, Hertz MI. The Registry of the International Society for Heart and Lung Transplantation: Twentieth Official Adult Heart Transplant Report—2003. J Heart Lung Transplant 2003; 22(6): 616–624.
4. Narula J, Haider N, Virmani R, et al. Apoptosis in myocytes in end-stage heart failure. N Engl J Med 1996; 335:1182–1189.
5. Swain SL. T cell subsets and the recognition of MHC class. Immunol Rev 1983; 74:129–142.
6. Pietra BA, Wiseman A, Bolwerk A, Rizeq M, Gill RG. CD4 T cell-mediated cardiac allograft rejection requires donor but not host MHC call II. J Clin Invest 2000; 106:1003–1010.
7. Finkel MS, Oddis CV, Jacob TD, Watkins SC, Hattler BG, Simmons RL. Negative inotropic effects of cytokines on the heart mediated by nitric oxide. Science 1992; 257(5068):387–389.
8. Day JD, Rayburn BK, Gaudin PB, et al. Cardiac allograft vasculopathy: the central pathogenetic role of ischemia-induced endothelial cell injury. J Heart Lung Transplant 1995; 14(6 Pt 2):S142–S149.
9. Pietra BA, Boucek MM. Coronary artery vasculopathy in pediatric cardiac transplant patients: the therapeutic potential of immunomodulators. Pediatr Drugs 2003; 5(8):513–524.
10. Jackson KA, Majka SM, Wang HG, Pocius J, Hartley CJ, Majesky MW, Entman ML, Michael LH, Hirschi KK, Goodell MA. Regenera-

tion of ischemic cardiac muscle and vascular endothelium by adult stem cells. J Clin Invest 2001; 107:1395–1402.

11. Fogt F, Beyser KH, Poremba C, Zimmerman RL, Ruschoff J. Evaluation of host stem cell-derived cardiac myocytes in consecutive biopsies in long-term cardiac transplant patients. J Heat Lung Transplant 2003; 22(12):1314–1317.

12. Pietra BA. Transplantation immunology 2003: simplified approach. Pediatr Clin North Am 2003; 50(6):1233–1259.

13. Kung L, Batiuk TD, Palomo-Pinon S, Noujaim J, Helms LM, Halloran PF. Am J Transplant 2001; 1(4):325–333.

14. O'Connell J, Bennett MW, O'Sullivan GC, Collins JK, Shanahan F. Fas counter-attack—the best form of tumor defense? Nat Med 1999; 5(3):267–268.

15. Kasiske BL. Epidemiology of cardiovascular disease after renal transplantation. Transplantation 2001; 72:S5–S8.

16. Kawauchi M, Boucek MM, Gundry SR, Kanakriyeh MS, de Begona JA, Razzouk AJ, Bailey LL. Changes in left ventricular mass with rejection after heart transplantation in infants. J Heart Lung Transplant 1992; 11(1 Pt 1):99–102.

17. Wilhem MJ, Pratschke J, Laskowski IA, et al. Brain death and its impact on the donor heart-lessons from animal models. J Heart Lung Transplant 2000; 19(5):414–418.

18. Millar DG, Garza KM, Odermatt B, Elford AR, Ono N, Li Z, Ohashi PS. Hsp70 promotes antigen-presenting cell function and converts T-cell tolerance to autoimmunity in vivo. Nat Med 2003; 9(12):1469–1476.

19. Halloran PF, Miller LW. In vivo immunosuppressive mechanisms. J Heart Lung Transplant 1996; 15:959–971.

20. Putzer GJ, Cooper D, Keehn C, Asante-Korang A, Boucek MM, Boucek RJ Jr. An improved echocardiographic rejection-surveillance strategy following pediatric heart transplantation. J Heart Lung Transplant 2000; 19(12):1166–1174.

21. Pahl E, Miller SA, Griffith BP, Fricker FJ. Occult restrictive hemodynamics after pediatric heart transplantation. J Heart Lung Transplant 1995; 14(6 Pt 1):1109–1115.

22. Kirklin JK, Naftel DC, Bourge RC, White-Williams C, Caulfield JB, Tarkka MR, Holman WL, Zorn GL Jr. Rejection after cardiac transplantation. A time-related risk factor analysis. Circulation 1992; 86(5 suppl):II236–II241.

23. Rodriguez ER. The pathology of heart transplant biopsy specimens: revisiting the 1990 ISHLT working formulation. J Heart Lung Transplant 2003; 22(1):3–15.

24. Chin C, Naftel DC, Singh TP, Blume ED, Luikart H, Bernstein D, Gamberg P, Kirklin JK, Morrow WR. Risk factors for recurrent rejection in pediatric heart transplantation: a multicenter experience. J Heart Lung Transplant 2004; 23(2):178–185.

25. Mills RM, Naftel DC, Kirklin JK, et al. Heart transplant rejection with hemodynamic compromise: a multi-institutional study of the role of endomyocardial cellular infiltrate. J Heart Lung Transplant 1997; 16:813–821.

26. Pahl E, Naftel DC, Canter CE, Frazier EA, Kirklin JK, Morrow WR. Pediatric heart transplant study. Death after rejection with severe hemodynamic compromise in pediatric heart transplant recipients: a multi-institutional study. J Heart Lung Transplant 2001; 20(3): 279–287.

27. Pahl E, Crawford SE, Cohn RA, Rodgers S, Wax D, Backer CL, Mavroudis C, Gidding SS. Reversal of severe late left ventricular failure after pediatric heart transplantation and possible role of plasmapheresis. Am J Cardiol 2000; 85(6):735–739.

28. McGown FX Jr, Takeuchi K, del Nido PJ, Davis PJ, Lancaster JR Jr, Hattler BG. Myocardial effects of interleukin-2. Transplant Proc 1994; 26(1):209–210.

29. Yamani MH, Yang J, Masri CS, Ratliff NB, Bond M, Starling RC, McCarthy P, Plow E, Young JB. Acute cellular rejection following human heart transplantation is associated with increased expression of vitronectin receptor (integrin alphavbeta3). Am J Transplant 2002; 2(2):129–133.

30. Behr TM, Feucht JE, Ricther K, et al. Detection of humoral rejection in human cardiac allografts by assessing the capillary deposition of complement fragment C4d in endomyocardial biopsies. J Heart Lung Transplant 1999; 18:904–912.

31. Zales VR, Crawford S, Backer CL, Lynch P, Benson DW, Mavroudis C. Spectrum of humoral rejection after pediatric heart transplantation. J Heart Lung Transplant 1993; 12:563–572.

32. Bowles NE, Ni J, Kearney DL, Pauschinger M, Schulttheiss HP, McCarthy R, Hare J, Bricker JT, Bowles KR, Towbin JA. Detection of viruses in myocardial tissues by polymerase chain reaction: evidence of adenovirus as a common cause of myocarditis in children and adults. JACC 2003; 42(3):466–472.

33. Suciu-Foca N, Manavalan JS, Cortesini R. Generation and function of antigen-specific suppressor and regulatory T cells. Transpl Immunol 2003; 11:235.

34. Wood KJ, Sakaguchi S. Regulatory T cells in transplantation tolerance. Nat Rev Immunol 2003; 3:199.

35. Ringewald JM, Gidding SS, Crawford SE, Backer CL, Mavroudis C, Pahl E. Nonadherence is associated with late rejection in pediatric heart transplant recipients. J Pediatr 2001; 139(1):75–78.

36. Hosenpud JD, Everett JP, Morris TE, et al. Cardiac allograft vasculopathy: association with cell-mediated but not humoral alloimmunity to donor-specific vascular endothelium. Circulation 1995; 92(2):205–211.

37. Poston RS, Billingham M, Hoyt EG, et al. Rapamycin reverses chronic graft vascular disease in a novel cardiac allograft model. Circulation 1999; 100(1):67–74.

38. Miller L. Cardiovascular toxicities of immunosuppressive agents. Am J Transplant 2002; 2:807–818.

39. Groth CG, Bäckman L, Morales JM, et al. Sirolimus (Rapamycin)-based therapy in human renal transplantation. Transplantation 1999; 67:1036–1042.

40. Hetzer R, Albert W, Hummel M, et al. Status of patients presently living 9–13 years after orthotopic heart transplantation. Ann Thorac Surg 1997; 64:1661–1668.

41. Chan MCY, Giannetti N, Kato T, et al. Severe tricuspid regurgitation after heart transplantation. J Heart Lung Transplant 2001; 20: 709–717.

42. Murphy DA, Thompson GW, Ardell JL, McCraty R, Stevenson RS, Sangalang VE, Cardinal R, Wilkinson M, Craig S, Smith FM, Kingma JG, Armour JA. The heart reinnervates after transplantation. Ann Thorac Surg 2000; 69(6):1769–1781.

43. Braith RW, Clapp L, Brown T, Brown C, Schofield R, Mills RM, Jill JA. Rate-responsive pacing improves exercise tolerance in heart transplant recipients: a pilot study. J Cardiopulm Rehabil 2000; 20(6): 377–382.

18

Cancer Treatment-Related Cardiotoxicities

SVJETLANA TISMA-DUPANOVIC,
WILLIAM G. HARMON, M. JACOB
ADAMS, GUL H. DADLANI, AMY
KOZLOWSKI, SARAH DUFFY, LARISSA
HERBOWY, KAROLINA ZAREBA,
CAROL FRENCH, and KATHARINE
MCLAUGHLIN

Division of Pediatric Cardiology,
University of Rochester Medical Center
and Golisano Children's Hospital at
Strong, University of Rochester School
of Medicine and Dentistry,
Rochester, New York, U.S.A.

STEVEN E. LIPSHULTZ
Department of Pediatrics, University
of Miami School of Medicine and
Holtz Children Hospital,
Miami, Florida, U.S.A.

INTRODUCTION

Cancer therapy has greatly improved the survival and quality of life for patients with childhood malignancies. Adult survivors of childhood cancer represent an ever-increasing population. By the year 2010, one of every 540 young adults in the United States, aged 20–45 years, is estimated to be a survivor of some form of childhood cancer. As these children progress into young adulthood and beyond, primary care givers must remain vigilant for the many potential long-term complications that these survivors may face.

In addition to the risk of secondary malignancies, cardiovascular complications are clearly becoming an increasingly defined source of morbidity and mortality. Unlike adult cancer patients, children undergo somatic and cardiac growth surrounding their cancer treatment. Heart growth generally occurs via myocardial cell hypertrophy, not by myocyte division. Loss of myocytes from cancer therapy during childhood may have permanent implications for subsequent adult cardiac structure and function. Children can survive for many decades after their initial cancer treatment; therefore, cardiovascular health needs to be a primary consideration when designing anticancer strategies.

This chapter reviews the common anticancer therapies and describes their potential cardiovascular side effects. Preventive techniques and heart failure management are also discussed.

THE PATHOPHYSIOLOGY OF CARDIOTOXICITY

The cardiac myocyte is critical to human survival. Postnatal myocardiocytes are generally unable to divide or regenerate. After early infancy, cardiac growth occurs via myocardial cell hypertrophy, not by cell division. Some myocyte loss occurs through apoptosis during the normal development. The remaining myocyte population is responsible for an individual's life-long cardiac workload. Conceptually, a minimal critical mass of myocardiocytes is required for adequate cardiac growth and to supply the increased cardiovascular demands of adult life. Childhood cardiac myocyte loss can be without manifestations until somatic growth increases myocardial demand. Thus, an adolescent or young adult cancer survivor may develop cancer-treatment-related heart failure years after receiving cardiotoxic cancer therapy.

Cancer therapy may induce acute myocyte injury directly and indirectly. Mitochondrial injury, free radical damage, apoptosis, and inflammatory or autoimmune responses are some of the mechanisms implicated in directly damaging myocardial cells. Indirect mechanisms include endocrine abnormalities (growth hormone deficiency), as well as well as autonomic and endothelial dysfunctions. Vascular injury may lead to increased systemic vascular resistance and ventricular afterload. Small- to medium-sized arteries can also be affected, raising the concern for coronary involvement and the development of ischemic heart disease.

Cardiomyopathy can be defined as any disease process affecting the heart muscle. Cardiomyopathies have vast origins. Most patients can be classified as having dilated, hypertrophic, or restrictive disease. A patient may have a disease that progresses from one classification to another, or a given patient may have characteristics that blend between classifications (e.g., dilated, hypertrophic disease).

Dilated cardiomyopathy results from myocardiocyte loss or functional impairment. Loss of myocyte function results in decreased contractility and, typically, ventricular dilation. Systolic dysfunction is the main clinical feature that leads to a spectrum of symptoms ranging from asymptomatic left ventricular dysfunction to florid congestive heart failure. Dilated cardiomyopathies are a recognized complication of many cancer therapies. Hypertrophic cardiomyopathies result in symmetric or asymmetric ventricular hypertrophy secondary to genetic defects of sarcomere proteins; they are not caused by cancer therapies. Restrictive cardiomyopathies impair diastolic ventricular filling. Diastolic dysfunction leads to elevated pulmonary arteriolar and systemic venous pressures, thereby causing dyspnea or symptoms of right-sided heart failure.

The development of cardiotoxicity after cancer therapy has been associated with both modifiable and nonmodifiable risk factors. Decisions regarding the class of chemotherapy agents used, cumulative dosing, rates of administration, the use of cardioprotectants and concomitant radiation therapy are just some of the many variables to be considered when designing modern treatment protocols. Nonmodifiable risk factors include age, sex, race, genetic predisposition, length of follow-up, and existing medical or surgical conditions. Specific risk factors for anthracyclines, other chemotherapeutic agents, and radiation are discussed separately below.

TYPES OF ANTICANCER THERAPIES

Anthracyclines

Anthracyclines are highly effective against a wide range of solid tumors and leukemias. They were introduced as chemotherapeutic agents in the late 1960s (daunorubicin) and early 1970s (doxorubicin). The most commonly used drugs in this class today are doxorubicin (Adrianiycin), daunorubicin (Cerubidine), epirubicin (Pharmorubicin), and idarubicin (Idamycin) (1). Protocols from the Pediatric Oncology Group (POG) show that more than 50% of 12,680 patients treated between 1974 and 1990 received an anthracycline agent (2). Increased anthracycline dose correlates directly with remission rates and event-free survival (3). However, anthracyclines are the most widely recognized cardiotoxic agents, and this toxicity is the major factor limiting their use. Childhood cancer survivors have an increased all-cause mortality following the cure of their cancer. In a large cohort of American patients who had survived at least 5 years from a diagnosis of pediatric cancer, the standardized mortality ratio for overall mortality was 10.8 (4). A large proportion of the described morbidity and mortality was cardiac in nature (the standardized cardiac mortality ratio was 8.2) (4). Mortality from anthracycline-induced cardiac failure is substantial, with mortality rates as high as 20% once symptoms of heart failure develop (5). Anthracycline-treated patients have a higher risk of cardiac death than those treated with anthracycline-free regimens (6).

Definition and Natural History of Anthracycline Cardiotoxicity

Anthracycline-induced cardiotoxicity has been categorized as an acute, early-onset chronic progressive, or late-onset chronic progressive disease based on the time of presentation in relation to anthracycline administration (1). Cardiotoxicity can often be identified by echocardiographic abnormalities long before clinical signs of congestive heart failure develop. Acute symptomatic congestive heart failure is indicative of severe myocardial injury and is more likely to be associated with lasting cardiac compromise (7). Figure 1 illustrates different patterns of anthracycline associated cardiac injury and ventricular dysfunction in the acute and long-term setting. These theoretical data were based on follow-up 6 years after completion of anthracycline therapy. Patients in Group 1 completed anthracycline administration with no evidence of cardiac injury or dysfunction. Patients in Group 2 experienced

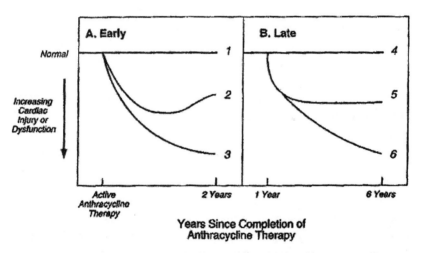

Figure 1 Theoretical presentation of anthracycline-induced cardiotoxicity during and after therapy. (A) Differences in early cardiomyopathy: some patients show no abnormality (Group 1). Cardiac dysfunction may be transient (Group 2) or persistent (Group 3). Patients with persistent changes may remain abnormal but stable, or they may deteriorate further. (B) Late cardiac effects on anthracycline therapy: some patients show no evidence of cardiac dysfunction (Group 4). Other patients (Groups 5 and 6) have cardiac dysfunction 6 years after therapy. Group 5 represents patients withcardiac dysfunction but who remain stable 6 years after the therapy. Group 6 represents patients with progressive cardiac dysfunction during the same period. (From Ref. 8.)

an acute, but transient dysfunction. These patients had normal clinical findings and left ventricular function at 1-year follow-up. Patients in Group 3 had early left ventricular dysfunction that remained abnormal or progressively worsened during anthracycline therapy. Patients in Group 4 showed no evidence of long-term cardiac injury or dysfunction. Cardiac dysfunction had a late-onset, but was stable in Group 5. Patients in Group 6 had late-onset, progressive ventricular dysfunction. These patients progress to end-stage disease and may ultimately be evaluated for cardiac transplantation.

Acute Anthracycline Toxicity

Acute anthracycline-induced cardiotoxicity manifests as a characteristically reversible episode of cardiac dysfunction after an initial infusion of an anthracycline agent. Cardiac dysfunction is usually attenuated or markedly improved by discontinuing the offending drug. Acute anthracycline toxicity occurs in less than 1% of patients treated with current front-line chemotherapy protocols (1). Clinical manifestations may occur during the first week of treatment and often result in clinical symptoms of congestive heart failure (8). Electrophysiologic abnormalities may be evident, including nonspecific ST segment and T wave changes, decreased QRS amplitude and QTc prolongation. Sinus tachycardia is nearly universal. ECG abnormalities may arise from alterations of autonomic tone, rather than representing direct anthracycline-induced effects. Acute life-threatening ventricular or supraventricular tachycardias (9–11) and myocarditis–pericarditis syndrome (12) have been reported. Rare reports have implicated anthracycline administration as inducing coronary vasospasm with resultant myocardial ischemia and sudden death (13,14).

Early-Onset Chronic Progressive Anthracycline-Induced Cardiotoxicity

Early-onset chronic progressive cardiomyopathy develops within 1 year after completion of anthracycline treatment

(Fig. 1, Group 3). Electrophysiologic changes, left ventricular dysfunction, decreased exercise capacity, and clinical congestive heart failure (CHF) may develop (7). These children tend to show combined dilated and restrictive pathophysiology (1). Adult patients typically display purely dilated disease (5,15).

Late-Onset Cardiotoxicity

Late-onset Cardiotoxicity occurs at least 1 year after the completion of anthracycline therapy. By definition, there must be a latency period before cardiac dysfunction develops (16). Some patients may report easy fatigability or dyspnea before being diagnosed as having cardiac dysfunction. Late-onset asymptomatic disease is common; severe disease causing symptomatic heart failure is less frequent. Late-onset dysfunction results from early myocyte loss which leads to progressive left ventricular dilation and left ventricular wall thinning. These changes produce a chronic elevation in left ventricular wall stress, thereby promoting further left ventricular compromise (7).

Echocardiographic parameters such as fractional shortening, left ventricular end diastolic dimension, left ventricular afterload (determined by end systolic wall stress), contractility (determined by the stress–velocity index) (16–18), and diastolic filling phases are abnormal (17). Electrocardiographic (19) and exercise stress results (20,21) may be abnormal. Noninvasive monitoring of long-term cancer survivors treated with anthracyclines generally reveals increasing abnormalities over time; some of these patients eventually experience symptomatic heart failure.

Risk Factors for the Development of Anthracycline Cardiotoxicity

Several factors affect the development of anthracycline toxicity. These include the cumulative dose administered, rate of administration, age, race, length of follow-up, sex, and the use of concomitant chemotherapy agents (Fig. 2).

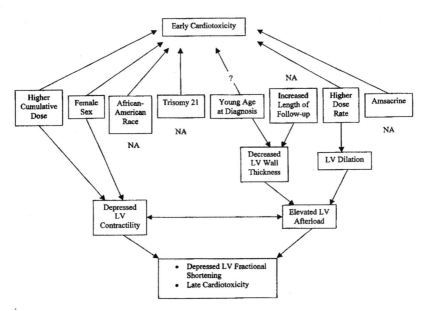

Figure 2 Risk factors for the development of late anthracycline-associated cardiotoxicity. (From Ref. 189.)

Cumulative Anthracycline Dose

In both children and adults, the risk of cardiotoxicity increases as the cumulative dose of anthracycline rises (22). Cumulative dose remains the most significant predictor for the development of cardiac dysfunction, but no safe dosing threshold can be defined for a specific individual. Despite attempts to reduce cardiotoxicity by limiting the cumulative dose of anthracycline, abnormalities of cardiac structure and function still occur. Cardiac abnormalities were found in 65% of survivors of childhood acute lymphoblastic leukemia (ALL) 6 years after the completion of anthracycline therapy. Children receiving a total dose of $550\,mg/m^2$ of doxorubicin or more had a risk of cardiotoxicity five times greater than that of those receiving a lower cumulative dose. Furthermore, 20% of these children died from cardiac causes during the follow-up period (1,22). Higher anthracycline dosage is also associated with an increased rate of early cardiac dysfunction. Although individual patients have tolerated doses above

$1000 \, \text{mg/m}^2$, some patients who received doses as low as $300 \, \text{mg/m}^2$ have experienced substantial myocardial dysfunction (23). Thus, no "safe" dose of anthracycline therapy has been established.

Rate of Administration

The rate of administration of anthracycline therapy is significantly associated with the development of left ventricular dysfunction (7). Rapid administration of a single anthracycline dose above $50 \, \text{mg/m}^2$ has been associated with a nearly threefold risk of cardiac embarrassment, almost three times higher than that associated with divided, lower dosing regimens (dosing strategies are discussed below, under preventive techniques) (7).

Age

Children appear to be more vulnerable than adults to anthracycline-induced myocardial impairment (24–26). Age below 4 years at the time of anthracycline exposure is a risk factor for abnormal cardiac function (16). This relationship has been documented in 120 children and adults who received cumulative doxorubicin doses of between 244 and $550 \, \text{mg/m}^2$ during the treatment of childhood acute lymphoblastic leukemia and osteosarcoma (17). Younger age at diagnosis was predictive of the eventual development of left ventricular dysfunction. Young age is one of the strongest predictors of left ventricular wall thinning and subsequent elevated afterload in anthracycline-exposed childhood cancer survivors (27,15).

Length of Follow-Up

Longer periods of follow-up after completion of anthracycline chemotherapy have higher detection rates of cardiac abnormalities (28,29). Presumably, this relationship is explained by the development of new cases of late-onset cardiac toxicity and by worsening of previously undetected, early-onset chronic progressive disease (1). Abnormalities of left ventricular mass, mass index, and compliance have been newly found in anthracycline-treated survivors of childhood cancer followed 7 years beyond completion of chemotherapy (30,31).

These data support the need for long-term cardiac follow-up for anthracycline-exposed childhood cancer survivors.

Sex

Female sex is a significant risk factor for an early clinical cardiac toxicity. Sex-related differences in body composition may explain this effect by altering anthracycline distribution and metabolism (32,33). Anthracyclines show relatively poor fat solubility. Females have a higher body fat content, leading to higher anthracycline concentrations in nonadipose tissue, such as the heart (32–37). Other possible explanations may include sex-based differences in gene expression. For example, the multidrug-resistance gene that governs the excretion of anthracyclines may differ by sex (38). Additionally, population studies have suggested an increased susceptibility of females to myocardial damage in other pathological settings (39–41).

*Concomitant Radiation and Other
Chemotherapy Agents*

Concomitant radiation is believed to increase the risk of anthracycline-induced cardiotoxicity (6,42). Endomyocardial biopsies have revealed increased histopathological changes in patients pretreated with radiation, as compared to nonirradiated individuals. However, much of the evidence linking radiation therapy to enhanced anthracycline cardiotoxicity is anecdotal and inconclusive (23). Children undergoing radiation therapy involving the heart do not have a significantly increased risk of early anthracycline cardiotoxicity (43). Late cardiotoxic effects of concurrent radiation therapy are unknown (7).

Race

Black race has been linked to the development of early anthracycline cardiotoxicity (22). This link is consistent with the increased morbidity and mortality found in patients of African American ancestry with other forms of cardiomyopathy (44). The risk of idiopathic dilated cardiomyopathy is 2–3 times higher in blacks than in other groups. Blacks are more likely to die within the first two years after diagnosis.

Other Risk Factors

Certain types of cancer increase the risk of cardiotoxicity (22). These cancers include Ewing's sarcoma, acute nonlymphoblastic leukemia, and T-cell leukemia. Occult late-onset anthracycline cardiac dysfunction is believed to manifest clinically in patients who remain in a compensated state for many years. Acute viral infection and cardiovascular stressors such as pregnancy, surgery or heavy isometric exercise (weightlifting) leave the weakened heart vulnerable (44,45). The risk of cardiotoxicity is also higher in children with trisomy 21, even when children with congenital cardiovascular malformations are excluded (46).

Other Chemotherapeutic Agents

As discussed, anthracycline chemotherapy is clearly associated with a risk of early cardiotoxicity and later cardiomyopathy. Research is ongoing, and much has been learned regarding the pathophysiology and epidemiology of anthracycline-related cardiovascular disease. Other antineoplastic drugs are also potentially cardiotoxic, but have been studied in considerably less depth. Cancer patients often suffer multiorgan complications of their disease, including relatively frequent cardiac manifestations. Direct causation of a specific agent with a specific cardiovascular effect can be difficult to determine in chronically debilitated patients undergoing multiple drug chemotherapy, radiation therapy, and often bone marrow transplantation. Nevertheless, a number of chemotherapy agents have specific cardiac toxicities that can lead to severe cardiovascular complications, including life-threatening arrhythmias and severe ventricular failure. This section reviews the acute and chronic cardiovascular complications of key nonanthracycline antineoplastic drugs. Alkylating agents, antimetabolites, antimicrotubules agents, and nonanthracycline antibiotics, as well as some newly evolving antineoplastic therapies are discussed.

Alkylating Agents

Alkylating agents were among the first anticancer drugs, and they remain the most common agents in use today. Alkylating agents are a group of synthetic compounds containing alkyl groups that combine readily with other molecules. They act independently of a specific cell phase, directly targeting nuclear DNA in a wide variety of malignant and normal cells. These drugs bind to DNA and interrupt transcription and repair mechanisms nonselectively, although they primarily affect rapidly proliferating cells (47). They are carcinogenic in humans, and can induce secondary urinary tract cancers and leukemias.

Alkylating agents are useful treating many cancers, especially lymphomas, Hodgkin's disease, breast cancers, and multiple myelomas. As with any chemotherapy drug, alkylating agents are used to cure cancer, thus the benefits of their use far outweigh the far lower risk of developing a second malignancy. Alkylating agents are polyfunctional compounds belonging to several different chemical classes (nitrogen mustards, ethylenimines, alkylsulfonates, triazenes, and nitrosoureas). The most commonly used alkylating agents are cyclophosphamide, ifosfamide, cisplatin, busulfan, carmustine, carboplatin, mechlorethamine, dacarbazine, thiotepa, melphalan, lomustine, chloromethane, and oxaliplatin. The alkylating agents commonly associated with cardiotoxicity are discussed below and are summarized in Table 1.

Cyclophosphamide

Cyclophosphamide, the most commonly used alkylating agent, shows a broad spectrum of antitumor activity. Cyclophosphamide prevents cell division primarily by crosslinking DNA strands. Cardiac toxicity has been associated with cyclophosphamide use, especially at the higher doses used in preparation for bone marrow transplantation. Clinically, cyclophosphamide-induced cardiotoxicity presents as a syndrome of CHF or myocarditis that may be severe. The incidence of myocarditis after high-dose treatment ($> 150\,mg/kg$) is estimated to be 7–25% in adults and 5% in children (48,49). Combined data from these reports reveal a 22% incidence of symptomatic cardiotoxicity, 11% of which resulted in cardiac mortality (48,50). ECG abnormalities are often associated with cyclophosphamide administration, even in the absence of clinical cardiomyopathy. These abnormalities include decreased QRS amplitude and nonspecific ST changes. These ECG changes are believed to result from damage to the cardiac endothelium and conduction system. Decreased QRS amplitude was observed in 50–90% of patients demonstrating cyclophosphamide-related cardiotoxicity. Nonspecific ST segment elevation and T wave inversion were found in 25–33% of patients. For most patients, these ECG changes are generally transient and return to baseline 1–7 days after drug infusion.

Echocardiographic monitoring in patients receiving high-dose cyclophosphamide therapy (48,51,52) has identified a dose-dependent acute, but reversible, decrease in systolic function in more than 50% of these patients. Myocardial hypertrophy, left ventricular wall thickening, hemorrhagic necrosis, and endothelial injury have been found at autopsy in patients dying from cyclophosphamide cardiotoxicity (48,49,53,54).

Cyclophosphamide toxicity increases with increasing dose, as calculated using body surface area measurements (54). Patients receiving more than $1.5\,g/m^2/day$ had a 25% incidence of cardiotoxicity as compared to a 3% incidence in those receiving dosages below this threshold. A lower incidence of cardiotoxicity was observed in children, which may be attributable to altered childhood dosing or pharmacokinetic characteristics.

Ifosfamide

Ifosfamide is a structural analog of cyclophosphamide with a similar mechanism of action (47). It is most commonly used as third-line therapy, in combination with other antineoplastic drugs in the treatment of some testicular cancers. Cardiovascular toxicity, including CHF, has been observed with ifosfamide use. Cardiovascular events were identified in 17% of bone marrow transplant patients with ifosfamide-containing conditioning regimens (55). A variety of arrhythmias (ventricular tachycardia, re-entrant supraventricular tachycardia) and ST segment abnormalities have also been reported with ifosfamide use. Coincident renal insufficiency

Table 1 Antineoplastic Agents Commonly Associated with Cardiotoxicity

Antineoplastic drug class	Drug generic (trade)	Acute toxicity	Chronic toxicity
Antimicrotubule agents—current and investigational			
Taxane	Paclitaxel (Taxol)	Sudden death, sinus bradycardia, and bradyarrhythmias, hypotension, trial and ventricular arrhythmias, myocardial dysfunction, MI, supraventricular tachycardia, AV or left bundle branch block	
Taxane	Docetaxel (taxotere)	CHF, hypertension, hypotension, anemia, fluid retention, chest tightness, dyspnea	
Vinca alkaloid	Vinblastine sulfate (Velban, Velsar)	Acute MI, dyspnea, tachypnea, pulmonary edema, ECG changes, T wave inversion, ST segment changes, atrial fibrillation, Raynaud's phenomenon	
Vinca alkaloid	Vincristine sulfate (Oncovin, Vincasar PFS, Vincrex)	Acute MI, hypotension, dyspnea, tachypnea, pulmonary edema, ECG changes, T wave inversion, ST segment changes, atrial fibrillation, acute CHF, cardiovascular autonomic neuropathy	
Vinca alkaloid–synthetic	Vindesine (Eldisine)	No known cardiac or respiratory toxicities	

Vinca alkaloid	Vinflunine	No known cardiac or respiratory toxicities	
Vinca alkaloid—semi synthetic	Vinorelbine (Navelbine)	Tachycardia, anemia, hypertension or hypotension, MI, myocardial ischemia, thromboembolic events (pulmonary embolus, deep vein thrombosis), chest pain, dyspnea, bronchospasm, pulmonary edema	CM, CHF
Topoisomerase inhibitor	Amsacrine (Amsa P-D) in Canada only	Atrial and ventricular tachyarrhythmias, CHF, hypotension, cardiopulmonary arrest	
Topoisomerase II inhibitor	Etoposide, VP-16 (VePesid)	Hypotension, (rarely) hypertension, acute MI, ECG changes	
Topoisomerase I inhibitor	Irinocan (Camptosar)	No known cardiac or respiratory toxicities	
Topoisomerase I inhibitor	Teniposide, VM-26 (Vumon)	Arrhythmias, hypotension	
Topoisomerase II inhibitor	Topotecan (Hycamtin)	No known cardiac or respiratory toxicities	
Alkylating agents—current			
Alkylating agent	Busulfan (Busulfex, Myleran)	CHF, palpitations, ndocardial/pulmonary fibrosis, pulmonary hypertension, congestion, and insufficiency, dyspnea, rales, cardiac tamponade, cardiomegaly, pericardial effusion, ECG changes	
Alkylating agent	Carboplatin	No known cardiac or respiratory	

(Continued)

Table 1 Antineoplastic Agents Commonly Associated with Cardiotoxicity (*Continued*)

Antineoplastic drug class	Drug generic (trade)	Acute toxicity	Chronic toxicity
	(Paraplatin)	toxicities	
Alkylating agent	Carmustine; BCNU (BiCNU, Gliadel)	Myocardial ischemia, chest pain, hypotension, sinus tachycardia, ECG changes, pulmonary interstitial pneumonitis	
Alkylating agent	Cisplatin, cisplatinum (Platinol)	Myocardial ischemia, palpitations, left-sided chest pain, nausea, vomiting, dyspnea, hypotension, arrhythmias, interventricular blocks, MI, ST segment/T wave changes, T wave inversions, Raynaud's phenomenon	
Alkylating agent	Cyclophosphamide (Cytoxan, Neosar)	Hemorrhagic cardic necrosis, reversible systolic dysfunction, loss of QRS voltage on ECG, ECG changes, CHF, pleural and pericardial effusion, pericardial friction rub, chest pain, cardiac tamponade, dyspnea	Chronic pulmonary fibrosis
Alkylating agent	Dacarbazine; DTIC (DTIC-Dome)	No known cardiac or respiratory toxicities	
Alkylating agent	Ifosfamide (Ifex)	CHF, pleural effusion, re-entrant ventricular tachycardia, pulseless tachycardia, ST segment/T wave abnormalities, decreased QRS complex on ECG, arrhythmias	

Alkylating agent	Lomustine (Cee Nu)	Pulmonary infiltrates and/or fibrosis	
Alkylating agent	Mechlorethamine, nitrogen mustard (Mustargen)	Vein irritation (sclerosis), transient cardiac arrhythmias	
Alkylating agent	Melphalan, phenylalanine mustard (Alkeran)	Bronchopulmonary dysplasis, pulmonary interstitial fibrosis, dyspnea, cyanosis	
Alkylating agent	Procarbazine hydrochloride (Matulane, Natulan)	Acute infiltrate, edema, pleural effusion, dyspnea	
Alkylating agent	Temozolomide (Temodar, Temodal)	Edema, pulmonary embolism, pleural or pericardial effusion, pulmonary edema, chest discomfort, ascites	
Alkylating agent	Thiotepa (Thioplex)	No known cardiac or respiratory toxicities	
Anthracycline antibiotics—current			
Antibiotic	Daunorubicin hydrochloride (Cerubidine)	Acute or subacute: ECG changes, sinus tachycardia, arrhythmias, pericarditis–myocarditis syndrome, MI, sudden cardiac death, CHF, cardiomyopathy	CM, early and late-onset chronic CHF
Antibiotic	Doxorubicin (Adriamycin RDF, Doxil, Rubex)	Acute or subacute: ECG changes, sinus tachycardia, arrhythmias, pericarditis–myocarditis syndrome, MI, sudden cardiac death, CHF, cardiomyopathy	CM, early and late-onset chronic CHF
Antibiotic	Epirubicin	CHF, transiet arrhythmias, dose-related cardiomyopathy	CM, early and late-onset chronic CHF

(Continued)

Table 1 Antineoplastic Agents Commonly Associated with Cardiotoxicity (*Continued*)

Antineoplastic drug class	Drug generic (trade)	Acute toxicity	Chronic toxicity
Antibiotic	Idarubicin (Idamycin)	Arrhythmias, CHF, decrease in left ventricular ejection fraction, angina, MI	CM, early and late-onset chronic CHF
Anthracenedione Antibiotic	Mitoxantrone (Novantrone)	CHF, decrease in left ventricular ejection fraction, MI, ECG changes, arrhythmias	CM, early and late-onset chronic CHF
Antimetabolities—current and investigational			
Antimetabolite	5-Azacytidine; 5-AZA	No known cardiac or respiratory toxicities	
Purine nucleoside analog	Cladribine (Leustatin)	No known cardiac or respiratory toxicities	
Antimetabolite	Cytarabine, ara-C, cytosine arabinoside (Cytosar-U)	CHF, pericarditis, pericardial friction rub, pulsus paradoxus, pleural/pericardial effusions, arrhythmias, and late chest pain	CM, early and late-onset chronic CHF
Antimetabolite	Fludarabine phosphate (Fludara)	No known cardiac or respiratory toxicities	
Antimetabolite	Fluorouracil, 5-FU (Adrucil, Efudex)	MI, angina, hypotension, cardiogenic shock/sudden death, dilated cardiomyopathy, asymptomatic ECG changes	
Antimetabolite	Hydroxyurea (Hydrea)	None: cardiac or respiratory	
Antimetabolite	Mercaptopurine 6-MP (Purinethol)	None: cardiac or respiratory	

Antimetabolite	Methotrexate; MTX amethopterin (Folex, Mexate, Mexate-AQ, Rheumatrex)	Pulmonary edema, pleuritic chest pain, interstitial pneumonitis	
Antimetabolite	Pentostatin, 2'-deoxycoformycin; DCF (Nipent)	Angina, MI, CHF, acute arrhythmias	CHF
Antimetabolite	Thioguanine 6-TG	None: cardiac or respiratory	
Nonanthracycline antibiotic—current			
Antibiotic	Actinomycin-d, dacrinomycin (Cosmegen)	None: cardiac or respiratory	
Antibiotic	Bleomycin sulfate (Blenoxane)	Raynaud's phenomenon, interstitial pneumonitis, chronic pulmonary fibrosis, dyspnea, cyanosis	
Antibiotic	Mitomycin, mitomycin-C; MTC (Mutamycin)	CHF, interstitial pneumonitis, chronic pulmonary fibrosis, dyspnea	CHF, progressive pulmonary dysfunction
Other chemotherapies—current			
Enzyme	(1-) Asparaginase colaspase, crasnitin (Elspar, Kidrolase)	Acute MI, ECG changes, thrombus formation	
Enzyme-modified	PEG-l-asparaginase; PEG-l-asparaginase (Oncaspar)	Acute MI, ECG changes, thrombus formation	

(Continued)

Table 1 Antineoplastic Agents Commonly Associated with Cardiotoxicity (*Continued*)

Antineoplastic drug class	Drug generic (trade)	Acute toxicity	Chronic toxicity
Biological response modifier	Interferon alpha-2A (Roferon-A)	Exacerbates underlying cardiac disease, hypotension, arrhythmias	CM
Retinoid	Isotretinoin (Accutane)	No known cardiac or respiratory toxicities	
Monoclonal antibody	Trastuzumab (Hercentin)	Ventricular dysfunction, CHF, tachycardia, dyspnea, hypotension, bronchospasm, wheezing	CM
Retinoid	Tretinoin-systemic (Vesanoid)	Retinoic acid syndrome (including: dyspnea, respiratory distress, hypotension, peripheral edema, pericardial or pleural effusions, pulmonary infiltrates, CHF), impaired myocardial contractility, MI	
Arsenic	Arsenic trioxide (Trisenox)	Arrhythmias, pericardial or pleural effusions, dyspnea, prolonged QT interval, complete AV block, torsades de pointes, electrolyte imbalances, sudden death	
Liposomal encapsulated anthracycline	DaunoXome containing daunorubicin	Risk of cardiac injury not adequately evaluated to date: observe warnings of conventional doxorubicin toxicity	Unknown

Liposomal encapsulated anthracycline	Doxil (ALZA, Evacet)(containing doxorubicin)	Risk of cardiac injury not adequately evaluated to date: observe warnings of conventional doxorubicin toxicity	Unknown
Monoclonal antibody	Gemuzumab ozogamicin (Mylotarg)	Dyspnea, pulmonary edema, pleural effusions, chest discomfort, hypotension, acute respiratory distress syndrome, tumor lysissyndrome	
Protein-tyrosine kinase inhibitor	Imatinib (Gleevac)	Pleural effusion, pericardiac effusion, pulmonary edema, dyspnea, ascites, chest discomfort	
Lymphokine	Interleukin-2; IL-2, aldesleukin (Proleukin)	Myocardial injury/myopericarditis, bacterial endocarditis, sepsis, MI, CHF, ventricular arrhythmias, hypotension, respiratory insufficiency requiring intubation, GI bleeding, coma, sudden death	Dilated CM
EGFR inhibitor	PKI-166	No known cardiac or respiratory toxicities	
FTI	R115777 (Zarnestra)	No known cardiac or respiratory toxicities	
Monoclonal antibody	Rituximab (Rituxan)	Cytokine release syndrome and/or tumor lysis syndrome may occur with high tumor cell counts. Dyspnea, bronchospasm, arrhythmia, edema, chest pain, hypotension, or hypertension	
Angiogenesis inhibitor	Thalidomide	No known cardiac or respiratory toxicities	

AV, atrioventricular; CHF, congestive heart failure; CM, cardiomyopathy; ECG, electrocardiogram; EGFR, epidermal growth factor receptor; FTI, farnesyltransferase inhibitor; MI, myocardiai infarction. Modified and adapted from Ref. 202.

(increasing serum creatinine) has been associated with the development of cardiac issues.

Cisplatin

Cisplatin is another alkylating agent in widespread use since the 1970s. Cisplatin covalently binds to DNA and produces inter- and intrastrand crosslinks, thereby inhibiting DNA synthesis and transcription. Cisplatin appears to enhance the effects of radiation therapy (56). Cisplatin has a wide spectrum of antineoplastic activity against pediatric brain tumors, osteosarcomas, ovarian cancer, and head and neck cancer.

Cisplatin-induced cardiac events include atrial fibrillation, supraventricular tachycardia, myocardial infarction, intraventricular conduction delay, T wave inversion, and ST segment or T wave changes (57–64). These events, however, do not seem to be dose-related and have been reported hours to months after cisplatin infusion. Cisplatin infusion has been reported to induce palpitations. Substernal chest hypomagnesemia have also been associated with cisplatin therapy. These mechanisms may potentiate vasospasm and promote ischemic physiology in susceptible individuals, and perhaps may lead to the cardiac symptoms described (65,66).

Carmustine and busulfan are two other alkylating agents that are used to treat refractory Hodgkin's disease and some leukemias. These agents have also been associated with ECG changes, potential vasospasm, and pericardial effusion (67–69). The incidence and mechanism of these effects are unknown.

Antimetabolites

Antimetabolites are structural analogs of normal metabolic components (47). These agents undergo normal cellular processing before inhibiting some vital function necessary for cell survival and proliferation. Many of the antimetabolites in current use interfere with the production of RNA and DNA. Antimetabolites are cell-cycle specific and primarily act on cells undergoing rapid DNA synthesis. The most common antimetabolites include cytarabine, floxuridine, fludarabine, fluorouracil, mercaptopurine, methotrexate, trimetrexate, and thioguanine.

Fluorouracil

Fluorouracil, developed in 1957, inhibits DNA synthesis by interfering with the normal production of thymidine base pairs. Fluorouracil is used to treat a number of solid tumors, including those of the gastrointestinal tract and breast. Fluorouracil has been associated with a wide variety of cardiac symptoms, from benign chest pain to severe myocardial infarction with fatal cardiogenic shock (70–72). Infusion-related hypotension, arrhythmias, and dilated cardiomyopathy have also been attributed to fluorouracil. Retrospective studies of patients receiving fluorouracil have been inconsistent, reporting incidences of clinically apparent cardiotoxicity from 1.6% to 68% (73). Others report up to a 10% incidence of clinically important events in association with high-dose fluorouracil therapy ($>800\,\mathrm{mg/m^2/day}$) (74). Fluorouracil cardiotoxicity is typically described early in the course of therapy, and is more common after high-dose continuous infusion than after bolus administration (72,75–77). In a prospective study of 367 patients, cardiac events occurred in 7.6% during the first cycle of fluorouracil treatment, resulting in 2.2% cardiac mortality (72).

Electrocardigraphic changes reported with fluorouracil include ST segment elevation or depression, decreased QRS amplitude, new Q waves suggestive of myocardial infarction, peaked T waves, T wave inversion, and sinus tachycardia (71,78). QT prolongation, atrial fibrillation, ventricular extra systoles, sustained, and nonsustained ventricular tachycardia, and ventricular fibrillation have also been reported, but less frequently (71). In most patients, ECG changes return to normal within several hours to several days after fluorouracil discontinuation.

Existing ischemic heart disease or arrhythmias are associated with increased risk of fluorouracil-associated cardiac complications. In 1083 patients receiving fluorouracil, a history of cardiac disease was associated with a significantly increased risk (4.5% vs. 1.1%) of chest pain during treatment, as compared to patients without such risk factors (70). Prior mediastinal irradiation, concurrent administration of other chemotherapeutic agents, and prolonged fluorouracil administration may also influence the development of fluorouracil-associated symptoms.

The exact cause of these interactions remains unknown. However, fluorouracil and its metabolites may interfere with myocardial energy metabolism (23). In addition, plasma endothelin concentrations have been elevated in patients treated with fluorouracil who experienced fluorouracil-related cardiac events (79). Endothelin is a potent vasoconstrictor produced by endothelial cells that may help precipitate or worsen ischemic disease in at-risk individuals. Other mechanisms may certainly be involved, but have yet to be elucidated.

Clinicians should be aware of these potential cardiovascular issues and screen patients for predisposing risk factors. Prophylactic administration of nitroglycerin, nifedipine, diltiazem, or verapamil has been attempted to decrease cardiovascular risk in susceptible adult cancer patients. None of these interventions have shown a markedly reduced rate of on-treatment ischemic cardiac events (71). Fluorouracil infusion should be discontinued if cardiac symptoms develop. If further treatment with fluorouracil is warranted, it should be administered in an environment with appropriate monitoring and medical resources.

Cytarabine

Cytarabine, a pyrimidine antagonist, interferes with the function of DNA polymerase. This agent is used to treat acute myeloblastic leukemia. Cardiac events associated with cytarabine include supraventricular and ventricular arrhythmias, pericarditis, acute respiratory distress, and recurrent CHF (80–85). Cardiomyopathy has been reported as a chronic toxicity of prolonged cytarabine use. Cytarabine-associated pericarditis has been described, and tends to occur between 3 and 28 days after drug initiation. Affected patients manifest the classic signs and symptoms of pericarditis including dyspnea, chest pain, pericardial friction rubs and ST changes.

Induced pulmonary dysfunction, including the acute respiratory distress syndrome (ARDS), has been attributed to cytarabine. These reactions may represent a hypersensitivity response; corticosteroid therapy has been associated with symptomatic improvement.

Antimicrotubule Agents

Antimicrotubule agents (Table 1) disrupt the metabolism of intracellular microtubules, thereby inhibiting cellular replication and transport mechanisms. Taxanes such as Taxol® and paclitaxel stabilize normal microtubule depolymerization, interrupting cellular mitosis (56). Vinca alkaloids such as vincristine disrupt microtubule depolymerization and inhibit mitotic spindle formation. Cardiovascular implications of antimicrotubule therapy are discussed below.

Taxanes

Taxol, a plant alkaloid, was isolated from the Pacific Yew tree (Taxus brevifolia) in 1967. A similar drug, paclitaxel, is used for a variety of adult cancers, and it is an investigational agent for children with solid tumors. Cardiovascular events associated with Taxol and paclitaxel infusion began to be reported during phase II trials in the late 1980s. Such concerns led to intense monitoring during protocol development with later, wider use. Paclitaxel, with its antimicrotubule properties, may mediate cardiac muscle damage by adversely affecting subcellular organelle function (86).

Taxine is a known alkaloid fraction (containing at least 10 separate alkaloid compounds) present in the yew tree and has well-recognized toxicities (87). Taxines adversely affect cardiac conduction and automaticity (88–91). Some taxine fractions have chemical structures in common with those of paclitaxel. Yew poisoning and paclitaxel toxicity have similar clinical effects. With these similarities in mind, protocols have been designed to limit the inclusion of patients with known cardiovascular risk factors. Cardiovascular symptoms associated with Taxol infusion consist of mainly symptomatic bradycardia and hypotension (23). Ventricular and supraventricular arrhythmias were reported less frequently, and tended to resolve 4–72 hr after drug discontinuation. Some patients briefly experienced episodes of supraventricular tachycardia or premature ventricular contractions up to 10 days after paclitaxel infusion. Myocardial infarction or ischemia was reported during and up to 14 days after paclitaxel therapy (92).

Adverse reaction data from more than 3400 adult patients have been collected by a variety of sources. The cumulative data show an approximate 0.5% incidence of life-threatening, adverse cardiac events related to treatment with paclitaxel with no apparent cumulative dose effect. Most patients with known cardiovascular risk factors were excluded from these trials, making it difficult to definitively identify any specific risk factors that may potentiate paclitaxel-induced cardiotoxicity. The following patients may have an elevated risk of a cardiac event while receiving paclitaxel therapy and should be carefully monitored:

– Patients not expected to tolerate bradycardia such as those with a history of myocardial infarction, angina, CHF or coronary artery disease.
– Patients with a history of altered cardiac conduction such as bundle branch blocks or first-degree atrioventricular (AV) block.
– Patients on medications that alter cardiac conduction such as beta-blockers, calcium antagonists, or digoxin.

Patients already taking cardiac medications should continue their medications without change in dose or schedule throughout paclitaxel therapy. Paclitaxel dosing should not be altered or discontinued in cases of asymptomatic bradycardia. Severe bradycardia or signs of developing heart block should be evaluated with a 12-lead ECG and monitored thereafter. Pacemaker therapy (temporary or permanent) should be based on the need to continue paclitaxel therapy and on the severity of the symptoms. Of note, combination doxorubicin and paclitaxel therapy may be associated with unexpectedly high level of cardiotoxicity and warrants close cardiovascular monitoring.

Vinca Alkaloids

The vinca alkaloids are created from alkaloids in the periwinkle plant *Catharanthus roseus*. Several naturally occurring, semisynthetic or synthetic forms are in this class. All have similar chemical properties but their clinical activities and toxicities differ.

Vincristine is a commonly used agent to treat a variety of pediatric tumors. Its use is associated with a peripheral and autonomic neuropathy that can severely limit vagal tone and chronotropic function (93). Orthostatic symptoms are commonly attributed to these mechanisms.

Myocardial infarction represents a more serious complication of vinca alkaloid use (94–103). In a large group of patients treated for malignant lymphoma, 25% showed some evidence of cardiac involvement, although only 10% had the corresponding clinical symptoms (104). Decreased left ventricular function was postulated to result from ongoing subclinical ischemic heart disease not necessarily related to the malignancy or course of therapy. The definite mechanism by which the vinca alkaloids lead to cardiotoxicity is not known, although a variety of mechanisms (similar to those described above) have been proposed (96,98–102). Most authors focus on induced vasospasm and progressive microvascular ischemia. More research is needed to definitively link myocardial infarction to the administration of vinca alkaloids and to clearly define the associated risk factors. Case reports suggest that patients with coexisting heart disease and those previously exposed to mediastinal irradiation may be at a higher risk for a coronary event (94,95–97). If a patient has experienced a therapy-induced myocardial infarction, decisions for further treatment should be based on the individual's clinical condition, ECG analysis and laboratory evaluation (105,106). Cardiac treatment should be based on institutional guidelines or the American College of Cardiology or American Heart Association guidelines for the management of acute myocardial infarction. The decision to continue vinca alkaloid therapy should be based on the potential benefits vs. the potential risk of further cardiac compromise.

Topoisomerase Inhibitors

Derived from the podophyllotoxin from the mandrake plant, topoisomerase inhibitors have also been useful in combination with other therapies in treating various cancers. Topoisomerase inhibitors, like the microtubule inhibitors, disrupt chromosomal dynamics necessary for DNA replication and mitosis. These agents tend not to be as damaging to the heart as some of the other agents in this section.

Etoposide and teniposide are semisynthetic podophyllotoxins in current clinical use. These agents cause hypotension in 1–2% of patients. Hypotension occurs less frequently with slow infusion (over 30 min), and typically responds to bolus fluid administration. Teniposide has caused high-grade arrhythmias, in rare case reports (107,108). Cardiac events associated with etoposide again include myocardial ischemia or infarction; these events are typically reported during combination chemotherapy with cisplatin, vinblastine, and bleomycin (62,97,109). Etoposide-induced cardiac events are thought to arise from induced coronary artery spasm, direct myocardial injury, or to be secondary to an autoimmune/ inflammatory mechanism (109,110). Again, patients with previous myocardial disease seem to be at greatest risk. The need to clarify these issues is clear.

Amsacrine is a topoisomerase inhibitor with more clearly defined cardiac interactions (56). Unlike etoposide, patients treated with amsacrine have experienced acute arrhythmias and chronic cardiomyopathies similar to those associated with anthracycline use. Toxicities are rare in naive patients, occurring in only 1% of those who have not received prior chemotherapy. There were no reports of amsacrine-induced adverse cardiac events in a number of phase II trials (111–117). We have reported (18) concurrent amsacrine administration to be a defined risk factor for anthracycline-related cardiomyopathy in children. The onset of CHF or cardiomyopathy has not been conclusively related to an increased cumulative dose (118–120). Hypokalemia has been suspected to contribute to amsacrine-induced arrhythmia. In one series of 45 patients treated with amsacrine chemotherapy, 37% of patients (14 of

45) demonstrated high-grade arrhythmia (frequent premature ventricular contractions and ventricular tachycardia, ventricular fibrillation, or both) or cardiac arrest (121,122). QT prolongation was found in a majority of these patients, which may explain their apparent susceptibility to induced fatal arrhythmias. Continuous cardiac monitoring has been advocated during amsacrine administration, but is not universally accepted. Serum potassium levels should be monitored daily before and during therapy (56). As with etoposide, any chest pain, shortness of breath or arrhythmia during amsacrine therapy should prompt an evaluation for ischemic cardiac injury (105,106). At the time of publishing, amsacrine is no longer available in the United States; it may still be available in some European countries (23).

Nonanthracycline Antibiotics

Nonanthracycline antitumor antibiotics are derived from a variety *Streptomyces species* (56). This category includes mitomycin, bleomycin and a variety of other agents currently used against a wide variety of pediatric cancers (Table 1). Cardiac interactions are rare, and when reported occur mainly in patients who have received anthracycline therapy or mantle irradiation. No studies have reported cardiotoxicity in patients who only received mitomycin. Many of these agents (e.g., mitomycin) have the potential to enhance radiation injury to tissues—a "radiation recall" response. Such a response can be rather unpredictable and quite remote from chemotherapy administration.

Other Chemotherapies

Alpha Interferon

Alpha interferon is a central mediator of immune function with antiviral, antiproliferative and widespread immunomodulatory effects. Alpha interferon induces a range of proinflammatory gene expression, while simultaneously inhibiting a variety of other cellular gene and oncogene expressions (56). Interferons can act directly on tumor cells and modulate natural killer cell, T-cell, and macrophage function. Interferon slows division of selected tumors and enhances natural activity of the immune system (47). It is most useful in treating renal tumors, melanoma, multiple myeloma, and some types of lymphoma and leukemia; wider uses are under investigation. Alpha interferon can induce a number of adverse cardiovascular events, especially in patients with existing disease. Hypotension and arrhythmia are most frequently reported (56) and may occur several days after interferon administration. An increased risk of ischemia and myocardial infarction were reported when high-dose alpha interferon was used in animals or adults with malignancies (123).

Tretinoin

Tretinoin is a retinoid derivative structurally related to vitamin A that induces terminal differentiation in several hemopoietic cell lines. It is used to treat acute promyelocytic leukemia (APL). A variety of mild cardiac events have been associated with tretinoin therapy, including arrhythmias and hypo- or hypertension (124). Severe events are reported much less frequently, and include cardiac arrest, myocardial infarction, cardiomegaly, stroke, myocarditis, pericarditis, pulmonary hypertension, and cardiomyopathy. Retinoic acid syndrome has been associated with tretinoin use. This syndrome results from tretinoin-induced leukocytosis and is characterized by a generalized and vigorous inflammatory response. Fever, dyspnea, hypotension, bone pain, pulmonary infiltrates, pericardial effusion, peripheral edema, CHF, and multiorgan failure may result (125). Once the syndrome is identified, early treatment with high-dose corticosteroids is mandatory. Vitamin A derivatives affect cardiac morphogenesis and may be teratogenic toward cardiovascular tissue (126).

Asparaginase

Asparaginase acts by deaminating extracellular L-asparagine, which is an essential amino acid for some tumor cells lacking adequate levels of asparagine synthetase. It is primarily used in the treatment of acute lymphoblastic leukemia, as well as other types of lymphomas and solid tumors.

Asparaginase has been associated with severe thrombotic complications such as pulmonary emboli and superior vena cava obstruction. Reduced fibrinogen levels and antithrombin III, protein C and plasminogen activity have been documented during asparaginase therapy (127,128). Parsons et al.(129) have documented transient increases in serum triglyceride levels during asparaginase therapy.

New Directions in Cancer Treatment

A wide variety of new drugs and focused delivery systems are on the horizon. Ideally, these new agents will have increased antitumor efficacy, with markedly decreased systemic and cardiovascular side effects. Liposomal encapsulation of anthracycline agents represents one such approach under current evaluation. Early data suggest that liposomal delivery attenuates, but does not eliminate, anthracycline-induced cardiotoxicity. Liposomal delivery seems to retain or even enhance the antitumor efficacy of the parent drug (130). However, experience with large cumulative doses is limited, and will be needed to evaluate fully any protective effect of these new delivery systems (131). In one study of over 700 AIDS-related Kaposi sarcoma patients treated with liposomally encapsulated anthracycline, 9.6% of patients experienced cardiac-related adverse events (131). Approximately, one-half of these events (4.3%) were thought to arise from a direct anthracycline effect. Nine cases of cardiomyopathy, CHF or both were reported, seven (1%) of which were classified as severe.

Other new drugs under investigation include arsenic (Trisenox) for the treatment of acute promyelocytic leukemia (131). This intriguing therapy is currently available only for use in refractory or recurrent settings. Striking QT prolongation has been documented in up to 40% of patients undergoing arsenic therapy. The QTc interval was found to be above 500 msec in the majority patients with QT prolongation. The QT interval lengthened 1–5 weeks after arsenic infusion and generally returned to baseline after 8 weeks. Routine ECG monitoring and electrolyte replacement is warranted for any patient undergoing arsenic therapy. Additionally, other drugs known to prolong the QT interval should be avoided during this course of therapy. An updated list of drug affecting myocardial repolarization is maintained at www.qtdrugs.org.

Aldesleukin (Proleukin®) is another investigational agent with marked cardiovascular effects. Aldesleukin is a recombinant human interleukin-2 (rIL-2) analog approved to treat metastatic melanoma and renal cell carcinoma. Treatment of cancer patients with rIL-2 reveals its substantial antitumor effects, but it is associated with life-threatening toxicity. Patients treated with rIL-2 may experience a profound inflammatory response characterized by severe capillary leak, loss of intravascular volume, and profound circulatory collapse. Other effects of aldesleukin administration include impaired neutrophil function resulting in increased risk of sepsis and bacterial endocarditis. Management strategies similar to those used to treat early septic shock with copious volume resuscitation and titrated vasopressor support may be required. An awareness of these pathophysiologic findings should help the cardiologist contribute to the care of these high-risk patients.

Radiation

Therapeutic irradiation is frequently used in the treatment of pediatric cancer. Although modern techniques attempt to minimize exposure, the heart often remains in the treatment field and is vulnerable to radiation damage. Radiotherapy is frequently used to treat Hodgkin's disease, seminoma, central nervous system tumors, prophylaxis, or treatment of leukemia in the central nervous system; whole-body irradiation may be used in preparation for bone marrow transplantation.

The spectrum of radiation-induced cardiac injury is broad and includes direct and indirect cardiovascular effects. Direct effects to the heart include acute myocardial infarction, restrictive cardiomyopathy, pericardial disease, arrhythmias, and damage to the valves, and the conduction system (Table 2). Indirect effects include injury to the great vessels, thyroid, pulmonary, and musculoskeletal systems. Injury to any of these systems may have cardiovascular implications.

Table 2 Radiation-Associated Cardiovascular Disease Injuries

Manifestation	Comments
Pericarditis	During therapy—associated with mediastinal tumor and some chemotherapy agents, such as cyclophosphamide
	Posttherapy—acute effusion, chronic effusion, pericarditis, constrictive pericarditis
Myocardial fibrosis	Fibrosis secondary to microvasculature changes
	Frequently with normal left ventricular dimensions, ejection fraction, and fractional shortening, as measured by radionuclide scan or echocardiography
	Progressive, restrictive cardiomyopathy with fibrosis may occur and can lead to pulmonary vascular disease and pulmonary hypertension
	Diastolic dysfunction may occur alone as well as with systolic dysfunction
Coronary artery disease	Structural changes in coronary arteries associated with radiation therapy are essentially the same as those of ordinary atherosclerosis
	Premature fibrosis may accelerate atherosclerosis
	Distribution of arteries affected tends to be anterior with anterior-weighted therapy
	Lesions tend to be proximal and even ostial
	Increased rates of silent ischemia (see autonomic effects)
Valvular disease	Predominantly mitral valve and aortic valve
	Increased regurgitation and stenosis with time since therapy
Conduction system/ arrhythmia	Complete or incomplete right bundle branch block suggests right bundle branch fibrosis
	Initial conduction abnormalities may progress to complete heart block and cause congestive heart failure, requiring a pacemaker
	Complete heart block rarely occurs without other radiation-associated abnormalities of the heart

(Continued)

Table 2   Radiation-Associated Cardiovascular Disease Injuries
(*Continued*)

Manifestation	Comments
	Increased left ventricular fibrosis associated with increased high-grade ventricular ectopic activity
	Increased right atrial pressure associated with increased risk of atrial arrhythmia
Autonomic dysfunction	Frequent cardiac dysfunction with tachycardia, loss of circadian rhythm, and repsiratory phasic heart rate variability
	The above signs are similar to a denervated heart, raising the question of whether such changes in survivors are related to autonomic nervous system damage
	Reduced perception of anginal pain
Vascular changes	Marked pulmonary artery stenosis and hypoplasia in some patients, especially in those treated in early childhood
	Carotid artery, aortic artery, and renal artery fibrosis and arteriosclerosis

Modified from Fig. 3, Chapter 8.15, Ref. 212.

Pathophysiology of Radiation-Associated Cardiotoxicity

Myocardial injury after irradiation develops in three phases (132,133). Damage to the small vessels of the myocardium is the first pathophysiologic response. An acute inflammation of the small- and medium-sized arteries, followed by neutrophilic infiltration that involves all layers of the heart, develops about 6 hr after exposure. The latent phase, beginning about 2 days after exposure, is notable for a remarkably healthy pericardium and myocardium, which typically shows only mild, if any, fibrosis. However, electron microscopy of the myocardial capillary endothelial cells reveals progressive injury. Endothelial damage leads to fibrin and platelet activation with subsequent capillary obstruction. Although the remaining healthy endothelial cells respond by replicating, this process, when severe, may be inadequate to provide sufficient capillary blood flow. Ischemia occurs and leads to myocardial cell death and extensive myocardial fibrosis, as the hallmark of the late phase. Whether free radicals produced by irradiation directly damage the myocardium, is unclear (134).

Myocardial injury is marked by nonspecific, diffuse interstitial fibrosis (135). Lesions can measure from a few millimeters to several centimeters in diameter but they usually do not involve the entire myocardium. Severity of fibrosis can differ markedly from one region to another. These changes are thought to alter the compliance of the myocardium, and thus, they contribute to diastolic dysfunction (136). Conductive tissue cells appear to be sensitive to radiation-induced fibrosis as well, appearing as arrhythmias after chest radiotherapy (137–139).

The pathology and pathophysiology of coronary artery disease after radiotherapy appears to differ, but only slightly, from that of coronary artery disease in the general population. Coronary arterial disease is directly related to radiation dose distribution; where the left anterior descending and the right coronary arteries are most often affected after anterior-weighted radiotherapy (140–142). In this setting and population, disease of the left main coronary artery occurs more often than in the general population, as well (140). However, due to modern radiotherapy techniques, it is found that the sites of disease are distributed similarly to those found in the general population. Narrowing generally occurs proximally and involves the coronary ostia (140,141,143,144). An autopsy study of 16 patients with radiation-associated heart disease found that medial smooth muscle tended to be greatly decreased in radiation-exposed individuals (143).

Media and adventitia were also more densely thickened with fibrous tissue compared to generic coronary lesion (143). These same investigators have found intimal plaques to be largely composed of fibrous tissues with little lipid present (143,145). Others have found plaques to be quite lipid-laden as well as fibrotic (144). Therefore, although certain features such as plaque location and fibrous replacement of the smooth muscle suggest disease caused by irradiation, definitive histological discrimination of a radiation-induced lesion from typical arteriosclerosis may be difficult in any one particular case.

Similarly, it is unclear to what degree the pathophysiology of coronary artery disease after irradiation is different from that of typical coronary artery disease. After irradiation, coronary artery endothelial cells are probably damaged by a mechanism similar to the process of injury described above (146). This damage causes fibrointimal hyperplasia and thrombus formation with potential lipid deposition, which is similar to the typical mechanism of coronary artery disease. However, animal studies have disagreed whether radiation-associated coronary disease can occur without lipid deposition (146). Evidence supports the conclusion that irradiation, combined with a high-fat diet, accelerates arteriosclerosis (146–148).

Radiation therapy has also been implicated as a cause of valvular heart disease. Fibrosis of the heart valve leaflets can occur with or without calcification (143,144). The pathophysiology of the valvular changes is not well understood. Left-sided valves are more commonly and severely affected than those on the right side, most probably as a result of the higher systemic ventricular pressures (144,149).

Radiation-Associated Cardiac Sequelae

Heart disease is the leading cause of noncancer mortality among survivors of Hodgkin's disease. The risk of fatal cardiovascular disease among these patients is about three times that of the general population (150), with estimates ranging from 2.2% to 7.2% (151,152). The absolute risk of cardiac-related death in survivors of Hodgkin's disease is estimated to be between 9.3 and 28 per 10,000 patient years (150,151). Fatal ischemic heart disease is the primary contributor to this increase in cardiac-related deaths, with myocardial infarction causing over two-thirds of the cardiac mortality observed in irradiated Hodgkin's disease patients (153,154). Furthermore, survivors of childhood Hodgkin's disease are at highest risk for fatal myocardial infarction in comparison to their age-matched population. One study of survivors treated between

1961 and 1991 found a relative risk of 41.5 in comparison to their age-matched population (155).

As in other populations, nonfatal myocardial infarction can lead to a chronic ischemic cardiomyopathy. Mediastinal radiotherapy may lead to a higher frequency of clinically silent ischemic events than that in the general population, due to radiation-induced sensory nerve damage (156).

Radiation can cause long-term systolic and diastolic left ventricular dysfunction (157). This dysfunction differs from the common, acute transient decrease in left ventricular ejection fraction that occurs soon after therapy. The relationship between these acute changes and the long-term effects is unknown (157). The significance of long-term changes may relate in part to concurrent chemotherapy (i.e., overlying anthracycline cardiotoxicity) and the individual's baseline cardiac condition. Restrictive cardiomyopathy, characterized by diastolic dysfunction, is more common in survivors who have not received an anthracycline (158). In contrast, dilated cardiomyopathy, characterized by systolic dysfunction, is more common in those who also received an anthracycline.

Clinically evident heart failure is rare in survivors treated with radiotherapy alone, but subclinical, progressive changes are common. Prevalence varies depending on treatment, length of follow-up, and method of screening. In 21 asymptomatic adults treated with 20 to 76 Gy (mean 35.9 Gy) for Hodgkin's disease before 1983, 12 had an abnormal left ventricular ejection fraction, 7–20 years after treatment (mean 14.1 years) (159). Constine et al.(160) evaluated 50 Hodgkin's disease survivors who had been treated with 18.5–47.5 Gy (mean 35.1 Gy), 1–30 years previously (mean 9.1 years), with modern radiotherapy techniques. On evaluation with radionuclide ventriculography, two had an abnormal left ventricular ejection fraction, but eight had an abnormal peak filling rate, an indirect measure of diastolic function.

Two recent studies of survivors of left-sided breast cancer treated with adjuvant irradiation to the chest wall help confirm that diastolic dysfunction is a manifestation of radiation injury to the heart (161,162). Perfusion defects found in these two studies likely represent microvascular damage to the myocardium, which over time leads to myocardial fibrosis and diastolic dysfunction (163). These studies suggest that diastolic dysfunction associated with radiotherapy continues to occur, even though modern techniques appear to have decreased the rate of systolic dysfunction. This continuing damage is of concern, because diastolic dysfunction usually worsens over time and may lead to symptomatic heart failure (Fig. 3).

Reports from the 1970s (164–166) first suggested that radiation to the heart in conjunction with anthracyclines, such as doxorubicin, is associated with greater cardiac toxicity than either modality alone (163). Radiation and doxorubicin may ultimately result in fibrosis, with an additive combined effect (167).

Valvular dysfunction can exacerbate any existing cardiomyopathy. Valvular insufficiency is more commonly reported; valvar stenosis occurs less often, but with more pronounced hemodynamic effects (149). In prospective studies of survivors treated with radiotherapy, the frequency of left-sided valvular regurgitation greater than Grade 1+ has ranged between 16% and 40% (168–170). Evidence supports a progressive nature for radiation-associated valvular disease. A review of 38 cases calculated a mean interval to asymptomatic valvular dysfunction of 11.5 years after therapy, with a mean time to symptomatic dysfunction of 16.5 years (149). Sequential echocardiograms in a single patient reveal progressive thickening of the aortic and mitral valves. Signs and symptoms of valve dysfunction remain similar to those in the general population.

Life-threatening arrhythmia and conduction disturbances may occur years after radiation exposure. They are different from the frequent, asymptomatic, nonspecific, and transient repolarization abnormalities seen soon after irradiation (19). Serious abnormalities reported after radiotherapy include atrioventricular nodal bradycardia, all levels (including complete) heart block (137,171), and sick sinus syndrome (171,172). Infranodal blocks were reported more often than nodal blocks, with the right bundle branch block as one of the more commonly reported abnormalities (137). Unfortunately, only a few prospective studies have reported

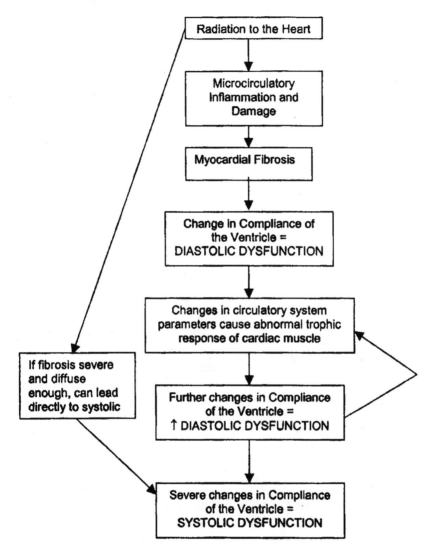

Figure 3   How radiation affects ventricular function.

the incidence of conduction abnormalities. In a study of 134 survivors of childhood cancer treated with anthracyclines and/or chest irradiation, ventricular tachycardia was significantly more common in those treated with chest radiotherapy than in a group of historical controls after 5-year follow-up

(19). This increased rate was not seen in anthracycline survivors who were not treated with radiotherapy. The frequency of patients in whom the QTc interval was prolonged more than 0.44 sec was 12.5% in those treated with chest irradiation alone, and 18.9% ($n = 25$) in those treated with irradiation and anthracyclines. In a recent study of 48 survivors of childhood Hodgkin's disease who received mediastinal irradiation between 1970 and 1991 and screened 6–28 years after diagnosis, 28 had a conduction abnormality on electrocardiogram (173).

Persistent tachycardia at a fixed rate and loss of circadian variability in heart rate was also common in the above study (173). This picture is similar to those found in heart transplant recipients who have a surgically denervated heart. These findings strongly suggest autonomic nervous system dysfunction in Hodgkin's disease survivors. Such denervation may explain the decreased perception of anginal chest pain observed in some of these patients (150). Symptoms from conduction abnormalities are uncommon but range from palpitations and syncope to rare sudden death.

Pericarditis was historically the most common cardiac complications of mediastinal irradiation. Pericarditis rarely occurs with the lower total doses and modern techniques currently used. The incidence of pericarditis was reported to be decreased from 20% to 2.5% with the implementation of modern methods of radiotherapy (160).

MANAGEMENT OF TREATMENT-RELATED CARDIOTOXICITIES

As discussed earlier in this chapter, treatment-related cardiotoxicity manifests as subclinical cardiomyopathy, CHF, arrhythmias, or sudden death. Longitudinal data have shown no safe level of anthracycline exposure, especially for children who have a life expectancy of many decades after cure of their cancer. Current medical therapy for heart failure provides symptomatic relief and prolongs life, but is not curative. Heart transplantation for end-stage cardiac disease is often a valid option, but it does open the door to chronic immunotherapy and to many transplant-related complications. Prevention represents the best therapy against treatment-related cardiotoxicity. A variety of preventive strategies have been examined including the modification of drug administration, dosing, and agent selection. To date, the concurrent administration of cardioprotective agents such as dexrazoxane seems to offer some promise of limiting at least anthracycline-related cardiotoxic effects.

Primary Prevention of Anthracycline Cardiotoxicity

Anthracycline agents (daunorubicin, doxorubicin, and epirubicin) remain central components for the treatment of numerous cancers. They are administered to cure cancer, with higher cumulative doses intended to lead to higher cure rates. Cardiotoxicity is also dose-related, but, as discussed above, may occur regardless of the cumulative dose of anthracycline administered. The Pediatric Oncology Group examined more than 6400 children and found that the risk of early congestive heart failure was five times higher when a cumulative anthracycline exposure exceeded $550\,\mathrm{mg/m^2}$ (22), than when it did not. This $550\,\mathrm{mg/m^2}$ dose has been used as the empiric maximal exposure to limit the onset of acute heart failure, with a typical antileukemic protocol scheduling $300\,\mathrm{mg/m^2}$ of doxorubicin during an initial course of therapy. Female sex, black race, trisomy 21, concurrent amsacrine exposure, and rate of anthracycline administration ($>50\,\mathrm{mg/kg/week}$) are also risk factors for acute heart failure. Late-onset cardiac dysfunction is common and progressive, with early cardiotoxicity being the strongest risk factor associated with later onset heart failure. Late-onset cardiotoxicity is related to diminish left ventricular contractility and to inappropriately thin left ventricular wall architecture. These conditions result in chronically elevated wall stress and progressive left ventricular dysfunction. Myocardiocyte loss is thought to be the general mechanism of these structural alterations. The majority of children receiving $400 \, \text{mg/m}^2$, or more, demonstrate some echocardiographic abnormalities on late follow-up (17). Despite their cardiotoxic effects, any modification of anthracycline use must be weighed against the risk of diminished remission and survival. The patient will be poorly served if anthracyclines are withheld in an attempt to limit cardiotoxicity, but then suffers a fatal cancer recurrence. Clinical success of a therapeutic agent is determined by the overall balance between oncologic efficacy and late effects.

Prevention Techniques: Modified Rate of Administration

Several dose-modification strategies have been proposed to limit anthracycline cardiotoxicity. Doxorubicin cellular toxicity depends on drug concentration and length of exposure (an area-under-the-curve phenomenon) (174,175). Continuous anthracycline infusion (typically over 48–96 hr) leads to lower peak plasma levels, as compared to similar dose given by bolus infusion. A cardioprotective benefit of continuous infusion has been documented in adult cancer patients (176). As a result of these findings, the majority of anthracycline therapy is now given as smaller weekly dosages, as opposed to monthly bolus administration.

Unfortunately, anthracycline dose-modification may not be as effective for children. This issue has been examined in a prospective, randomized manner in children with high-risk acute lymphoblastic leukemia treated on the Dana-Farber Childhood Leukemia Consortium protocol (177). All children with high-risk ALL in this study received doxorubicin to $360 \, \text{mg/m}^2$ given every 3 weeks at $30 \, \text{mg/m}^2$ doses and administered as either a bolus (over 1 hr), or as a continuous 48-hr infusion. Both groups were similar at baseline, showing some abnormalities of left ventricular structure and function as compared to healthy controls. These abnormalities included increased fractional shortening and left ventricular mass, which may have developed secondary to the anemia, increased adrenergic tone and preload induced by their malignancy. Similar baseline abnormalities have been documented in other studies of newly diagnosed children with acute lymphoblastic leukemia (17). After doxorubicin administration, both the bolus and continuous infusion groups showed similarly depressed left ventricular function and contractility, as well as increased end-systolic left ventricular dimensions. Late findings of inadequate left ventricular hypertrophy leading to progressively abnormal peak systolic wall stress were also found, and were not affected by mode of anthracycline administration. Thus, 48-hr continuous doxorubicin infusion was not found to be cardioprotective for children, emphasizing the need to develop further cardioprotective strategies.

Prevention Techniques: Myocardial Protectants

Late cardiotoxicity is likely related to acute myocardial cell injury that occurs during anthracycline administration. Prevention of the initial cellular insult may represent the best means of limiting treatment-related cardiotoxicity. Oxidative stress is thought to be central to the development of anthracycline-induced myocardial cell damage. Free radical generation stems primarily from doxorubicin's iron and copper chelating properties, as well its binding effects in the NADPH/Cytochrome P-450 system. Oxidant-induced myocardial injury can be detected by measuring serum cardiac troponin T (cTnT), which accurately reflects the degree of acute myocardial cell injury in children (178). Coadministration of anthracyclines with an antioxidant compound aimed at scavenging reactive oxygen species (ROS) is a potentially promising approach that has undergone both bench-top and clinical evaluation. A variety of agents have been proposed, including the classic antioxidants vitamins C and E, *N*-acetyl cysteine, coenzyme-Q, L-carnitine, and carvedilol (179,180). Beta-adrenergic blockade has been proven beneficial in treating adult heart failure. Carvedilol has antioxidant properties that are not shared by all beta-adrenergic antagonists (181). Carvedilol's ability to scavenge reactive oxygen species makes it an attractive agent to potentially reduce anthracycline-related oxidant injury. Carvedilol has indeed been cardioprotective in several murine models of anthracycline cardiotoxicity (182,183).

Several innate antioxidant proteins have also been identified in cardiac tissue. These proteins include several forms of superoxide dismutase and thioredoxin, a multifunctional stress-inducible protein that protects cells from oxidative and postischemic injury. A novel gene therapy leading to thioredoxin overexpression was cardioprotective in anthracycline-exposed mice (184). These, as well as other protective strategies, are currently undergoing intense investigation to define their clinical applicability.

Dexrazoxane (Zinecard; Pfizer, New York, NY, U.S.A.) is a free radical scavenger, which has met FDA approval for the prophylaxis of anthracycline cardiotoxicity in adult cancer patients (185,186). Pediatric reports also suggest that dexrazoxane provides some benefit in preventing short-term, subclinical cardiac dysfunction (187). Dexrazoxane is an iron-chelating agent with similar chemical structure to ethylene diamine tetra acetic acid (EDTA). When coadministered with anthracycline agents, dexrazoxane metabolites rapidly displace Fe^{3+} complexes from doxorubicin, as well as from intracellular ferritin and transferrin (179). Dexrazoxane–iron binding markedly decreases anthracycline-induced free radical formation, lipid peroxidation, and progressive oxidative myocyte injury. Current evidence in adults supports delayed dexrazoxane use during treatment of metastatic breast cancer only after a woman has received a cumulative doxorubicin dose of $300 \, \mathrm{mg/m^2}$ (188). However, this type of delayed administration may not be cardioprotective for children. We have found low-level cTnT elevation with initial anthracycline therapy, and that this cTnT elevation predicts late-onset cardiac dysfunction in children (189). Thus, dexrazoxane may need to be administered early in the course of chemotherapy to prevent the subclinical myocardial injury associated with late-onset cardiac dysfunction in children.

Early, concurrent dexrazoxane administration has been examined in randomized trials in a cohort of children with high-risk ALL being treated on the Dana-Farber Cancer Institute 95–001 protocol (190). These children received a total of $300\,mg/m^2$ of doxorubicin divided into 10 doses given every 3 weeks. Dexrazoxane ($300\,mg/m^2$/dose, a 10:1 dexrazoxane to anthracycline ratio) was infused immediately before all doxorubicin infusions. Significant cardioprotection was found. Concurrent dexrazoxane administration eliminated or markedly reduced anthracycline-associated myocardial injury, as assessed by elevation of serum cTnT. Importantly, no detrimental anticancer effect of dexrazoxane use was identified in these children in the short term. We reported that the degree of early cardiac injury correlates with the development of later-onset echocardiographic abnormalities. Thus, although longer-term follow-up is needed, prevention of early anthracycline-induced cardiomyocyte injury by concurrent dexrazoxane administration may be expected to decrease the incidence of late-onset cardiac dysfunction.

Similar findings have been described with dexrazoxane in pediatric solid tumor (i.e., sarcoma, PNET) protocols (187,191). These smaller series showed intact antitumor efficacy with decreased early adverse cardiac events with the addition of dexrazoxane to anthracycline-containing chemotherapy regimens. The optimal dosing, timing, and mode of dexrazoxane administration remain to be determined, but it does appear that this agent provides substantial myocardial protection for children undergoing anthracycline chemotherapy. Longer-term monitoring is also needed to confirm that the cardioprotective effects are achieved without reducing antileukemic efficacy. Ongoing research is expected to answer some of the questions regarding the use of dexrazoxane. If validated, current data support the use of dexrazoxane as a major advance in improving the quality of life and longevity for the ever-increasing population of childhood cancer survivors.

Treating Cancer-Related Cardiomyopathy

Cancer-related cardiotoxicity results from the complex interplay of physiologic, pharmacologic, and lifestyle interactions imposed by cancer and its treatment. Anthracyclines are the most frequently described causes of myocardial injury, but late-onset heart failure has been associated with radiation therapy and a variety of other chemotherapy drugs (Table 1). Patients, families, and care providers must be cognizant of the potential for subclinical and late-onset cardiac compromise after successful cancer treatment. Accordingly, cancer survivors should be considered "Stage A" patients at risk for the development of heart failure, as described in published American Heart Association/American College of Cardiology treatment guidelines (192). Screening strategies and "heart-healthy" lifestyle modifications are discussed below. Once abnormalities of cardiac function have been identified, the risks and benefit of therapeutic interventions must be weighed.

Cancer survivors show an increasing incidence of cardiac abnormalities over time (17). By definition, late subclinical cardiotoxicity is not associated with CHF; however, many of these patients do show some degree of easy fatigability or shortness of breath (16). Screening measures aim to detect early subclinical left ventricular dysfunction to guide medical intervention and to prevent the likely progression to overt cardiac failure.

Typical changes identified after anthracycline exposure include left ventricular wall thinning with associated chronically elevated afterload (peak wall stress) and decreased fractional shortening. Therapeutic goals after identifying asymptomatic left ventricular dysfunction include the prevention of further myocyte loss, as well as normalization of ventricular filling and afterload values. As detailed early in this text, pediatric heart failure management has generally been extrapolated from the vast clinical trial data generated on adults. Diuretics, digoxin, angiotensin-converting enzyme (ACE) inhibitors, angiotensin receptor blockers, beta-adrenergic receptor antagonists, and aldosterone antagonists represent the current pharmacologic armamentarium against heart failure. Evidence-based guidelines support the near universal use of beta-blockade and ACE inhibitors in adults with asymptomatic left ventricular dysfunction (192). These recommendations are being evaluated for their appropriateness in children with anthracycline-related cardiotoxicity.

ACE Inhibitors

Large randomized controlled trials in adults have demonstrated ACE inhibitors to slow the progression from asymptomatic left ventricular dysfunction to overt congestive heart failure. Success in adults has led to widespread use of ACE inhibitors in children with myocardial compromise, despite a paucity of data regarding their long-term safety and efficacy for treatment of pediatric disease (193–196). During the 1990s, upwards of 68% of children with dilated cardiomyopathy began treatment with ACE inhibitors within a month after the diagnosis of cardiac dysfunction (Lipshuitz 2003, unpublished data). As discussed elsewhere in this book, the long-term use of ACE inhibitors in children raises some potential concerns. In particular, ACE inhibitors limit cardiomyocyte hypertrophy, which is the major mechanism for cardiac growth in a normal child. Chronic ACE inhibitor administration has at least a theoretical risk of impeding cardiac growth, leading to a phenotypically smaller, thinner-walled and less-compliant adult left ventricle. These changes represent the pathophysiologic hallmarks of restrictive cardiomyopathy that are commonly described in children with late-onset doxorubicin related cardiotoxicity. Thus, the benefits of afterload reduction induced by ACE inhibitor use must be evaluated against their potential adverse effects on a child's cardiac growth.

Long-term ACE inhibitor use was examined in childhood cancer survivors with anthracycline-related cardiac dysfunction followed at the Children's Hospital, Boston (197). This retrospective study examined serial echocardiograms from 18 children treated with enalapril over a 10-year period. Enalapril was begun after asymptomatic left ventricular dysfunction was identified (12 patients), or after symptomatic heart failure developed (six patients). At the institution of enalapril therapy, ventricular function was decreased (mean shortening fraction, Z-score $= -5.89$) with markedly increased measures of left ventricular afterload (end systolic wall stress Z-score $= 6.31$). The increased wall stress is attributed to abnormally thin left ventricular wall thickness in the setting of baseline subnormal blood pressure, which fell further following ACE inhibitor initiation. Enalapril was well tolerated, and no serious adverse events were reported. The mean final enalapril dose was 18 mg/day (range 5–40 mg/day) in these young adults.

Over the first six years of enalapril therapy left ventricular dimension, afterload, fractional shortening and mass continued to improve. Unfortunately, all parameters worsened after 6–10 years. After 10 years on enalapril, all six of the symptomatic and three of the asymptomatic patients suffered cardiac deaths or required cardiac transplantation. Of the remaining nine patients, CHF developed in four, and only five (28%) of these 18 patients remained asymptomatic. Left ventricular wall thickness remained subnormal and thinned progressively, raising the concern of enalapril-induced interference of a potentially beneficial hypertrophic response. Thus, enalapril therapy for doxorubicin-related cardiac dysfunction provided a marked, but transient, benefit for 6–10 years. ACE inhibitor use for the treatment of doxorubicin-related heart failure and subclinical left ventricular dysfunction can be expected to provide short- and medium-term benefit and can be recommended based on the current level of evidence. However, clinicians must be aware of the likely transient nature of left ventricular improvement, and of the possible pitfalls associated with inadequate left ventricular hypertrophy. Further research is required to address these issues.

Beta-Adrenergic Blockade

Beta-adrenergic blockade is effective treatment for subclinical left ventricular dysfunction (198), mild symptomatic (199), and severe chronic heart failure (200) in adults. Preliminary pediatric carvedilol experience supports similar short- and medium-term benefit in children (201,202). Carvedilol provides combined alfa- and beta-adrenergic blockade, as well as antioxidant properties as discussed above. Benefits of beta-adrenergic blockade in heart failure include symptomatic improvement, increased ejection fraction, and decreased mortality in adults with congestive heart failure secondary to left ventricular dysfunction. Beta-blockade is thought to prevent and reverse adrenergically mediated intrinsic myocardial dysfunction and remodeling. Other potential benefits of beta-adrenergic blockade include antiarrhythmic, coronary vasodilatory, negative chronotropic, and antioxidant effects (see Chapter 15 for a complete discussion of beta-adrenergic antagonist therapy).

Beta-blockade is beneficial in treating cardiomyopathy of diverse origins, including anthracycline-induced disease (203). The pediatric experience using beta-blockade for anthracycline-induced cardiomyopathy was first reported in the late 1990s. Shaddy et al.(204) applied metoprolol to three children (mean age 14.3 years) with doxorubicin-related cardiomyopathy (mean cumulative doxorubicin dose $= 437 \pm 32 \, \mathrm{mg/m^2}$) with severe CHF. Metoprolol was initially administered at 6.25 mg twice daily with some report of short-lived fatigue and decreased exercise tolerance. Thereafter, mean metoprolol dose was gradually increased to $92 \pm 52 \, \mathrm{mg/day}$. The rate of increase was individualized and based on the absence of worsening CHF or marked bradycardia. These patients demonstrated symptomatic improvement within 2 months of beginning metoprolol therapy, with a markedly improved left ventricular shortening fraction (mean FS increased from 14.3 to 27.0). The authors concluded that children could be palliated for extended periods with metoprolol, thereby delaying or preventing the need for heart transplantation. A similar beneficial response was subsequently reported for individual children with myocarditis, congenital heart disease (D-TGA), Duchenne's muscular dystrophy, and idiopathic dilated cardiomyopathy (205). These preliminary data support the need for larger studies to determine the appropriateness of widespread use of beta-adrenergic-blockers in children.

Wider data regarding the pediatric use of carvedilol use are becoming available (201). Bruns et al. reported a retrospective, open-label carvedilol study of 46 children (age range 3 months to 19 years) with heart failure, spanning the years 1998–2000. Five of these children had chemotherapy-related cardiomyopathy. Carvedilol was administered in tablet or suspension form at an initial dose of 0.08 mg/kg (range 0.03–0.21 mg/kg) twice daily. The dose was slowly increased over 12-week period to an average maintenance dose of 0.46 mg/kg (range 0.04–0.75 mg/kg). Titration to a higher dose was limited by side effects, which were common, but tended to be transient. Dizziness (19%), hypotension (14%), and headache (14%) were most frequently described, but side effects forced the discontinuation of carvedilol therapy in only 3 (6.5%) of the 46 patients. Left ventricular fractional shortening was recorded at baseline and at 6 and 12-month follow-up in those patients with a morphologic left ventricle (38/46 patients). These 38 patients experienced a statistically significant increase of fractional shortening from baseline ($16.2 \pm 5.2\%$) measured after 6 months ($19.0 \pm 8.0\%$), and after 12 months ($21.8 \pm 8.0\%$) of carvedilol therapy. Clinical improvement was seen 3–6 months after the initiation of carvedilol, a time-course similar to that described in adults. Most of these patients (67%) showed an improvement in their modified New York Heart Association functional class during the observation period. Despite these improvements, adverse outcomes (transplantation in 12, death in 1, mechanical support in 1) occurred in 14 (30%) patients. The specific impact of carvedilol therapy could not be determined in this study because it was retrospective and lacked a control group. However, this study does provide evidence that carvedilol is relatively well tolerated in children and that its use is associated with improved symptoms and left ventricular function. A prospective, placebo-controlled study of pediatric carvedilol use is underway to address these important questions (204).

Further study is also needed to define carvedilol's role specifically in the treatment of chemotherapy-related cardiomyopathy. As discussed above, carvedilol has unique antioxidant properties not shared by other widely used beta-blockers. Carvedilol may prove to have cardioprotectant properties when administered with anthracyclines (182,183). It is unknown whether this antioxidant effect will provide added benefit when applied to children with either early- or late-onset anthracycline-related cardiac dysfunction. These questions are just a few of the many that need to be answered to improve the outcome for this challenging group of children.

The above text summarizes some of the issues inherent in managing pediatric heart failure. Enalapril significantly improved echocardiographically determined cardiac function in children with anthracycline-related left ventricular dysfunction. This improvement lasted as long as a decade; however, eventual cardiac failure was not prevented in the majority of these young patients. Most of these children declined to undergo transplantation or suffered a cardiac death following a period of transient improvement. Few would argue that a several year delay in heart failure progression, although a very positive result, represents the ultimate therapeutic goal for these young people. Current heart failure management strategies cannot restore a normal life expectancy for the children or young adults with serious heart failure. Prevention represents the best medicine. In the interim, the future holds the promise of new drugs, refined transplantation techniques, and eventual gene therapy to promote myocyte restoration and repair.

Evaluating the Pediatric Cancer Survivor

Screening Strategies

Childhood cancer survivors should be considered at risk for the early development of heart disease. Cardiotoxin-exposed individuals are classified as "Stage A" patients in the American Heart Association/American College of Cardiology consensus guidelines for the treatment of chronic heart failure in the adult (192). Stage A patients are considered to be at high risk for developing cardiomyopathy without concurrent evidence of structural heart disease or ongoing symptoms. The time from treatment of the malignancy to the onset identifiable cardiac dysfunction is variable, but increases over with length of follow-up. The cumulative dose of anthracycline is the most important risk factor for the development of the chronic cardiac disease. Other contributory factors include high ranges of individual anthracycline dose, younger age at diagnosis, female sex, trisomy 21, concurrent amsacrine use, and irradiation (1). Added cardiac stress such as pregnancy, infection, cocaine use, or an unsupervised exercise program can lead to the heart failure (1,16). These factors should be considered when evaluating cancer survivors. Early detection and appropriate treatment of cardiac abnormalities can prevent or minimize morbidity and mortality.

National evidence-based standards to guide the long-term follow-up of cancer survivors have yet to be developed, so we will describe our approach (Fig. 4). Currently, we monitor patients with ECG and echocardiography at a baseline off therapy, at 1 year off therapy, and every 1–5 years thereafter. Those patients with cardiac abnormalities or who received higher cumulative anthracycline doses or cardiac irradiation are followed most frequently. Further evaluations, including Hotter monitoring and/or stress testing are recommended when abnormalities are detected by echocardiography and/or ECG, when the patient has symptoms (chest pain or syncope) or has a history of radiation to the heart. Competitive athletes are also monitored with regular exercise testing and ambulatory ECGs. We also recommend echocardiography and ECG monitoring during the first and third trimesters of pregnancy and postpartum. Cardiac evaluation is recommended surrounding the pubertal growth spurt and for those undergoing growth hormone therapy. Patients are counseled regarding the long-term benefits of appropriate aerobic exercise, and are advised to avoid heavy isometric activity (as well as weight lifting, with weights greater that 20 lb). For patients wanting to pursue more rigorous weight lifting, cardiovascular consultation and more frequent evaluations are recommended. Lipid profiles, markers of cardiovascular inflammation, and thyroid function screening are also performed annually. A global cardiovascular risk profile is performed annually; pulmonary function tests are performed periodically. We do not routinely perform radionuclide ventriculography; however, this test has been proposed as an appropriate screen for radiation-induced silent coronary ischemia (162).

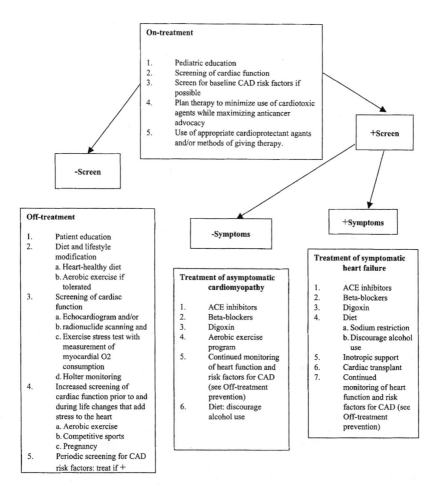

Figure 4 A protocol for screening and treating cardiomyopathy in survivors of cardiotoxic cancer therapy. ACE, angiotensin-converting enzyme; CAD, coronary artery disease. (From Ref. 212.)

As discussed, radiation-exposed children remain at risk for developing serious cardiovascular compromise. These children are also monitored longitudinally, as described above. Similarly, women who received mediastinal radiotherapy are advised to see a cardiologist at the time (or contemplation) of pregnancy and should be monitored serially throughout gestation (206). The wide range of possible cardiac abnormalities associated with therapeutic chest irradiation suggests the potential usefulness of multiple screening tests. High-risk survivors should be screened regularly for myocardial dysfunction, valvular disease, conduction abnormalities, and coronary artery disease. Other survivors treated with chest radiotherapy may also benefit from increased surveillance.

All cancer survivors should be monitored regularly for risk factors such as obesity, hypertension, dyslipidemia, and insulin resistance. Screening should begin soon after therapy is completed, no matter the age of the patient and should continue throughout life, because fatal myocardial infarctions have occurred in survivors during childhood. The recently revised national Cholesterol Educational Panel recommendations provide a well thought out minimum of care that should be applied to the screening and treatment of dyslipidemia. Radiation exposure should be counted as a risk factor, along with the standard risk factors listed in the guidelines, in determining the LDL-cholesterol goal of therapy. Several studies have suggested that survivors of childhood ALL are at increased risk for developing targeted cardiovascular risk factors and metabolic syndrome (207,208). Metabolic syndrome involves a complex milieu of endocrine, morphometric, and lipid abnormalities associated with increased cardiovascular risk. These patients are typically overweight and have elevated serum triglycerides, elevated LDL, and decreased HDL concentrations. Similar abnormalities are associated with decreased growth hormone levels, which have been described in survivors of ALL as a consequence of cranial irradiation (209). The decision to treat children and women of childbearing potential with lipid-lowering medications should be made in consultation with dyslipidemia experts, because the teratogenicity and the long-term safety in children of the most commonly used drugs have not been well studied.

Specific Screening Techniques

Life-long cardiac monitoring including regular echocardiographic assessment is recommended for anthracycline-exposed children (210). We suggest a similar assessment for radiation-exposed individuals. Serial echocardiography and radionuclide angiography are useful for monitoring myocardial function: both provide reliable measures of left ventricular systolic performance. Echocardiography has the advantages of being noninvasive and of providing assessment of valvular diseases. The most commonly used indices of left ventricular systolic functions are fractional shortening (FS) and ejection fraction (EF). These widely used measurements are easily obtained, but are not sensitive to early myocardial dysfunction. Both measurements vary with changes in the cardiac preload and afterload. Chronic heart failure, concurrent infections, and various drug responses are just some of the many conditions known to affect cardiac loading parameters (1).

Several load-independent variables that can be measured echocardiographically are sensitive and specific indicators of early myocardial dysfunction. These include measurements of the left ventricular afterload (end systolic wall stress) and load-independent contractility (the stress–velocity index) (211). Unfortunately, transthoracic echocardiograms are of poor quality in many adults because of body habitus and bone density issues. Radionuclide imaging may therefore be necessary for repeated quantitative analysis of systolic function in some patients. However, diastolic function may be difficult to measure with the radionuclide technology found in many hospitals. Myocardial function should therefore be assessed with echocardiography, with or without radionuclide studies, depending on the quality of each technique in a particular patient. Of note, chest radiography is neither sensitive, nor specific for detection of early cardiomyopathy, cardiomegaly, or pulmonary edema (1).

Physiologic or pharmacologic (e.g., dobutamine) stress testing augments the diagnosis of ischemic heart disease and cardiac dysfunction. Traditional exercise stress testing assesses ischemia noninvasively. However, the prognostic value of stress echocardiography and stress myocardial perfusion scanning in this population has not been well studied. Radionuclide myocardial perfusion scanning during exercise is 90% sensitive and specific for ischemic heart disease in the general population, but it also appears to detect radiation-induced microvascular damage in radiation-exposed individuals (148). Maximal myocardial oxygen consumption has prognostic significance in patients with cardiomyopathy (133) and may provide additional prognostic information in cancer survivors. Myocardial oxygen consumption is surprisingly low in many patients with prior mediastinal irradiation, including those who did not have symptoms of cardiac dysfunction (212). Hypotension, syncope, and rate-related conduction changes and rhythm abnormalities have also been unexpectedly found on exercise testing.

Electrical conduction abnormalities and rhythm disturbances may remain silent until fatal. The most important of these abnormalities are prolonged QTc interval, atrioventricular conduction delay, and ventricular ectopy. Thus, EGG screening is important for cancer survivors treated with chemotherapy or mediastinal irradiation. These potentially serious complications may progress from nonspecific changes that are commonly found on cancer survivor's ECGs. The prognostic value of nonspecific conduction abnormalities remains unknown, as does the usefulness of repeatedly screening asymptomatic survivors. Nevertheless, routine EGG monitoring is clearly indicated for those patients with identified left ventricular dysfunction or symptomatic heart failure. In these patients, a 24-hr Holter monitor may detect silent arrhythmias amenable to therapeutic interventions (213).

Measurements of cardiac troponin (cTnT) potentially detect cardiotoxicity in the following settings: (1) during front-line chemotherapy; (2) during anthracycline therapy for relapse or second malignancy; (3) during bone marrow transplantation; (4) when using experimental therapy that might potentiate cardiotoxicity; and (5) in intercurrent illness, which may precipitate a cardiac event (178). New generation troponin assays are specific indicators of even low-level cardiac injury. Our group (214) has determined prospectively that serum troponin T (cTnT) is elevated in 15–18% of newly diagnosed ALL patients before chemotherapy. This subclinical myocardial injury appears to arise from the acute illness that typically surrounds the diagnosis of pediatric cancer. In addition, troponin T continued to rise in 35% of these patients during doxorubicin therapy. The elevations were more frequent in patients who received more than $60\,\mathrm{mg/m^2}$ of doxorubicin. Thus, troponin measurement can detect the subtle myocardial injury seen with anthracycline-related inflammatory heart disease (214).

Angiography and cardiac catheterization are appropriate to evaluate symptoms of angina and heart failure. Some experts believe angiography should be performed if any other clinically important cardiac lesions are found, because coronary artery disease is often concurrent and in this population, often asymptomatic (215). However, no evidence exists for the use of these invasive methods for routine screening of asymptomatic survivors. Endomyocardial biopsy is expensive, invasive, and not recommended for routine monitoring in children. Abnormal biopsy results that may correlate with increased anthracycline dose but do not predict symptomatic cardiomyopathy. The relevance to left ventricular dysfunction may be limited since only the apical portion of the right ventricular septum is sampled (1). Nevertheless, biopsy is useful to determine etiology of cardiomyopathy.

In conclusion, chemotherapy and radiotherapy for cancer can lead to a broad range of cardiac abnormalities, many of which may be progressive. Childhood cancer survivors should be counseled as to the presence of this risk, and be encouraged to follow a preventive "heart-healthy" lifestyle. Survivors should be periodically screened with multiple tests to identify subclinical cardiovascular disease. Once identified, standard therapies should be instituted against myocardial dysfunction to increase survival and improve the quality of life for these patients. Advances in pediatric cancer treatment are one of the triumphs of modern medicine. Treatment strategies continue to increase in efficacy. With this success, cardiac care providers need to recognize their increasing responsibility to prevent, diagnose, and manage treatment-related heart disease.

REFERENCES

1. Giantris A, Abdurrahman L, Hinkle A, Asselin B, Lipshultz SE. Anthracycline-induced cardiotoxicity in children and young adults. Crit Rev Oncol Hematol 1998; 27:53–68.

2. Tracy RP, Lemaitre RN, Psaty BM, Ives DG, Evans RW, Cushman M, Meilahn EN, Kuller LH. Relationship of C-reactive protein to risk of cardiovascular disease in the elderly. Results from the cardiovascular health study and the rural health promotion project. Arterioscler Thromb Vasc Biol 1997; 17:1121–1127.

3. Hitchcock-Bryan S, Gelber R, Cassady JR, Sallan SE. The impact of induction anthracycline on long-term failure-free survival in childhood acute lymphoblastic leukemia. Med Pediatr Oncol 1986; 14:211–215.

4. Mertens AC, Yasui Y, Neglia JP, Potter JD, Nesbit ME, Jr, Ruccione K, Smithson WA, Robison LL. Late mortality experience in five-year survivors of childhood and adolescent cancer: the childhood cancer survivor study. J Clin Oncol 2001; 19:3163–3172.

5. Von Hoff DD, Layard MW, Basa P, Davis HL Jr, Von Hoff AL, Rozencweig M, Muggia FM. Risk factors for doxorubicin-induced congestive heart failure. Ann Intern Med 1979; 91:710–717.

6. Praga C, Beretta G, Vigo PL, Lenaz GR, Pollini C, Bonadonna G, Canetta R, Castellani R, Villa E, Gallagher CG, von Melchner H, Hayat M, Ribaud P, De Wasch G, Mattsson W, Heinz R, Waldner R, Kolaric K, Buehner R, Bokkel-Huyninck W, Perevodchikova NI, Manziuk LA, Senn HJ, Mayr AC. Adriamycin cardiotoxicity: a survey of 1273 patients. Cancer Treat Rep 1979; 63:827–834.

7. Grenier MA, Lipshultz SE. Epidemiology of anthracycline cardiotoxicity in children and adults. Semin Oncol 1998; 25:72–85.

8. Solymar L, Marky I, Mellander L, Sabel KG. Echocardiographic findings in children treated for malignancy with chemotherapy including adriamycin. Pediatr Hematol Oncol 1988; 5:209–216.

9. Bristow MR, Thompson PD, Martin RP, Mason JW, Billingham ME, Harrison DC. Early anthracycline cardiotoxicity. Am J Med 1978; 65:823–832.

10. Steinberg JS, Cohen AJ, Wasserman AG, Cohen P, Ross AM. Acute arrhythmogenicity of doxorubicin administration. Cancer 1987; 60:1213–1218.

11. Lenaz L, Page JA. Cardiotoxicity of adriamycin and related anthracyclines. Cancer Treat Rev 1976; 3:111–120.

12. Harrison DT, Sanders LA. Letter: pericarditis in a case of early daunorubicin cardiomyopathy. Ann Intern Med 1976; 85:339–341.

13. Wortman JE, Lucas VS, Jr, Schuster E, Thiele D, Logue GL. Sudden death during doxorubicin administration. Cancer 1979; 44:1588–1591.

14. Mancuso L, Marchi S, Canonico A. Dynamic left ventricular outflow obstruction and myocardial infarction following doxorubicin administration in a woman affected by unsuspected hypertrophic cardiomyopathy. Cancer Treat Rep 1985; 69:241–244.

15. Lefrak EA, Pitha J, Rosenheim S, Gottlieb JA. A clinicopathologic analysis of adriamycin cardiotoxicity. Cancer 1973; 32:302–314.

16. Lipshultz SE, Colan SD, Gelber RD, Perez-Atayde AR, Sallan SE, Sanders SP. Late cardiac effects of doxorubicin therapy for acute lymphoblastic leukemia in childhood. N Engl J Med 1991; 324: 808–815.

17. Lipshultz SE, Lipsitz SR, Mone SM, Goorin AM, Sallan SE, Sanders SP, Orav EJ, Gelber RD, Colan SD. Female sex and drug dose as risk factors for late cardiotoxic effects of doxorubicin therapy for childhood cancer. N Engl J Med 1995; 332:1738–1743.

18. Steinherz LJ, Steinherz PG, Tan CT, Heller G, Murphy ML. Cardiac toxicity 4 to 20 years after completing anthracycline therapy. JAMA 1991; 266:1672–1677.

19. Larsen RL, Jakacki RI, Vetter VL, Meadows AT, Silber JH, Barber G. Electrocardiographic changes and arrhythmias after cancer therapy in children and young adults. Am J Cardiol 1992; 70:73–77.

20. Klewer SE, Goldberg SJ, Donnerstein RL. Exercise assessment of cardiac function in children and young adults before and after bone marrow transplantation. Pediatrics 1992; 19:394–401.

21. Larsen RL, Barber G, Heise CT, August CS. Exercise assessment of cardiac function in children and young adults before and after bone marrow transplantation. Pediatrics 1992; 89:722–729.

22. Krischer JP, Cuthbertson SE, Epstein S, Goorin AM, Epstein ML, Lipshultz SE. Risk factors for early anthracycline clinical cardiotoxicity in children: the pediatric oncology group experience. Progr Pediatr Cardiol 1998; 8:83–90.

23. Pai VB, Nahata MC. Cardiotoxicity of chemotherapeutic agents: incidence, treatment and prevention. Drug Safety 2000; 22:263–302.

24. Von Hoff DD, Rozencweig M, Layard M, Slavik M, Muggia FM. Daunomycin-induced cardiotoxicity in children and adults. Am J Med 1977; 62:200–208.

25. Dearth J, Osborn R, Wilson E, Kelly D, Mantle J, Rogers E, Malluh A, Crist W. Anthracycline-induced cardiomyopathy in children—a report of 6 cases. Med Pediatr Oncol 1984; 12:54–58.

26. Pratt CB, Ransom JL, Evans WE. Age-related adriamycin cardiotoxicity in children. Cancer Treat Rep 1978; 62:1381–1385.

27. Fisher B, Redmond C, Wickerham DL, Bowman D, Schipper H, Wolmark N, Sass R, Fisher ER, Jochimsen P, Legault-Poisson S. Doxorubicin-containing regimens for the treatment of stage II breast cancer: the national surgical adjuvant breast and bowel project experience. J Clin Oncol 1989; 7:572–582.

28. Musci M, Loebe M, Grauhan O, Weng Y, Hummel M, Lange P, Hetzer R. Heart transplantation for doxorubicin-induced congestive heart failure in children and adolescents. Transplant Proc 1997; 29: 578–579.

29. Moreb JS, Oblon DJ. Outcome of clinical congestive heart failure induced by anthracycline chemotherapy. Cancer 1990; 70:2637–2641.

724   *Lipshultz et al.*

30. Leandro J, Dyck J, Poppe D, Shore R, Airhart C, Greenberg M, Gilday D, Smallhorn J, Benson L. Cardiac dysfunction late after cardiotoxic therapy for childhood cancer. Am J Cardiol 1994; 74: 1152–1156.
31. Lipshultz SE, Lipsitz SR, Mone SM, Sallan SE, Colan SD. Left ventricular structure and function eleven years after doxorubicin treatment for childhood leukemia; is this a restrictive cardiomyopathic process?. Am Coll Cardiol 1995; 25:54A.
32. Frisancho AR. Triceps skin fold and upper arm muscle size norms for assessment of nutrition status. Am J Clin Nutr 1974; 27:1052–1058.
33. Tanner JM, Whitehouse RH. Revised standards for triceps and subscapular skinfolds in British children. Arch Dis Child 1975; 50: 142–145.
34. Sibler JH, Jakacki RI, Larsen RL, Goldwein JW, Barber G. Increased risk of cardiac dysfunction after anthracyclines in girls. Med Pediatr Oncol 1993; 21:477–479.
35. Lee YTN, Chan KK, Harris PA. Tissue disposition of doxorubicin in experimental-animals. Med Pediatr Oncol 1982; 10:259–267.
36. Piazza E, Natale N, Trabattoni A, Mariscotti C, Mosca L, Libretti A, Ottolenghi L, Morasca L. Plasma and tissue distribution of adriamycin in patients with pelvic cancer. Tumori 1981; 67:533–537.
37. Rodvold KA, Rushing DA, Tewksbury DA. Doxorubicin clearance in the obese. J Clin Oncol 1988; 6:1321–1327.
38. Bradley G, Georges E, Ling V. Sex-dependent and independent expression of the P-glycoprotein isoforms in Chinese hamster. J Cell Physiol 1990; 145:398–408.
39. Eysmann SB, Douglass PS. Cardiovascular health and disease in women. In: Douglass PS, ed. Coronary Heart Disease: Therapeutic Principles. Philadelphia: W.B. Saunders, 1993:57.
40. The SOLVD Investigators. Effect of enalapril on survival in patients with reduced left ventricular ejection fractions and congestive heart failure. N Engl J Med 1991; 325:293–302.
41. Wenger NK, Speroff L, Packard B. Cardiovascular health and disease in women. N Engl J Med 1993; 329:247–256.
42. Pihkala J, Saarinen UM, Lundstrom U, Virtanen K, Virkola K, Siimes MA, Pesonen E. Myocardial function in children and adolescents after therapy with anthracyclines and chest irradiation. Eur J Cancer 1996; 32A:97–103.
43. Krischer JP, Epstein S, Cuthbertson DD, Goorin AM, Epstein ML, Lipshultz SE. Clinical cardiotoxicity following anthracycline treatment for childhood cancer: the pediatric oncology group experience. J Clin Oncol 1997; 15:1544–1552.
44. Ali MK, Ewer MS, Gibbs HR, Swafford J, Graff KL. Late doxorubicin-associated cardiotoxicity in children: the possible role of intercurrent viral infection. Cancer 1994; 74:182–188.

45. Steinherz LJ, Steinherz PG, Tan C. Cardiac failure and dysrhythmias 6–19 years after anthracycline therapy: a series of 15 patients. Med Pediatr Oncol 1995; 24:352–361.
46. Khoury MJ, Erickson JD. Improved ascertainment of cardiovascular malformations in infants with Down's syndrome, Atlanta, 1968 through 1989. Implications for the interpretation of increasing rates of cardiovascular malformations in surveillance systems. Am J Epidemiol 1992; 136:1457–1464.
47. Emory University. Cancerquest. Cancerquest 2002.
48. Gottdiener JS, Appelbaum FR, Ferrans VJ, Deisseroth A, Ziegler J. Cardiotoxicity associated with high-dose cyclophosphamide therapy. Arch Intern Med 1981; 141:758–763.
49. Dow E, Schulman H, Agura E. Cyclophosphamide cardiac injury mimicking acute myocardial infarction. Bone Marrow Transplant 1993; 12:169–172.
50. Steinherz LJ, Steinherz PG, Mangiacasale D, O'Reilly R, Allen J, Sorell M, Miller DR. Cardiac changes with cyclophosphamide. Med Pediatr Oncol 1981; 9:417–422.
51. Kupari M, Volin L, Suokas A, Timonen T, Hekali P, Ruutu T. Cardiac involvement in bone marrow transplantation: electrocardiographic changes, arrhythmias, heart failure and autopsy findings. Bone Marrow Transplant 1990; 5:91–98.
52. Braverman AC, Antin JH, Plappert MT, Cook EF, Lee RT. Cyclophosphamide cardiotoxicity in bone marrow transplantation: a prospective evaluation of new dosing regimens. J Clin Oncol 1991; 9: 1215–1223.
53. Cazin B, Gorin NC, Laporte JP, Gallet B, Douay L, Lopez M, Najman A, Duhamel G. Cardiac complications after bone marrow transplantation. A report on a series of 63 consecutive transplantations. Cancer 1986; 57:2061–2069.
54. Goldberg MA, Antin JH, Guinan EC, Rappeport JM. Cyclophosphamide cardiotoxicity: an analysis of dosing as a risk factor. Blood 1986; 68:1114–1118.
55. Quezado ZM, Wilson WH, Cunnion RE, Parker MM, Reda D, Bryant G, Ognibene FP. High-dose ifosfamide is associated with severe, reversible cardiac dysfunction. Ann Intern Med 1993; 118:31–36.
56. BC Cancer Agency. BC Cancer Agency 2003.
57. Talley RW, O'Bryan RM, Gutterman JU, Brownlee RW, McCredie KB. Clinical evaluation of toxic effects of cis- diamminedichloroplatinum (NSC-119875)—phase I clinical study. Cancer Chemother Rep 1973; 57:465–471.
58. Wiltshaw E, Carr B. Cis-platinum (II) diamminedichloride: clinical experience of the royal marsden hospital and institute of cancer research in platinum coordination complexes. Connors and Roberts, ed. Cancer Chemotherapy. London: Springer, 1974:178–182.

59. Hashimi LA, Khalyl MF, Salem PA. Supraventricular tachycardia: a probable complication of platinum treatment. Oncology 1984; 41: 174–175.
60. Shaeppi U, Hayman IA, Fleschman RW. Cis-diamminedichloroplatinum (II) preclinical evaluation of intravenous injection in dogs, monkeys and mice. Toxicol Appl Pharmacol 1973; 25:230.
61. Canobbio L, Fassio T, Gasparini G, Caruso G, Barzan L, Comoretto R, Brema F, Villani F. Cardiac arrhythmia: possible complication from treatment with cisplatin. Tumori 1986; 72:201–204.
62. Doll DC, List AF, Greco FA, Hainsworth JD, Hande KR, Johnson DH. Acute vascular ischemic events after cisplatin-based combination chemotherapy for germ-cell tumors of the testis. Ann Intern Med 1986; 105:48–51.
63. Talcott JA, Herman TS. Acute ischemic vascular events and cisplatin. Ann Intern Med 1987; 107:121–122.
64. Berliner S, Rahima M, Sidi Y, Teplitsky Y, Zohar Y, Nussbaum B, Pinkhas J. Acute coronary events following cisplatin-based chemotherapy. Cancer Invest 1990; 8:583–586.
65. Rosenfeld CS, Broder LE. Cisplatin-induced autonomic neuropathy. Cancer Treat Rep 1984; 68:659–660.
66. Turlapaty PD, Altura BM. Magnesium deficiency produces spasms of coronary arteries: relationship to etiology of sudden death ischemic heart disease. Science 1980; 208:198–200.
67. Kanj SS, Sharara AI, Shpall EJ, Jones RB, Peters WP. Myocardial ischemia associated with high-dose carmustine infusion. Cancer 1991; 68:1910–1912.
68. Littler WR, Kay JH, Hasleton PS, Heath D. Busulpan lung. Thorax 1969; 24:639–655.
69. Oliner H, Schwartz R, Kubio F, Jr. Interstitial pulmonary fibrosis following busulphan therapy. Am J Med 1961; 31:134–139.
70. Labianca R, Beretta G, Clerici M, Fraschini P, Luporini G. Cardiac toxicity of 5-fluorouracil: a study on 1083 patients. Tumori 1982; 68:505–510.
71. Patel B, Kloner RA, Ensley J, Al Sarraf M, Kish J, Wynne J. 5-Fluorouracil cardiotoxicity: left ventricular dysfunction and effect of coronary vasodilators. Am J Med Sci 1987; 294:238–243.
72. de Forni M, Malet-Martino MC, Jaillais P, Shubinski RE, Bachaud JM, Lemaire L, Canal P, Chevreau C, Carrie D, Soulie P. Cardiotoxicity of high-dose continuous infusion fluorouracil: a prospective clinical study. J Clin Oncol 1992; 10:1795–1801.
73. Rezkalla S, Kloner RA, Ensley J, Al Sarraf M, Revels S, Olivenstein A, Bhasin S, Kerpel-Fronious S, Turi ZG. Continuous ambulatory EGG monitoring during fluorouracil therapy: a prospective study. J Clin Oncol 1989; 7:509–514.
74. Gradishar WJ, Yokes EE. 5-Fluorouracil cardiotoxicity: a critical review. Ann Oncol 1990; 1:409–414.

75. Collins C, Weiden PL. Cardiotoxicity of 5-fluorouracil. Cancer Treat Rep 1987; 71:733–736.
76. Sanani S, Spaulding MB, Masud AR, Canty R. 5-FU cardiotoxicity. Cancer Treat Rep 1981; 65:1123–1125.
77. Ensley JF, Patel B, Kloner R, Kish JA, Wynne J, Al Sarraf M. The clinical syndrome of 5-fluorouracil cardiotoxicity. Invest New Drugs 1989; 7:101–109.
78. Pottage A, Holt S, Ludgate S, Langlands AO. Fluorouracil cardiotoxicity. Br Med J 1978; 1:547.
79. Thyss A, Gaspard MH, Marsault R, Milano G, Frelin C, Schneider M. Very high endothelin plasma levels in patients with 5-FU cardiotoxicity. Ann Oncol 1992; 3:88.
80. Willemze R, Zwaan FE, Colpin G, Keuning JJ. High dose cytosine arabinoside in the management of refractory acute leukaemia. Scand J Haematol 1982; 29:141–146.
81. Conrad ME. Cytarabine and cardiac failure. Am J Hematol 1992; 41:143–144.
82. Andersson BS, Cogan BM, Keating MJ, Estey EH, McCredie KB, Freireich EJ. Subacute pulmonary failure complicating therapy with high-dose Ara-C in acute leukemia. Cancer 1985; 56:2181–2184.
83. Haupt HM, Hutchins GM, Moore GW. Ara-C lung: noncardiogenic pulmonary edema complicating cytosine arabinoside therapy of leukemia. Am J Med 1981; 70:256–261.
84. Donehower RC, Karp JE, Burke PJ. Pharmacology and toxicity of high-dose cytarabine by 72-hour continuous infusion. Cancer Treat Rep 1986; 70:1059–1065.
85. Chiche D, Pico JL, Bernaudin JF, Chouaib S, Wollman E, Arnoux A, Denizot Y, Nitenberg G. Pulmonary edema and shock after high-dose aracytine-C for lymphoma; possible role of TNF-alpha and PAF. Eur Cytokine Netw 1993; 4:147–151.
86. McGuire WP, Rowinsky EK, Rosenshein NB, Grumbine FC, Ettinger DS, Armstrong DK, Donehower RC. Taxol: a unique antineoplastic agent with significant activity in advanced ovarian epithelial neoplasms. Ann Intern Med 1989; 111:273–279.
87. Burke MJ, Siegel D, Davidow B. Anaphylaxis; consequence of yew (Taxus) needle ingestion. NY State J Med 1979; 79:1576–1578.
88. Bryan-Brown T. The pharmacological actions of Taxane. Q J Pharmacol 1932; 5:205–219.
89. Schulte T. Lethal intoxication with leaves of the yew tree (*Taxusbaccata*) (author's transl). Arch Toxicol 1975; 34:153–158.
90. Veatch JK, Reid FM, Kennedy GA. Differentiating yew poisoning from other toxicioses. Vet Med 1988; 81:298–300.
91. Tekol Y. Negative chronotropic and atrioventricular blocking effects of taxine on isolated frog heart and its acute toxicity in mice. Planta Medica 1985:357–360.

92. Arbuck SG, Strauss H, Rowinsky E, Christian M, Suffness M, Adams J, Oakes M, McGuire W, Reed E, Gibbs H. A reassessment of cardiac toxicity associated with Taxol. J Natl Cancer Inst Mono 1993; 15:117–130.
93. Roca E, Bruera E, Politi PM, Barugel M, Cedaro L, Carraro S, Chacon RD. Vinca alkaloid-induced cardiovascular autonomic neuropathy. Cancer Treat Rep 1985; 69:149–151.
94. Cargill RI, Boyter AC, Lipworth BJ. Reversible myocardial ischaemia following vincristine containing chemotherapy. Respir Med 1994; 88:709–710.
95. Somers G, Abramov M, Witter M, Naets JP. Letter: myocardial infarction: a complication of vincristine treatment?Lancet 1976; 2:690.
96. Mandel EM, Lewinski U, Djaldetti M. Vincristine-induced myocardial infarction. Cancer 1975; 36:1979–1982.
97. Samuels BL, Vogelzang NJ, Kennedy BJ. Severe vascular toxicity associated with vinblastine, bleomycin, and cisplatin chemotherapy. Cancer Chemother Pharmacol 1987; 19:253–256.
98. Subar M, Muggia FM. Apparent myocardial ischemia associated with vinblastine administration. Cancer Treat Rep 1986; 70:690–691.
99. Vogelzang NJ, Frenning DH, Kennedy BJ. Coronary artery disease after treatment with bleomycin and vinblastine. Cancer Treat Rep 1980; 64:1159–1160.
100. Blijham GH, Fiolet HH, van Deijk WA, Hupperets PS, Janssen JH. Angina pectoris associated with infusions of 5-FU and vindesine. Cancer Treat Rep 1986; 70:314–315.
101. Yancy RS, Talpaz M. Vindesine associted angina and ECG changes. Cancer Treat Rep 1982; 66:587–589.
102. Bedikian AY, Valdivieso M, Maroun J, Gutterman JU, Hersh EM, Bodey GP. Evaluation of vindesine and MER in colorectal cancer. Cancer 1980; 46:463–467.
103. Bergeron A, Raffy O, Vannetzel JM. Myocardial ischemia and infarction associated with vinorelbine. J Clin Oncol 1995; 13:531–532.
104. Roberts WC, Glancy DL, DeVita VT, Jr. Heart in malignant lymphoma (Hodgkin's disease, lymphosarcoma, reticulum cell sarcoma and mycosis fungoides). A study of 196 autopsy cases. Am J Cardiol 1968; 22:85–107.
105. Guidelines for cardiopulmonary resuscitation and emergency cardiac care. Emergency cardiac care committee and subcommittees, American heart association. part III. Adult advanced cardiac life support. JAMA 1992; 268:2199–2241.
106. Ryan TJ, Anderson JL, Antman EM, Braniff BA, Brooks NH, Califf RM, Hillis LD, Hiratzka LF, Rapaport E, Riegel BJ, Russell RO, Smith EE, Jr, Weaver WD. ACC/AHA Guidelines for the Management of Patients with Acute Myocardial Infarction. A Report of the American College of Cardiology/American Heart Association Task

Force on Practice Guidelines (Committee on Management of Acute Myocardial Infarction). J Am Coll Cardiol 1996; 28:1328–1428.

107. O'Dwyer PJ, King SA, Fortner CL, Leyland-Jones B. Hypersensitivity reactions to teniposide (VM-26): an analysis. J Clin Oncol 1986; 4:1262–1269.

108. Vumon in Physician's Desk Reference. Montvale, NJ: Medical Economics Company Inc., 1999:810–812.

109. Schwarzer S, Eber B, Greinix H, Lind P. Non-Q-wave myocardial infarction associated with bleomycin and etoposide chemotherapy. Eur Heart J 1991; 12:748–750.

110. Airey CL, Dodwell DJ, Joffe JK, Jones WG. Etoposide-related myocardial infarction. Clin Oncol (Royal Coll Radiol) 1995; 7:135.

111. Ratanatharathorn V, Drelichman A, Sexon-Porte M, Al Sarraf M. Phase II evaluation of 4'-[9-acridinylamino]-methanesulfon-m-anisidine (AMSA) in patients with advanced head and neck cancers. Am J Clin Oncol 1982; 5:29–32.

112. Ettinger DS, Day R, Ferraro JA, Ruckdeschel JC, Well JE, Creech RH, Vogl SE. A randomized phase II study of m-AMSA (NSC 249992) and neocarzinostatin (NSC 157365) in non-small cell bronchogenic carcinoma. An eastern cooperative group study. Am J Clin Oncol 1983; 6:167–170.

113. Legha SS, Blumenschein GR, Buzdar AU, Hortobagyi GN, Bodey GP. Phase II study of 4'-[9-acridmylamino]methanesulfon-m-anisidide (AMSA) in metastatic breast cancer. Cancer Treat Rep 1979; 63:1961–1964.

114. Schneider RJ, Woodcock TM, Yagoda A. Phase II trial of 4'-[9-acridinylamino]methanesulfon-m-anisidide (AMSA) in patients with metastatic hypernephroma. Cancer Treat Rep 1980; 64:183–185.

115. Legha SS, Hall SW, Powell KC, Burgess MA, Benjamin RS, Gutterman JU, Bodey GP. Phase II study of 4'-[9-acridinylamino] methanesulfon-m-anisidide (AMSA) in metastatic melanoma. Cancer Clin Trials 1980; 3:111–114.

116. Bukowski RM, Leichman LP, Rivkin SE. Phase II trial of m-AMSA in gallbladder and cholangiocarcinoma: a southwest oncology group study. Eur J Cancer Clin Oncol 1983; 19:721–723.

117. De Jager R, Siegenthaler P, Cavalli F, Klepp O, Bramwell V, Joss R, Alberto P, van Glabbeke M, Renard J, Rozencweig M, Hansen HH. Phase II study of amsacrine in solid tumors: a report of the EORTC early clinical trial-group. Eur J Cancer Clin Oncol 1983; 19:289–293.

118. Weiss RB, Grillo-Lopez AJ, Marsoni S, Posada JG Jr, Hess F, Ross BJ. Amsacrine-associated cardiotoxicity: an analysis of 82 cases. J Clin Oncol 1986; 4:918–928.

119. Vorobiof DA, Iturralde M, Falkson G. Amsacrine cardiotoxicity: assessment of ventricular function by radionuclide angiography. Cancer Treat Rep 1983; 67:1115–1117.

120. Legha SS, Gutterman JU, Hall SW, Benjamin RS, Burgess MA, Valdivieso M, Bodey GP. Phase 1 clinical investigation of 4'-[9-acridinylamino]methanesulfon-m-anisidide (NSC 249992), a new acridine derivative. Cancer Res 1978; 38:3712–3716.

121. Von Hoff DD, Elson D, Polk G, Coltman C Jr. Acute ventricular fibrillation and death during infusion of 4'-[9-acridinylamino]methanesulfon-m-anisidide (AMSA). Cancer Treat Rep 1980; 64:356–358.

122. Legha SS, Latreille J, McCredie KB, Bodey GP. Neurologic and cardiac rhythm abnormalities associated with 4'-[9-acridinylamino]-methanesulfon-m-anisidide (AMSA) therapy. Cancer Treat Rep 1979; 63:2001–2003.

123. Wong J, Lipshultz SE. Cardiovascular complications of pharmacotherapeutic agents (excluding the antiretrovirals) in pediatric HIV infection. In: Lipshultz SE, ed. Cardiology in AIDS. New York: Chapman and Hall, 1998:331–344.

124. Vesanoid in Physicians Desk Reference. Montvale, NJ: Medical Economics Company Inc., 1999:2726–2728.

125. Frankel SR, Eardley A, Heller G, Berman E, Miller WH Jr, Dmitrovsky E, Warrell RP Jr. All-trans retinoic acid for acute promyelocytic leukemia. Results of the New York study. Ann Intern Med 1994; 120:278–286.

126. Mone SM, Gillman MW, Miller TL, Herman EH, Lipshultz SE. Effects of environmental exposures on the cardiovascular system: prenatal period through adolescence. Pediatrics (accepted 9/02). In press.

127. Cairo MS, Lazarus K, Gilmore RL, Baehner RL. Intracranial hemorrhage and focal seizures secondary to use of L-asparaginase during induction therapy of acute lymphocytic leukemia. J Pediatr 1980; 97:829–833.

128. Conard J, Cazenave B, Maury J, Horellou MH, Samama M. L-asparaginase, antithrombin III, and thrombosis. Lancet 1980; 1:1091.

129. Parsons SK, Skapek SX, Neufeld EJ, Kuhlman C, Young ML, Donnelly M, Brunzell JD, Otvos JD, Sallan SE, Rifai N. Asparaginase-associated lipid abnormalities in children with acute lymphoblastic leukemia. Blood 1997; 89:1886–1895.

130. Muggia M. Liposomal encapsulated anthracyclines: new therapeutic horizons. Curr Oncol Rep 2001; 3:156–162.

131. The Internet Drug Index. RxList, 2002.

132. Stewart JR, Fajardo LF. Radiation-induced heart disease. Clinical and experimental aspects. Radiol Clin North Am 1971; 9:511–531.

133. Stewart JR, Fajardo LF, Gillette SM, Constine LS. Radiation injury to the heart. Int J Radiat Oncol Biol Phys 1995; 31:1205–1211.

134. Walden TL, Farzaneh NK. Biochemical response of normal tissue to ionizing radiation. In: Gutin PH, Leibel SA, Sheline GE, eds.

Radiation Injury to the Nervous System. New York: Raven Press, 2003:17–36.

135. Fajardo LF, Stewart JR, Cohn KE. Morphology of radiation-induced heart disease. Arch Pathol 1968; 86:512–519.

136. Chello M, Mastroroberto P, Romano R, Zofrea S, Bevacqua I, Marchese AR. Changes in the proportion of types I and III collagen in the left ventricular wall of patients with post-irradiative pericarditis. Cardiovasc Surg 1996; 4:222–226.

137. Orzan F, Brusca A, Gaita F, Giustetto C, Figliomeni MC, Libero L. Associated cardiac lesions in patients with radiation-induced complete heart block. Int J Cardiol 1993; 39:151–156.

138. Cohen SI, Bharati S, Glass J, Lev M. Radiotherapy as a cause of complete atrioventricular block in Hodgkin's disease. An electrophysiological-pathological correlation. Arch Intern Med 1981; 141:676–679.

139. La Vecchia L. Physiologic dual chamber pacing in radiation-induced atrioventricular block. Chest 1996; 110:580–581.

140. McEniery PT, Dorosti K, Schiavone WA, Pedrick TJ, Sheldon WC. Clinical and angiographic features of coronary artery disease after chest irradiation. Am J Cardiol 1987; 60:1020–1024.

141. King V, Constine LS, Clark D, Schwartz RG, Muhs AG, Henzler M, Hutson A, Rubin P. Symptomatic coronary artery disease after mantle irradiation for Hodgkin's disease. Int J Radiat Oncol Biol Phys 1996; 36:881–889.

142. Annest LS, Anderson RP, Li W, Hafermann MD. Coronary artery disease following mediastinal radiation therapy. J Thorac Cardiovasc Surg 1983; 85:257–263.

143. Brosius FC III, Waller BF, Roberts WC. Radiation heart disease: analysis of 16 young (aged 15 to 33 years) necropsy patients who received over 3,500 rads to the heart. Am J Med 1981; 70:519–530.

144. Veinot JP, Edwards WD. Pathology of radiation-induced heart disease: a surgical and autopsy study of 27 cases. Hum Pathol 1996; 27:766–773.

145. McReynolds RA, Gold GL, Roberts WC. Coronary heart disease after mediastinal irradiation for Hodgkin's disease. Am J Med 1976; 60:39–45.

146. Joensuu H. Myocardial infarction after irradiation in Hodgkin's disease: a review. Recent Results Cancer Res 1993; 130:157–173.

147. Bradley EW, Zook BC, Casarett GW, Rogers CC. Coronary arteriosclerosis and atherosclerosis in fast neutron or photon irradiated dogs. Int J Radiat Oncol Biol Phys 1981; 7:1103–1108.

148. Artom C, Lofland HB Jr, Clarkson TB. Ionizing radiation, atherosclerosis, and lipid metabolism in pigeons. Radiat Res 1965; 26:165–177.

149. Carlson RG, Mayfield WR, Normann S, Alexander JA. Radiation-associated valvular disease. Chest 1991; 99:538–545.

150. Hancock SL, Tucker MA, Hoppe RT. Factors affecting late mortality from heart disease after treatment of Hodgkin's disease. JAMA 1993; 270:1949–1955.

151. Aisenberg AC. Problems in Hodgkin's disease management. Blood 1999; 93:761–779.

152. Lee CK, Aeppli D, Nierengarten ME. The need for long-term surveillance for patients treated with curative radiotherapy for Hodgkin's disease: university of Minnesota experience. Int J Radiat Oncol Biol Phys 2000; 48:169–179.

153. Mauch PM, Kalish LA, Marcus KC, Shulman LN, Krill E, Tarbell N, Silver B, Weinstein H, Come S, Canellos GP, Coleman CN. Long-term survival in Hodgkin's disease. Cancer J Sci Am 1995; 1:33.

154. Hoppe RT. Hodgkin's disease: complications of therapy and excess mortality. Ann Oncol 1997; 8(suppl 1):115–118.

155. Hancock SL, Donaldson SS, Hoppe RT. Cardiac disease following treatment of Hodgkin's disease in children and adolescents. J Clin Oncol 1993; 11:1208–1215.

156. Adams MJ, Hardenbergh PH, Constine LS, Lipshultz SE. Radiation-associated cardiovascular disease. Grit Rev Oncol Hematol 2003; 45:55–75.

157. Cameron EH, Lipshultz SE, Tarbell NJ, Mauch P. Cardiovascular disease in long- term survivors of pediatric Hodgkin's disease. Prog Pediatr Cardiol 1998; 8:139–144.

158. Tolba KA, Deliargyris EN. Cardiotoxicity of cancer therapy. Cancer Invest 1999; 17:408–422.

159. Burns RJ, Bar-Shlomo BZ, Druck MN, Herman JG, Gilbert BW, Perrault DJ, McLaughlin PR. Detection of radiation cardiomyopathy by gated radionuclide angiography. Am J Med 1983; 74:297–302.

160. Constine LS, Schwartz RG, Savage DE, King V, Muhs A. Cardiac function, perfusion, and morbidity in irradiated long-term survivors of Hodgkin's disease. Int J Radiat Oncol Biol Phys 1997; 39:897–906.

161. Hardenbergh PH, Munley MT, Bentel GC, Kedem R, Borges-Neto S, Hollis D, Prosnitz LR, Marks LB. Cardiac perfusion changes in patients treated for breast cancer with radiation therapy and doxorubicin: preliminary results. Int J Radiat Oncol Biol Phys 2001; 49: 1023–1028.

162. Gyenes G, Fornander T, Carlens P, Glas U, Rutqvist LE. Myocardial damage in breast cancer patients treated with adjuvant radiotherapy: a prospective study. Int J Radiat Oncol Biol Phys 1996; 36: 899–905.

163. Fajardo LF, Stewart JR. Pathogenesis of radiation-induced myocardial fibrosis. Lab Invest 1973; 29:244–257.

164. Billingham ME, Bristow MR, Glatstein E, Mason JW, Masek MA, Daniels JR. Adriamycin cardiotoxicity: endomyocardial biopsy evidence of enhancement by irradiation. Am J Surg Pathol 1977; 1: 17–23.

165. Merrill J, Greco FA, Zimbler H, Brereton HD, Lamberg JD, Pomeroy TC. Adriamycin and radiation: synergistic cardiotoxicity. Ann Intern Med 1975; 82:122–123.
166. Kinsella TJ, Ahmann DL, Giuliani ER, Lie JT. Adriamycin cardiotoxicity in stage IV breast cancer: possible enhancement with prior left chest radiation therapy. Int J Radiat Oncol Biol Phys 1979; 5: 1997–2002.
167. Eltringham JR, Fajardo LF, Stewart JR, Klauber MR. Investigation of cardiotoxicity in rabbits from adriamycin and fractionated cardiac irradiation: preliminary results. Front Radiat Ther Oncol 1979; 13: 21–35.
168. Glanzmann C, Huguenin P, Lutolf UM, Maire R, Jenni R, Gumppenberg V. Cardiac lesions after mediastinal irradiation for Hodgkin's disease. Radiother Oncol 1994; 30:43–54.
169. Gustavsson A, Eskilsson J, Landberg T, Svahn-Tapper G, White T, Wollmer P, Akemian M. Late cardiac effects after mantle radiotherapy in patients with Hodgkin's disease. Ann Oncol 1990; 1:355–363.
170. Lund MB, Ihlen H, Voss BM, Abrahamsen AF, Nome O, Kongerud J, Stugaard M, Forfang K. Increased risk of heart valve regurgitation after mediastinal radiation for Hodgkin's disease: an echocardiographic study. Heart 1996; 75:591–595.
171. Slama MS, Le Guludec D, Sebag C, Leenhardt AR, Davy JM, Pellerin DE, Drieu LH, Victor J, Brechenmacher C, Motte G. Complete atrioventricular block following mediastinal irradiation: a report of six cases. Pacing Clin Electrophysiol 1991; 14:1112–1118.
172. Pohjola-Sintonen S, Totterman KJ, Kupari M. Sick sinus syndrome as a complication of mediastinal radiation therapy. Cancer 1990; 65: 2494–2496.
173. Adams MJ, Lipsitz SR, Colan S, Mauch PM, Diller L, Treves ST, Tarbell NJ, Greenbaum N, Lipshultz SE. Late cardiotoxicity of mediastinal irradiation [abstr]. Proc ASCO 2003. In press.
174. Eichholtz-Wirth H. Dependence of the cytostatic effect of adriamycin on drug concentration and exposure time in vitro. Br J Cancer 1980; 41:886–891.
175. Haskell CM, Sullivan A. Comparative survival in tissue culture of normal and neoplastic human cells exposed to adriamycin. Cancer Res 1974; 34:2991–2994.
176. Steinherz PG, Redner A, Steinherz L, Meyers P, Tan C, Heller G. Development of a new intensive therapy for acute lymphoblastic leukemia in children at increased risk of early relapse: the memorial sloan-kettering-New York-II protocol. Cancer 1993; 72:3120–3130.
177. Lipshultz SE, Giantris AL, Lipsitz SR, Kimball Dalton V, Asselin BL, Barr RD, Clavell LA, Hurwitz CA, Moghrabi A, Samson Y, Schorin MA, Gelber RD, Sallan SE, Colan SD. Doxorubicin administration by continuous infusion is not cardioprotective: the dana-farber

91–01 acute lymphoblastic leukemia protocol. J Clin Oncol 2002; 20:1677–1682.

178. Ottlinger ME, Pearsall L, Rifai N, Lipshultz SE. New developments in the biochemical assessment of myocardial injury in children: troponins T and I as highly sensitive and specific markers of myocardial injury. Progr Pediatr Cardiol 1998; 8:71–81.

179. Darussi I, Indolfi P, Casale F, Coppolino P, Tedesco MA, DiTullio MT. Recent advances in the prevention of anthracycline cardiotoxicity in childhood. Cur Med Chem 2001; 8:1649–1660.

180. Andrieu-Abadie N, Jaffrezou JP, Hatem S, Laurent G, Levade T, Mercaider JJ. L-carnitine prevents doxorubicin-induced apoptosis of cardiac myocytes: role of inhibition of ceramide generation. FASEB J 1999; 13:1501–1510.

181. Yue TL, Cheng HY, Lysko PG, McKenna PJ, Feuerstein R, Gu JL, Lysko KA, Davis LL, Feuerstein G. Carvedilol, a new vasodilator and beta adrenoceptor antagonist, is an antioxidant and free radical scavenger. J Pharmacol Exp Ther 1992; 263:92–98.

182. Santos DL, Moreno AJ, Leino RL, Froberg MK, Wallace KB. Carvedilol protects against doxorubicin-induced mitochondrial cardiomyopathy. Toxicol Appl Pharmacol 2002; 185:218–227.

183. Matsui H, Morishima I, Nurnaguchi Y, Toki Y, Okumura K, Hayakawa T. Protective effects of carvedilol against doxorubicin-induced cardiomyopathy in rats. Life Sci 1999; 65:1265–1274.

184. Shioji K, Kishimoto C, Nakamura H, Masutani H, Yuan Z, Oka S, Yodoi J. Overexpression of thioredoxin-1 in transgenic mice attenuates adriamycin-induced cardiotoxicity. Circulation 2002; 106: 1403–1409.

185. Swain SM. Adult multicenter trials using dexrazoxane to protect against cardiac toxicity. Semin Oncol 1998; 25:43–47.

186. Seymour L, Bramwell V, Moran LA. Use of dexrazoxane as a cardioprotectant in patients receiving doxorubicin or epirubicin chemotherapy for the treatment of cancer. Cancer Care Ontario Practice Guidelines Initiative CPG 2002:12–15.

187. Wexler LH, Andrich MP, Venzon D, Berg SL, Weaver-McClure L, Chen CC, Dilsizian V, Avila N, Jarosinski P, Balis FM, Poplack DG, Horowitz ME. Randomized trial of the cardioprotective agent ICRF-187 in pediatric sarcoma patients treated with doxorubicin. J Clin Oncol 1996; 14:362–372.

188. Schuchter LM, Hensley ML, Meropol NJ, Winer EP. 2002 update of recommendations for the use of chemotherapy and radiotherapy protectants: clinical practice guidelines of the American Society of Clinical Oncology. J Clin Oncol 2002; 20:2895–2903.

189. Lipshultz SE, Rifai N, Sallan SE, Lipsitz SR, Dalton V, Sacks DB, Ottlinger ME. Predictive value of cardiac troponin T in pediatric patients at risk for myocardial injury. Circulation 1997; 96: 2641–2648.

190. Lipshultz SE, Colan SD, Silverman LB, Levy DE, Dalton VK, Rifai N, Lipsitz SR, Gelber R, Sallan SE. Dexrazoxane reduces incidence of doxorubicin-associated acute myocardiocyte injury in children with acute lymphoblastic leukemia (ALL). Proc ASCO 2002; 21:390A.

191. Bu'Lock FA, Gabriel HM, Oakhill A, Mott MG, Martin RP. Cardioprotection by ICRF187 against high dose anthracycline toxicity in children with malignant disease. Br Heart 1993; 170:185–188.

192. Hunt SA, Baker DW, Chin MH, Cinquegrani MP, Feldmanmd AM, Francis GS, Ganiats TG, Goldstein S, Gregoratos G, Jessup ML, Noble RJ, Packer M, Silver MA, Stevenson LW, Gibbons RJ, Antman EM, Alpert JS, Faxon DP, Fuster V, Gregoratos G, Jacobs AK, Hiratzka LF, Russell RO, Smith SC Jr. ACC/AHA Guidelines for the Evaluation and Management of Chronic Heart Failure in the Adult: Executive Summary A Report of the American College of Cardiology/American Heart Association Task Force on Practice Guidelines (Committee to Revise the 1995 Guidelines for the Evaluation and Management of Heart Failure): Developed in Collaboration with the International Society for Heart And Lung Transplantation; Endorsed by the Heart Failure Society of America. Circulation 2001; 104:2996–3007.

193. Lipshultz SE. Ventricular dysfunction clinical research in infants, children and adolescents. Prog Fed Cardiol 2000; 12:1–28.

194. Kay JD, Colan SD, Graham TP Jr. Congestive heart failure in pediatric patients. Am Heart J 2001; 142:923–928.

195. Shaddy RE. Optimizing treatment for chronic congestive heart failure in children. Crit Care Med 2001; 29:S237–S240.

196. Grenier MA, Fioravanti J, Tniesdell SC, Mendelsohn AM, Vermilion RP, Lipshultz SE. Angiotensin-converting enzyme inhibitor therapy for ventricular dysfunction in infants, children and adolescents: a review. Prog Fed Cardiol 2000; 12:91–111.

197. Lipshultz SE, Lipsitz , Sallan SE, Simbre VC, Shaikh SL, Mone SM, Gelber RD, Colan SD. Long-term enalapril therapy for left ventricular dysfunction in doxorubicin-treated survivors of childhood cancer. J Clin Oncol 2002; 20:4517–4522.

198. Colucci WS, Packer M, Bristow MR, Gilbert EM, Cohn JN, Fowler MB, Krueger SK, Hershberger R, Uretsky BF, Bowers JA, Sackner-Bernstein JD, Young ST, Holcslaw TL, Lukas MA. Carvedilol inhibits clinical progression in patients with mild symptoms of heart failure: US Carvedilol Heart Failure Study Group. Circulation 1996; 94:2800–2806.

199. Packer M, Bristow MR, Cohn JN, Colucci WS, Fowler MB, Gilbert EM, Shusterman NH. The effect of carvedilol on morbidity and mortality in patients with chronic heart failure: U.S. Carvedilol Heart Failure Study Group. N Engl J Med 1996; 334:1349–1355.

200. Packer M, Fowler MB, Roecker EB, Coats AJ, Katus HA, Krum H, Mohacsi P, Rouleau JL, Tendera M, Staiger C, Holcslaw TL,

Amann-Zalan I, DeMets DL. Effect of carvedilol on the morbidity of patients with severe chronic heart failure: results of the carvedilol prospective randomized cumulative survival (COPERNICUS) study. Circulation 2002; 106:2194–2199.

201. Bruns LA, Chrisant, Lamour JM, Shaddy RE, Pahl E, Blume ED, Hallowell S, Addonizio LJ, Canter CE. Carvedilol as therapy in pediatric heart failure: an initial multicenter experience. J Pediatr 2001; 138:505–511.

202. Williams RV, Tani LY, Shaddy RE. Intermediate effects of treatment with metoprolol or carvedilol in children with left ventricular systolic dysfunction. J Heart Lung Transplant 2002; 21:906–909.

203. Noori A, Lindenfeld J, Wolfel E, Ferguson D, Bristow, Lowes BD. Beta-blockade in adriamycin-induced cardiomyopathy. J Card Fail 2000; 6:115–119.

204. Shaddy RE, Olsen SL, Bristow MR, Taylor DO, Bullock EA, Tani LY, Renlund DG. Efficacy and safety of metoprolol in the treatment of doxorubicin-induced cardiomyopathy in pediatric patients. Am Heart J 1995; 129:197–199.

205. Shaddy RE. Beta-blocker therapy in young children with congestive heart failure under consideration for heart transplantation. Am Heart J 1998; 136:19–21.

206. Morton DL, Glancy DL, Joseph WL, Adkins PC. Management of patients with radiation-induced pericarditis with effusion: a note on the development of aortic regurgitation in two of them. Chest 1973; 64:291–297.

207. Oeffmger KC, Buchanan GR, Eshelman DA, Denke MA, Andrews TC, Germak JA, Tomlinson GE, Snell LE, Foster BM. Cardiovascular risk factors in young adult survivors of childhood acute lymphoblastic leukemia. J Pediatr Hematol Oncol 2001; 23:424–430.

208. Didi M, Didcock E, Davies HA, Ogilvy-Stuart AL, Wales JK, Shalet SM. High incidence of obesity in young adults after treatment of acute lymphoblastic leukemia in childhood. J Pediatr 1995; 127:63–67.

209. Talvensaari KK, Lanning M, Tapanainen P, Knip M. Long-term survivors of childhood cancer have an increased risk of manifesting the metabolic syndrome. J Clin Endocrinol Metab 1996; 81:3051–3055.

210. Sung RY, Huang GY, Shing MK, Oppenheimer SJ, Li CK, Lau J, Yuen MP. Echocardiographic evaluation of cardiac function in paediatric oncology patients treated with or without anthracycline. Int J Cardiol 1997; 60:239–248.

211. Lipshultz SE, Orav EJ, Sanders SP, McIntosh K, Golan SD. Limitations of fractional shortening as an index of contractility in pediatric patients infected with human immunodeficiency virus. J Pediatr 1994; 125:563–570.

212. Lipshultz SE, Sallan SE. Cardiovascular abnormalities in long-term survivors of childhood malignancy. J Clin Oncol 1993; 11:1199–1203.

213. Warda M, Khan A, Massumi A, Mathur V, Klima T, Hall RJ. Radiation-induced valvular dysfunction. J Am Coll Cardiol 1983; 2: 180–185.
214. Lipshultz SE, Sallan SE, Dalton V, Arslanian S, Zou, Shaikh S, Asselin B, Gelber R, Rifai N. Elevated serum cardiac troponin T as a marker for active cardiac injury during therapy for childhood lymphoblastic leukemia. Proc Am Soc Clin Oncol 1999; 18:568A.
215. Adams MJ, Constine L, Lipshultz SE. Radiation effects on the heart. In: Crawford MH, DiMarco JP, eds. Cardiology. 2nd ed. London: Mosby International, 2002. In press.

19

Coronary Artery Abnormalities

ELFRIEDE PAHL and STEPHEN G. POPHAL
Department of Pediatrics, Children's Memorial
Hospital, Northwestern University,
Feinberg School of Medicine,
Chicago, Illinois, U.S.A.

INTRODUCTION

Structural abnormalities of the coronary arteries in children occur rarely. Congenital coronary anomalies may occur in isolation, as in anomalous left coronary artery from the pulmonary artery (ALCAPA), single coronary artery, or coronary artery fistula (CAF). Coronary anomalies may also be associated with certain congenital heart defects, such as tetralogy of Fallot (TOF), transposition of the great arteries, truncus arteriosus (TA), and pulmonary atresia. Although acquired abnormalities of the coronary vessels in children are also rare, they have been identified in Kawasaki disease (KD),

739

as well as in cardiac transplant recipients (i.e., allograft vasculopathy), familial hyperlipidemia, children with chronic renal failure, and patients with acquired immunodeficiency disorder.

NORMAL CORONARY ANATOMY

Angelini (1)summarized normal coronary anatomy. In the setting of normally related great arteries, the aorta is right and posterior, and the normal ostia of the coronary arteries are in the right and the left facing aortic sinuses. They arise from the center of each sinus close to the sinotubular ridge. Two coronary ostia are the minimum requirements, however, 3–4 ostia are considered normal variants; separate coronary ostia for either a conal vessel or separate ostia for the left anterior descending (LAD) and circumflex branches (Cx) are common (2,3).

The left coronary artery (LCA) usually divides into LAD and Cx branches. An intermediate artery (Ramus intermedius) often arises as a trifurcation of the left main or may come from a proximal aspect of either the Cx or LAD and is a normal variant. The right coronary artery (RCA) often gives a conal branch (in 30–50% of humans) to the infundibulum of the right ventricle as well as a posteriorly directed vessel to the SA node. The RCA continues with an AV nodal branch and then supplies the posterointerventricular septum via the posterior descending vessel. The majority of the population has a dominant RCA system with a posterior descending branch from the RCA (1). Angiographically, coronary artery anatomy can usually be defined with standard views. However, in certain circumstances, such as in d-transposition of the great arteries, special views are necessary to optimally define anatomy (4,5).

The incidence of coronary anomalies detected by angiography is 0.3–1% of the general population based on two large series (6,7). Since autopsy is not routinely performed, the true incidence of coronary anomalies in the general population remains unknown since angiographic series represent a "select" population. A prospective 3-year study of echocardiograms in 2388 children sought to determine the incidence of coronary artery anomalies (CAA) in young patients with structurally normal hearts referred for echo usually because of heart murmur. This study found only four cases (0.17%) of abnormal coronary origins and included anomalous origin of the LCA from the right sinus in two, and the converse, i.e., anomalous RCA from a single left CA in two others (8).

In a European study, 62,320 children had routine echocardiographic assessment of the coronary ostia and the course of the initial segment of the coronary arteries (9). CAA were found in only 29 children aged 1 day to 12 years. Abnormalities were isolated in 18, including ALCAPA in 13, anomalous RCA from the PA in one, and four with CAF. Nine other children with CAA had congenital heart defects and two had Kawasaki syndrome.

Coronary anomalies must be characterized by features such as number and location of ostia, proximal course, pattern and size of main vessels; and branching patterns of vessels. A large table with classification of coronary anomalies was reported recently (7). These authors define an anomaly as a morphologic feature seen in less than 1% of the population. Thus, "normal" refers to any anatomic or morphologic feature observed in greater than 1% of an unselected population and "normal variant" is a "relatively unusual morphologic feature" that is seen in greater than 1% of the population.

Culham (10) defines "anomalous origin" as occurring when a LCA, RCA, LAD, or Cx vessel arises abnormally from the aorta or another vessel. The term "aberrant" is applied to the course of a vessel. The term "accessory" is used when two or more vessels supply a segment of myocardium that is typically supplied by a single vessel.

The Congenital Heart Surgery Database Project reviews the existent nomenclature for CAA in a recent report (11). Table 1 is a modification of major categories of coronary anomalies in children that may be associated with congestive heart failure.

Table 1 Types of Coronary Artery Abnormalities

Congenital anomalies—isolated
A. Anomalous pulmonary artery origins of the coronaries
B. Anomalous aortic origins of the coronary arteries
C. Congenital atresia of the left main coronary artery
D. Coronary artery fistulas
E. Coronary artery bridging
Coronary artery abnormalities associated with congenital heart disease
Coronary artery aneurysms
Coronary artery stenosis—acquired
a. Postoperative etiology
b. Atherosclerosis

CONGENITAL ANOMALIES—ISOLATED

Anomalous Left Coronary Artery Connected to the Pulmonary Artery (ALCAPA)

There is extensive literature on ALCAPA (12); these patients often present with a dilated cardiomyopathy in infancy. However, adolescent patients have been identified who had excellent collateral vessels (Fig. 1A and B). Anomalous connection of the RCA to the pulmonary artery is much more rare, may have hemodynamic importance in some cases, and is amenable to surgical correction (13). These anomalies usually occur in isolation with an otherwise structurally normal heart. ALCAPA has rarely been reported in conjunction with congenital heart defects such as TOF or VSD (14).

Symptoms are uncommon in the first days to weeks of life due to the normal physiologic situation where diastolic pressures of the pulmonary trunk and aortic root are similar. The child does not develop symptoms until the pulmonary pressures drop and when ischemia (due to changes in coronary perfusion) leads ultimately to myocardial ischemia and/or infarction of the left ventricle often involving the papillary muscles. Retrograde flow from the RCA to the LCA via collateral channels occurs. The degree of cardiac dysfunction, ischemia, and infarction are variable based on the degree of collateral development. Mitral regurgitation is common and may be due to papillary muscle ischemia or infarction.

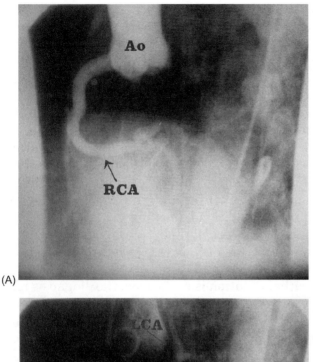

(A)

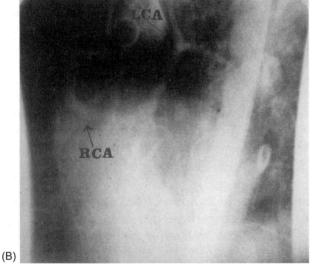

(B)

Figure 1 Eighteen-year-old with left coronary artery from the pulmonary artery. (A) Aortogram in left anterior oblique view demonstrates dilated right coronary artery with no origin of the left coronary artery. (B) Delayed filling of the left coronary artery occurred from a mesh of collaterals from the right coronary artery.

The anomalous LCA usually connects to a facing pulmonary sinus but the connection may be to the main or the proximal left pulmonary artery as well. Standard diagnosis in the current era is by two-dimensional echocardiography, although sensitivity is not 100%. With the addition of color flow Doppler, echo diagnosis has improved and is based on identifying retrograde flow in segments of the anomalous coronary artery and/or a diastolic flow jet in the pulmonary artery (15,16). Serial electron beam computer tomography (EBCT) nicely demonstrated ALCAPA in a 28-year-old woman who presented with exertional ischemic chest pain (17). Thus, in any patient where the diagnosis is unclear and the electrocardiogram suggests ischemia (18), additional imaging with either contrast CT, transesophageal echocardiography, or angiography should be performed since ALCAPA is one of the few treatable etiologies for dilated cardiomyopathy.

If cardiac catheterization is performed, the diagnosis may be confirmed by left ventriculography, aortic root angiography (Fig. 1), or selective coronary injections. The angiographic criteria for diagnosis include (1) retrograde filling of the abnormal vessel, (2) connection of the abnormal vessel to the pulmonary artery with pulmonary artery opacification, and (3) the absence of a connection to the aorta. Selective coronary angiography of the right coronary vessel usually demonstrates an enlarged vessel with retrograde filling of the LCA from collaterals. Although patients may be stabilized hemodynamically using inotropic support and diuretics, corrective surgery should be scheduled once the diagnosis is established.

Several different operations have been performed historically. Originally, simple ligation of the anomalous vessel was performed; however, the incidence of late death is unacceptable with this procedure and a two-coronary system should be established. Currently, the preferred method is an establishment of antegrade flow into the anomalous vessel usually by direct implantation if possible (19) (Fig. 2). In cases that are not favorable for reimplantation, a tunnel repair (20) or bypass grafting is advocated (21).

A recent study assessed mid-term functional outcome and time to left ventricular recovery (22). These authors reviewed

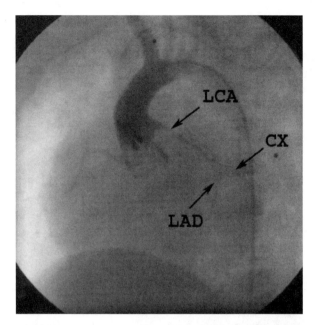

Figure 2 Postoperative aortogram (left anterior oblique) of infant with left coronary artery from the pulmonary artery shows direct anastomosis of proximal left coronary artery to ascending aorta. Note the long left main coronary artery (LCA) and the distal branching of the LAD and circumflex (Cx) arteries.

47 children with ALCAPA who had repair, by aortic reimplantation at a median age of 7.7 months with concomitant mitral repair in only one child. Hospital survival was 92% and five children required ECMO for 2–8 days. Ventricular recovery took 3–6 months. In another series of infants with severe LV dysfunction, mechanical left ventricular support using a centrifugal pump was successful in 5/7 infants operated for ALCAPA who could not be weaned from bypass (23).

Single Coronary Artery/Anomalous Coronary Origin

This group includes anomalies where the coronary artery does not arise from the usual position as well as abnormalities arising from a single coronary artery, which may have an aberrant course. The term "single coronary artery" is reserved for both right and left vessels arising from a single orifice. A single RCA traditionally refers to the right coronary arising appropriately from the right sinus with the LCA arising from the right coronary vessel and vice versa for a single LCA (Figs. 3 and 4). Additionally, the main trunk itself may have an anomalous aortic wall or sinus origin. Single coronary arteries are seen in 0.02–0.05% of adult angiographic series (10).

Coronary arteries normally arise at right angles to the wall of the aortic sinus; however, a more tangential origin may be associated with a slit-like orifice and cause vascular compromise; there may be further narrowing by aortic distention associated with exercise (24). Coronary anomalies are an

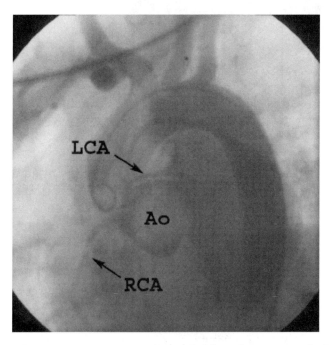

Figure 3 Aortogram from child with exertional chest pain with origin of single coronary artery from the right sinus with the left main coronary artery (LCA) taking off and coursing between the pulmonary artery and the aorta (Ao = aorta; RCA = right coronary artery).

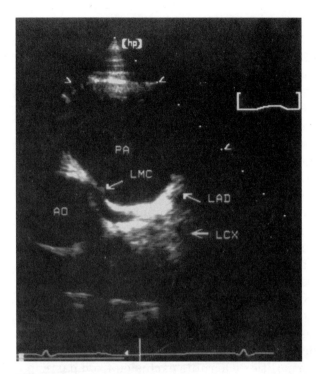

Figure 4 Transthoracic echocardiogram, short axis view of a teenage boy who collapsed during basketball and was resuscitated from ventricular fibrillation. Note the single coronary artery with the LCA arising from the RCA with intramural course of proximal left coronary artery: AO = aorta, LMC = left main coronary, PA = pulmonary artery, LAD = left anterior descending, CX = Circumflex. (Courtesy of Dr. Ernerio Alboliras, Rush Children's Heart Center.)

important cause of sudden death (25). In a report of young athletes, 11.8% of deaths were due to coronary anomalies (26). In another report, Maron et al. (27) found that 19% of the sudden deaths in athletes were from coronary anomalies.

Another study reported on congenital coronary anomalies with "origin of wrong aortic sinus" which led to sudden death in 27 young competitive athletes. Of these sudden deaths, 23 had a left main coronary artery arising from the right aortic sinus and four had an RCA arising from the left sinus (28). All athletes died during or immediately after intensive exertion on the athletic field. Although 15 (55%) had no prior cardiovascular manifestations during life, 12 of the remaining athletes reported prior symptoms including syncope and chest pain. None of these patients had congestive heart failure.

Frommelt et al. (29) recently identified 10 patients with anomalous origin of a coronary artery from the opposite sinus with an interarterial course between the great arteries. In seven patients, unroofing of the intramural portion was done surgically without need for bypass grafting.

Strategies for identification of these patients with non-invasive screening are difficult since routine evaluation of athletes is not performed. Certainly, it is appropriate to perform anatomic evaluation of patients with history of exertional syncope or chest pain either with transthoracic echo or MRI, even in the setting of a normal ECG. Imaging of the left and right coronary arteries with echocardiography was feasible and reliable in 95% of young athletes studied (30).

If screening fails to demonstrate that both proximal coronary arteries' origins are from the usual sinus, then further anatomic definition is indicated. Clinical identification of these abnormalities warrants exclusion from participation in competitive sports to reduce the risk of sudden death. More importantly, these patients should undergo surgical intervention with either coronary bypass grafting or reimplantation of the anomalous vessel into the proper sinus (31).

Ostial Stenosis/Atresia of Left Coronary Artery

Isolated ostial stenosis, hypoplasia, or atresia of the LCA is extremely rare (32). In the absence of congenital heart disease, there may be a wide clinical spectrum, which is reflected by the degree and quality of the collateral circulation, as well as the degree of development of the involved coronary artery (Fig. 5).

Ostial lesions are difficult to demonstrate angiographically. An aortic root injection should indicate whether or not there is antegrade flow into the involved coronary. Additional injections in the left coronary sinus may be required to demonstrate an ostial lesion. The differential diagnosis would include an anomalous LCA arising from the pulmonary artery

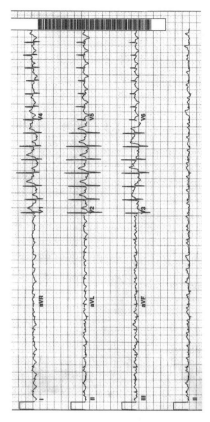

Figure 5 Initial EKG in a 3-week old infant with atresia of the orifice of the LCA presenting with dilated cardiomyopathy, demonstrating low voltage on limb leads.

as well as a single right coronary with extreme dominance and collateral flow to the distribution of the LCA. If an exact preoperative diagnosis cannot be made by angiography, surgical exploration is indicated, with plans to establish a two-coronary system.

Coronary Artery Fistula

Some authors distinguish two categories of fistula; that is of a coronary—cameral fistula referring to a direct connection to one of the cardiac chambers, and AV fistulas, where the coronary artery has a connection with venous plexi, such as to the coronary sinus, which drains the cardiac veins (1). Clinically, the features are similar and may be combined as CAF. These connections may be single and small or large and multiple. The true incidence of CAF is difficult to ascertain since many patients may have small fistula which are asymptomatic and without clinical signs on physical examination. With advances in echocardiography, a higher incidence of "silent" CAF has been noted (33). The majority of connections are to the right side of the heart. The dilation may be uniform or aneurysmal and may have a minimal left-to-right shunt (Fig. 6).

Whether or not incidental fistulas should be closed at all is controversial. A large study of adults with coronary fistulas showed a benign natural history. In adults undergoing diag-

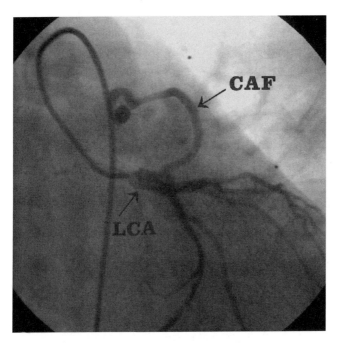

Figure 6 Selective left coronary artery angiogram (right anterior oblique view) with long tortuous coronary artery fistula from left main coronary artery ending in main pulmonary artery.

nostic cardiac catheterization, 34 (0.1%) of 33,600 patients had CAF (34). Nineteen fistulas originated from the RCA, 11 from the LAD, and 4 from the Cx. During a mean follow-up period of 6.3 years (range 2–14 years), there were no complications related to CAF.

Mavroudis et al. (35) report surgical intervention in 17 children age 6 weeks to 16 years who were diagnosed with CAF. The indications for surgery were to protect patients from the natural history of angina (36), endocarditis, syncope (37), rupture, or development of congestive heart failure. The majority of patients had isolated fistula, and all were asymptomatic. Anatomy was confirmed in all by angiography. All patients underwent epicardial and endocardial ligation, with 100% survival and 100% closure rate. Large CAFs produce left-to-right shunt with associated symptoms/signs of congestion, LV dilation and may present in infancy requiring early intervention.

Transcatheter occlusion with coils or other devices is a reasonable alternative to standard surgical closure; however, surgical results should be considered the standard against which catheter techniques are compared. Coronary artery fistula has been closed using coils (Fig. 7), balloons, polyvinyl alcohol foam, and double umbrella devices (38,39).

Acquired fistulas have been reported after trauma, cardiac surgery, and cardiac transplantation. Fistulas from coronary arteries into the right ventricle following endomyocardial biopsies are a relatively frequent finding after heart transplantation. Most of these fistulas are small and hemodynamically insignificant (40). However, if large, coronary fistulas can be closed percutaneously by a variety of devices including a detachable balloon (41).

MYOCARDIAL BRIDGE

Typically, the coronary arteries are epicardial structures and enter the myocardium at the distal end of the branches. Myocardial bridging is evident by the "intramyocardial course" of portions of the coronary arteries, often the mid-portion of the

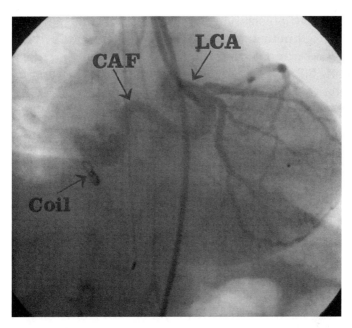

Figure 7   Selective left coronary artery angiogram after successful coil of fistula from left main coronary artery to right atrium. (Courtesy of Dr. David Wax, Children's Memorial Hosptial.)

LAD (42,43). The typical angiographic finding is "systolic milking" due to transient systolic compression of the involved branch of the coronary artery.

Majority of the myocardial bridges occur exclusively in the mid-LAD and may be located at a depth of 1–10 mm with a typical length of 10–30 mm (44). Atherosclerosis has been reported, particularly, in the segment proximal to the myocardial bridge (43). Subendocardial ischemia increases with the intramyocardial depth of the tunneled segment and may be associated with myocardial fibrosis. The clinical presentation of patients with myocardial bridges is generally with angina, myocardial ischemia, myocardial infarction, or exercise induced ventricular tachycardia. Rarely, patients may have left ventricular dysfunction. Rest ECGs are frequently normal, however, stress testing may induce nonspecific signs of ischemia. Myocardial bridging has been associated with increasing severity of septal thickness in patients with hypertrophic cardiomyopathy; however, its prognostic significance is debated (Fig. 8) (45,46).

Treatment of myocardial bridging in symptomatic patients has included the use of negative inotropic agents such as beta-adrenergic receptor antagonists or calcium antagonists, surgical myotomy or coronary artery bypass graft as well as endovascular stenting of the tunneled segment. Medication is first-line therapy; however, in the pediatric patient, more aggressive surgical type intervention may be undertaken if significant ischemia is demonstrated.

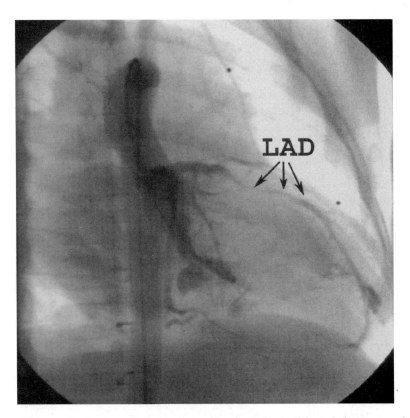

Figure 8 Left ventriculogram from a 2-year old with hypertrophic cardiomyopathy, and a myocardial bridge (view of systole) with marked compression of the mid LAD.

CONGENITAL CORONARY ANOMALY—WITH INTRACARDIAC DEFECT

Coronary artery abnormalities have been associated with specific types of congenital heart disease with variable frequency (Table 2).

In transposition of the great arteries, the aortic origin and epicardial distribution of the coronary branches has been extensively studied and reported and is of particular importance since the arterial switch procedure has become standard corrective therapy. The surgeon will be interested in the relationship of the great arteries, the location of the coronary artery origins, and their epicardial course. A review by Wernovsky and Sanders (5) reported that nine types of CAA account for 95% of all patients with transposition. Intramural coronary arteries in infants with TGA pose an additional technical challenge at arterial switch surgery. A recent review reported 27 intramural CAs of 435 infants with TGA; 20 were diagnosed preoperatively on transthoracic echocardiogram (47).

Intramural Coronary Course

"Intramural course" of a proximal coronary artery is defined as a coronary vessel lined within a wall of the aorta with shared adventitial covering. The intramural component may be compressed as the aorta dilates during exercise. An intramural

Table 2 Congenital Defects with Coronary Artery Abnormalities

1. D-Transposition of the great arteries—variations common
2. Tetralogy of Fallot (anomalous left anterior descending coronary artery, dual left anterior descending coronary artery, single coronary artery)
3. Pulmonary atresia and ventricular septal defect and coronary-artery-to-pulmonary-artery fistula
4. Truncus arteriosus
5. Pulmonary atresia with intact ventricular septum and coronary-artery-to-right-ventricular communication
6. Hypoplastic left heart syndrome
7. William syndrome with supravalvar aortic stenosis

course is of importance and significant in complete transposition when an arterial switch procedure is planned and technically difficult to transfer (47). Intramural course is difficult to diagnosis preoperatively; however, echocardiography may identify this abnormality.

In evaluating children with TOF, preoperative imaging must include a thorough assessment of coronary origins and course since 5% of patients with TOF have CAA. The types of CAA include dual LAD, accessory LAD from the RCA, and single coronary artery. All of these may lead to perioperative myocardial ischemia or infarction if the anomalous CA is inadvertently transected at surgery.

Pahl et al. (48) reported a series of four cases of TOF and pulmonary atresia in which a coronary-artery-to-pulmonary-artery fistula provided the majority of pulmonary flow. The report details anatomy and operative issues. Extremely rare cases of anomalous CA arising from a pulmonary trunk have been associated with TOF and should be suspected in the unoperated patient with LV dysfunction and/or ECG pattern to suggest ischemia or infarction. A child with TOF and acquired pulmonary valve atresia in whom the pulmonary blood flow was provided solely by retrograde flow from an anomalous RCA originating from the main pulmonary artery underwent surgery at our center. Complete repair with implantation of RCA into the ascending aorta is described (14).

Truncus arteriosus is associated with coronary abnormalities that contribute to high operative mortality rates and may be a cause of late sudden death (49). The origin and distribution of the coronary arteries are described in a review of 39 autopsy specimens of TA (50). The specimens were classified according to the number and the pattern of truncal cusps. Great variability in the origin of the coronary arteries was observed with a tendency for the RCA to arise from the anterior right quadrant and for the LCA to arise from the anterior and left quadrant. A single coronary artery was observed in seven cases (18%) (50).

Children with pulmonary atresia and intact ventricular septum may have CAA, which are associated with high mortality if two or more coronary arteries are obstructed (51).

Right ventricular decompression may cause myocardial ischemia in this group. Akagi et al. (52) reported on the influence of
ventriculocoronary arterial connections on ventricular performance and late outcome in this group of patients. The most
severe coronary pathology is associated with sudden death;
thus this group of patients is difficult to manage.

Aortic atresia has also been associated with CAA (53). In
this setting, CAA are more prominent in association with
mitral valve patency. A case of anomalous LCA and aortic
atresia is described.

Williams syndrome includes cardiovascular disease,
mental retardation, growth deficiency, and characteristic
"elfin" facies. Sudden death is a recognized complication of
this syndrome and has been attributed both to significant
supravalvar aortic stenosis as well as coronary artery stenosis
(54). The increased perfusion pressure in the setting of
supravalvar aortic stenosis leads to excessive dilatation of
the coronary arteries as well as tortuosity, occasional ostial
stenosis, and accelerated arteriosclerosis (55).

KAWASAKI DISEASE

Kawasaki disease is an acute vasculitis of unknown etiology
that predominantly affects children <5 years of age, although
cases have been reported in adolescents. Structural damage
to the coronary arteries (dilation/ectasia/aneurysm) after the
acute, self-limited illness is detected by echocardiography in
20–25% of untreated patients (56). Pathologic studies were
done on 20 hearts of patients who had typical clinical signs
and symptoms of KD and demonstrated diffuse cardiac inflammation during the acute state (57). The cardiac lesions were
classified according to the duration of illness at the time
of death. Stage I (0–9 days) was characterized by acute
perivasculitis of the microvessels as well as endarteritis of
the three major coronary arteries (MCAs). Pericarditis, myocarditis, inflammation of the atrioventricular conduction
system, and endocarditis with valvulitis were also present.
Stage II (12–25 days) was characterized by panvasculitis of

the MCAs and aneurysm with thrombus. By 28–31 days, granulation of the MCAs and disappearance of inflammation in the microvessels was noted. Patients who died 40 days to 4 years after KD had scarring with severe stenosis in the MCAs. Fibrosis of the myocardium, coagulation necrosis, lesions of the conduction system, and endocardial fibroelastosis were also present.

Clinically, the acute presentation includes both pericarditis and myocarditis, at times with depressed cardiac function. Supportive therapy for CHF in addition to early use of intravenous gamma globulin and high dose aspirin is routine (58). Patients with giant aneurysms (>8 mm) are restricted from sports and anticoagulated, usually, with warfarin and aspirin to reduce the risk of late myocardial infarction.

The long-term effects of acute coronary arteritis are unknown. Typical early findings are coronary ectasia and coronary artery aneurysms in up to 10% of treated patients despite use of IVIG and aspirin (58) (Fig. 9). A retrospective survey of cases of adult coronary artery disease attributed to antecedent KD was reported (59). In this series of 74 adults, the mean age at presentation with presumed late cardiac sequelae of KD was 24.7 ± 8.4 years (range 12–39). Symptoms included chest pain/myocardial infarction (60.8%), arrhythmia (10.8%), and sudden death (16.2%). These symptoms were precipitated by exercise in 82% of patients. Autopsy findings included coronary artery aneurysms in all and coronary artery occlusion in 72.2%. Thus, a history of antecedent KD should be sought in all young adults who present with ischemic cardiomyopathy, acute myocardial infarction, or sudden death.

Left ventricular systolic function was assessed in 75 children with coronary arterial lesions following KD. Quantitative left ventricular cineangiography was used to obtain left ventricular ejection fraction (LVEF) (60). Children with no or small coronary artery aneurysms (<8 mm) were compared to patients with giant aneurysms. The average values of LVEF were markedly lower in the giant coronary artery aneurysms group whereas LV function was normal in patients with minimal residual coronary involvement.

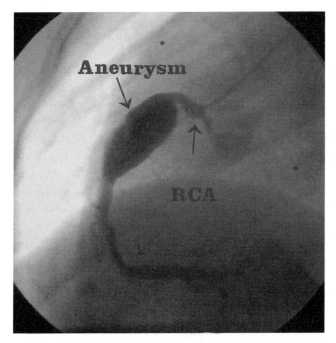

Figure 9 Selective right coronary angiogram (long axial oblique view) of a 4-year-old boy with history of KD; note the marked diffuse dilated giant fusiform aneurysm EKG demonstrating myocardial injury in a 10-year-old boy with acute KD.

Long-term follow-up of patients with KD and prior myocardial infarction is difficult. New modalities such as magnetic resonance imaging using gadolinium diethylene-triamine pentaacetic acid (Gd-DTPA) as a contrast medium can evaluate myocardial thinning noninvasively and may be useful for long-term follow evaluation (61).

Kitamura et al. (62) reported a long-term outcome of myocardial revascularization by coronary artery bypass grafting in KD in 168 patients from numerous centers in Japan. Obstructive CAD affected the left main trunk in 11.8%, the RCA in 77.6%, the LAD in 87.6%, and the Cx in 25.9%. Old myocardial infarction was noted in 46%. Fifty-four patients (32%) underwent saphenous vein grafts alone. The remaining 114 patients received at least one internal mammary graft to the LAD. The actuarial patency rate was significantly higher for arterial grafts than for vein grafts 85 months after operation ($p < 0.003$) (Fig. 10).

In rare situations, patients with severe sequelae of KD may be inoperable. A worldwide experience for cardiac transplantation for KD published several years ago reported 13 known cases, with clinical data in 10 (63). The timing of transplantation was within 6 months after diagnosis of KD in four, 1–5 years after diagnosis in three, and 9–12 years after diagnosis in three others. Indications for transplantation included coronary artery rupture (64), severe myocardial dysfunction, severe ventricular arrhythmias including cardiac arrest, and severe distal multivessel occlusive coronary artery disease. With up to 6 years posttransplant follow-up, 9 of the 10 patients were alive and well.

CORONARY STENOSIS/IATROGENIC

In children with prior surgery involving the coronary arteries, iatrogenic coronary injury must be excluded if suspicious symptoms such as exertional chest pain or syncope occur. This category includes patients with a history of arterial switch procedure, history of coronary surgery for ALCAPA, as well as patients who have undergone the Ross procedure for aortic valve disease.

Some centers perform routine angiography of arterial switch patients. A report of 366 patients had a 3% incidence of unsuspected CAA discovered on routine postoperative angiography (65). Another center found an 8% incidence of coronary lesions in 278 patients with TGA who had postoperative coronary angiography (66). Since most of these patients are asymptomatic, one center advocates myocardial perfusion study of this group of patients (67). PET scanning has also been used; however, the clinical significance of abnormalities detected is unknown (68). In patients with ALCAPA who have had surgical repair, we perform serial stress testing, as well as echocardiography during follow-up. This type of serial follow-up may be relevant for patients after arterial switch and any other coronary surgery such as the Ross procedure (69).

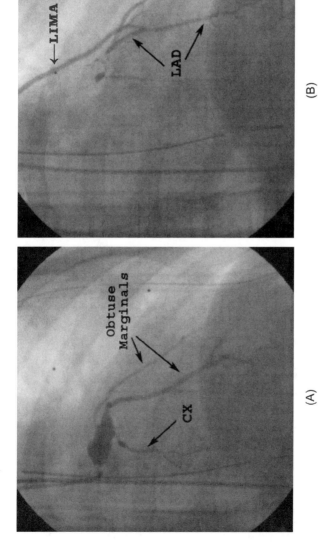

Figure 10 Selective coronary angiograms from a 10-year-old boy with KD. (A) Left coronary artery injection shows left anterior descending coronary artery occlusion (right anterior oblique view) and dilation of the proximal circumflex (Cx) extending into obtuse marginal branches. (B) Postoperative left internal mammary artery (LIMA) injection with adequate filling of the distal left anterior descending. Thrombus occludes the proximal left anterior descending. (Courtesy of Dr. David Wax, Children's Memorial Hospital.) This boy currently has improved LV function, and most recent exercise test was without inducible ischemia.

HEART TRANSPLANT CORONARY ARTERY DISEASE

Transplant coronary artery disease is an accelerated vasculopathy that occurs in adult and pediatric heart transplant recipients and is a leading cause of death among late survivors (70). This form of coronary artery disease, also known as graft coronary disease or coronary graft vasculopathy, differs from classical atherosclerosis in both histologic and angiographic features and generally progresses much more rapidly (Fig. 11). Both immune and nonimmune mechanisms appear to contribute to its pathogenesis, with a final common pathway of endothelial injury.

The incidence of TCAD in a multicenter survey of 17 pediatric transplant centers was 58 (7.2%) of 818 transplants, and >10% of patients who survive more than 1 year (71). In a more recent era, however, the incidence of severe TCAD was quite low in a multicenter angiographic series of over 2000 angiograms in 751 patients who survived greater than 1 year (72). In this study, the incidence of any TCAD at 1, 3, and 5 years by angiography was 2%, 9% and 17%, respectively. Angiography remains the gold standard for diagnosis and surveillance of TCAD although intracoronary ultrasound is being used at an increasing number of centers for surveillance (73). The types of clinical presentation of TCAD are summarized in Table 3.

At our center, we have retransplanted five patients with TCAD aged 9.6–21.2 years (mean = 12.9), who were 5.2–13.8 years (mean 8.7) after initial transplantation. They were listed for the following indications:

- Progressive coronary stenosis and left ventricle dysfunction in two.
- Resuscitation after cardiac arrest in one.
- Angina in two, intractable in one (angina is uncommon due to a relatively low incidence of cardiac reinnervation after heart transplantation).

Three additional patients with severe TCAD and left ventricle dysfunction died suddenly from 17 days to 1 year

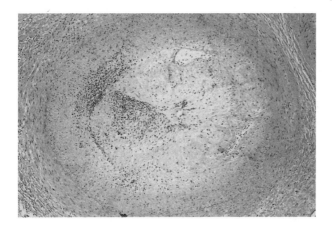

Figure 11 Path—microscopic section of the left anterior descending taken from explanted allograft of a 14-year old who was resuscitated after cardiac arrest and successfully retransplanted. Note the near complete obliteration of the lumen. (Courtesy of Dr. Hector Melin, Pathology, Children's Memorial Hospital.)

after diagnosis while considering retransplantation. In children with TCAD, the optimal treatment of heart failure is unknown, but may include routine therapy of ischemic cardiomyopathy as extrapolated from studies in adults. In addition to digitalis, diuretics, and angiotensin-converting enzyme inhibitors, if left ventricular dysfunction is significant, we have added low dose beta-blocker therapy. We have used nitrates in cases of either symptomatic angina or severe coronary stenosis. We routinely use statins in all patients >12 years of age, as well as any patient with TCAD or LDL >110 mg/dL (74).

Table 3 Types of Clinical Presentation of Transplant Coronary Artery Disease

1. Asymptomatic left ventricular dysfunction
2. Routine angiographic findings
3. Classic angina (if the transplanted heart has reinnervated)
4. Dysrhythmias
5. Sudden death

A few patients who underwent endovascular stent for palliation received Plavix in addition to aspirin.

Some authors advocate treatment/augmentation of
immunosuppression including lympholytic therapy for early
TCAD (75). Interventions in adults have included coronary
angioplasty, bypass surgery, and atherectomy (76). Despite
attempts at treatment, significant TCAD with >50% stenosis
is often rapidly progressive and ultimately fatal, thus listing
for retransplantation should be considered (77,78). Unfortunately, TCAD can recur in the second allograft (Fig. 12).

MISCELLANEOUS CAUSES OF PREMATURE
CORONARY DISEASE

Young children rarely present with atherosclerosis, unless
they have predisposing factors such as familial hypercholesterolemia or history of chronic renal failure. Homozygous type
familial hypercholesterolemia is associated with ischemic cardiomyopathy, and has been successfully treated with liver
transplant, as well as heart–liver transplant in a child with
severe ischemic cardiomyopathy (79,80). Significant coronary
artery disease may be present even in childhood, and these
children warrant serial cardiac evaluation, including coronary
angiography.

Cardiovascular morbidity and mortality are significant
in adults with end stage renal disease; however, data regarding cardiac morbidity have not been reported for children. We
evaluated an 18-year-old girl with history of ESRD who
underwent renal transplant at 13 years of age after several
years of dialysis. She developed transient intermittent chest
pain for 2 weeks prior to admission. She had mildly elevated
troponins. While undergoing a low level exercise test in
anticipation of hospital discharge, she became bradycardic,
had a full cardiac arrest, and could not be resuscitated.
Autopsy found severe diffuse coronary atherosclerosis, with
95% luminal occlusion of the left main coronary artery, 90%
occlusion of the Cx, an 80% of the RCA, with no evidence of
acute myocardial infarction.

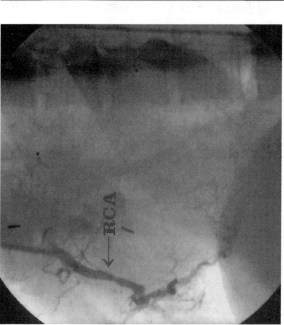

(A)

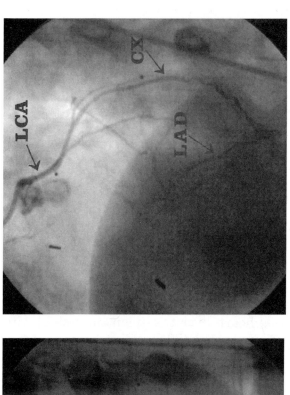

(B)

Figure 12 (A) Selective right coronary artery angiogram of 22-year-old man, 4 years after second allograft for transplant coronary artery disease; note the ragged appearance of the proximal RCA, and complete occlusion of distal vessel. (B) Selective left coronary artery angiogram from the same patient demonstrates occlusion of the LAD with retrograde filling through collateral vessels from the circumflex (Cx).

Advanced coronary arteriopathy was common in young adults with childhood-onset chronic renal failure, in a recent review of 39 patients aged 19–39 years (81). In this study, patients were screened with CT scan to assess coronary calcification burden. Routine screening with stress testing has not been advocated; however, cardiac investigation of adolescents with prolonged renal insufficiency may be appropriate for risk stratification.

Human immunodeficiency virus (HIV) infection leading to acquired immunodeficiency syndrome is associated with acquired cardiomyopathy. Several patterns of cardiovascular involvement have been reported, with a continuum from asymptomatic LV dysfunction to dilated cardiomyopathy with heart failure (82). Other reported cardiac problems include hemodynamic abnormalities, conduction abnormalities, dysrhythmias, and sudden death, as well as pericardial and vascular involvement. Although the pathophysiology is poorly understood, we believe coronary vasculopathy may have a role. In an autopsy series of 18 children who died of perinatally acquired HIV infection, coronary vasculopathy was common (83).

CONCLUSIONS

Although coronary artery abnormalities are rare in children, significant pathology can lead to congestive heart failure as well as sudden death. Improvements in imaging have been extended to include patients with potential coronary disease, and include early identification of asymptomatic lesions with noninvasive testing. Both congenital and acquired causes of coronary artery disease are discussed. Treatment includes medical therapy as well as surgical intervention with complete correction in the setting of anomalous LCA from the pulmonary artery, to coronary bypass grafting which offers palliation in cases of KD. Long-term follow-up is needed for all children with coronary artery abnormalities.

REFERENCES

1. Angelini P. Normal and anomalous coronary arteries: definitions and classification [Review] [314 Refs.]. Am Heart J 1989; 117:418–434.
2. Schlesinger MJ, Zoll PM, Wessler S. The conus artery: a third coronary artery. Am Heart J 1949; 38:823–836.
3. Dicicco BS, McManus BM, Waller BF, Roberts WC. Separate aortic ostium of the left anterior descending and left circumflex coronary arteries from the left aortic sinus of Valsalva (absent left main coronary artery). Am Heart J 1982; 104:153–154.
4. Mandell VS, Lock JE, Mayer JE, Parness IA, Kulik TJ. The "laidback" aortogram: an improved angiographic view for demonstration of coronary arteries in transposition of the great arteries. Am J Cardiol 1990; 65:1379–1383.
5. Wernovsky G, Sanders SP. Coronary artery anatomy and transposition of the great arteries. Coron Artery Dis 1993; 4:148–157.
6. Cieslinski G, Rapprich B, Kober G. Coronary anomalies: incidence and importance. Clin Cardiol 1993; 16:711–715.
7. Angelini P, Velasco JA, Flamm S. Coronary anomalies: incidence, pathophysiology, and clinical relevance. Circulation 2002; 105:2449–2454.
8. Davis JA, Cecchin F, Jones TK, Portman MA. Major coronary artery anomalies in a pediatric population: incidence and clinical importance. J Am Coll Cardiol 2001; 37:593–597.
9. Werner B, Wroblewska-Kaluzewska M, Pleskot M, Tarnowska A, Potocka K. Anomalies of the coronary arteries in children. Med Sci Monitr 2001; 7:1285–1291.
10. Culham J. Abnormalities of the coronary arteries. In: Robert M, Freedom M, John B, Mawson MCN, Shi-Joon Yoo M, Leland N, Benson M, eds. Congenital Heart Disease: Textbook of Angiocardiography. Armonk: Futura Publishing Company, 1997:849–878.
11. Dodge-Khatami A, Mavroudis C, Backer CL. Congenital Heart Surgery Nomenclature and Database Project: anomalies of the coronary arteries. Ann Thorac Surg 2000; 69(suppl):97.
12. Wesselhoeft H, Fawcett JS, Johnson AL. Anomalous origin of the left coronary artery from the pulmonary trunk. Its clinical spectrum, pathology, and pathophysiology, based on a review of 140 cases with seven further cases. Circulation 1968; 38:403–425.
13. Vairo U, Marino B, De Simone G, Marcelletti C. Early congestive heart failure due to origin of the right coronary artery from the pulmonary artery. Chest 1992; 102:1610–1612.
14. Moss RL, Backer CL, Zales VR, Florentine MS, Mavroudis C. Tetralogy of fallot with anomalous origin of the right coronary artery. Ann Thorac Surg 1995; 59:229–231.
15. Schmidt KG, Cooper MJ, Silverman NH, Stanger P. Pulmonary artery origin of the left coronary artery: diagnosis by two-dimensional

echocardiography, pulsed Doppler ultrasound and color flow mapping. J Am Coll Cardiol 1988; 11:396–402.

16. Karr SS, Parness IA, Spevak PJ, van der Velde ME, Colan SD, Sanders SP. Diagnosis of anomalous left coronary artery by Doppler color flow mapping: distinction from other causes of dilated cardiomyopathy. J Am Coll Cardiol 1992; 19:1271–1275.

17. Hamada S, Yoshimura N, Takamiya M. Images in cardiovascular medicine. Noninvasive imaging of anomalous origin of the left coronary artery from the pulmonary artery. Circulation 1998; 97:219.

18. Johnsrude CL, Perry JC, Cecchin F, Smith EO, Fraley K, Friedman RA, Towbin JA. Differentiating anomalous left main coronary artery originating from the pulmonary artery in infants from myocarditis and dilated cardiomyopathy by electrocardiogram. Am J Cardiol 1995; 75:71–74.

19. Dodge-Khatami A, Mavroudis C, Backer CL. Anomalous origin of the left coronary artery from the pulmonary artery: collective review of surgical therapy. Ann Thorac Surg 2002; 74:946–955.

20. Takeuchi S, Imamura H, Katsumoto K, Hayashi I, Katohgi T, Yozu R, Ohkura M, Inoue T. New surgical method for repair of anomalous left coronary artery from pulmonary artery. J Thorac Cardiovasc Surg 1979; 78:7–11.

21. Mavroudis C, Backer CL, Muster AJ, Pahl E, Sanders JH, Zales VR, Gevitz M. Expanding indications for pediatric coronary artery bypass. J Thorac Cardiovasc Surg 1996; 111:181–189.

22. Azakie A, Russell JL, McCrindle BW, Van Arsdell GS, Benson LN, Coles JG, Williams WG. Anatomic repair of anomalous left coronary artery from the pulmonary artery by aortic reimplantation: early survival, patterns of ventricular recovery and late outcome. Ann Thorac Surg 2003; 75:1535–1541.

23. Del Nido PJ, Duncan BW, Mayer JE, Jr., Wessel DL, LaPierre RA, Jonas RA. Left ventricular assist device improves survival in children with left ventricular dysfunction after repair of anomalous origin of the left coronary artery from the pulmonary artery. Ann Thorac Surg 1999; 67:169–172.

24. Barth CW III, Roberts WC. Left main coronary artery originating from the right sinus of Valsalva and coursing between the aorta and pulmonary trunk. J Am Coll Cardiol 1986; 7:366–373.

25. Roberts WC, Shirani J. The four subtypes of anomalous origin of the left main coronary artery from the right aortic sinus (or from the right coronary artery). Am J Cardiol 1992; 70:119–121.

26. Van Camp SP, Bloor CM, Mueller FO, Cantu RC, Olson HG. Nontraumatic sports death in high school and college athletes. Med Sci Sports Exerc 1995; 27:641–647.

27. Maron BJ, Thompson PD, Puffer JC, McGrew CA, Strong WB, Douglas PS, Clark LT, Mitten MJ, Crawford MH, Atkins DL, Driscoll DJ, Epstein AE. Cardiovascular preparticipation screening of

competitive athletes. A statement for health professionals from the Sudden Death Committee (clinical cardiology) and Congenital Cardiac Defects Committee (cardiovascular disease in the young), American Heart Association. Circulation 1996; 94:850–856.

28. Basso C, Maron BJ, Corrado D, Thiene G. Clinical profile of congenital coronary artery anomalies with origin from the wrong aortic sinus leading to sudden death in young competitive athletes. J Am Coll Cardiol 2000; 35:1493–1501.

29. Frommelt PC, Frommelt MA, Tweddell JS, Jaquiss RD. Prospective echocardiographic diagnosis and surgical repair of anomalous origin of a coronary artery from the opposite sinus with an interarterial course. J Am Coll Cardiol 2003; 42:148–154.

30. Pelliccia A, Spataro A, Caselli G, Maron BJ. Absence of left ventricular wall thickening in athletes engaged in intense power training. Am J Cardiol 1993; 72:1048–1054.

31. Ghosh PK, Agarwal SK, Kumar R, Chandra N, Puri VK. Anomalous origin of right coronary artery from left aortic sinus. J Cardiovasc Surg [Torino] 1994; 35:65–70.

32. Bedogni F, Castellani A, La Vecchia L, Menicanti L, Finocchi G, Dor V, Vincenzi M. Atresia of the left main coronary artery: clinical recognition and surgical treatment. Cathet Cardiovasc Diagn 1992; 25: 35–41.

33. Velvis H, Schmidt KG, Silverman NH, Turley K. Diagnosis of coronary artery fistula by two-dimensional echocardiography, pulsed Doppler ultrasound and color flow imaging. J Am Coll Cardiol 1989; 14: 968–976.

34. Vavuranakis M, Bush CA, Boudoulas H. Coronary artery fistulas in adults: incidence, angiographic characteristics, natural history. Cathet Cardiovasc Diagn 1995; 35:116–120.

35. Mavroudis C, Backer CL, Rocchini AP, Muster AJ, Gevitz M. Coronary artery fistulas in infants and children: a surgical review and discussion of coil embolization. Ann Thorac Surg 1997; 63:1235–1242.

36. Huang MH, Xavier L, Walsh TK, Morrison DA. Images in cardiology: a coronary-left ventricular fistula associated with myocardial ischemia. Clin Cardiol 2002; 25:441.

37. Braden DS, O'Neal KR, McMullan MR, Ebeid MR. Congenital coronary arteriovenous fistula presenting with syncope. Pediatr Cardiol 2002; 23:218–220.

38. Perry SB, Rome J, Keane JF, Baim DS, Lock JE. Transcatheter closure of coronary artery fistulas. J Am Coll Cardiol 1992; 20: 205–209.

39. Krabill KA, Hunter DW. Transcatheter closure of congenital coronary arterial fistula with a detachable balloon. Pediatr Cardiol 1993; 14: 176–178.

40. Pophal SG, Sigfusson G, Booth KL, Bacanu SA, Webber SA, Ettedgui JA, Neches WH, Park SC. Complications of endomyocardial biopsy in children. J Am Coll Cardiol 1999; 34:2105–2110.
41. Hartog JM, van den BM, Pieterman H, di Mario C. Closure of a coronary cameral fistula following endomyocardial biopsies in a cardiac transplant patient with a detachable balloon. Cathet Cardiovasc Diagn 1993; 30:156–159.
42. Hillman ND, Mavroudis C, Backer CL, Duffy CE. Supraarterial decompression myotomy for myocardial bridging in a child. Ann Thorac Surg 1999; 68:244–246.
43. Mohlenkamp S, Hort W, Ge J, Erbel R. Update on myocardial bridging. Circulation 2002; 106:2616–2622.
44. Angelini P, Trivellato M, Donis J, Leachman RD. Myocardial bridges: a review. Prog Cardiovasc Dis 1983; 26:75–88.
45. Mohiddin SA, Begley D, Shih J, Fananapazir L. Myocardial bridging does not predict sudden death in children with hypertrophic cardiomyopathy but is associated with more severe cardiac disease. J Am Coll Cardiol 2000; 36:2270–2278.
46. Yetman AT, McCrindle BW, MacDonald C, Freedom RM, Gow R. Myocardial bridging in children with hypertrophic cardiomyopathy—a risk factor for sudden death. N Engl J Med 1998; 339:1201–1209.
47. Pasquini L, Parness IA, Colan SD, Wernovsky G, Mayer JE, Sanders SP. Diagnosis of intramural coronary artery in transposition of the great arteries using two-dimensional echocardiography. Circulation 1993; 88:1136–1141.
48. Pahl E, Fong L, Anderson RH, Park SC, Zuberbuhler JR. Fistulous communications between a solitary coronary artery and the pulmonary arteries as the primary source of pulmonary blood supply in tetralogy of Fallot with pulmonary valve atresia. Am J Cardiol 1989; 63:140–143.
49. Lenox CC, Debich DE, Zuberbuhler JR. The role of coronary artery abnormalities in the prognosis of truncus arteriosus. J Thorac Cardiovasc Surg 1992; 104:1728–1742.
50. de la Cruz MV, Cayre R, Angelini P, Noriega-Ramos N, Sadowinski S. Coronary arteries in truncus arteriosus. Am J Cardiol 1990; 66: 1482–1486.
51. Gentles TL, Colan SD, Giglia TM, Mandell VS, Mayer JE Jr, Sanders SP. Right ventricular decompression and left ventricular function in pulmonary atresia with intact ventricular septum. The influence of less extensive coronary anomalies. Circulation 1993; 88:II183–II188.
52. Akagi T, Benson LN, Williams WG, Trusler GA, Freedom RM. Ventriculo-coronary arterial connections in pulmonary atresia with intact ventricular septum, and their influences on ventricular performance and clinical course. Am J Cardiol 1993; 72:586–590.

53. DeRose JJ Jr, Corda R, Dische MR, Eleazar J, Mosca RS. Isolated left ventricular ischemia after the Norwood procedure. Ann Thorac Surg 2002; 73:657–659.
54. Bird LM, Billman GF, Lacro RV, Spicer RL, Jariwala LK, Hoyme HE, Zamora-Salinas R, Morris C, Viskochil D, Frikke MJ, Jones MC. Sudden death in Williams syndrome: report of ten cases. J Pediatr 1996; 129:926–931.
55. Bischoff D, Fassbender D, Piper C, Hort W, Korfer R, Horstkotte D. Congenital tubular supravalvular aortic stenosis with massive coronary artery dilatation in a 35-year-old man. Z Kardiol 2000; 89:199–205.
56. Pahl E. Kawasaki disease: cardiac sequelae and management. Pediatr Ann 1997; 26:112–115.
57. Fujiwara H, Hamashima Y. Pathology of the heart in Kawasaki disease. Pediatrics 1978; 61:100–107.
58. Newburger JW, Takahashi M, Burns JC, Beiser AS, Chung KJ, Duffy CE, Glode MP, Mason WH, Reddy V, Sanders SP. The treatment of Kawasaki syndrome with intravenous gamma globulin. N Engl J Med 1986; 315:341–347.
59. Burns JC, Shike H, Gordon JB, Malhotra A, Schoenwetter M, Kawasaki T. Sequelae of Kawasaki disease in adolescents and young adults [Review] [76 Refs.]. J Am Coll Cardiol 1996; 28:253–257.
60. Nakano II, Ueda K, Saito A, Nojima K. Left ventricular systolic function in children with coronary arterial lesion following Kawasaki disease. Heart Vessels 1985; 1:89–93.
61. Fujiwara M, Yamada TN, Ono Y, Yoshibayashi M, Kamiya T, Furukawa S. Magnetic resonance imaging of old myocardial infarction in young patients with a history of Kawasaki disease. Clin Cardiol 2001; 24:247–252.
62. Kitamura S, Kawachi K, Nishii T, Taniguchi S, Inoue K, Mizuguchi K, et al. Internal thoracic artery grafting for congenital coronary malformations. Ann Thorac Surg 1992; 53(3):513–516.
63. Checchia PA, Pahl E, Shaddy RE, Shulman ST. Cardiac transplantation for Kawasaki disease. Pediatrics 1997; 100:695–699.
64. Koutlas TC, Wernovsky G, Bridges ND, Suh EJ, Godinez RI, Nicolson SC, Spray TL, Gaynor JW. Orthotopic heart transplantation for Kawasaki disease after rupture of a giant coronary artery aneurysm. J Thorac Cardiovasc Surg 1997; 113:217–218.
65. Tanel RE, Wernovsky G, Landzberg MJ, Perry SB, Burke RP. Coronary artery abnormalities detected at cardiac catheterization following the arterial switch operation for transposition of the great arteries. Am J Cardiol 1995; 76:153–157.
66. Losay J, Touchot A, Serraf A, Litvinova A, Lambert V, Piot JD, Lacour-Gayet F, Capderou A, Planche C. Late outcome after arterial switch operation for transposition of the great arteries. Circulation 2001; 104: I121–I126.

67. Weindling SN, Wernovsky G, Colan SD, Parker JA, Boutin C, Mone SM, Costello J, Castaneda AR, Treves ST. Myocardial perfusion, function and exercise tolerance after the arterial switch operation. J Am Coll Cardiol 1994; 23:424–433.

68. Bengel FM, Hauser M, Duvernoy CS, Kuehn A, Ziegler SI, Stollfuss JC, Beckmann M, Sauer U, Muzik O, Schwaiger M, Hess J. Myocardial blood flow and coronary flow reserve late after anatomical correction of transposition of the great arteries. J Am Coll Cardiol 1998; 32: 1955–1961.

69. Pahl E, Duffy CE, Chaudhry FA. The role of stress echocardiography in children. Echocardiology 2000; 17:507–512.

70. Pahl E. Transplant coronary artery disease in children. Prog Pediatr Cardiol 2000; 11:137–143.

71. Pahl E, Zales VR, Fricker FJ, Addonizio LJ. Posttransplant coronary artery disease in children. A multicenter national survey. Circulation 1994; 90:II56–II60.

72. Pahl E, Naftel D, Kuhn M, Shaddy R, Morrow W, Kirklin J. The impact and outcome of transplant coronary artery disease in a pediatric population: a 9 year multi-institutional study. Presented at the American Heart Association Annual Scientific Sessions in Chicago. Circulation November 18, 2002. circulation 2002; 106:396.

73. Costello JM, Wax DF, Binns HJ, Backer CL, Mavroudis C, Pahl E. A comparison of intravascular ultrasound with coronary angiography for evaluation of transplant coronary disease in pediatric heart transplant recipients. J Heart Lung Transplant 2003; 22:44–49.

74. Seiplet I, Crawford S, Rodgers S, Backer C, Mavroudis C, Pahl E. Hypercholesterolemia is common after Pediatric heart transplantation: initial experience with pravastatin. J Heart Lung Transplant 2004; 23(3):317–322.

75. Lamich R, Ballester M, Marti V, Brossa V, Aymat R, Carrio I, Berna L, Camprecios M, Puig M, Estorch M, Flotats A, Bordes R, Garcia J, Auge, Padro JM, Caralps JM, Narula J. Efficacy of augmented immunosuppressive therapy for early vasculopathy in heart transplantation. J Am Coll Cardiol 1998; 32:413–419.

76. Halle AA III, DiSciascio G, Massin EK, Wilson RF, Johnson MR, Sullivan HJ, Bourge RC, Kleiman NS, Miller LW, Aversano TR. Coronary angioplasty, atherectomy and bypass surgery in cardiac transplant recipients. J Am Coll Cardiol 1995; 26:120–128.

77. Michler RE, Edwards NM, Hsu D, Bernstein D, Fricker FJ, Miller J, Copeland J, Kaye MP, Addonizio L. Pediatric retransplantation. J Heart Lung Transplant 1993; 12:S319–S327.

78. Razzouk AJ, Chinnock RE, Dearani JA, Gundry SR, Bailey LL. Cardiac retransplantation for graft vasculopathy in children: should we continue to do it?. Arch Surg 1998; 133:881–885.

79. Bilheimer DW, Goldstein JL, Grundy SM, Starzl TE, Brown MS. Liver transplantation to provide low-density-lipoprotein receptors and lower

plasma cholesterol in a child with homozygous familial hypercholesterolemia. N Engl J Med 1984; 311:1658–1664.

80. Hoeg JM, Starzl TE, Brewer HB Jr. Liver transplantation for treatment of cardiovascular disease: comparison with medication and plasma exchange in homozygous familial hypercholesterolemia. Am J Cardiol 1987; 59:705–707.

81. Oh J, Wunsch R, Turzer M, Bahner M, Raggi P, Querfeld U, Mehls O, Schaefer F. Advanced coronary and carotid arteriopathy in young adults with childhood-onset chronic renal failure. Circulation 2002; 106:100–105.

82. Lipshultz SE, Sleeper LA, Towbin JA, Lowe AM, Orav EJ, Cox GF, Lurie PR, McCoy KL, McDonald MA, Messere JE, Colan SD. The incidence of pediatric cardiomyopathy in two regions of the United States. N Engl J Med 2003; 348:1647–1655.

83. Chadwick EG, Crawford SE, McShae CT, Pahl E, Backer CL, Das L, Crussi FG. Coronary vasculopathy (CV) is common in children with end-stage perinatally-acquired HIV infection: A study of 18 autopsy cases. Presented at the 4th Conference on Retro viruses and Opportunistic Infections, December, 1996.

20

Heart Failure in the Postoperative Patient

CHITRA RAVISHANKAR and GIL WERNOVSKY

Department of Pediatrics,
Division of Pediatric Cardiology,
Children's Hospital of Philadelphia,
University of Pennsylvania School of Medicine,
Philadelphia, Pennsylvania, U.S.A.

As the survival of infants and children with all forms of congenital heart defects has dramatically improved over the last three decades, the focus of care has now shifted toward reducing short and long-term morbidity. The field of perioperative care is rapidly evolving with nearly simultaneous advances in surgical techniques and adjunctive therapies, respiratory care, intensive care technology and monitoring, pharmacologic research and development, and computing and electronics. Despite these advances, there remains a predictable fall in cardiac output after cardiopulmonary bypass (CPB) particularly in the neonate and young infant. This chapter will mostly focus on early identification and aggressive treatment of the "low cardiac output syndrome" (LCOS) peculiar to these patients.

FREQUENCY AND RISK FACTORS

Despite improvements in myocardial protection, surgical and CPB techniques, many young patients will experience a fall in cardiac output with associated tissue edema and end-organ dysfunction (referred to as LCOS) after surgery for congenital heart disease. Low cardiac output syndrome typically occurs between 6 and 18 hr after surgery (1,2). In a study of 139 children undergoing biventricular repair, 25% had cardiac index (CI) less than 2.0 L/min per m^2 (1). In this study, CI of less than 2.0 L/min per m^2 strongly correlated with mortality. Similarly, in the Boston circulatory arrest study, 25% of neonates had CI < 2.0 L/min per m^2 on the first postoperative night after the arterial switch operation (2). Low cardiac output syndrome was associated with an elevated systemic vascular resistance of 25% and a rise in pulmonary vascular resistance of nearly 40% from baseline values (Fig. 1). Similarly, in the PRIMACORP trial (Prophylactic Intravenous use of Milrinone After Cardiac Operation in Pediatrics), the incidence of LCOS in the placebo group was 25.9% and occurred in the first 6–18 hr after surgery (3,4). Nearly half of the patients with clinical LCOS had a widened ($> 30\%$) arterial-mixed venous oxygen difference. Consistent with previous studies, the lowest mixed venous saturations occurred in the first 6–18 hr after surgery (3,5,6). Compared to neonates and infants, LCOS is less commonly seen in older children, but may occur following any complex operation with long myocardial ischemic times or in patients of any age with pre-existing ventricular dysfunction, atrioventricular valve regurgitation, arrhythmias, or following operations which adversely change loading conditions of the myocardium (see also Chapter 2).

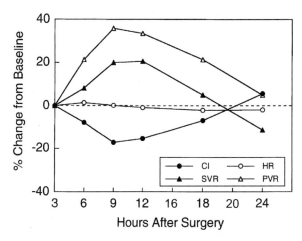

Figure 1 Decrease in cardiac index (CI) associated with a rise in systemic (SVR) and pulmonary vascular resistance (PVR) in newborns after an arterial switch operation. During the study period, heart rate (HR) remained unchanged, and inotropic support (mean dose dopamine 7 mcg/kg/min) and sedation (mean dose fentanyl 10 mcg/kg/hr) were held constant. (Modified with permission from Ref. 2.)

ETIOLOGY

Causes of LCOS after cardiac surgery are multifactorial. They include factors related to CPB such as myocardial ischemia during aortic cross clamping, hypothermia, reperfusion injury, activation of inflammatory and complement cascades, and alterations in systemic and pulmonary vascular reactivity (7–18). Nonspecific and lesion specific causes of LCOS are listed in Tables 1 and 2. However, before implicating myocardial

Table 1 Nonspecific Causes of LCOS

Inflammation
Ischemia–reperfusion injury
Lack of atrioventricular synchrony
Brady or tachyarrhythmia
Hypothyroidism

Table 2 Lesion Specific Causes of LCOS

1. Changes in loading conditions
   Decreased preload and increased afterload (after repair of systemic
   atrioventricular valve regurgitation)
   Increased volume load (systemic-to-pulmonary artery shunt, pulmonary
   regurgitation)
2. Ventriculotomy
3. Coronary reimplantation (after the arterial switch operation or Ross)
4. Denervation (orthotopic heart transplantation)

dysfunction as the cause of LCOS, it is imperative to rule out residual surgically remedial structural defects, as medical management is unlikely to reverse the low cardiac output state in the presence of an anatomical problem. Specific examples include residual aortic arch obstruction after the Norwood operation, presence of a significant left-to-right shunting due to a residual VSD, or previously unrecognized muscular VSD after repair of tetralogy of Fallot, etc.

DIAGNOSIS/DETECTION OF LCOS

Clinical and Laboratory Data

Anticipation and early identification of LCOS are central to the critical care of children with heart disease (19). A variety of clinical and laboratory parameters may help estimate the adequacy of cardiac output and oxygen delivery in the pediatric patient (20–22). Peripheral pulse volume, capillary refill, blood pressure, urine output, and blood gas analysis provide an indirect assessment of cardiac output and oxygen delivery. Capillary refill and core-peripheral temperature difference are useful markers, however, they may be obscured by factors such as fever, use of vasoactive medications, and deliberate hypothermia [in postoperative junctional ectopic tachycardia (JET), for instance]. Nevertheless, capillary refill is an easy, noninvasive bedside test to estimate cardiac output and its value cannot be overemphasized. In the postoperative patient after congenital cardiac surgery, cardiac output is rarely directly measured using thermodilution catheters, and is usually estimated using surrogate markers of adequate oxygen delivery such as mixed venous saturation and serum lactate.

Mixed Venous Oxygen Saturation

Mixed venous oxygen saturation is an indicator of oxygen extraction and has a useful clinical role (23–27). In patients without any intracardiac left-to-right shunt, the pulmonary artery oxygen saturation is the true "mixed" venous oxygen saturation. However, the pulmonary artery saturation is not easily accessible in young infants and children and cannot be used in children with residual intracardiac communications with left-to-right shunting. The saturation in the superior vena cava (SVC) approximates the pulmonary artery saturation closely enough that we routinely use the SVC saturation as a surrogate for the mixed venous saturation. In patients with biventricular repair, saturations obtained from a right atrial catheter provide an indirect assessment of cardiac output and oxygen delivery and are a useful trend to follow. In patients with single ventricle physiology, a catheter in the SVC is required to measure a "mixed" venous saturation (28,29). Some centers use an optical catheter in the superior vena cava to continuously monitor systemic venous oxygen saturation after the Norwood operation (5,29).

Serum Lactate

Serum lactate is another surrogate marker of adequate oxygen delivery. Several studies have suggested the usefulness of serum lactate in predicting outcome after open-heart surgery (30–33). An elevated serum lactate represents anaerobic metabolism, which occurs with inadequate oxygen delivery or impaired oxygen utilization. Although absolute values of serum lactate vary from lesion to lesion, and are dependant on a host of intraoperative factors (e.g., DHCA, blood transfusion, etc.), a steadily falling lactate is a reassuring finding, while elevations in serum lactate may suggest inadequate oxygen delivery.

TREATMENT OF POSTOPERATIVE LCOS

Intraoperative Strategies

We recently celebrated the 50th anniversary of the first success-ful open-heart operation performed with the use of Gibbon's heart-lung machine. On the basis of the pioneering work of Bar-ratt-Boyes and others, congenital heart defects in newborns and infants have been corrected by using deep hypothermic circula-tory arrest (DHCA) (34,35). DHCA provides unparalleled surgi-cal exposure in the small heart by eliminating the need for multiple cannulas within the surgical field. Because of the asso-ciated neurologic morbidity with prolonged periods of DHCA, many centers favor hypothermia and low-flow CPB (6–8). Improvements in the technology of CPB have significantly reduced morbidity after repair of complex congenital heart defects. However, use of CPB may expose infants to extremes of hemodilution and hypothermia, often in association with tissue ischemia, as well as a systemic inflammatory response comprising complement activation, leukocyte stimulation and cytokine synthesis (9–17). Proinflammatory cytokines such as tumor necrosis factor alpha, interleukin (IL) 6, and IL-8 cause myocardial cell damage and myocardial dysfunction as a result of increased leukocyte–endothelial cell interactions leading to impaired microcirculation in the myocardium.

Use of Modified Ultrafiltration (MUF)

Ultrafiltration is a technique that removes plasma water and low molecular weight solutes using hydrostatic forces across a semipermeable membrane (Fig. 2). Elliott et al. (36,37) intro-duced a technique of ultrafiltration after separation from CPB, which they termed modified ultrafiltration. Early stu-dies on the use of MUF reported a decrease in the amount of total body water that accumulates after CPB. Modified ultrafiltration removes not only plasma water, but also solutes of less than 50 kDa, including a number of inflammatory mediators such as IL-6 and endothelin-1, thus attenuating the inflammatory cascade activated by CPB. Use of MUF has been shown to decrease total body water accumulation

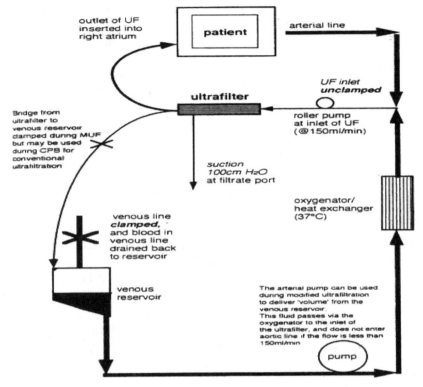

Figure 2 Diagram of ultrafiltration process. (From Ref. 37.)

and postoperative blood loss, decrease the incidence of pleural effusions after cavopulmonary connection and the Fontan procedure, improve left ventricular systolic function, improve lung compliance, and decrease the duration of postoperative ventilation (38–41).

RULE OUT RESIDUAL LESIONS

It is imperative to rule out any residual anatomical lesion utilizing echocardiography (transthoracic or transesophageal) and/or cardiac catheterization. In the postoperative patient with LCOS, this cannot be emphasized enough. In the presence of a surgically remedial residual structural lesion, escalation of medical therapy is not only futile but can also be detrimental to the patient. After CPB, factors that influence cardiac output, preload, afterload, myocardial contractility, heart rate, and rhythm must be assessed and manipulated.

PRELOAD

Right atrial pressure provides a valuable measure of the preload conditions of the right heart. Fluid boluses in quantities of 5–10 mL/kg should be used judiciously to optimize preload. By infusing volume and observing right atrial pressure along with blood pressure and heart rate, the clinician determines the optimal filling pressure for the patient. Patients with poorly compliant ventricles require additional preload, particularly in the early postoperative period. Specific examples include infant repair of tetralogy of Fallot, bidirectional Glenn or Fontan procedure, and operations complicated by pulmonary hypertension such as repair of obstructed total anomalous pulmonary venous connection.

PHARMACOLOGICAL SUPPORT

Failure to improve cardiac output after volume adjustments requires the additional use of pharmacological agents that provide inotropy and/or afterload reduction (Table 3). Traditionally, catecholamines such as dopamine, dobutamine, epinephrine, norepinephrine, phenylephrine, and isoproterenol have been used as inotropic support after cardiac surgery (42–47). Dopamine is commonly used to support cardiac output after CPB. Epinephrine is occasionally useful in the immediate postoperative period when high systemic blood pressures are sought. Isoproterenol is often used in the immediate postoperative period after heart transplantation for its chronotropic and vasodilatory effects. The adverse effects of high-dose catecholamines include an increase in myocardial oxygen consumption, heart rate, systemic afterload, and the risk of arrhythmia. Arginine vasopressin is another potent vasoconstrictor that has been advocated for

Table 3 Usual Dose Range for Vasoactive Agents Used in the Postoperative Period After Cardiac Surgery

Agent	Usual dose range (IV)
Dopamine	2–20 μ/kg/min
Dobutamine	2–20 μ/kg/min
Epinephrine	0.01–0.5 μ/kg/min
Norepinephrine	0.1–0.5 μ/kg/min
Phenylephrine	0.1–0.5 μ/kg/min
Isoproterenol	0.01–0.5 μ/kg/min
Sodium nitroprusside	0.5–5 μ/kg/min
Amrinone	1–3 mg/kg loading dose[a], 5–20 μ/kg/min
Milrinone	100–250 μ/kg load on CPB
	25–75 μ/kg load off CPB
	0.25–1.0 μ/kg/min
Vasopressin	0.0003–0.002 units/kg/min
T3 (triiodothyronine)	0.05–0.15 μ/kg/hr

CPB: cardiopulmonary bypass.
[a]Based on blood pressure.

states of refractory vasodilatation associated with low circulating vasopressin levels as may rarely occur after CPB in children (48).

Transient hypothyroidism is well described in adults and children after CPB. The mechanism of hypothyroidism is not fully characterized but is likely related to hemodilution, endogenous release of mediators such as glucocorticoids, tumor necrosis factor, and cytokines such as IL-6, and exogenous factors such as dopamine infusion and iodine skin preparations (49,50). Some investigators have recently evaluated the role of tri-iodothyronine (T3) infusion as an inotrope after cardiac surgery in children and the initial experience appears favorable (51–55). Larger multicenter trials seem warranted at this time to evaluate the efficacy and safety of routine T3 in the prevention and treatment of LCOS.

Phosphodiesterase Type III Inhibitors

Because of the undesirable side effects associated with the use of high-dose catecholamines, afterload reducing agents such as amrinone and milrinone are being increasingly used in the postoperative period (56). They are nonglycoside, noncatecholamine inotropic agents with additional vasodilatory and lusitropic properties. These drugs inhibit phosphodiesterase type III, the enzyme that metabolizes cyclic adenosine monophosphate (cyclic AMP). By increasing intracellular cyclic AMP, they increase intracellular calcium, thus enhancing myocardial contractility. In addition, they also enhance diastolic relaxation of the myocardium by increasing the rate of reuptake of calcium after systole, thus providing a "lusitropic" effect. These drugs also act synergistically with beta-agonists and have fewer side effects (Fig. 3).

Phosphodiesterase type III inhibitors have been used extensively in adults and more recently introduced to pediatric practice (57–61). In a pharmacodynamic study evaluating the

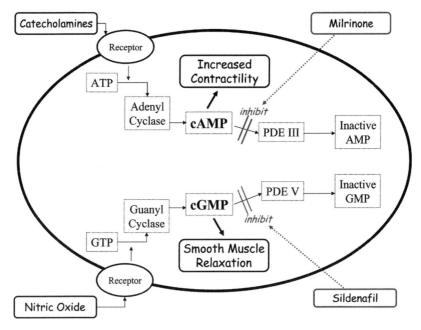

Figure 3 This figure depicts the mechanism of action of phosphodiesterase inhibitors at the cellular level and the synergistic effects of catecholamines and phosphodiesterase type III inhibitors (PDE III). ATP, adenosine triphosphate; cAMP, cyclic adenosine monophosphate; GTP, guanosine triphosphate; cGMP, guanosine monophosphate.

hemodynamic effects of intravenous milrinone in 10 neonates with established LCOS after cardiac surgery (mean CI of 2.0 L/min/m^2), Chang and colleagues showed that milrinone lowered filling pressures, systemic and pulmonary artery pressures, and systemic and pulmonary vascular resistances, while improving CI (Fig. 4). The results of the PRIMACORP trial were recently published (3,4). In this multicenter pediatric trial, patients were randomly assigned, in a 1:1:1 ratio within 90 min after arriving in the intensive care unit, to receive either low-dose intravenous milrinone (25 μ/kg bolus over 60 min followed by 0.25 μ/kg per min infusion for 35 hr), or placebo. The prophylactic use of high-dose milrinone resulted in a 64% relative risk reduction in the development of LCOS (Fig. 5). Consistent with previous studies, the lowest mixed venous saturations and highest lactate values occurred in the first 12 hr after surgery. Patients who developed LCOS had a significantly lower urine output (1.9 vs. 1.4 days, $p = 0.002$), longer duration of mechanical ventilation, (3.1

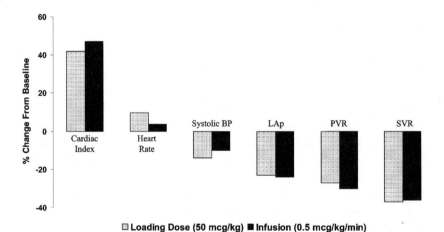

☐ Loading Dose (50 mcg/kg) ■ Infusion (0.5 mcg/kg/min)

Figure 4 Hemodynamic effects of milrinone in 10 children with LCOS. Cardiac index rose significantly following the loading dose, and was maintained during the continuous infusion. Improved cardiac index was associated with a significant fall in systemic vascular resistance (SVR) and left atrial pressure (LAp) and pulmonary vascular resistance (PVR). (Modified with permission from Ref. 61.)

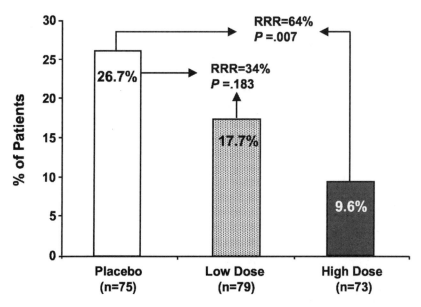

Figure 5 Development of LCOS/death in the first 36 hr after placebo, low-dose and high-dose milrinone. RRR, relative risk ratio. See text for details. (From Ref. 4.)

versus 1.4 days, $p = 0.01$) and longer length of stay (11.3 vs. 8.9 days, $p = 0.016$). There were no significant differences in the incidence of adverse events (hypotension, arrhythmia, and thrombocytopenia) with milrinone compared with placebo. In many centers, milrinone is the first line of therapy for children with LCOS following cardiac surgery, as well as for children with cardiomyopathy awaiting heart transplantation. A combination of dopamine (typically 3–5 mcg/kg/min) and milrinone (typically 0.5–1.0 mcg/kg/min) has become standard therapy for all neonates and young infants undergoing bypass, and for many older children following complex biventricular repair or staged reconstruction (e.g., Fontan procedure). In the majority of cases, this intravenous inotropic support can be rapidly weaned and discontinued within 24–48 hr of surgery, with the need for enteral cardiac medications decided upon on a case-by-case basis.

Phenoxybenzamine is a potent, long acting alpha-blocker that has been advocated as part of the postoperative management of infants after the Norwood operation. It is used to lower the systemic vascular resistance and produce a more "balanced" circulation (5,29). In a sequential, nonrandomized trial by Tweddell et al., infants who received phenoxybenzamine after the Norwood operation had higher systemic oxygen delivery and a more stable postoperative course compared with historical controls.

MANAGEMENT OF PULMONARY HYPERTENSION

Pulmonary hypertension complicates the postoperative course of many forms of congenital heart disease. Several factors peculiar to CPB may raise pulmonary vascular resistance: microemboli, atelactasis, endothelial dysfunction, vasoconstriction, and adrenergic events (62,63). Pulmonary hypertension is frequently assumed if there is right ventricular hypertension, however, the critical care physician must always exclude anatomical factors that impose either obstruction to pulmonary blood flow or residual left-to-right shunting. Elevated left atrial pressure due to mitral valve disease or left ventricular dysfunction, pulmonary venous obstruction, branch pulmonary artery stenosis, or decreased pulmonary vascular cross-sectional area (surgically related or congenital) all will raise right ventricular pressure and impose a burden on the right heart. Similarly, a significant residual left-to-right shunt will raise pulmonary artery pressure postoperatively and should be surgically addressed.

Management strategies for postoperative elevations in pulmonary vascular resistance include sedation, moderate hyperventilation (maintaining pCO_2 between 30 and 35 Torr), moderate alkalosis, increased inspired oxygen, positive end expiratory pressure (to maximize functional residual capacity), pulmonary vasodilators (e.g., nitric oxide), and creating or maintaining an intracardiac right-to-left shunt to maintain cardiac output (at the expense of hypoxemia).

Inhaled Nitric Oxide

The use of nonspecific vasodilators such as tolazaline, dobutamine, milrinone, and prostacyclin is often limited by their systemic vasodilatory effects (64,65). On the other hand, nitric oxide (NO) is a vasodilator that can be delivered selectively by inhalation and distributed across the alveoli to the pulmonary vascular smooth muscle (66,67). Because of its rapid inactivation by hemoglobin, inhaled NO can achieve selective pulmonary vasodilatation and lower pulmonary artery pressure in a number of diseases without the unwanted effect of systemic hypotension. Inhaled NO has had a dramatic impact in a number of complex heart defects in children (68–74). Descriptions of the use of NO after the Fontan procedure and after ventricular septal defect repair have been reported, along with a variety of other anatomical lesions. In a study by Atz and colleagues, 20 infants presenting with isolated TAPVR were monitored for pulmonary hypertension in the postoperative period. A mean percentage decrease of 42% in pulmonary vascular resistance and 32% in mean pulmonary artery pressure was demonstrated with 80 ppm of NO (Fig. 6). There was no significant change in heart rate, systemic blood pressure, or vascular resistance. Possible toxicities of inhaled NO include methemoglobinemia, production of excess nitrogen dioxide, peroxynitrite, or injury to the pulmonary surfactant system. Importantly, abrupt withdrawal of NO can lead to rebound pulmonary hypertension (75). Appreciation of the transient characteristics of withdrawal of NO may facilitate weaning from NO. The withdrawal response to NO may be attenuated by pretreatment with the phosphodiesterase type 5 inhibitor sildenafil (76).

Sildenafil is a selective phosphodiesterase type V inhibitor. Phosphodiesterase type V breaks down cyclic guanosine monophosphate (cyclic GMP); cyclic GMP relaxes smooth muscle in the pulmonary vascular bed. Sildenafil thus produces acute and relatively selective pulmonary vasodilatation and acts synergistically with NO (76–81, Fig 3), Preliminary reports suggest that sildenafil may have useful effects in pulmonary hypertension particularly in attenuating rebound effects after discontinuing inhaled NO and in the chronic

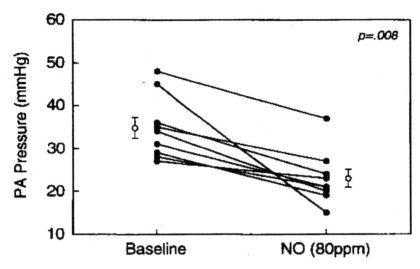

Figure 6 Effect of a 15-min trial of inhaled nitric oxide (NO) on mean pulmonary artery (PA) pressure. Open circles: changes for the group. (From Ref. 75.)

therapy of pulmonary hypertension (76). Sildenafil is well tolerated and available as an oral preparation, which makes it particularly attractive in patients with pulmonary hypertension whose symptoms do not warrant a continuous intravenous infusion. At the current time, use of sildenafil in the immediate postoperative period is limited by the lack of an intravenous preparation.

ARRHYTHMIA AFTER CPB

Arrhythmias occur in >25% of patients after CPB. Risk factors include longstanding volume overload, ventricular hypertrophy, myocardial ischemia, ventriculotomy, multiple suture lines, and electrolyte disturbances. A majority of arrhythmias occur within the first 48 hr of surgery and include bradyarrhythmias such as sinus bradycardia and complete heart block, and tachyarrhythmias such as supraventricular tachycardia, atrial flutter, atrial fibrillation, junctional ectopic tachycardia, and ventricular tacycardia. Junctional ectopic tachycardia is quite common after pediatric cardiac surgery, particularly in young infants after repair of tetralogy of Fallot, closure of ventricular septal defects, and atrioventricular canal defects (82–88). Strategies for management of JET include adequate analgesia and sedation, avoidance of hyperthermia and induced hypothermia, minimizing exogenous catecholamines, using medications such as amiodarone and procainamide, and atrial pacing. Atrioventricular synchrony using atrial and/or atrioventricular sequential pacing augments cardiac output and it is particularly important in the treatment of arrhythmias such as JET and complete heart block.

FLUID OVERLOAD AFTER CPB

Despite the advances in intraoperative strategies, including the routine use of MUF after CPB, fluid overload and renal dysfunction are major contributors to morbidity after neonatal and infant surgery. The relative increase in total body water accumulation is more significant in neonates, and is directly proportional to the duration of CPB (2); the etiology includes both capillary leak and transient postoperative renal dysfunction. In the PRIMACORP trial, the creatinine clearance (mL/min per 1.73 m^2) was significantly less in neonates (mean 37.2) compared with infants aged 1.0–4.8 months (mean 59.2) and older children aged 4.8 months through 6 years (mean 84.5). In neonates, diuresis typically peaks on the second–fourth postoperative day (Fig. 7). Intermittent diuretic therapy is perhaps just as efficient as a continuous infusion, though the latter may be better tolerated in the hemodynamically unstable patient (89,90). "Renal dose dopamine" is commonly used in clinical practice, however, according to a recent meta-analysis, the renal protective effect of dopamine is equivocal (91).

Recent animal and clinical studies in adults suggest a role for fenoldopam, a dopamine 1 receptor agonist, in improving renal function after ischemia and reperfusion (92,93). It has been used in adults as antihypertensive therapy; however, there is minimal experience in pediatrics. Clinical trials

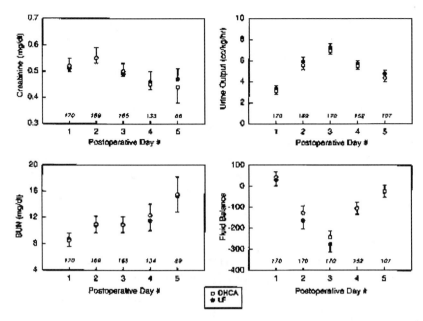

Figure 7 This figure shows renal function, urine output, and fluid balance during the first 5 days after cardiac surgery. Numbers above the postoperative day indicate the number of patients with measurements on that particular day. DHCA, deep hypothermic circulatory arrest; LF, low-flow cardiopulmonary bypass. (Modified with permission from Ref. 2.)

are underway evaluating the pharmacokinetics of fenoldopam in children (Laussen PC, personal communication).

CREATION OF A RIGHT-TO-LEFT SHUNT

Select children with LCOS may benefit from right-to-left shunting at the atrial level. This is particularly helpful in children with single ventricle undergoing the Fontan procedure, as well as following biventricular repairs (especially with ventriculotomy) performed in patients with right ventricular hypertrophy (e.g., young patients with tetralogy of Fallot or truncus arteriosus) and those with labile pulmonary vascular resistance. A typical example is the patient following complete repair of tetralogy of Fallot in infancy, when the moderately hypertrophied, noncompliant right ventricle has undergone extensive muscle resection (with or without a ventriculotomy) and has a new volume load from pulmonary regurgitation secondary to a transannular patch or valvotomy. Although left ventricular function is intrinsically normal, LCOS is a common finding in the first postoperative night, as there is inadequate filling of the LV secondary to the dysfunction on the right side of the circulation. In these situations, cardiac output may be augmented (at the expense of hypoxemia) by leaving a right-to-left shunt at the atrial level at the completion of surgery. This strategy is also useful in the postoperative patient with pulmonary hypertension and may be lifesaving in patients with primary pulmonary hypertension with right heart failure. This concept has been modified from the principle used in patients with single ventricle physiology who are at risk for LCOS following the Fontan operation (94,95). Fenestration allows right-to-left shunting, preserving cardiac output and oxygen delivery.

MECHANICAL SUPPORT

When conventional measures such as fluid resuscitation, inotropic support, and afterload reduction fail, institution of mechanical support may be lifesaving (96). Mechanical support in children is usually limited to extracorporeal membrane oxygenation (ECMO) or centrifugal ventricular assist devices.

Indications for ECMO are as follows:

- Inability to wean off CPB
- Ventricular dysfunction
- Respiratory failure
- Pulmonary hypertension refractory to medical therapy
- Occluded systemic-to-pulmonary artery shunt
- Intractable arrhythmias with hemodynamic compromise
- Cardiopulmonary arrest

Several centers report survival rates of 40–50% for children requiring ECMO after cardiac surgery (97–99). In a recently published large series of 137 patients supported with ECMO over a 6-year period, 89 (65%) had undergone cardiac surgery during the same hospital admission (99). These patients represented 3.4% of the cardiac surgeries performed with CPB during that period. The survival for these patients was 40% and similar to the survival rate of the nonsurgical patients. Risk factors for mortality were age < 1 month, male gender, longer duration of mechanical ventilation before ECMO, and development of renal or hepatic dysfunction while on ECMO. Single ventricle physiology and failure to separate from CPB were not associated with increased mortality. Survival rates were similar following the use of rapid resuscitation ECMO for cardiopulmonary arrest. The effect of ECMO on hospital mortality postcardiotomy is unequivocal, and even more obvious when used as rescue therapy during cardiopulmonary resuscitation. Children with cardiac disease represent a heterogeneous group and it is not prudent to impose strict indications or contraindications for ECMO support.

OTHER STRATEGIES

Cardiac resynchronization therapy (CRT) through biventricular pacing is being increasingly used in the treatment of adults with heart failure and has been shown to improve ventricular remodeling, decrease the severity of mitral regurgitation, and improve cardiac output (99). Some centers are using this technique to improve hemodynamics in patients with heart failure and selected dysarrhythmias after congenital heart surgery (100). Finally, anti-inflammatory agents such as monoclonal antibodies, competitive receptor blockers, C1-esterase inhibitors, and preoperative preparation with steroids are being investigated to mitigate the inflammatory response provoked by CPB (101–107).

CONCLUSION

Postoperative LCOS should be anticipated, transient, and self-limited, especially in neonates and young infants.

Emphasis has shifted from escalation of inotropy to escalation of lusitropy and afterload reduction. The strategy of anticipation, early identification, and aggressive treatment of LCOS has led to a dramatic decline in the postoperative mortality of congenital cardiac defects with shorter length of stay and decreased incidence of nosocomial complications.

REFERENCES

1. Parr GVS, Blackstone EH, Kirklin JW. Cardiac performance and mortality early after intracardiac surgery in infants and young children. Circulation 1975; 51:867–877.
2. Wernovsky G, Wypji D, Jonas RA, Mayer JE, Hanley FL, Hickey PR, Walsh AZ, Chang AC, Castenada AR, Newburger JW, Wessel DL. Postoperative course and hemodynamic profile after the arterial switch operation in neonates and infants: a comparison of low-flow cardiopulmonary bypass and circulatory arrest. Circulation 1995; 92: 2226–2235.
3. Hoffman TM, Wernovsky G, Atz AM, Bailey JM, Akbary A, Kocsis JF, Nelson DP, Chang AC, Kulik TJ, Spray TL, Wessel DL. Prophylactic intravenous use of milrinone after cardiac operation in pediatrics (PRIMACORP) study. Am Heart J 2002; 143:15–21.
4. Hoffman TM, Wernovsky G, Atz AM, Kulik TJ, Nelson DP, Chang AC, Bailey JM, Akbary A, Kocsis JF, Kaczmarek R, Spray TL, Wessel DL. Efficacy and safety of milrinone in preventing low cardiac output syndrome in infants and children after corrective surgery for congenital heart disease. Circulation 2003; 107:996–1002.
5. Tweddell JS, Hoffman GM, Fedderly RT, Berger S, Thomas JP Jr, Ghanayem NS, Kessel MW, Litwin SB. Phenoxybenzamine improves systemic oxygen delivery after the Norwood procedure. Ann Thorac Surg 1999; 67:161–168.
6. Pesonen EJ, Peltola KI, Korpela RE, Sairanen HI, Leijala MA, Raivio KO, Andersson SHM. Delayed impairment of cerebral oxygenation after deep hypothermic circulatory arrest in children. Ann Thorac Surg 1999; 67:1765–1770.
7. Newburger JW, Jonas RA, Wernovsky G, Wypij D, Hickey PR, Kuban K, Farrell DM, Holmes GL, Helmers SL, Constantinou J, Carrazana E, Barlow JK, Walsh AZ, Lucius KC, Share JC, Wessel DL, Hanley FL, Mayer JE, Castaneda AR, Ware JH. A comparison of the perioperative neurologic effects of hypothermic circulatory arrest versus low-flow cardiopulmonary bypass in infant heart surgery. N Engl J Med 1993; 329:1057–1064.

8. Bellinger DC, Jonas RA, Rappaport LA, Wypij D, Gil Wernovsky G, Kuban K, Barnes PD, Holmes GL, Hickey PR, Strand RD, Walsh AZ, Helmers SL, Constantinou JE, Carrazana EJ, Hanley FL, Castaneda AR, Ware JH, Newburger JW. Developmental and neurologic status of children after heart surgery with hypothermic circulatory arrest or low-flow cardiopulmonary bypass. N Engl J Med 1995; 332:549–555.

9. Bellinger DC, Wypij D, Kuban KC, Rappaport LA, Hickey PR, Wernovsky G, Jonas RA, Newburger JW. Developmental and neurologic status of children at 4 years of age after heart surgery with hypothermic circulatory arrest or low-flow cardiopulmonary bypass. Circulation 1999; 100:526–532.

10. Kirklin JK, Westaby S, Blackstone EH, Kirklin JW, Chenoweth DE, Pacifico AD. Complement and the damaging effects of cardiopulmonary bypass. J Thorac Cardiovasc Surg 1983; 86:845–857.

11. Wan S, LeClerc JL, Vincent JL. Inflammatory response to cardiopulmonary bypass: mechanisms involved and possible therapeutic strategies. Chest 1997; 112:676–692.

12. Edmunds LH Jr. Inflammatory response to cardiopulmonary bypass. Ann Thorac Surg 1998; 66:S12–S16.

13. Menasche P. The inflammatory response to cardiopulmonary bypass and its impact on postoperative myocardial function. Curr Opin Card 1995; 10:597–604.

14. Taggart DP, Hadjinikolas L, Wong K, Yap J, Hooper J, Kemp M, Hue D, Yacoub M, Lincoln JC. Vulnerability of paediatric myocardium to cardiac surgery. Heart 1996; 76:214–217.

15. Butler J, Pathi VL, Paton RD, Logan RW, MacArthur KJD, Jamieson MPG, Pollock JCS. Acute-phase responses to cardiopulmonary bypass in children weighing less than 10 kilograms. Ann Thorac Surg 1996; 62:538–542.

16. Hirsch R, Dent CL, Wood MK, Huddleston CB, Mendeloff EN, Balzer DT, Landt Y, Parvin CA, Landt M, Ladenson JH, Canter CE. Patterns and potential value of cardiac troponin I elevations after pediatric cardiac operations. Ann Thorac Surg 1998; 65:1394–1399.

17. Immer FF, Stocker F, Seiler AM, Pfammatter JP, Bachmann D, Printzen G, Carrel T. Troponin I for prediction of early postoperative course after pediatric cardiac surgery. J Am Coll Cardiol 1999; 33: 1719–1723.

18. Hovels-Gurich HH, Vazquez-Jimenez JF, Silvestri A, Schumacher K, Minkenberg R, Duchateau J, Messmer BJ, von Bernuth G, Seghaye MC. Production of proinflammatory cytokines and myocardial dysfunction after arterial switch operation in neonates with transposition of the great arteries. J Thorac Cardiovasc Surg 2002; 124: 811–820.

19. Wessel DL. Managing low cardiac output syndrome after congenital heart surgery. Crit Care Med 2001; 29(suppl):220–230.

20. Tibby SM, Hatherill M, Murdoch IA. Capillary refill and core-peripheral temperature gap as indicators of hemodynamic status in pediatric intensive care patients. Arch Dis Child 1999; 80:163–166.

21. Tibby SM, Murdoch IA. Monitoring cardiac function in intensive care. Arch Dis Child 2003; 88:46–52.

22. Tibby SM, Murdoch IA. Measurement of cardiac output and tissue perfusion. Curr Opin Pediatr 2002; 14:303–309.

23. Wippermann CF, Huth RG, Schmidt FX, Thul J, Betancor M, Schranz D. Continuous measurement of cardiac output by the Fick principle in infants and children: comparison with the thermodilution method. Intensive Care Med 1996; 22:467–471.

24. Reddy PS, Curtiss EL, Bell B. Determinants of variation between Fick and indicator dilution estimates of cardiac output during diagnostic catheterization: Fick vs. dye cardiac outputs. J Lab Clin Med 1976; 87:568–576.

25. Hillis LD, Firth BG, Winniford MD. Analysis of factors affecting the variability of Fick versus indicator dilution measurements of cardiac output. Am J Cardiol 1985; 56:764–768.

26. Rudolph AM, Cayler GG. Cardiac catheterization in infants and children. Pediatr Clin North Am 1958; 5:907–943.

27. Rudolph AM. Complications occurring in children. Circulation 1968; 37:59–66.

28. Rossi AF, Sommer RJ, Lotvin A, Gross RP, Steinberg LG, Kipel G, Golinko RJ, Griepp RB. Usefulness of intermittent monitoring of mixed venous oxygen saturation after stage 1 palliation for hypoplastic left heart syndrome. Am J Cardiol 1994; 73:1118–1123.

29. Hoffman GM, Ghanayem NS, Kampine JM, Berger S, Mussatto KA, Litwin SB, Tweddell JS. Venous saturation and anaerobic threshold in neonates after the Norwood procedure for hypoplastic left heart syndrome. Ann Thorac Surg 2000; 70:1515–1521.

30. Siegel LB, Dalton HJ, Hertzog JH, Hopkins RA, Hannan RL, Hauser GJ. Initial postoperative serum lactate levels predict survival in children after open-heart surgery. Intensive Care Med 1996; 22:1418–1423.

31. Hatherill M, Sajjanhar T, Tibby SM, Champion MP, Anderson D, Marsh MJ, Murdoch IA. Serum lactate as a predictor of mortality after pediatric cardiac surgery. Arch Dis Child 1997; 77:235–238.

32. Duke T, Butt W, South M, Karl TR. Early markers of major adverse events in children after cardiac operations. J Thorac Cardiovasc Surg 1997; 114:1042–1051.

33. Cheifetz IM, Kern FH, Schulman SR, Greeley WJ, Ungerleider RM, Meliones JN. Serum lactates correlate with mortality after operations for complex congenital heart disease. Ann Thorac Surg 1997; 64:735–738.

34. Barratt-Boyes BG, Simpson M, Neutze JM. Intracardiac surgery in neonates and infants using deep hypothermia with surface cooling

and limited cardiopulmonary bypass. Circulation 1971; 43(suppl):I-25–I-30.

35. Castaneda AR, Lamberti J, Sade RM, Williams RG, Nadas AS. Open-heart surgery during the first three months of life. J Thorac Cardiovasc Surg 1974; 68:719–731.

36. Naik SK, Knight A, Elliott MJ. A randomized study of a modified technique of ultrafiltration during pediatric open-heart surgery. Circulation 1991; 84(suppl 3):422–431.

37. Elliott MJ. Ultrafiltration and modified ultrafiltration in pediatric open heart operations. Ann Thorac Surg 1993; 56:1518–1522.

38. Koutlas TC, Gaynor JW, Nicolson SC, Steven JM, Wernovsky G, Spray TL. Modified ultrafiltration reduces postoperative morbidity after cavopulmonary connection. Ann Thorac Surg 1997; 64:37–42.

39. Chaturvedi RR, Shore DF, White PA, Scallan MH, Gothard JW, Redington AN, Lincoln C. Modified ultrafiltration improves global left ventricular systolic function after open-heart surgery in infants and children. Eur J Cardiothorac Surg 1999; 15:742–746.

40. Darling D, Nanry K, Shearer I, et al. Technique of paediatric modified ultrafiltration: 1996 survey results. Perfusion 1998; 13:93–103.

41. Thompson LD, McElhinney DB, Findlay P, Miller-Hance W, Chen MJ, Minami M, Petrossian E, Parry AJ, Reddy VM, Hanley FL. A prospective randomized study comparing volume-standardized modified and conventional ultrafiltration in pediatric open-heart surgery. J Thorac Cardiovasc Surg 2001; 122:220–228.

42. Friedman WF, George BL. Treatment of congestive heart failure by altering loading conditions of the heart. J Pediatr 1985; 106:697.

43. Bohn DJ, Poirer CS, Demonds JF. Efficacy of dopamine, dobutamine and epinephrine during emergence from cardiopulmonary bypass in children. Crit Care Med 1980; 8:367.

44. Habib DM, Padbury JF, Anas NG. Dobutamine pharmacokinetics and pharmacodynamics in pediatric intensive care patients. Crit Care Med 1992; 20:601.

45. Berg RA, Donnerstein RL, Padbury JF. Dobutamine infusions in stable, critically ill children: pharmacokinetics and hemodynamic actions. Crit Care Med 1993; 21:678–686.

46. Caspi J, Coles JG, Benson LN, Herman SL, Augustine J, Tsao P, Brezina A, Kolin A, Wilson GJ. Effects of high plasma epinephrine and Ca^{2+}concentrations on neonatal myocardial function after ischemia. J Thorac Cardiovasc Surg 1993; 105:59–67.

47. Caspi J, Coles JG, Benson LN, Herman SL, Diaz RJ, Augustine J, Brezina A, Kolin A, Wilson GJ. Age-related response to epinephrine-induced myocardial stress: a functional and ultrastructural study. Circulation 1991; 84(suppl III):III-394–III-399.

48. Rosenzweig EB, Starc TJ, Chen JM, Cullinane S, Timchak DM, Gersony WM, Landry DW, Galantowicz ME. Intravenous arginine-

vasopressin in children with vasodilatory shock after cardiac surgery. Circulation 1999; 100:182–186.

49. Murzi B, Iervasi G, Masini S, Moschetti R, Vanini V, Zucchelli G, Biagini A. Thyroid hormones homeostasis in patients during and after cardiopulmonary bypass. Ann Thorac Surg 1995; 59:481–485.

50. Bettendorf M, Schmidt KG, Tiefenbacher U, Grulich-Henn J, Heinrich UE, Schonberg DK. Transient secondary hypothyroidism in children after cardiac surgery. Pediatr Res 1997; 41:375–379.

51. Mainwaring RD, Capparelli E, Schell K, Acosta M, Nelson JC. Pharmacokinetic evaluation of triiodothyronine supplementation in children after modified Fontan procedure. Circulation 2000; 101: 1423–1429.

52. Bettendorf M, Schmidt KG, Grulich-Henn J, Ulmer HE, Heinrich UE. Triiodothyronine treatment in children after cardiac surgery: a double-blind, randomized, placebo-controlled study. Lancet 2000; 356:529–534.

53. Portman MA, Fearneyhough C, Ning XH, Duncan BW, Rosenthal GL, Lupinetti FM. Triodothyronine repletion in infants during cardiopulmonary bypass for congenital heart disease. J Thorac Cardiovasc Surg 2000; 120:604–608.

54. Chowdhury D, Ojamaa K, Parnell VA, McMahon C, Sison CP, Klein I. A prospective randomized clinical study of thyroid hormone treatment after operations for complex congenital heart disease. J Thorac Cardiovasc Surg 2001; 122:1023–1025.

55. Carrel T, Eckstein F, Englberger L, Mury R, Mohacsi P. Thyronin treatment in adult and pediatric heart surgery: clinical experience and review of literature. Eur J Heart Fail 2002; 4:577–582.

56. Dupuis JY, Bondy R, Cattran C, Nathan HJ, Wynands JE. Amrinone and dobutamine as primary treatment of low cardiac output syndrome following coronary artery surgery: a comparison of their effects on hemodynamics and outcome. J Cardiothorac Vasc Anesth 1992; 6:542–553.

57. Robinson BW, Gelband H, Mas MS. Selective pulmonary and systemic vasodilator effects of amrinone in children. New therapeutic implications. J Am Coll Cardiol 1993; 21:1461–1465.

58. Berner M, Jaccard C, Oberhansli I. Hemodynamic effects of amrinone in children after cardiac surgery. Intensive Care Med 1990; 16:85–88.

59. Bailey JM, Miller BE, Lu W, Tosone SR, Kanter KR, Tam VK. The pharmacokinetics of milrinone in pediatric patients after cardiac surgery. Anesthesiology 1999; 90:1012–1018.

60. Ramamoorthy C, Anderson GD, Williams GD, Lynn AM. Pharmacokinetics and side effects of milrinone in infants and children after open heart surgery. Anesth Analg 1998; 86:283–289.

61. Chang AC, Atz AM, Wernovsky G, Burke RP, Wessel DL. Milrinone: systemic and pulmonary hemodynamic effects in neonates after cardiac surgery. Crit Care Med 1995; 23:1907–1914.
62. Hickey PR, Hansen DD. Pulmonary hypertension in infants: Postoperative management. In: Yacoub M, ed. Annual of Cardiac Surgery. London: Current Science, 1989:16–22.
63. Wheller J, George BL, Mulder DG, Jarmakani JM. Diagnosis and management of postoperative pulmonary hypertensive crisis. Circulation 1979; 70:1640–1644.
64. Jones OD, Shore DF, Rigby ML, Leijala M, Scallan J, Shinebourne EA, Lincoln JC. The use of tolazoline hydrochloride as a pulmonary vasodilator in potentially fatal episodes of pulmonary vasoconstriction after cardiac surgery in children. Circulation 1981; 64:134–139.
65. Drummond WH, Gregory GA, Heymann MA, Phibbs RA. The independent effects of hyperventilation, tolazoline, and dopamine on infants with persistent pulmonary hypertension. J Pediatr 1981; 98: 603–611.
66. Furchgott RF. The role of endothelium in the responses of vascular smooth muscle to drugs. Annu Rev Pharmacol Toxicol 1984; 24: 175–197.
67. Ignarro LJ, Buga GM, Wood KS, Byrns RE, Chaudhuri G. Endothelium-derived relaxing factor produced and released from artery and vein is nitric oxide. Proc Natl Acad Sci USA 1987; 84:9265–9269.
68. Wessel DL, Adatia I, Giglia TM, Thompson JE, Kulik TJ. Use of inhaled nitric oxide and acetylcholine in the evaluation of pulmonary hypertension and endothelial function after cardiopulmonary bypass. Circulation 1993; 88:2128–2138.
69. Journois D, Pouard P, Mauriat P, Malhere T, Vouhe P, Safran D. Inhaled nitric oxide as a therapy for pulmonary hypertension after operations for congenital heart defects. J Thorac Cardiovasc Surg 1994; 107:1129–1135.
70. Luciani GB, Chang AC, Starnes VA. Surgical repair of transposition of the great arteries in neonates with persistent pulmonary hypertension. Ann Thorac Surg 1996; 61:800–805.
71. Adatia I, Perry S, Landzberg M, Moore P, Thompson JE, Wessel DL. Inhaled nitric oxide and hemodynamic evaluation of patients with pulmonary hypertension before transplantation. J Am Coll Cardiol 1995; 25:1652–1664.
72. Wessel DL, Adatia I, Van Marter LJ, Thompson JE, Kane JW, Stark AR, Kourembanas S. Improved oxygenation in a randomized trial of inhaled nitric oxide for persistent pulmonary hypertension of the newborn. Pediatrics 1997; 100:1–7.
73. Yahagi N, Kumon K, Tanigami H, Watanabe Y, Ishizaka T, Yamamoto F, Nishigaki K, Matsuki, Yagihara T. Inhaled nitric oxide for the postoperative management of Fontan-type operations. Ann Thorac Surg 1994; 57:1371–1372.

74. Atz AM, Munoz RA, Adatia I, Wessel DL. Diagnostic and therapeutic uses of inhaled nitric oxide in neonatal Ebstein's anomaly. Am J Card 2003; 91:906–908.

75. Atz AM, Adatia I, Wessel DL. Rebound pulmonary hypertension after inhalation of nitric oxide. Ann Thorac Surg 1996; 62:1759–1764.

76. Atz AM, Wessel DL. Sildenafil ameliorates effects of inhaled nitric oxide withdrawal. Anesthesiology 1999; 91:307–310.

77. Prasad S, Wilkinson J, Gatzoulis MA. Sildenafil in primary pulmonary hypertension. N Eng J Med 2000; 343:1342–1343.

78. Abrams D, Schulze-Nieck I, Magee AG. Sildenafil as a selective pulmonary vasodilator in childhood primary pulmonary hypertension. Heart 2000; 84:e4–e5.

79. Zhao L, Mason NA, Morrell NW. Sildenafil inhibits hypoxia-induced pulmonary hypertension. Circulation 2001; 104:424–428.

80. Atz AM, Lefler AK, Fairbrother DC. Sildenafil augments the effect of inhaled nitric oxide for postoperative pulmonary hypertensive crises. J Thorac Cardiovasc Surg 2002; 124:628–629.

81. Schulze-Neick I, Hartenstein P, Li J, Stiller B, Nagdyman N, Hubler M, Butrous G, Petros A, Lange P, Redington AN. Sildenafil is a potent pulmonary vasodilator in children after heart surgery. Circulation 2003; 108(suppl 1):167–173.

82. Braunstein PW, Sade RM, Gillette PC. Life-threatening postoperative junctional ectopic tachycardia. Ann Thorac Surg 1992; 53:726–728.

83. Pfammatter JP, Paul T, Ziemer G, Kallfelz HC. Successful management of junctional tachycardia by hypothermia after cardiac operations in infants. Ann Thorac Surg 1995; 60:556–560.

84. Perry JC, Fenrich AL, Hulse JE, Triedman JK, Friedman RA, Lamberti JJ. Pediatric use of intravenous amiodarone: efficacy and safety in critically ill patients from a multicenter protocol. J Am Coll Cardiol 1996; 27:1246–1250.

85. Walsh EP, Saul P, Sholler GF, Triedman JK, Jonas RA, Mayer JE. Evaluation of a staged treatment protocol for rapid automatic junctional ectopic tachycardia after operation for congenital heart disease. J Am Coll Cardiol 1999; 29:1046–1053.

86. Dodge-Khatami A, Miller OI, Anderson RH, Goldman AP, Gil-Jaurena JM, Elliott MJ, Tsang VT, De Leval MR. Surgical substrates of postoperative junctional ectopic tachycardia in congenital heart defects. J Thorac Cardiovasc Surg 2002; 123:624–630.

87. Hoffman TM, Wernovsky G, Wieand TS, Cohen MI, Jennings AC, Vetter VL, Godinez RI, Gaynor JW, Spray TL, Rhodes LA. The incidence of arrhythmias in a pediatric intensive care unit. Pediatr Cardiol 2002; 23:598–604.

88. Hoffman TM, Bush DM, Wernovsky G, Cohn MI, Wieand TS, Gaynor JW, Spray TL, Rhodes LA. Postoperative junctional ectopic tachycardia in children: incidence, risk factors, and treatment.

Postoperative junctional ectopic tachycardia in children: incidence, risk factors, and treatment. Ann Thorac Surg 2002; 74:1607–1611.

89. Klinge JM, Scharf J, Hofbeck M, Gertlig S, Bonakdar S, Singer H. Intermittent administration of furosemide versus continuous infusion in the postoperative management of children following open heart surgery. Intensive Care Med 1997; 23:693–697.

90. van der Vorst MM, Ruys-Dudok van Heel I, Kist-van Holthe JE, den Hartigh J, Schoemaker RC, Cohen AF, Burggraaf J. Continuous intravenous furosemide in hemodynamically unstable children after cardiac surgery. Intensive Care Med 2001; 27:711–715.

91. Marik PE. Low-dose dopamine: a systematic review. Intensive Care Med 2002; 28:877–883.

92. Hughes AD, Sever PS. Action of fenoldopam, a selective dopamine (DA1) receptor agonist, on isolated human arteries. Blood Vessels 1989; 26:119–127.

93. Strauser LM, Pruitt RD, Tobias J. Initial experience with fenoldopam in children. Am J Ther 1999; 6:283–288.

94. Bridges ND, Mayer JE Jr, Lock JE, Jonas RA, Hanley FL, Keane JF, Perry SB, Castaneda AR. Effect of baffle fenestration on outcome of the modified Fontan operation. Circulation 1992; 86:1762–1769.

95. Lemler MS, Scott WA, Leonard SR, Stromberg D, Ramaciotti C. Fenestration improves clinical outcome of the Fontan procedure: a prospective randomized study. Circulation 2002; 105:207–212.

96. Duncan BW, Bohn DJ, Atz AM, French JW, Laussen PC, Wessel DL. Mechanical circulatory support for the treatment of children with acute fulminant myocarditis. J Thorac Cardiovasc Surg 2001; 122:440–448.

97. Duncan BW. Mechanical circulatory support for infants and children with cardiac disease. Ann Thorac Surg 2002; 73:1670–1677.

98. Kolovos NS, Bratton SL, Moler FW, Bove EL, Ohye RG, Bartlett RH, Kulik TJ. Outcome of pediatric patients treated with extracorporeal life support after cardiac surgery. Ann Thorac Surg 2003; 76: 1435–1442.

99. Morris MC, Ittenbach RF, Godinez RI, Portnoy JD, Tabbutt S, Hanna BD, Hoffman TM, Gaynor JW, Connelly JT, Helfaer MA, Spray TL, Wernovsky G. Risk factors for mortality in 137 pediatric cardiac intensive care unit patients managed with extracorporeal membrane oxygenation. Crit Care Med 2004; 32:1061–1069.

100. Young JB, Abraham WT, Smith AL, Leon AR, Lieberman R, Wilkoff B, Canby RC, Schroeder JS, Liem LB, Hall S, Wheelan K. Multicenter InSync ICD Randomized Clinical Evaluation (MIRACLE ICD) Trial Investigators. Combined cardiac resynchronization and implantable cardioversion defibrillation in advanced chronic heart failure. JAMA 2003; 289:2685–2694.

101. Janousek J, Vojtovic P, Chaloupecky V, Hucin B, Tlaskal T, Kostelka M, Reich O. Hemodynamically optimized temporary cardiac pacing

after surgery for congenital heart defects. Pacing Clin Electrophysiol 2000; 23:1250–1259.

102. Bronicki RA, Backer CL, Baden HP, Mavroudis C, Crawford SE, Green TP. Dexamethasone reduces the inflammatory response to cardiopulmonary bypass in children. Ann Thorac Surg 2000; 69:1490–1495.

103. Lodge AJ, Chai PJ, Daggett CW, Ungerleider RM, Jaggers J. Methylprednisolone reduces the inflammatory response to cardiopulmonary bypass in neonatal piglets: timing of dose is important. J Thorac Cardiovasc Surg 1999; 117:515–522.

104. Kawamura T, Inada K, Nara N, Wakusawa R, Endo S. Influence of methylprednisolone on cytokine balance during cardiac surgery. Crit Care Med 1999; 27:545–548.

105. Jansen NJ, van Oeveren W, van Vliet M, Stoutenbeek CP, Eysman L, Wildevuur CR. The role of different types of corticosteroids on the inflammatory mediators in cardiopulmonary bypass. Eur J Cardiothorac Surg 1991; 5:211–217.

106. Checchia PA, Backer CL, Bronicki RA, Baden HP, Crawford SE, Green TP, Mavroudis C. Dexamethasone reduces postoperative troponin levels in children undergoing cardiopulmonary bypass. Crit Care Med 2003; 31:1742–1745.

107. Tassani P, Kunkel R, Richter JA, Oechsler H, Lorenz HP, Braun SL, Eising GP, Haas F, Paek SU, Bauernschmitt R, Jochum M, Lange R. Effect of C1-esterase inhibitor on capillary leak and inflammatory response syndrome during arterial switch operations in neonates. J Cardiothorac Vasc Anesth 2001; 15:469–473.

21

Ventricular Assist Devices

PEDRO J. DEL NIDO

Department of Cardiac Surgery,
Children's Hospital, Harvard Medical School,
Boston, Massachusetts, U.S.A.

Mechanical circulatory support for management of ventricular dysfunction after surgery or acute decompensation of chronic heart failure in children has become an important tool to achieve hemodynamic stability as part of surgical management in most pediatric cardiac units. When combined with an active transplantation program, mechanical circulatory support can have a significant impact on overall mortality. Despite the limited types of devices available for pediatric use, mechanical circulatory support with a conventional roller pump or centrifugal pump has been applied widely with substantial success. Unlike the application of mechanical support in adults, the most common indications in children is for short-term support (less than 2 weeks) as bridge to recovery following acute decompensation. Bridge to transplantation as an indication for support remains limited in the pediatric setting due to the limitations of the circulatory support systems, and the relatively high incidence of complications with conventional extracorporeal life support systems (ECLS). In this section, we will review current systems available for pediatric support, indications for support and results, and new types of systems including new devices currently under design.

TYPES OF PUMPS

A wide variety of pumps have been developed for circulatory support in adults and children. The simplest type is a peristaltic or roller pump that compresses a length of tubing to displace the volume inside the tube, occluding the lumen of the tube to maximize forward flow and to prevent retrograde flow. A typical roller pump consists of a length of tubing inside a circular metal raceway, and a series of rollers mounted on the ends of rotating arms. The position of the rollers is adjustable to account for different size tubing and to permit near complete occlusion of the lumen inside the tubing. The rollers are offset by 180° so that a roller is occluding the tubing at all times as the arms rotate. Flow out of this system is therefore governed by the volume inside the tubing and the revolutions per minute of the pump (minus the residual volume inside the tubing when the roller is not completely occlusive). Due to the compression by the roller, the tubing must be of resistant material that does not fracture or release microparticles (spallation). Polyvinylchloride (PVC) is such a material and newer forms of PVC have become the standard for both cardiopulmonary bypass circuits and for long-term support. The roller pump has also become the standard for clinical open-heart surgery and, along with a membrane oxygenator, is the most commonly used mechanical circulatory assist system for temporary support of children, also called extracorporeal life support (ECLS).

The next most common type of pump used as a pediatric ventricular assist device is a centrifugal pump, which consists of a rapidly spinning impeller containing veins to create a vortex, housed inside a smooth conical plastic housing. This type of pump, unlike the roller pump, has limited durability in its commonly used design, requiring changing of the pump head after 24 or 48 hr of use. Centrifugal pumps have been used for conventional bypass surgery in adults and children. There is a limited experience with its use as an assist device for ventricular failure in children when the dysfunction is confined primarily to the left ventricle. Newer versions of this type of pump have now been designed for longer-term support.

Diaphragm type pulsatile pumps are commonly used for chronic support in adults as heart replacement systems and as ventricular assist devices, but there are few such systems specifically designed for pediatric use. These pumps consist of an inlet port with one-way, or check valve, a chamber lined with a distensible bladder or a diaphragm that serves as a "ventricle," and an outlet port, also containing a one-way valve. The main advantage is that they provide pulsatile flow and a more physiologic arterial waveform. The main disadvantages are size, and the limited range of flows, which are governed primarily by bladder size and pump rate.

A useful way to classify pumps is by their mechanism of action or how they create movement of a fluid. Using this classification, two types of pumps are available for clinical use. These are *positive displacement* pumps and *centrifugal* pumps. Each has its inherent advantages and disadvantages and there are now a wide variety of systems available clinically and in development, which maximize the particular advantages of the type of pump. It is helpful to categorize the clinical systems according to the mechanism of blood displacement since this way one can more easily understand the limitations of the clinical systems and the potential sources of complications.

Positive displacement pumps: A positive displacement pump is one in which a definite volume of liquid is delivered for each cycle of pump operation. This volume is constant regardless of the resistance to flow offered by the circulatory system the pump is supporting, provided the capacity of the power unit driving the pump or pump component strength limits are not exceeded. Stated another way, a positive displacement pump is any pump mechanism that seals water in a chamber, then forces it out by reducing the volume of the chamber. Examples include diaphragm, piston, and peristaltic (roller) pumps (Fig. 1).

A positive displacement pump has an expanding cavity on the suction side of the pump and a decreasing cavity on the discharge side. Liquid is allowed to flow into the pump as the cavity on the suction side expands and the liquid is forced out of the discharge as the cavity collapses. A positive displacement pump, unlike a centrifugal pump, will produce the same flow at a given cycle or rpm, no matter what the discharge pressure

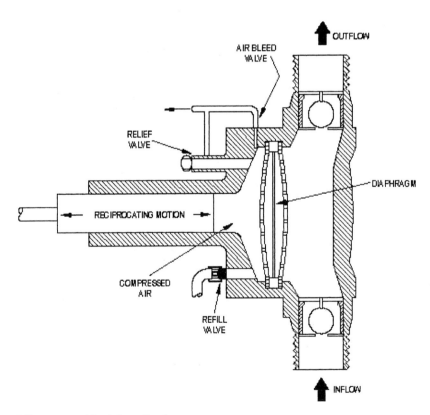

Figure 1 Positive displacement pump.

is. Control of flow in a positive displacement pump can be achieved by varying the number of cycles/revolutions per minute, changing the degree of diaphragm displacement, and ultimately by varying the size of the bladder and housing. For practical purposes, however, in most clinical pump systems, changing the pump rate is the most readily available method of altering flow, with a few systems permitting control over the extent of diaphragm displacement. Clinical systems that are commercially available in Europe provide two or three sizes of bladder and housing for pediatric use.

Centrifugal pumps: These pumps contain a mechanism that spins water in order to push it out by means of centrifugal force. Centrifugal pumps consist of a fanned impeller that sits inside a housing. The impellers or cones are mechanically or magnetically coupled with an electric motor and, when rotated rapidly, generate a pressure differential that may cause the movement of blood. Unlike roller pumps, they are nonocclusive and are therefore afterload-dependent; i.e., an increase in downstream resistance decreases forward flow delivered to the patient. This has both favorable and unfavorable consequences. Flow is not determined by rotational rate alone, so a flow meter must be incorporated in the arterial outflow to quantitate pump flow. Furthermore, when the pump is connected to the patient's arterial system but is not running, blood will flow backward through the pump unless the arterial line is clamped. The two main components of a centrifugal pump are the impeller and the volute. The impeller produces liquid velocity and the volute forces the liquid to discharge from the pump converting velocity to pressure (see Fig. 2). This is accomplished by offsetting the impeller in the volute and by maintaining a close clearance between the impeller and the volute, at the edge of the impeller vane (cut-water). Three of the more common types of centrifugal pumps used in medical devices are:

- Radial flow—a centrifugal pump in which the pressure is developed wholly by centrifugal force (Fig. 2).
- Mixed flow—a centrifugal pump in which the pressure is developed partly by centrifugal force and

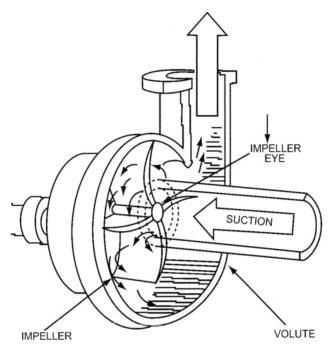

Figure 2 Axial flow pump.

partly by the lift of the vanes of the impeller on the liquid.

– Axial flow—a centrifugal pump in which the pressure is developed by the propelling or lifting action of the vanes of the impeller on the liquid (Fig. 3).

TYPES OF CIRCULATORY SUPPORT SYSTEMS

Extracorporeal Life Support (ECLS)

The most common circulatory support system in use for pediatric patients is an ECLS system (also termed extracorporeal membrane oxygenator or ECMO system), which is comprised of a roller pump, oxygenator, and control systems to prevent cavitation or excessive negative pressure in the venous side, and excessively high pressure on the arterial side. The major

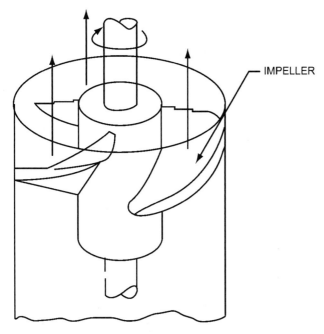

IMPELLER

Figure 3   Axial flow pump.

advantages of this system are its durability, familiarity (since it is similar to conventional cardiopulmonary bypass), relative simplicity, and low cost. Additional advantages include the capacity for biventricular support and to treat pulmonary dysfunction, which are frequently seen in pediatric patients with acute hemodynamic decompensation. The disadvantages of the ECLS system include: high priming volume, which causes dilution of not only red cells but also platelets and clotting factors; large surface area, which promotes activation of platelets and clotting factors; it is a relatively open system due to the multiple access ports, which can permit introduction of bacteria; and it requires immobilization of the patient due to the extracorporeal circuit and cannula design (Table 1).

Cannulas: Cannulas for ECLS systems have been designed primarily for peripheral cannulation via neck or groin vessels. Ideally the cannula is thin walled (maximal inner to outer diameter ratio), reinforced to prevent kinking,

Table 1   Extracorporeal Membrane Oxygenation (ECMO)

Advantages	Disadvantages
Durability	Large prime volume
Inexpensive	Open system
Simplicity	Use of oxygenator
Familiar system	Immobilizes patient
Biventricular support	Large artificial surface
Pulmonary support	High rate of platelet and clotting factor consumption
Versatility	—

and is available in a variety of sizes to accommodate the large range of flow rates required for pediatric patients. Most commercially available cannulas are modifications of conventional cannulas used for cardiopulmonary bypass. They are made of flexible plastic material, polyurethane, or polyvinyl chloride, with no mechanism to prevent infection along the shaft of the cannula such as the felt cuff used in a VAD cannula. ECMO cannulas are inexpensive compared to VAD cannulas and usually come prepared for rapid insertion and connection to a circuit. Most have an obturator to facilitate insertion into a small vessel, and have the connector for the circuit tubing already incorporated into the cannula.

Oxygenators: Two types of membrane oxygenators are available for the bypass circuit and although equally effective, there are fundamental differences in design that determine ease of priming and longevity. Hollow fiber oxygenators consist of a large number of fibers with a central lumen and semiporous walls with holes large enough to let water through but small enough so that proteins, particularly plasma proteins, can cover these holes creating a thin film. The protein film then becomes the semipermeable membrane through which gas exchange occurs but water does not readily leak out. Sheet type membrane oxygenators do not have holes in the membrane wall and depend on the permeability of the plastic material that makes up the membrane to permit gas transfer. Since hollow fiber membrane oxygenators have holes that can allow gas to escape, deairing the fibers with the priming solution is easy and can be done rapidly. For this reason, they have been incorporated in some ECLS circuits for support following cardiac arrest as a rapid response system. Sheet membrane oxygenators require flushing the air out of the membrane with a very soluble gas, such as carbon dioxide, to prevent air trapping in the section that will contain the blood. Therefore the preparation time for a sheet membrane oxygenator is substantially longer than a hollow fiber type of membrane oxygenator.

Hollow fiber oxygenators, however, are not designed for use for longer than 6 hrs before replacement. There are reports, however, of ECLS systems with a hollow fiber oxygenator that were used for periods up to 48 hrs, but there is a significant risk of leakage of serum into the compartment carrying the gases, resulting in rapid loss of gas transfer capacity. Sheet membrane oxygenators have a much longer usable life span with approval for use up to 14 days, and some reports indicate that longer periods of use can be achieved with little risk of dysfunction.

Ventricular Assist Devices (VADs)

Cannulas: Aside from the type of pump used for circulatory support, cannula design and size availability are important features of VAD system since these systems are designed for longer-term support compared to ECLS systems. For pulsatile systems, cannulas need to be larger than the size of cannula used for continuous flow pumps. With pulsatile devices, too small an arterial cannula for the required flow will increase the pressure in the pump housing, potentially increasing damage to red cells and platelets, and will also dampen the pulse pressure limiting the potential advantages of pulsatile flow in children. The inflow cannula size should also be appropriate to the patient size, but its diameter is often less critical as this cannula is usually inserted in the apex of the ventricle and the systems rely on ventricular contraction for filling. Another important design characteristic is the flexibility of the cannula and the exit angle for the inflow cannula inserted into the apex of the ventricle. The cannulas must be rigid enough to prevent kinking as they exit from the ventricle towards the pump, but should also have the proper geometric curvature to exit directly from the ventricle and aim towards the pump without distorting the heart or shifting the inflow nozzle against the ventricular wall, thereby potentially obstructing pump inflow. Since the VAD systems currently available for children are all paracorporeal, infection is a significant risk particularly at the entry points of cannulas through the skin. Most cannulas have an external felt cuff, similar to that used in chronic indwelling tubes such as a Broviac or Tenckoff catheter, to prevent bacteria from migrating along the wall of the cannula into the mediastinum.

Valves: Pulsatile VADs require valves to ensure forward flow during pump activation and prevent retrograde flow during pump filling. Most systems have incorporated commercially available mechanical valves for the inflow and outflow circuit. Some devices, however, have valves designed specifically for that pump system. The MEDOS-HIA and Berlin heart pumps are examples of the latter with a custom designed tri-leaflet polyurethane valve for both the inflow and outflow valves. The valves of any system are key components since they must withstand the forces generated by the assist device, and must also have a low thrombogenic potential. In some of the early assist devices, the valves used were commercially available valves used clinically, however, some of these valves proved to be inadequate for use in an assist device.

INDICATIONS FOR SUPPORT

The majority of children placed on mechanical circulatory support require it for acute decompensation following a cardiac surgical procedure, or for acute decompensation of chronic heart failure (1–3). In many of these, the expectation is that there will be recovery of contractile function and therefore circulatory support as a bridge to transplantation accounts for less than half of children placed on some form of circulatory support system. This experience is different than with adult patients with hemodynamic compromise where bridge to transplantation is the most common indication for insertion of a VAD (4). This difference is in great part due to the ready availability, in children, of a support system that is temporary in nature (ECLS) and therefore is not viewed as commitment to long-term support. In the adult patients, the Food and Drug Administration requires that a patient be approved for transplantation prior to VAD implantation since the currently available devices only have approval as a bridge to transplantation as opposed to bridge to recovery or permanent replacement which require experimental protocols. In children, indications for longer-term support (over 10 days) have been primarily as a bridge to transplantation with the exception of the acute myocarditis patients where there is evidence that full recovery can occur late, despite several days of severe contractile dysfunction. It is therefore useful in children to group the indications for mechanical support into those requiring short-term support (<10 days) and those where there will likely be a need for longer-term support (2–6 weeks, or longer in teenagers).

The most common uses of mechanical circulatory support in children are to treat acute hemodynamic decompensation, to prevent end-organ injury, and to allow a more complete evaluation to determine the hemodynamic cause of the deterioration and the probability of recovery (5,6). For this reason, the ECLS systems, which include a pump (usually a roller pump) and an oxygenator, have gained widespread acceptance since they are readily available in most pediatric centers, are easily adaptable for any patient size, and are relatively inexpensive (7). Since the expectation in most of these patients is that they will not require support for longer than 1–2 weeks, it is reasonable to use this type of system as an initial method of support for the majority of children suffering from circulatory collapse or severe ventricular dysfunction (1,2). The alternative support systems that have been used in children include centrifugal pumps (8,9), and pneumatic pumps that are paracorporeal, with the pump housing and drive lines outside the patient (10–12).

In adults, patients with acute heart failure from myocardial infarction, postcardiotomy failure, and acute myocarditis represent a large percentage of the population receiving VAD support as a bridge to transplantation (4). Patients with chronic heart failure who suffer acute decompensation requiring VAD support make up the other group. Much less common indications include bridge to recovery (13,14), and intractable ventricular arrhythmias. In children, the indications for VAD have not been as well worked out. There are a number of reports describing use of VAD for isolated ventricle dysfunction such as LV dysfunction in infants with anomalous left coronary arising from the pulmonary artery (ALCAPA) (8,15), retraining the LV following an arterial switch operation for transposition (16), and for support of the single ventricle patient following initial palliation (17). There is also a small but growing experience with adult assist devices implanted in adolescents, with some modifications, for chronic support as a bridge to heart transplantation (18).

Indications for Short-Term Support in Children (<10 Days)

Postcardiotomy Cardiac Arrest

In the current era, ECLS systems are used widely as a tool for resuscitation in children refractory to conventional cardiopulmonary resuscitation (3,19–21). Although the overall results with this approach have resulted in limited improvement in outcome, as indicated by a 26% long-term survival reported in the Extracorporeal Life Support Organization Registry, centers that have developed rapid response systems report significantly better results. Long-term survival rates as high as 58% have been reported when ECMO type systems are used as part of a rapid response program, with the perfusion system primed and ready for use and the ready availability of trained personnel that can initiate resuscitation with mechanical circulatory support within a relatively short period of time (20). Several reports have confirmed the utility of such a system particularly when combined with an active transplant program since some of these children do not have return of adequate cardiac function (3).

For the vast majority of the ECLS systems described for resuscitation, however, a conventional ECMO circuit is used, with a roller pump and membrane oxygenator making up the key components of the system. Although some centers have modified the circuit with the use of a centrifugal pump to avoid the need for a regulatory mechanism such as a bladder box to control pump speed, the concept of total cardiopulmonary support has not changed (21). This is due in part to the ease of use of the available ECMO circuit, the perceived need for biventricular support, and the lack of available alternatives. True VADs have seldom been used for postcardiotomy support in children and even less frequently for resuscitation. Even in adults, initial stabilization is best accomplished with a conventional bypass circuit since cannulation is easier and, once on cardiopulmonary bypass, there is time to evaluate the patient for chronic support with a VAD. Since a VAD system is meant for chronic support (i.e., >2 weeks) proper position of inflow and outflow cannulas is required, along with a sterile environment and well-prepared surgical field. This is seldom available in an ICU setting.

Postcardiotomy Failure

Inability to wean from bypass represents the highest risk group for children requiring mechanical circulatory support. The reasons for failure of the native heart to adequately support the systemic circulation post-bypass are many but in most cases are due to either poor myocardial protection during cardiac arrest, or inadequate hemodynamic repair with residual anatomic defects, or anatomic limitations preventing adequate ventricular function. These and other potential causes for postcardiotomy contractile dysfunction are listed in Table 2.

The initial step required when a patient is unable to wean from conventional bypass is to rule out residual or unrecognized anatomic defect that requires repair. This step is often aided by the use of echocardiography with a transesophageal or epicardial probe. Oximetry of samples obtained

Table 2   Potential Factors Responsible for Postcardiotomy Low
Cardiac Output

Unrecognized residual anatomic defect[a]
Inadequate myocardial protection[a]
Severe hypoxemia
Pulmonary hypertension
Refractory arrhythmias

[a]Most common causes of low cardiac output.

from various anatomic chambers permits evaluation of
residual shunts and often can be the first indication of a residual defect. If a residual defect is identified, then the best
chance for survival is usually immediate repair. Frequently
this requires additional ischemic time for the myocardium,
but, if repair relieves a significant hemodynamic load, the
improvement is usually sufficient to allow discontinuation
from bypass. In cases where myocardial function has not fully
recovered, then a short period of circulatory support
(24–48 hr) is usually sufficient for recovery of "stunned myocardium" in children. If no defect is identified or a lesion is
found that cannot be readily repaired, then mechanical circulatory support can be used to maintain perfusion and end-
organ function pending evaluation of alternatives such as
transplantation. It is important in this case to ensure that
the residual or uncorrected defect does not interfere with adequate perfusion, even on mechanical circulatory support.
Examples where an anatomic defect impacts on the effectiveness of support include aortic valve regurgitation, and large
aorto-pulmonary collaterals. These lesions should be
addressed, in the operating room or in the catheterization
laboratory, within a relatively short time period as inadequate organ perfusion may result in irreversible injury (22).

Posttransplant Graft Dysfunction

Posttransplant graft dysfunction is most commonly due to
either prolonged ischemic time with inadequate protection

of the myocardium, or graft failure from too great a hemodynamic load, such as elevated pulmonary vascular resistance. Mechanical circulatory support in these patients is
often very helpful and should be initiated early to avoid com-
pounding the injury with high-dose inotropic drugs. The long-
term results are dependent primarily on the indication for
support rather than the timing, i.e., early or late after transplantation. Patients with graft dysfunction from prolonged
ischemia or from rejection generally have better long-term
survival than patients who require support for elevated
pulmonary vascular resistance or pulmonary infection (23)
(Fig. 4).

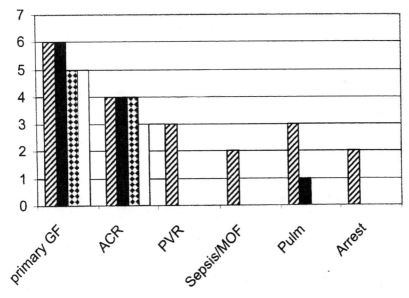

Figure 4 Effect of indication for extracorporeal membrane
oxygenation (ECMO) on outcome. Slashed bars = total; solid
bars = decannulated; dotted bars = discharged; open bars = alive
5.6 months to 9.8 years after ECMO; ACR = acute cellular rejection;
Arrest = sudden cardiac arrest; GF = graft failure; MOF =
multiorgan failure; Pulm = pulmonary failure; PVR = elevated
pulmonary vascular resistance. (From Ref. 23.)

Uncontrolled Arrhythmias

Ventricular arrhythmia, or supraventricular tachycardia with rapid conduction that is refractory to medical therapy, represent a potential indication for short-term circulatory support. Reports describing good results with this indication exist mostly in the adult literature but anecdotal experience in pediatric centers also exists (24). Here the indication for circulatory support is not for inadequate cardiac contractile function since in most cases, contractility is relatively well preserved. Instead, the indications are to maintain adequate cardiac output in the face of inefficient ventricular function and also to decrease oxygen consumption and improve perfusion of the myocardium. In adults, biventricular support is required due to the effects of the rhythm abnormality on filling and coordinated contraction of both ventricles. In children, ECLS with a conventional ECMO circuit makes more sense since cannulation can be achieved peripherally, when there is no thoracic incision, and biventricular support is achieved automatically, avoiding the complexity of bi-VAD.

Indications for Longer-Term Support in Children (2–6 Weeks)

Bridge to Transplantation

The most common indication in adults for the use of ventri-VADs is for long-term support as a bridge to transplantation. Chronic support with a device that permits patient mobility, and requires less anticoagulation is more conducive to long-term support and enables rehabilitation of the patient prior to transplantation. Thus, VAD support is viewed, in adults, as a way to improve patients who are candidates for transplantation and to decrease the morbidity and mortality in high-risk patients undergoing heart transplantation, as well as maintaining organ perfusion in patients who otherwise would not survive to transplantation. In children, most of the experience with mechanical circulatory support as a bridge to transplantation has been with ECLS using a conventional ECMO circuit (3,25,26). Although the experience is limited, reasonably good results have been reported with about 50% of children listed for transplantation receiving an organ and surviving to hospital discharge. This is in spite of the fact that the ECMO circuit immobilizes the patient, requires full anticoagulation with heparin, and has many access ports where bacteria can be introduced. Thus, for many centers, conventional ECMO circuits provide adequate support for a significant number of children requiring circulatory support as a bridge to transplantation. What is not known, however, is whether additional patients who are never considered for transplantation would become candidates if a pediatric VAD system were readily available, or whether survival to transplant and hospital discharge would be improved with the use of a VAD, as has been shown in adults.

In adults, ECLS with a conventional ECMO circuit is seldom used. Instead, patients requiring a VAD are placed on cardiopulmonary bypass, emergently or semielectively, depending on hemodynamic status. Once on bypass, VAD cannula are inserted and once the VAD circuit is connected and primed, bypass is discontinued and VAD support initiated. In children and adolescents, the sequence is the same except that more often an ECMO circuit is used for support, except in cases where postcardiotomy support of single ventricle dysfunction is required such as in children with LV dysfunction post-repair of ALCAPA. Conversion to VAD, which requires a sternotomy, can be accomplished much the same way as in adults. The main advantages of VAD support over ECMO, for long-term support, are the fact that it is a simpler system to run and maintain, and VADs have less adverse effects on platelets and clotting factors due to the smaller surface area compared to ECMO circuits. Additional advantages, as discussed above, include smaller size, greater potential for patient mobility, lower infection risk, and better LV decompression compared to ECMO circuits.

Acute Myocarditis

Acute fulminant myocarditis resulting in rapid hemodynamic deterioration is one indication for mechanical support where recovery of contractile function can be expected in the majority of children. The rate of recovery, however, can be quite slow and therefore longer-term support may be required. Because of the unpredictable nature of the disease and our inability to foretell which patients will recover in a relatively short period of time (<2 weeks), ECLS with conventional ECMO circuit is usually the initial system used for circulatory support. Also, in many patients, there is biventricular dysfunction at first so that ECLS is the least complicated system for early management. Frequently, the degree of contractile dysfunction is so severe that active decompression of the left ventricle is necessary to prevent distention and further injury to the myocardium, LV decompression is best achieved with the use of an LV vent cannula that is connected to the venous return line of the ECLS circuit. If contractile function has not returned after 3–5 days, then consideration should be given to converting to VAD support, since recovery without transplantation, although still possible, will likely take more than 10–14 days. At this stage, frequently there is sufficient recovery of right ventricular function to consider LVAD alone but careful assessment of RV function should be made prior to conversion.

This can be done in the operating room with transesophageal echocardiography to monitor RV function and visual inspection of the RV once the LVAD has been implanted and activated.

PATIENT MANAGEMENT ON CIRCULATORY SUPPORT

The management of children placed on circulatory support varies as the duration of support increases. It is useful, therefore, to separate management strategies depending on the phase of support the patient is in.

- In the *initial stabilization phase*, shortly after initiation of support, emphasis must be placed on evaluating the effectiveness of support, and determining the cause of the hemodynamic deterioration.

- In the *intermediate phase*, the emphasis is on management of anticoagulation, prevention of infection, optimizing nutrition, and a decision must be made regarding the likelihood of recovery vs. the need to consider transplantation and longer-term circulatory support.
- In the *weaning phase*, in patients where there has been substantial recovery, weaning from support requires specific steps to optimize hemodynamics and end-organ function to permit adequate evaluation of cardiac function.

Initial Stabilization Phase

In the first few hours after initiation of circulatory support, emphasis must be placed on assessing the adequacy of perfusion and end-organ function. Achieving flow rates that are appropriate for the size of the child along with indicators of end-organ function such as urine output, serum lactate levels, and acid–base status are indices that help to determine the adequacy of tissue perfusion. In cases where perfusion is felt to be inadequate, circuit flow must be determined accurately. With an ECMO circuit, the circuit flow can be easily established by knowing the pump speed (rpm) and tubing size. Similarly, with any positive displacement pump, the circuit flow is determined by multiplying the assist device chamber volume by the number of cycles per minute. In nonocclusive pumps such as centrifugal or axial flow pumps, a flow meter is required to measure circuit flow accurately since flow is governed only in part by pump speed, with afterload on the pump being another important determinant. Initial steps to improve flow when perfusion is deemed inadequate include:

- Ensure that cannula position is optimal, ideally in the center of a large chamber or central vessel.
- Optimize preload by treating hypovolemia.
- Search for possible shunts between the systemic and pulmonary circulation that could be diverting flow away from the systemic circuit.

Once adequate perfusion is achieved, the next step must be evaluation of the adequacy of left ventricular decompression. In cases where the sternum is open, visual inspection of the heart can provide immediate assessment of decompression. If there is any doubt, however, echocardiography should be done to confirm decompression. If the left ventricle is distended, then a vent cannula must be inserted in the left ventricle to achieve decompression. In patients with a closed sternum, this can be accomplished by creation or enlargement of an atrial septal defect in the cardiac catheterization laboratory (27).

Anticoagulation is in almost all cases achieved initially with a continuous infusion of heparin. The goal is to maintain an activated clotting time (ACT) between 200 and 240 sec. At high flow rates, this level of anticoagulation should prevent clot formation and limit consumption of clotting factors. Even with VAD support, anticoagulation with heparin is required initially and only after full support is achieved and the patient stabilized, should oral anticoagulation with coumadin be considered. Other factors must also be considered, particularly with VAD support, when deciding on the degree of anticoagulation including: operative site bleeding, ventricular function, and the presence of prosthetic valves. Early after initiation of support, operative site bleeding is an important consideration and often the ACT is allowed to fall below 200 sec. With a VAD system, the ACT may be allowed to fall below 180 sec for a few hours until hemostasis is achieved. With an ECMO circuit, however, this level of anticoagulation runs a significant risk of clot formation in the membrane, particularly if flows are relatively low with respect to the membrane size. Once hemostasis is achieved, the level of anticoagulation should be raised. Once the patient has stabilized, anticoagulation should be maintained within a therapeutic range with heparin for an ECMO circuit, and coumadin for chronic anticoagulation with a VAD system.

Intermediate Support Phase

Once stabilized on circulatory support, emphasis shifts towards assessment of potential for recovery and a search for treatable causes of the acute decompensation. If a residual anatomic defect is detected by echocardiography or cardiac catheterization, then repair of the defect is imperative, otherwise successful weaning from mechanical circulatory support is very unlikely. The timing of repair depends in great part on the nature of the residual defect and the degree of recovery of contractile function. In the case where the residual defect impacts on systemic or coronary perfusion, such as with aortic regurgitation or obstructed coronary artery, then urgent repair of the defect must undertaken to prevent irreversible injury. If a residual defect is ruled out, or the cause of the decompensation is resolved, then assessment of contractile function can be done by weaning from support while monitoring function noninvasively with echocardiography. In most cases, children successfully weaned from mechanical support showed significant improvement in ventricular function within two to three days after initiation of support (28). Exceptions include patients with acute viral myocarditis where recovery can be delayed for several days but complete recovery is still possible.

If recovery of contractile function is not seen within a few days of initiation of support, then evaluation for transplantation should be undertaken. At this stage, if the child is deemed a transplant candidate, then circulatory support should be continued and closely monitored to maintain the patient as a good candidate for transplantation. This implies that mechanical circulatory support may be required for days to weeks while awaiting availability of an organ, and emphasis must now be placed on maintaining end-organ function and avoiding infection as these can affect eligibility for a transplant. Efforts at weaning from support must therefore be discontinued unless there is strong evidence for recovery, since further organ injury can occur during unsuccessful attempts at discontinuing circulatory support. In adolescents who are candidates for a VAD, the decision to list for transplantation should go hand in hand with the decision to convert to chronic support with a VAD. There are significant advantages of a VAD system over and ECMO circuit for long-term support including less bleeding complications, need for blood products and platelets, lower risk of infection, and the potential for permitting physical rehabilitation while on circulatory support. The latter is most evident in adolescents who are able to return to near normal activity thus regaining muscle strength and improved nutritional status. Due to the current lack of available assist devices appropriate for young children and infants in North America, these benefits cannot be realized in the youngest patients. Ventricular support with a conventional centrifugal pump does not permit patient mobility due to the type of cannulas available, tubing connections required, and the size of the devices available with respect to the patient size. Therefore, one of the major advantages of a VAD system cannot be readily realized with currently available centrifugal pumps either.

Meticulous antiseptic technique must be maintained during ECMO support to prevent nosocomial infections. Routine use of broad-spectrum antibiotic prophylaxis is to be discouraged since resistant organisms are likely to arise, particularly as the period of support is prolonged. Usually narrow spectrum prophylactic coverage for gram-positive bacteria is indicated at least the first few days of circulatory support. Cephalosporins are the most commonly used antibiotics for this purpose, although some centers prefer a combination of ampicillin or vancomycin and gentamycin, particularly in infants less than 1 month of age. Antibiotic prophylaxis is usually discontinued after three to five days of support and antibiotic use thereafter should be reserved for suspected infections with fever and leukocytosis.

Nutritional support must also be maintained during this period of support and is usually achieved via a parenteral route. Enteral feeding should be avoided if the circulatory support system is an ECMO type circuit since there is a significant risk of inducing necrotizing enterocolitis with enteral feeding particularly in infants. The need for adequate calories must be balanced against efforts to maintain fluid balance and prevent third space fluid accumulation. If renal function is adequate, then achieving this balance is not difficult and adequate calorie intake can be maintained even while correcting fluid overload. In cases where renal function is marginal, ultrafiltration or peritoneal dialysis should be considered.

In adolescents who receive circulatory support with a VAD, management during this intermediate phase has, as one of its goals, return of the patient to as close to normal activity as possible. Once stabilized on VAD support, muscle relaxant drugs should be discontinued and sedation weaned to promote return of motor function. Enteral nutrition should be started as soon as gastrointestinal motility returns, and parenteral nutrition discontinued to decrease the risk of intravenous line infection. Prophylactic antibiotics are managed much the same as in children on ECMO support and should be discontinued after the first few days of support. Specific antibiotic therapy for suspected infections should be guided by the likely source of infection and once an organism is identified, antibiotic coverage should be targeted to that organism. During the intermediate phase, anticoagulation is usually maintained with coumadin and close monitoring of the level of anticoagulation is maintained.

Neurologic complications: Although most complications resulting in transient organ dysfunction can be well managed during circulatory support and usually do not have more than a transient impact on the patient's eligibility for transplantation, neurologic complications often result in irreversible injury and ultimately impact transplant status. The most common complication is a thromboembolic event and multiple areas of infarction are usually detected when cerebral perfusion is evaluated. Intra-ventricular or intra-cerebral bleeding can occur, although much less common, and usually are seen in neonates or very young infants.

Weaning Phase of Support

If ventricular function recovers, then weaning from support should be initiated. Echocardiography is indispensable in this phase to assess adequacy of recovery and to detect residual or new intracardiac defects that may affect weaning. In most cases, adequate ejection is easily detected by observing the degree of pulsatility in the arterial pressure tracing. If atrial pressure lines are in place, this facilitates weaning. In cases where intracardiac lines are not available, central venous pressure can be used as a substitute although these are not ideal particularly in cases where left ventricular dysfunction is the main pathology. Consideration should be given to inserting intracardiac lines especially if weaning is difficult. In children supported with ECLS where biventricular support is achieved, assessment of pulmonary function prior to weaning is also necessary. With ECLS, weaning is usually done by gradually decreasing flow, monitoring end-organ perfusion and function as well as cardiac contractile function by echocardiography. Gradual weaning over several days may be required in cases where recovery has been slow, such as with viral myocarditis, or where ventricular "retraining" is required. During this time, anticoagulation must be carefully monitored and maintained at relatively high levels (ACT of 220–240 sec) since the risk of thrombus formation in the circuit is higher during periods of low flow. The child should be sedated and muscle relaxant drugs used to facilitate evaluation of perfusion and pulmonary function. Once flow is discontinued for one or two hours, if the child is deemed stable, decannulation is performed, repairing peripheral vessels such as the common carotid if the period of support has lasted less than 7–10 days.

A similar protocol is followed for weaning from a VAD, although this is less common an occurrence since the indications for a VAD are for chronic support as a bridge to transplant. In the case where recovery of ventricular function occurs, then weaning from support can proceed. Evaluation of ventricular function should be performed noninvasively with echocardiography, and as with ECMO support in younger children, intracardiac pressures should be monitored. The method of weaning depends on the type of device used for support. In children on a centrifugal pump, gradual decrease in pump flow, as determined by a flow meter, is done monitoring end-organ perfusion and function. A period of clamping of the circuit is also done, similar to weaning from ECMO, prior to decannulation. With adolescents on a pulsatile assist device, weaning is done by decreasing the number of cycles per minute of the device, synchronizing the pump cycles with the native heart. In most pulsatile assist devices, there is an option to decrease the stroke volume by partial compression of the bladder. Due to the risk of thrombus formation, anticoagulation is increased during weaning from a VAD, and the patient should be converted to heparin. Unlike an ECMO or centrifugal pump system, a VAD system cannot be "clamped" therefore careful assessment of ventricular function must be done prior to deciding to remove the device and the period of weaning is usually longer. Due to the chronic nature of support and design of the cannulas, removal of an assist device is a procedure of significant magnitude, requiring the use of cardiopulmonary bypass for removal of the cannulas from the cardiac structures.

RESULTS WITH VAD SYSTEMS

The results with VADs in adult patients have significantly improved over the last decade with new designs having improved outcome with respect to survival and complication rate. A variety of total artificial heart (TAH) systems are now available for severe biventricular failure. Systems such as the CardioWest TAH (CardioWest Laboratories, Tucson, AZ, U.S.A.) which is currently the only FDA approved device have proven to be very successful with over 60% of the patients surviving to heart transplantation and over 90% of these surviving to hospital discharge (29). Other TAH systems including the Penn State Heart and the Berlin Heart have been developed but are not currently available worldwide. Clinical trials are currently underway to evaluate a new TAH device, the AbioCor implantable replacement heart (ABIOMED Inc, Danvers, MA, U.S.A.). This electrohydraulically actuated device is designed as a permanent heart replacement and utilizes the new transcutaneous energy transfer technology as opposed to other TAH devices which use percutaneous cables in order to provide energy and device control.

Unlike the total artificial heart systems, VADs were developed for single chamber support, with a second device being added in cases of right ventricular dysfunction. The main advantage of the VAD system over a TAH is its versatility. Since a cardiectomy is unnecessary, they can be used as a bridge to recovery in addition to the usual indication of bridge to transplantation. For these reasons, VADs have gained much wider use than TAH systems. There are a number of devices available for clinical use and even more under development. The Thoratec VAD (Thoratec Laboratories Corp., Pleasanton, CA, U.S.A.) is a paracorporeal pulsatile device that can be used for short- as well as medium-term support. About 1700 patients worldwide have had this device implanted with approximately 60% survival to hospital discharge. The importance of the Thoratec system is that it can be implanted in smaller patients. The HeartMate LVAD (Thoratec Laboratories Corp., Pleasanton, CA, U.S.A.) is an intracorporeal pulsatile device designed for long-term left ventricular support as a bridge to heart transplant, and was recently approved for permanent support in the United States. The recently completed REMATCH trial demonstrated some superiority of this device in end-stage heart failure patients compared to medical therapy alone (30). The 2-year survival, however, was only 26% in the HeartMate group compared to 8% in the medically treated group, underscoring the need to have transplantation as the main indication for VAD use. Another device available is the Novacor LVAS (WorldHeart Corporation, Ottawa, Canada) which is also undergoing evaluation as destination therapy (INTREPID trial). The Novacor LVAS is considered to be the most reliable system on the market and some patients have been supported with this device for more than 4 years. New devices that are implantable and use transcutaneous energy transduction are currently in clinical trials including the Arrow LionHeart, which potentially could decrease the risk of infections.

Because of the relatively high complication rate with pulsatile devices including thromboembolic events, infection, and the lack of clinical evidence that pulsatility affords significant benefit, there has been a growing interest in the use of non-pulsatile devices for short- and long-term support (31). Although there are several advantages of these devices over pulsatile systems, and they have been proposed as the "next generation" of implantable systems, for pediatric use the most relevant advantage is their small size. Clinically available systems include axial flow pumps (DeBakey MicroMed, Jarvik 2000, Heart Mate II, Incor Berlin Heart) and centrifugal pumps (HeartMate III, CorAide, Medquest, Kriton). The devices that are currently undergoing clinical evaluation are axial flow devices including the MicroMed DeBakey pump (MicroMed Technology, Houston, TX, U.S.A.) and the Jarvik 2000 (Jarvik Heart Inc, New York, New York, U.S.A.). Initial reports have indicated a relatively high hemolysis rate, and some instances of device failure. However, the 30-day survival in the study group is approaching 80% (32,33). The Jarvik 2000 pump has had less clinical use compared to the MicroMed device but has been implanted for longer periods of up to 1 year. Currently, there is an NIH sponsored development effort to design and perform clinical testing of new pediatric devices with most of the proposed systems utilizing the axial flow design.

Experience with VAD systems in children is much more limited with most of the implants in North America being centrifugal pump systems, and a few reports describing results with pulsatile systems such as the Thoratec device and the HeartMate system in adolescents (18,34). Reports describing the results with pulsatile systems specifically designed for pediatric use have come from Europe and the experience with these systems has been similar to slightly worse than with adults supported with pulsatile pumps. A relatively high rate of thromboembolic complications has been described for both the MEDOS HIA (MEDOS Medizintechnik AG, Stolberg, Germany) and the Berlin Heart (Berlin Heart AG, Berlin, Germany) VADs. In the bridge to transplant experience, over two-thirds of the patient survived to transplantation, but of those, only half survived to hospital discharge for an overall survival of 36% (35). Similar results were seen with the patients that were bridged to recovery.

FUTURE DIRECTIONS

Advances in assist device technology have evolved in two directions. Although the goal has always been to develop a small, totally implantable device, pumps available and being developed are of two types: pulsatile devices which require a bladder reservoir, inlet and outflow valves, as well as cannulas; and continuous flow pumps that depend on centrifugal forces to move blood. The latter have the advantage of not requiring valves to maintain forward flow, have fewer moving parts, require much less energy, and can be miniaturized for use in pediatric patients. Both types of pumps have been developed for pediatric use and there is a sufficient experience with both systems to make conclusions regarding the most appropriate system for children.

The pulsatile systems that have been developed for children have the advantage of providing true pulsatility but the drawbacks include availability of only paracorporeal systems with no totally implantable device either available or in development. Furthermore, the relatively high incidence of thrombosis and thromboembolic complications seen with current systems raises concerns that these types of devices for pediatric use will always be more prone to this complication. Thus simply scaling the pump down to the size required for infants and children may be too simplistic an approach.

The main drawback of the centrifugal pumps, however, is the potential for greater damage to red cells. This is related to the high rate of rotation in these pumps, particularly the axial flow systems that rotate at over 10,000 rpm as compared to 2000 to 4000 for centrifugal pumps. Rotor and blade design in the case of the axial flow pump is critical, as is the clearance between impeller or turbine and the pump housing. With advances in computer simulation, improvements in turbine and blade design may overcome the problem of hemolysis seen in continuous flow pumps.

Reliability is also a concern with current rotary pump systems. The limiting factor seems to be the bearings, which must perform under high rotor speed conditions and can generate significant heat, further accelerating wear, and potentially leading to pump failure. Current clinically available systems use blood or blood components to lubricate the bearings, but this in turn can lead to platelet activation, thrombus generation, and a higher risk of infection. "Third generation" rotary pump systems use a magnetically suspended rotor that avoids the problems with bearings. These devices, such as the Heart Mate III, are under development with preclinical evaluation going on now. If these studies confirm the lower thromboembolic rate predicted, clinical trials will likely follow in short order.

Another limitation of centrifugal pumps is the lack of feedback control with inability to adapt to the body's needs and interacting ventricular contraction. Flow through the pump is affected by the pressure difference between the inflow and outflow and control algorithms to compensate for this effect are not available yet. Also avoidance of negative pressure at the inflow side is important, particularly when running at high flows with an empty ventricle and pulseless flow. This problem requires frequent manual adjustments, which obviates some of the advantages of an implantable system. Thus reliable control mechanisms based on electric motor sensors and specific algorithms need to be developed. Finally, a mechanism needs to be incorporated to prevent backflow in case of pump failure.

In parallel with advances in centrifugal pumps, smaller pulsatile pumps are now being designed with new biomaterials and components aimed at minimizing the risk of infection and thrombus formation, which are important limitations of current systems (12). Given that reliability and the ability to adapt to the patient' physiologic needs are some of the strengths of pulsatile pumps, research on new generation pulsatile systems, particularly systems designed for pediatric use, should continue.

REFERENCES

1. Black MD, Coles JG, Williams WG, et al. Determinants of success in pediatric cardiac patients undergoing extracorporeal membrane oxygenation. Ann Thorac Surg 1995; 60(1):133–138.
2. Kulik TJ, Moler FW, Palmisano JM, et al. Outcome-associated factors in pediatric patients treated with extracorporeal membrane oxygenator after cardiac surgery. Circulation 1996; 94 (9 suppl):II63–68.
3. Morris MC, Ittenbach RF, Godinez RI, et al. Risk factors for mortality in 137 pediatric cardiac intensive care unit patients managed with

extracorporeal membrane oxygenation. Crit Care Med 2004; 32(4): 1061–1069.

4. Williams MR, Oz MC. Indications and patient selection for mechanical ventricular assistance. Ann Thorac Surg 2001; 71(3 suppl):S86–S91. Discussion S114–S115.

5. del Nido PJ. Extracorporeal membrane oxygenation for cardiac support in children. Ann Thorac Surg 1996; 61(1):336–339. Discussion 40–41.

6. Duncan BW, Hraska V, Jonas RA, et al. Mechanical circulatory support in children with cardiac disease. J Thorac Cardiovasc Surg 1999; 117(3):529–542.

7. Duncan BW. Mechanical circulatory support for infants and children with cardiac disease. Ann Thorac Surg 2002; 73(5):1670–1677.

8. Karl TR, Horton SB, Mee RB. Left heart assist for ischemic postoperative ventricular dysfunction in an infant with anomalous left coronary artery. J Card Surg 1989; 4(4):352–354.

9. Thuys CA, Mullaly RJ, Horton SB, et al. Centrifugal ventricular assist in children under 6 kg. Eur J Cardiothorac Surg 1998; 13(2): 130–134.

10. Hetzer R, Loebe M, Potapov EV, et al. Circulatory support with pneumatic paracorporeal ventricular assist device in infants and children. Ann Thorac Surg 1998; 66(5):1498–1506.

11. Konertz W, Hotz H, Schneider M, Redlin M, Reul H. Clinical experience with the MEDOS HIA-VAD system in infants and children: a preliminary report. Ann Thorac Surg 1997; 63(4):1138–1144.

12. Asfour B, Weyand M, Kececioglu D, et al. A novel paracorporeal mechanical assist device for newborns and infants allows bridging to transplantation. Transplant Proc 1997; 29(8):3330–3332.

13. Hetzer R, Muller J, Weng Y, Wallukat G, Spiegelsberger S, Loebe M. Cardiac recovery in dilated cardiomyopathy by unloading with a left ventricular assist device. Ann Thorac Surg 1999; 68(2):742–749.

14. Chang AC, Hanley FL, Weindling SN, Wernovsky G, Wessel DL. Left heart support with a ventricular assist device in an infant with acute myocarditis. Crit Care Med 1992; 20(5):712–715.

15. del Nido PJ, Duncan BW, Mayer JE Jr, Wessel DL, LaPierre RA, Jonas RA. Left ventricular assist device improves survival in children with left ventricular dysfunction after repair of anomalous origin of the left coronary artery from the pulmonary artery. Ann Thorac Surg 1999; 67(1):169–172.

16. Mee RB, Harada Y. Retraining of the left ventricle with a left ventricular assist device (Bio-Medicus) after the arterial switch operation. J Thorac Cardiovasc Surg 1999; 101(1):171–173.

17. Aharon AS, Drinkwater DC Jr, Churchwell KB, et al. Extracorporeal membrane oxygenation in children after repair of congenital cardiac lesions. Ann Thorac Surg 2001; 72(6):2095–2101. Discussion 101–102.

18. Helman DN, Addonizio LJ, Morales DL, et al. Implantable left ventricular assist devices can successfully bridge adolescent patients to transplant. J Heart Lung Transplant 2000; 19(2):121–126.

19. del Nido PJ, Dalton HJ, Thompson AE, Siewers RD. Extracorporeal membrane oxygenator rescue in children during cardiac arrest after cardiac surgery. Circulation 1992; 86(suppI):II300–304.

20. Duncan BW, Ibrahim AE, Hraska V, et al. Use of rapid-deployment extracorporeal membrane oxygenation for the resuscitation of pediatric patients with heart disease after cardiac arrest. J Thorac Cardiovasc Surg 1998; 116(2):305–311.

21. Jacobs JP, Ojito JW, McConaghey TW, et al. Rapid cardiopulmonary support for children with complex congenital heart disease. Ann Thorac Surg 2000; 70(3):742–749. Discussion 9–50.

22. Booth KL, Roth SJ, Perry SB, del Nido PJ, Wessel DL, Laussen PC. Cardiac catheterization of patients supported by extracorporeal membrane oxygenation. J Am Coll Cardiol 2002; 40(9):1681–1686.

23. Fenton KN, Webber SA, Damford PA, et al. Long-term survival after pediatric cardiac transplantation and post-operative ECMO support. Ann Thorac Surg. 2003; 76:843–847.

24. Swartz MT, Lowdermilk GA, McBride LR. Refractory ventricular tachycardia as an indication for ventricular assist device support. J Thorac Cardiovasc Surg 1999; 118(6):1119–1120.

25. del Nido PJ, Armitage JM, Fricker FJ, et al. Extracorporeal membrae oxygenation support as a bridge to pediatric heart transplantation. Circulation 1994; 90(5 Pt 2):II66–69.

26. Gajarski RJ, Mosca RS, Ohye RG, et al. Use of extracorporeal life support as a bridge to pediatric cardiac transplantation. J Heart Lung Transplant 2003; 22(1):28–34.

27. Seib PM, Faulkner SC, Erickson CC, et al. Blade and balloon atrial septostomy for left heart decompression in patients with severe ventricular dysfunction on extracorporeal membrane oxygenation. Catheter Cardiovasc Interv 1999; 46(2):179–186.

28. Ibrahim AE, Duncan BW, Blume ED, Jonas RA. Long-term follow-up of pediatric cardiac patients requiring mechanical circulatory support. Ann Thorac Surg 2000; 69(1):186–192.

29. Copeland JG III, Arabia FA, Banchy ME, et al. The CardioWest total artificial heart bridge to transplantation: 1993 to 1996 national trial. Ann Thorac Surg 1998; 66(5):1662–1669.

30. Rose EA, Gelijns AC, Moskowitz AJ, et al. Long-term mechanical left ventricular assistance for end-stage heart failure. N Engl J Med 2001; 345(20):1435–1443.

31. Mesana TG. Rotary blood pumps for cardiac assistance: a "must"? Artif Organs 2004; 28(2):218–225.

32. Noon GP, Morley DL, Irwin S, Abdelsayed SV, Benkowski RJ, Lynch BE. Clinical experience with the MicroMed DeBakey ventricular

assist device. Ann Thorac Surg 2001; 71(3 suppl):S133–S138. Discussion S44–S46.
33. Grinda JM, Latremouille CH, Chevalier P, et al. Bridge to transplantation with the DeBakey VAD axial pump: a single center report. Eur J Cardiothorac Surg 2002; 22(6):965–970.
34. Ashton RC Jr, Oz MC, Michler RE, et al. Left ventricular assist device options in pediatric patients. Asaio J 1995; 41(3):M277–M280.
35. Ishino K, Loebe M, Uhlemann F, Weng Y, Hennig E, Hetzer R. Circulatory support with paracorporeal pneumatic ventricular assist device (VAD) in infants and children. Eur J Cardiothorac Surg 1997; 11(5): 965–972.

22

Psychosocial Aspects of Acute and Chronic Heart Failure in Children

KATHY MUSSATTO

Herma Heart Center,
Children's Hospital and Health System,
Milwaukee, Wisconsin, U.S.A.

Out of clutter, find simplicity. From discord, find harmony. In the middle of difficulty lies opportunity.

Albert Einstein

The impact of illness in a child extends far beyond the affected organ itself. When the illness is potentially life threatening, as in acute or chronic heart failure, there are important psychosocial implications for both the child and family. Dramatic improvements in survival for children with complex congenital heart disease (CHD) and success with new modes of congestive heart failure (CHF) management mean that greater numbers of children are living with heart failure

833

(1). These tremendous accomplishments, although bringing hope to many that previously would not have survived their illness, have created a new set of challenges for children who receive care for CHF and their families. As health care providers it has become increasingly important that we acknowledge and explore not only the medical aspects of the illnesses our patients are facing but also the short and long-term psychosocial implications.

Children diagnosed with a significant illness like CHF may experience challenges in multiple areas of their lives. Health-related quality of life (HRQL), neurocognitive, psychological and behavioral functioning, and relationships with family and friends may all be affected. In addition, when illness occurs in a dependent child, the impact on the family must not be underestimated. The family will experience several sources of stress associated with caring for a child with CHF that may include financial impacts, changes in familial and social networks, personal strain (e.g., fatigue, day-to-day practical limitations), and effects on siblings. There is also potential that mastery of the illness and its associated demands may provide positive benefits to a family, e.g., bringing family members closer together or establishing a deeper sense of faith (2).

Several factors will influence how the affected child and his or her family experience the psychosocial impact of acute or chronic CHF. Aspects of the child, the family, and the community work together to help the child and family bring meaning to their experience. Child-related factors include the developmental stage of the child, his or her baseline temperament and personality, the degree of limitations imposed by the illness, and the disease management trajectory, i.e., medical management vs. transplant. Family variables of importance include the developmental stage of the family, family configuration, previous experience with stress, communication patterns and coping skills utilized, as well as socioeconomic resources, religious and cultural background. All families also rely on community and social resources for some degree of support. The availability of both formal and informal support networks, child-care assistance, access to care for children with special needs, and respite care may play a role in how a child and family adapt to living with CHF. Finally, the health care systems, school systems, and legal and political systems with which a family must contend affect the ability to adjust to serious illness (3) (Fig. 1).

Society as a whole also bears a significant responsibility as increasing numbers of children survive with complex medical issues. The American Heart Association currently estimates that over 1,000,000 Americans are living with CHD and approximately 40,000 new infants will be affected each year (4). It is well recognized that many children living with

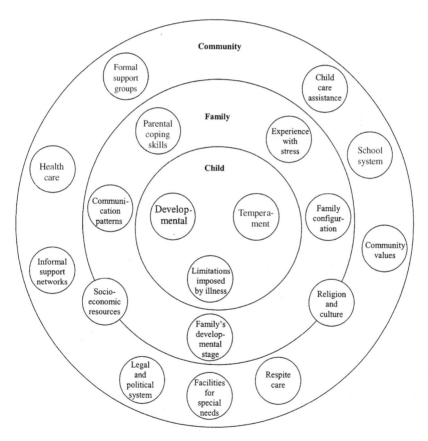

Figure 1 Factors affecting family and child adjustment to chronic illness. (From Ref. 3.)

palliated defects and even some with anatomically corrected problems remain at risk for the development of CHF during the course of their lives (5). Combined with the incidence of acquired heart diseases such as cardiomyopathies and myocarditis, this places a large population at risk for the development of CHF. Heart disease consumes a larger portion of health care resources than any other illness entity in the United States (4). The societal burden of CHF in children is not only represented in health care dollars spent, however; there are other impacts such as lost productivity from parents who leave the workforce to care for an ill child, resources needed to provide special therapies, i.e., physical therapy, occupational therapy, or special education services and the long-term issues of insurance and employment in children surviving with CHF.

MEASUREMENT ISSUES

Many studies have explored the psychosocial implications of CHF in adult populations, however research in pediatric populations has been limited. Recently, increased attention has been directed to this area; however, further investigation is certainly warranted. Several pitfalls are inherent to research involving psychosocial variables. One principal problem is that many psychosocial variables are decidedly subjective in nature and difficult to quantify. They are measured from the patient's perspective and unlike objective measures such as cardiac function, we are forced to directly ask the subject how they feel about a particular aspect of their life and/or treatment and take their response as true. As researchers, we must put aside our own internal value judgments and interpretation of the subject's situation and accept that only the person living the experience can truly tell us what it is like. Consistently, it has been found that clinical severity of disease does not correlate well with the patient's subjective interpretation of the overall impact on quality of life (6,7). In fact, the perception of the illness (8) and psychosocial issues such as effects on relationships with peers and activity restrictions have been found to be more predictive of subjective health status than medical variables (9). Other studies have found that health professionals identify different issues of importance (10) and rate quality of life for given health states lower than subjects and parents (11). Therefore, it is increasingly important that we ask not just how *we* think these subjects are doing but how *they* think they are doing.

Although we are not able to clinically validate how satisfied someone may be with their life situation, a growing number of instruments have evolved that are designed to measure these sorts of psychosocial variables. Arising initially from work in adult populations, instruments are now available to assess HRQL, psychological and behavioral functioning, and the impact of chronic illness on a family system in pediatric samples. It is important to remember that psychosocial outcomes are not static. As children and their families' progress through normal developmental stages, their perception of the impact of a disease is likely to evolve.

HEALTH-RELATED QUALITY OF LIFE

Health-related quality of life has been defined as "a person's perception of the impact of a disease and its treatment functioning in a variety of dimensions, including physical, psychological, and social domains" (12). As focus has shifted to morbidity and long-term outcomes in children with heart disease, HRQL has received increased attention as a measure potentially useful in evaluating treatment effectiveness and burden, differences between diagnostic groups, and changes in status over time. Unfortunately, inconsistency in definitions and variations in instruments designed to measure the concept of HRQL have produced studies with sometimes contradictory findings and a lack of broad generalizability (13). Developmental considerations and concerns regarding the accuracy and acceptability of caregiver-proxy ratings of HRQL in young children further complicate the assessment of a child's HRQL (14). In general, it is agreed that HRQL represents one subset of global quality of life and that it is primarily subjective in nature. Several generic instruments designed to measure HRQL in pediatric samples are available. They offer the benefit of a broad assessment of HRQL and allow comparison with the general population. Disease-specific instruments are designed to measure HRQL with a specific focus on areas of concern that may be unique to a given disease, e.g., exercise tolerance in CHF (15). A combination of both generic and disease-specific measures likely offers the most comprehensive assessment of HRQL. A few instruments specifically designed to measure HRQL in subjects with heart failure have evolved (16–18), however, these have not been adapted for use in pediatric samples. Recently, a disease-specific measure for children with heart disease has become available (19) and others are in development (10,20). To be acceptable, instruments designed to measure HRQL should possess adequate reliability, validity, and responsiveness (21).

In adult samples of subjects with CHF, quality of life has been found to be significantly affected in several dimensions including psychologic distress, activity limitations, and altered social interactions with both family and friends (22). Others have found that poor HRQL is associated with higher rates of mortality and rehospitalization in CHF patients (23,24). NYHA functional class and physical activity level have been found to be closely correlated with HRQL scores (25–27), however clinical measures of disease severity, i.e., ejection fraction are not reliable predictors of HRQL (22,28,29). Health-related quality of life has been included as a secondary end point in many clinical trials evaluating various pharmacologic CHF management strategies. While β-blockers have demonstrated consistent efficacy in reducing mortality and hospitalizations for patients with CHF, their impact on HRQL has been inconsistent (30). Improved function may be outweighed by clinically significant side effects of the medications. Recent trials reporting results of biventricular pacing for CHF have demonstrated improvements in functional class, exercise capacity, and overall well being of subjects (31). In a comparison of CHF patients treated with transplantation vs. medical management, Walden et al.

(32,33) found that both groups demonstrated adjustment problems and that HRQL was not significantly different between groups.

Health-related quality of life has also become more common as an outcome measure in samples of children with congenital and acquired heart disease. Although degree of CHF is not typically included as a variable, these studies represent children from a wide variety of diagnostic backgrounds many of whom have symptomatic heart disease requiring long-term surgical and/or medical intervention. These reports shed light on the burden of pediatric heart disease in relation to its impact on HRQL.

We recently reported results from a survey on functional status and HRQL in a sample of subjects that had undergone surgical treatment of CHD (34). Fifty-one subjects ages 8–27 years and 81 parents of children ages 2–18 years completed interviews. All subjects had anatomy that was amenable to a two-ventricle repair and each had required replacement of an absent or abnormal valve. The 100 subjects represented had undergone a total of 271 cardiac surgical procedures including previous palliative and corrective operations. The Health Utilities Index Mark 2 (HUI-2) (35) was used to categorize functional status. Age-appropriate measures including the Short-Form 36 (SF-36) (36) and both the parent and child reports of the Pediatric Quality of Life Inventory (PedsQL) (37) were employed to quantify HRQL. The reports from the CHD subjects themselves did not differ significantly from the reports of healthy individuals provided by the instrument's normative samples on any of the domains assessed including overall, physical, emotional, social, and school functioning (Fig. 2). Parents reported a more negative impact on HRQL with scores on overall ($p < 0.01$), physical ($p < 0.01$), social ($p < 0.001$), and school (p < 0.01) functioning falling significantly lower than those of the healthy reference group (Fig. 3). These results provide testimony to the incredible resilience of children living with a chronic illness. It appears that their perception of "normal" is reset to their individual life experience. Parents, on the other hand, may not be able

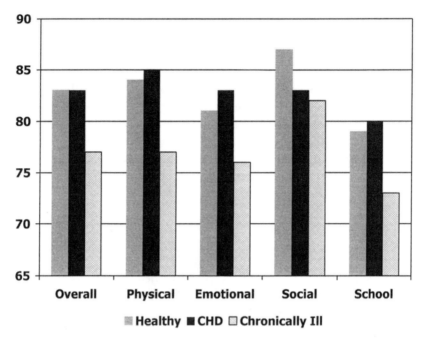

Figure 2 PedsQL child report results. $n = 32$; ages 8–18 years. Child self-report of HRQL: no statistically significant differences between CHD and healthy samples.

to completely separate from their wishes of what they had hoped their child to be, thereby reflecting lower quality of life reports.

Subjects reporting poorer HRQL also identified significantly greater levels of disability on the HUI-2 functional categories including deficits in mobility, cognition, sensation, self-care, and emotional functioning. For all respondents, HRQL reports did not vary by the subject's primary cardiac diagnosis, the age or sex of the respondent, or the elapsed time from the subject's last cardiac operation. Socioeconomic status (SES) demonstrated minimal relationships to any of the domains assessed. Several subjects had implanted valves in place at the time of the interview that met echocardiographic criteria for dysfunction. "Dysfunction" was defined as valves with moderate or greater regurgitation or a steno-

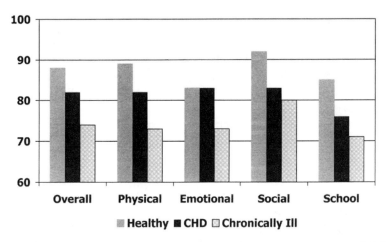

Figure 3 PedsQL parent report results. $n = 81$ parents of children aged 2–18 years. Parents reported HRQL scores that were significantly lower than those of healthy controls for overall, physical, social, and school functioning ($p < 0.05$). Scores for emotional functioning were not different from those of the healthy controls. Scores were similar to those of children with other chronic illnesses for social and school functioning but higher than those of the chronically ill group for overall, physical, and emotional functioning ($p < 0.05$).

tic gradient of 40 mmHg or greater. These were subjects experiencing some degree of CHF with an expected need for surgical intervention in their future. In these subjects, emotional functioning was reported as significantly lower on parent reports ($p < 0.01$) and there was a trend toward lower scores for school functioning ($p = 0.07$) on the child reports. Also of interest, we found that children who had undergone more than one cardiac operation reported lower HRQL scores for overall, physical, and social function than those who had only a single procedure. This suggests a cumulative impact of repeated interventions.

Other studies have reported similar results with findings indicating quality of life in subjects with CHD similar to healthy controls (38,39) suggesting effective normalization and use of healthy coping mechanisms in the populations surveyed. Uzark has done extensive work in the area of HRQL assessment in children with heart disease. She has concluded that HRQL reports are independent of disease severity and are perceived differently by parents vs. children (40). Using a disease-specific measure, the New York University Children's Heart Health Survey, Connolly et al. (20) found that parents reported their children to have psychological well-being similar to healthy controls but to experience more symptom-related distress ($p = 0.001$), be less able to fulfill their role functions ($p < 0.001$), and to utilize more healthcare resources ($p=0.001$). In contrast, the adolescents surveyed did not perceive themselves to differ from their healthy counterparts on any of the instrument's subscales per self-report. In this study, degree of heart failure was quantified using the NYU Pediatric Heart Failure Index (PHFI) (41). The authors found no significant correlation between PHFI scores and psychological function but lower heart failure scores did correlate with better role function ($p = 0.001$), less healthcare utilization ($p = 0.001$), and less symptom-related distress ($p < 0.05$). In a recent report by Kendall et al. (9), 66% of adolescents with CHD considered themselves "the same" as, or only very slightly "different" from, their peers. Reports of adults with CHD have identified poorer physical functioning and lower overall general health perception than the general population (6,42). However, in one study, adult (17–49 years) survivors with single ventricle heart disease reported HRQL similar to the healthy population with higher education correlating with improved scores (43).

In one of the only studies specifically targeting psychosocial outcomes in children with hypoplastic left heart syndrome (HLHS), a group known to be at risk for CHF, Williams et al. (44) sampled a cross-sectional cohort of children in various stages of surgical palliation. They found that after stage I repair, parents reported quality of life similar to a healthy reference population despite significant developmental delays. After stage II, scores were significantly worse in the areas of physical ability, growth and development, pain, temperament, general health perception, and parental impact. Eight subjects with a mean age of 3.8 years had completed stage III palliation and responded to the Infant/Toddler version of the Child Health Questionnaire (CHQ). In this group, parents reported HRQL scores similar to the reference sample falling significantly lower on only the general health perception scale. In contrast, a slightly older sample s/p stage III (mean age 7.3 years) reported lower scores on the following subscales of the CHQ: role/social limitations due to emotional or behavioral difficulty; behavior; self-esteem; global health; parental impact—emotional; family activities; and psychosocial summary score. Interestingly, scores reported by this group were not different from the healthy reference sample in the areas of physical function; role/social limitations due to physical health; bodily pain; mental health; parental impact—time; family cohesion or the physical summary score. This important study, although involving a relatively small sample, emphasizes the importance of evaluating multiple aspects of HRQL. It also points out that what subjects or their parents report as troubling may not make sense clinically and that the perceived impact of heart disease on HRQL changes with the developmental stage of the child and family.

No study reported to date in the pediatric population has assessed HRQL on a longitudinal basis nor has HRQL yet been used as an outcome measure for comparing different treatment strategies. It is important to distinguish the effect of different treatment options on improving quantity of life vs. quality of life. For example, particularly in active children, the negative side effects of β-blocker therapy for CHF, e.g., dizziness and lethargy, may lead to a reduction in HRQL as reported from the subject's perspective regardless of a clinical improvement in cardiac function (30). Despite the limited information on the impact of CHF on quality of life in children, the reports highlighted here imply that children are able to incorporate the challenges of their disease and to live with a satisfying quality of life. However, the sometimes contradictory findings, differing perceptions of parents, and lack of a unified measurement strategy emphasize the need for ongoing assessment of HRQL in this population.

NEUROCOGNITIVE IMPACT

In adults with CHF, generalized cognitive impairment particularly in the area of memory and attention deficits has been
reported (45,46), however the confounding effects of widespread cerebrovascular disease and coexisting psychological
distress or depression are difficult to adequately control (47).
Congestive heart failure in children, both acute and chronic,
may also pose risks to normal neurological and cognitive
development. Altered cerebral blood flow, hormonal changes,
and reduced physical activity secondary to CHF may impact a
child's brain growth and developmental achievement (5).
Children with chronic CHF beginning in infancy are likely
to be at greatest risk of impairment.

The implications of heart disease in children on neurocognitive development have long been an important concern. It is recognized that children with significant heart
disease are exposed to multiple layers of risk including preoperative insults and comorbidities such as congenital brain
abnormalities or syndromes; operative variables such as
cardiopulmonary bypass (CPB) techniques; postoperative
physiologic vulnerability and low cardiac output; and the
potentially cumulative effects of long-term medication use,
multiple hospitalizations, altered growth, and the impact
of palliated anatomy (48,51). Several studies have identified
that neurological abnormalities and cognitive delays,
although typically not severe in nature, are relatively common (48–53). Infants with complex CHD have been found
to have a significant incidence of congenital brain abnormalities (54), genetic aberrations (55), and an incidence of
preoperative neurologic abnormalities greater than 50%
(56). Compared with healthy normative samples, studies
have identified lower IQ scores, microcephaly, gross and
fine motor delays, speech and language deficits, reduced
visual–motor integration and higher-level processing skills,
increased use of special education services, and neurologic
abnormalities such as hypotonia and attention deficits in
a variety of samples of children with heart disease
(49,53,57–66).

The Boston Circulatory Arrest Study Group, studying a cohort of patients with transposition of the great arteries (TGA) managed with either a predominantly low-flow CPB strategy vs. a technique employing deep hypothermic circulatory arrest (DHCA), has provided landmark data on neurocognitive outcomes with longitudinal assessments in over 150 subjects. In early reports, Bellinger et al. (67) identified higher prevalence of seizures and poorer motor function at 1 year of age and poorer expressive language development at 2.5 years of age (68) in children assigned to DHCA. By 4 years of age (53) delays in coordination and motor planning abilities particularly in oromotor function persisted in the group assigned to DHCA. Intellectual function and overall neurologic status were not significantly different between the two CPB strategies, however the group as a whole performed worse than normative samples on IQ, expressive language, visual–motor integration, motor function, and oromotor control. Most recently, neurodevelopmental assessments in the cohort at 8 years of age were reported (57,69). Scores for the cohort as a whole were lower than population norms on tests of memory, concept formation, visual–motor skills, and attention. Forty-three percent of the cohort was receiving special education services and over half had abnormalities on neurologic exam, most of which were mild in nature. A higher prevalence of motor and speech abnormalities persisted in the DHCA group. Perioperative seizures were found to be an independent risk factor for lower achievement and IQ. Although CHF is not a common finding either perioperatively or as a late complication since the adoption of the arterial switch procedure as the definitive treatment for TGA, these findings shed light on the neurologic sequelae of infant heart surgery and the importance of comprehensive, prospective neurocognitive assessment in populations considered at risk.

Those populations at greater risk for experiencing some degree of CHF such as survivors of single ventricle palliation (63,64), particularly HLHS (58,59,70–72) and cardiac transplantation (65,73–75), appear to be most susceptible to neurocognitive impairment. Neurocognitive outcomes in subjects with HLHS have received close attention because of the continued controversy over optimal management strategies, palliative surgery vs. transplant, and the relatively recent shift away from offering supportive care only. Studies of intellectual function in survivors of staged palliation of HLHS have reported mean IQ scores ranging from 86 to 94 (59,63,71,72). Interestingly, recent reports of subjects undergoing early cardiac transplantation for HLHS have reported similar findings with IQ scores ranging from 88 to 95 (58,75). Increased waiting time prior to transplant was found to have a negative impact on cognitive outcome (58). It appears that outcomes in this complex group may be significantly influenced by patient-related factors such as coexisting brain abnormalities, genetics, and socioeconomic class rather than by treatment regime alone. Ongoing assessment of this population will help to further clarify optimal treatment strategies and allow improved counseling and realistic expectations for new and existing families (48). Table 1 summarizes findings of studies exploring neurocognitive outcomes in survivors of some of the most complex forms of CHD and heart transplantation.

PSYCHOLOGICAL AND BEHAVIORAL FUNCTIONING

Closely related to both quality of life and neurodevelopment are psychological and behavioral functioning. Although few studies have explored these areas specific to CHF in children, the impact of CHF on psychologic and behavioral issues has received considerable attention in adults. Reports of higher than average symptoms of depression, anxiety, anger, social isolation, neuroticism, and altered coping have been reported (22,27,76). Self-reported symptoms of depression have been correlated with negative outcomes such as more frequent hospitalizations, recurrent cardiac events, and increased mortality from CHF (77–79). However, other important studies have found that neither depression nor anxiety were significantly associated with these outcomes (24,80). Unfortunately, symptoms of depression such as fatigue and insomnia are also common symptoms of CHF and may go undiagnosed in many patients. Anxiety would be expected in patients coping with a life-altering diagnosis of CHF; however, little research has been done regarding its contribution to long-term outcomes. A high level of concern or anxiety about taking part in physical activity has been shown to have a negative impact on rehabilitation efforts (81). The impact of anxiety on cardiac output must also be considered. The normal stress response causes an elevation of systemic vascular resistance raising the afterload on a failing ventricle. In extreme cases, stress has been linked to acute cardiopulmonary crisis (82). Social and emotional support as well as individual coping strategies are likely important mediators between the stress of CHF and resultant psychological outcomes. Lack of emotional support, particularly for women, was found to be significantly associated with adverse events in patients with CHF (80). In another study, unmarried patients had higher rates of rehospitalization and mortality (83). Coping strategies that resulted in disengagement and lack of acceptance also predicted higher mortality despite adjusting for disease severity, sex, and age (84).

The psychological and behavioral outcomes of children surviving CHD are also receiving increased attention. Many of these children, particularly those with palliated defects remain at risk for CHF (5). Psychiatric symptoms particularly internalizing disorders such as withdrawn behavior, depressed mood, increased somatic complaints, attention deficits, and higher total problem socres (38,85–89) have been demonstrated in children with poor cardiac function as well as poorer self-perception in CHD subjects prior to surgery (90). Generalized anxiety, feeling different from others, parental overprotectiveness, and greater medical fears (91,92) have also been found in subjects with CHD. Spurkland (93) compared adolescent subjects with severe CHD to those with repaired atrial septal defect and found higher rates of psychiatric disorders in the complex group. Level of function was significantly associated with both physical capabilities

Table 1 Neurocognitive Outcomes in Survivors of Complex Congenital Heart Disease

Study	Subjects	Dependent variables	Findings
Ref. 72	115 HLHS survivors born prior to 1992; mean age 9 ± 2 years	IQ, reading and math achievement, language skills, visual–motor integration, behavior (CBCL), general health status, activity limitations, school performance, medication use	Full scale IQ = 86/50–116[a] WJPB–Reading = 85/54–124[a] WJPB–Math = 87/47–132[a] Language = 74/52–117[a] VMI = 86/57–109[a] Behavior: 50% in normal range for all subsets Health status: 80% "excellent" or "good" Activity limitations: 51% "none" School performance (parental report): 83% "average" or "above average" Medication use: 64%
Ref. 58	26 HLHS survivors transplanted between 1993 and 1998; at assessment: 12 < 36 months, 14 > 36 months, range 1 year 11 months–6 years 7 months	BSID (subjects < 36 months), WPPSI-R and WISC-III (subjects > 36 months), VABS, CBCL	BSID-MDI = 88/ < 50–102[a] BSID-PDI = 87/50–113[a] Full scale IQ (mean ± SD) = 89 ± 13 Adaptive behavior (mean ± SD) = 89 ± 18 CBCL: mean scores within average range

Ref.	Sample	Measures	Results
Ref. 71	51 Fontan survivors with initial surgical palliation between December 1989 and February 1994, 26 HLHS, 25 non-HLHS; age 58 ± 5 months	WPPSI-R, WISC-III, VABS, CBCL	Full scale IQ (mean ± SD) 101 ± 5.4 (entire sample) 94 ± 7 (HLHS) 107 ± 7 (non-HLHS) Adaptive behavior (mean ± SD) 89 ± 4 (entire sample) 86 ± 7 (HLHS) 92 ± 6 (non-HLHS) CBCL: mean scores within average range (all groups)
Ref. 59	14 HLHS survivors with initial surgical palliation between 1990 and 1996; mean age 4.4 years	WPPSI-R, VABS, VMI PPVT	Full scale IQ = 88/46–93[a] Adaptive behavior (mean ± SD)= 91 ± 20 VMI (mean ± SD)= 82 ± 16 PPVT (mean ± SD)= 84 ± 12
Ref. 63	32 Fontan survivors (12.5% HLHS) with Fontan procedure performed betwee 1986 and 1994; age 6.3 ± 3.3 years, range 2–16 years	SBIS, VMI	Full scale IQ (mean ± SD) 98 ± 12 (entire sample) 88 (HLHS) VMI (mean ± SD)= 95 ± 15 School performance (parental report): 77% "average" or "above average"

(Continued)

Table 1 Neurocognitive Outcomes in Survivors of Complex Congenital Heart Disease (*Continued*)

Study	Subjects	Dependent variables	Findings
Ref. 64	133 Fontan survivors (7% HLHS) with Fontan procedure performed between April 1973 and July 1991; age 14 ± 9 years, range 3.7–41 years	WPPSI-R, WISC-III, K-ABC, WRAT-R, SES	Full scale IQ (mean ± SD) 96 ± 17 (entire sample) 70 (HLHS) 97 (non-HLHS) K-ABC Composite (mean ± SD)= 93 ± 12 WRAT-R Composite (mean ± SD)= 91 ± 16 SES was a very strong predictor of performance Health status: 92% "excellent" or "good" Medication use: 68%
Ref. 74	5 transplant survivors (4 CHD 1 CM) mean age at transplant 4.3 months; mean age at testing 15 months	BSID, gross and fine motor, expressive and receptive language	Cognition = 92 Gross motor = 72 Fine motor = 89 Expressive language = 89 Receptive language = 88
Ref. 65	49 heart or heart/lung transplant survivors (mean age at evaluation 9.4 years, range 0.6–16.6 years) vs. 52 conventional cardiac surgery patients (mean age 6.2 years) vs. healthy controls	IQ: British Ability Scales Behavior: Rutter A Scale	Full scale IQ (mean ± SD) 99 ± 14.5 (transplant) 110 ± 18 (cardiac surgery) 111 ± 14.8 (healthy) Behavior problems 24% (transplant) 17% (cardiac surgery) 6% (healthy)

| Ref. 75 | 18 transplant survivors (12 CHD, 6 CM)(mean age at transplant 7.4 months) vs. 14 cardiac surgery controls (mean age at surgery 7.1 months); age at testing 2.7–10.8 years | BSID, SBIS, PPVT, neurologic exam | BSID-MDI (median ±SD)
71 ± 20 (transplant)
97 ± 16 (cardiac surgery)
BSID-PDI (median ±SD)
69 ± 17 (transplant)
89 ± 13 (cardiac surgery)
SBIS full scale IQ
97.6 ± 10 (transplant)
101 ± 14 (cardiac surgery)
PPVT
88 ± 18 (transplant)
89 ± 15 (cardiac surgery)
Neurologic exam
72% normal (transplant)
93% normal (cardiac surgery) |

[a] Median/range values.

HLHS = Hypoplastic left heart syndrome; CBCL = Child Behavior Checklist; WJPB = Woodcock–Johnson Psychoeducational Battery; VMI = visual–motor integration; BSID = Bayley Scales of Infant Development; MDI = Mental Development Index; PDI = Psycho-motor Development Index; WPPSI-R = Weschler Preschool and Primary Scale of Intelligence Revised; WISC-III = Weschler Intelligence Scale for Children; VABS = Vineland Adaptive Behavior Scales; PPVT = Peabody Picture Vocabulary Test; SBIS = Stanford–Binet Intelligence Scale; K-ABC = Kaufman Assessment Battery for Children Achievement Scale; WRAT-R = Wide Range Achievement Test—Revised; SES = socioeconomic status; CHD = congenital heart disease; CM = cardiomyopathy.

and the degree of chronic family difficulties. In contrast, Utens et al.(88,94,95) have explored psychopathology in large samples of survivors of CHD and have generally found outcomes comparable to the normal population. Consistently, this group has noted that disease severity was not a reliable predictor of psychological outcomes. Another group of adolescents with CHD demonstrated lower state anxiety and a greater superego strength than healthy controls despite scoring lower on cognitive processing skills (96). Males in the sample reported self-concept that was significantly lower than normal. The authors conclude that challenges faced by children with CHD may result in development of better coping strategies and a higher degree of self-control. In addition, they emphasize the importance of helping children adjust to physical limitations imposed by the disease in order to promote a healthy self-concept.

IMPACT ON THE FAMILY

The diagnosis of a serious illness such as CHF in a child has a ripple effect on all that are involved in the care of that child, most particularly, parents, siblings, and even extended family. Uncertainty, anxiety, distress, hopelessness, and altered interactions among family members have been reported when faced with such a crisis (97–100). The needs of a child with CHF may require family members to extend their normal caregiving roles to include functions typically performed by health professionals, i.e., managing oxygen therapy or complex medication regimes. These tasks may be unpleasant, even frightening for family members and will frequently alter the normal familial and social roles of the caregiver (101). Although parents generally assume the majority of the caregiving burden, altered roles for siblings and other family members can also be expected.

The overall impact on the family is very difficult to generalize to a specific diagnosis, as it will be affected by many factors unrelated to the child's illness. The family's previous experiences with stressful events and their current level of functioning play an important role in how the diagnosis of CHF will be interpreted (102). For example, a family caring for a child with complex CHD who has undergone multiple surgical interventions may interpret the late onset of CHF as just one more phase of an illness that they have been coping with for a long time. Alternatively, the family of a previously healthy child diagnosed with an acute onset of CHF may find the diagnosis to be an overwhelming stressor for which they have not previously developed reliable coping skills. As health professionals, it is important that we evaluate the psychosocial functioning of the family during the critical phase of their child's illness. It has been demonstrated that maternal perceptions of stress have a strong relationship with the child's emotional adjustment; significantly greater than the mother's perceived severity of illness or their beliefs about their ability to control what happens to their child (103). Despite achieving outcomes within the normal range on measures of stress and emotional adjustment, parents of children with CHD have reported persistent high levels of vigilance with their children and conscious efforts to achieve normalization whenever possible (104,105). Social support has been identified as an important factor that influences the resiliency of families faced with chronic illness (100,104).

TRANSPLANTATION

For children with severe CHF, whether acute or chronic in nature, heart or heart–lung transplantation may be the definitive therapy. The transplantation process from evaluation through the transplant itself and subsequent follow-up poses unique stressors to psychosocial functioning. Unlike many other surgical or medical regimes, transplantation is typically presented as an option and potential recipients along with their parents are asked to make a choice to either proceed with this therapy or not. In addition, once the decision to pursue transplant is made, patients and families face a number of stressors including the waiting period, during which time the child's condition may be progressively deteriorating;

compliance with a complex medical regime both pre- and post-transplant; the surgical procedure itself; adaptation to life with a new organ; and long-term issues associated with constant monitoring for infection or rejection and the side effects of transplant medications. Maintaining a healthy psychological state throughout this process can be an extreme challenge for all family members involved.

In adult candidates for heart transplantation, psychiatric evaluation prior to listing is typically a routine part of the pretransplant evaluation process. In a review of the psychiatric evaluations of 246 heart transplant candidates, Phipps (106) found that greater than 90% of the subjects identified the following issues as being stressful:

- Having end-stage heart disease
- Symptoms of the illness: feeling worn out, no energy, sleeping poorly
- Waiting for a heart donor to be found
- Having family worrying about them
- Poor quality of life before transplantation
- Finding out that they needed a heart transplant
- Uncertainty regarding the future
- Decreased control over one's life
- Worrying how they will do after surgery
- Having to be dependent on others

Emotions may vacillate between hope and anticipation about receiving a new organ and fear that a suitable donor may not be found in time. In addition, there may be feelings of guilt over the realization that another person must die in order to undergo transplant. The prevalence of psychiatric morbidity in transplant candidates has been reported to range from 39% to 50% (107) with anxiety, depression, and sexual dysfunction being particularly common. A history of psychiatric dysfunction and illness-related factors such as duration of illness and degree of symptoms have been found to predict poorer psychosocial function and subjective reports of decreased pretransplant quality of life (106,107).

Similar findings of pretransplant psychological impact have been found in children awaiting transplantation

(108,109). Serrano-Ikkos et al. (109) evaluated a sample of 48 children ages 5–16 years prior to transplant and a control group of healthy siblings. Twenty-five percent of the subjects were found to meet ICD-9 criteria for diagnosis of an emotional disorder and 58% reported mild to moderate impairment of psychosocial functioning such as depressed mood and problems with friends or school performance. However, on subjective reports of depression, self-concept, and behavior problems at home or school that were completed by the children, parents, and school teachers, the ill children did not differ significantly from their healthy siblings. In the sample, 43% of families were found to be well adjusted but 57% demonstrated difficulties with family functioning including disagreements about child care, unresolved conflicts, and problems discussing the severity of their child's illness.

A number of factors have resulted in an increase in the average waiting time for transplant including a higher number of potential candidates despite a relatively stable number of organ donations and the increased application of assist devices as a bridge to transplant. Although one might speculate that stress levels would increase with the length of the waiting period, studies have not found this to be true (109,110). Rather, a negative perception of the transplantation process was found to be more strongly correlated to parent-reported stress. Parents typically viewed transplant more negatively in girls than in boys. Interestingly, in Suddaby's study of 26 parents of 18 children awaiting heart transplant, no correlation was found between how sick a parent perceived their child to be and their reported level of stress. In fact, despite significant intervention such as care in an ICU or use of a ventilator, parents reported a median score of 3 (1 = near death; 5 = healthy) when asked about their child's current state of health (110).

Successful transplantation provides a life saving therapy for many children with CHF and rapid improvements in physical health status are typically seen. However, ongoing physical and psychological stressors remain. The physical changes associated with transplant medications, e.g., acne, cushingoid features, hirsutism, gingival hypertrophy, and others, may be upsetting and may even impact long-term treatment compliance. This may be particularly true for previously healthy children who experience acute CHF and subsequent transplant. In a study comparing psychosocial outcome in subjects managed with transplant vs. those undergoing conventional cardiac surgery, it was found that preoperative psychological disorders were present in 26–28% of both groups. Postoperatively, the prevalence of psychiatric disorders persisted in the transplant group but decreased significantly in the group managed with conventional cardiac surgery (6.5%) (111). The transplant group, however, did demonstrate an overall improvement in psychosocial function post-transplant that was significantly related to improvements in physical ability. Lower social competence and behavior problems that correlated with low perceived popularity and were most commonly suggestive of depression were found in 33% of a cohort of 49 pediatric subjects after heart transplant (112). Wray et al. (113) and DeMaso (114) reported similar findings but demonstrated a significant decrease in behavior problems from pre- to post-transplant evaluation.

Because of the extreme medical, psychological, and socioeconomic consequences of heart transplantation, the familial impact may be significantly greater than that of other more conventional therapies. One major factor is that parents are asked to make an individual choice about transplantation for their children; a major challenge to their role as parents. Higgins et al. (115–117) have explored this decision-making process in depth and offer important insights into the processes used by parents to make informed choices regarding transplantation. Using qualitative interviews and observation with 24 parents of 15 children undergoing transplant evaluation, the decision to accept or reject the transplant option was explored. For the majority of families, familial factors such as the effect on family functioning and quality of life considerations were found to play the greatest role in parental decision making regarding transplant. For others, psychological/emotional issues such as the deteriorating condition of the child and complex social circumstances guided decision making. Physician endorsement for or against the transplant option played less of a role than anticipated. Although there was an initial disparity in opinions about transplant in 40% of the parent/physician groups, physician endorsement accounted for a change from the parents' original perspective in only two out of six situations (115). Parents varied in their approach to the decision-making process with 60% using logical, information based behaviors and the remaining 40% reaching a more spontaneous decision based on the facts immediately at hand. Style of decision making varied as well, ranging from a desire for an autonomous, independent choice, to a shared approach, to some who preferred an authoritarian, paternalistic choice that was directed by the medical team (117). Most importantly Higgins emphasized, "It is imperative that health professionals facilitate and support what the parent portrays as the best choice for them, a choice that they can live with in the future (115)."

Just as for the children, the consequences of transplant may be long-lived for parents as well. Fathers of children undergoing transplantation have reported considerable financial stress, disruption of family activities, and increased family burden despite reporting lower than normal scores on the Parenting Stress Index (118). These results may portray successful adaptation to the stress of the transplant experience or alternatively may reflect fathers' shift in focus from the uncontrollable situation of their child's illness to a desire to regain successful management of more concrete family affairs. In a recent study of 170 caregivers of pediatric transplant recipients, the cohort did not demonstrate increased levels of depression or anxiety when compared to the normative samples for the Beck Depression Inventory or the State-Trait Anxiety Inventory. However, the Posttraumatic Stress Diagnostic Scale revealed that 51% of the sample reported moderate to severe symptoms of posttraumatic stress disorder (PTSD) at 10–38 months (mean 18.2 months) after transplant. Of these, 45% had moderate to severe impairment of day-to-day functioning as a result of these symptoms (119). Avoidance, e.g., feeling distant or cut off from people around you, was the most common symptom of PTSD reported. While no demographic variables predicted the severity of PTSD, the impact on family and social functioning and the perceived benefits of the transplant experience did correlate with self-reported PTSD symptoms. Also the parents' appraisal of the child's current health state was significantly related to the degree of PTSD (119).

Overall, the literature supports that the transplant process, both pre- and post-transplant, presents unique and significant stressors to children and their families. It is extremely important for health care providers to acknowledge not only the medical issues associated with transplant but also to be realistic and forthcoming with families about the potential psychosocial implications (116). Ongoing assessment for symptoms of psychologic dysfunction should be incorporated into the transplant regime starting with a comprehensive pretransplant psychosocial assessment. Use of social support networks and effective coping mechanisms should be encouraged.

IMPLICATIONS FOR RESEARCH AND PRACTICE

Although evidence has been presented here highlighting the psychosocial impact of CHF in adults, CHD, and pediatric cardiac transplant, relatively little is known about these outcomes specific to CHF in children. Given the growing number of children at risk for the diagnosis of CHF, continued research on its psychosocial implications is imperative for comprehensive management of this disease. The facts supporting effects on HRQL, neurocognitive, psychological, behavioral, and family functioning are significant and warrant comprehensive psychosocial evaluations of both children diagnosed with CHF and their families. To produce generalizable results, psychosocial outcomes should be included in research evaluating varying treatment strategies, clinical trials, long-term outcomes, and longitudinal assessments of children receiving care for CHF. Whenever possible, instruments with well-defined reliability, validity, and sensitivity should be employed.

A multidisciplinary approach to management of the child with CHF must be emphasized. Too often, the medical aspects of the disease are prioritized with no one assigned to specifically and realistically address the psychosocial implications. Nurses, social workers, and child life specialists are members of the multidisciplinary team with unique insight and training in how to address these issues. The developmental changes inherent to children and families necessitate an individualized approach (120,121). No two individuals react to stress in exactly the same way and reactions do not always appear to reflect the clinical situation at hand. Children and families should be given opportunities to discuss their experiences and to identify how CHF has affected other aspects of their lives. Feelings of vulnerability, uncertainty, and changes in self-perception should be expected and subjects should be provided with anticipatory guidance for facing these challenges. Healthy coping mechanisms and use of social support networks should be fostered remembering that individual coping styles vary significantly. Providing opportunities to learn from the experiences of others in similar situations may help to reduce feelings of isolation, inspire optimism and improve understanding of the disease process (122). Most importantly, we must remember that a person's perception of psychosocial impact and level of function is inherently subjective in nature and cannot be predicted by the severity of their condition alone. In order to truly begin to understand what our patients are facing, beyond just their cardiac issues, we are obligated to ask, "How do *you* think you are doing?"

REFERENCES

1. Talner N, McGovern JJ, Carboni MP. Congestive heart failure. In: Moller JH, Hoffman JIE, eds. Pediatric Cardiovascular Medicine. Philadelphia: Churchill Livingstone, 2000:817–832.
2. Stein RE, Riessman CK. The development of an impact-on-family scale: preliminary findings. Med Care 1980; 18(4):465–472.
3. Mott S, James SR, Sperhac AM. Nursing Care of Children and Families 2nd ed Redwood City: Addison-Wesley, 1990.
4. American Heart Association. Congenital Cardiovascular Disease Statistics. Vol. 2002. Available at: http://www.americanheart.org Accessed January 29, 2003.

5. Morton M. Heart failure secondary to congenital heart disease. In: Hosenpud JD, Greenberg BH, eds. Congestive Heart Failure. New York: Springer-Verlag, 1994:246–257.

6. Kamphuis M, Ottenkamp J, Vliegen HW, et al. Health related quality of life and health status in adult survivors with previously operated complex congenital heart disease. Heart (British Cardiac Society). 2002; 87(4):356–362.

7. DeMaso DR, Beardslee WR, Silbert AR, Fyler DC. Psychological functioning in children with cyanotic heart defects. J Dev Behav Pediatr 1990; 11(6):289–294.

8. Van Horn M, DeMaso DR, Gonzalez-Heydrich J, Erickson JD. Illness-related concerns of mothers of children with congenital heart disease. J Am Acad Child Adolesc Psychiatry 2001; 40(7):847–854.

9. Kendall L, Lewin RJ, Parsons JM, Veldtman GR, Quirk J, Hardman GE. Factors associated with self-perceived state of health in adolescents with congenital cardiac disease attending paediatric cardiologic clinics. Cardiol Young 2001; 11(4):431–438.

10. Marino B, Wernovsky G, Shea J, Aquirre A, Helfaer M. Development of a research tool to assess quality of life in children and adolescents with heart disease: Preliminary data. Cardiol Young 2001; 11(suppl 1):33.

11. Saigal S, Stoskopf BL, Feeny D, et al. Differences in preferences for neonatal outcomes among health care professionals, parents, and adolescents [comment]. JAMA 1999; 281(21):1991–1997.

12. Varni JW, Seid M, Rode CA. The PedsQL: measurement model for the pediatric quality of life inventory. Med Care 1999; 37(2):126–139.

13. Frey M. Health-related quality of life: promises and pitfalls. J Child Family Nurs 2001; 4(1):63–67.

14. Kozinetz CA, Warren RW, Berseth CL, Aday LA, Sachdeva R, Kirkland RT. Health status of children with special health care needs: measurement issues and instruments. Clin Pediatr 1999; 38(9): 525–533.

15. Eiser C, Morse R. A review of measures of quality of life for children with chronic illness. Arch Dis Child 2001; 84(3):205–211.

16. Guyatt GH, Nogradi S, Halcrow S, Singer J, Sullivan MJ, Fallen EL. Development and testing of a new measure of health status for clinical trials in heart failure. J Gen Intern Med 1989; 4(2): 101–107.

17. Rector T, Kubo S, Chachques JC. Patient's self assessment of their congestive heart failure. Part 2: Content, reliability and validity of a new measure, the Minnesota Living With Heart Failure Questionnaire. Heart Fail 1987; 3:189–209.

18. al-Kaade S, Hauptman PJ. Health-related quality of life measurement in heart failure: challenges for the new millennium. J Card Fail 2001; 7(2):194–201.

19. Uzark K, Jones K, Burwinkle T, Varni JW. The pediatric quality of life inventory in children with heart disease: reliability and validity of a cardiac module. Prog Pediatr Cardiol 2003; 18(2):141–149.
20. Connolly D, Rutkowski M, Auslender M, Artman M. Measuring health-related quality of life in children with heart disease. Appl Nurs Res 2002; 15(2):74–80.
21. Nanda U, Andresen EM. Health-related quality of life. A guide for the health professional. Eval Health Prof 1998; 21(2):179–215.
22. Moser DK, Worster PL. Effect of psychosocial factors on physiologic outcomes in patients with heart failure. J Cardiovasc Nurs 2000; 14(4):106–115.
23. Bennett SJ, Pressler ML, Hays L, Firestine LA, Huster GA. Psychosocial variables and hospitalization in persons with chronic heart failure. Prog Cardiovasc Nurs 1997; 12(4):4–11.
24. Konstam V, Salem D, Pouleur H, et al. Baseline quality of life as a predictor of mortality and hospitalization in 5,025 patients with congestive heart failure. SOLVD investigations. Studies of left ventricular dysfunction investigators. Am J Cardiol 1996; 78(8):890–895.
25. Doba N, Tomiyama H, Nakayama T. Drugs, heart failure and quality of life: what are we achieving? What should we be trying to achieve? Drugs Aging 1999; 14(3):153–163.
26. Hobbs FD, Kenkre JE, Roalfe AK, Davis RC, Hare R, Davies MK. Impact of heart failure and left ventricular systolic dysfunction on quality of life: a cross-sectional study comparing common chronic cardiac and medical disorders and a representative adult population [comment]. Eur Heart J 2002; 23(23):1867–1876.
27. Westlake C, Dracup K, Creaser J, et al. Correlates of health-related quality of life in patients with heart failure. Heart Lung: J Acute Critical Care 2002; 31(2):85–93.
28. Shively M, Fox C, Brass-Mynderse NJ. Health-related quality of life as an outcome for patients with heart failure [erratum appears in J Cardiovasc Nurs 1996 Apr; 10(3):92–93]. J Cardiovasc Nurs 1996; 10(2):89–96.
29. Shephard RJ, Franklin B. Changes in the quality of life: a major goal of cardiac rehabilitation. J Cardiopulm Rehabil 2001; 21(4):189–200.
30. Reddy P, Dunn AB. The effect of beta-blockers on health-related quality of life in patients with heart failure. Pharmacotherapy 2000; 20(6):679–689.
31. Luck JC, Wolbrette DL, Boehmer JP, Ulsh PJ, Silber D, Naccarelli GV. Biventricular pacing in congestive heart failure: a boost toward finer living. Curr Opin Cardiol 2002; 17(1):96–101.
32. Walden JA, Stevenson LW, Dracup K, Wilmarth J, Kobashigawa J, Moriguchi J. Heart transplantation may not improve quality of life for patients with stable heart failure. Heart Lung: J Acute Critical Care 1989; 18(5):497–506.

33. Walden JA, Stevenson LW, Dracup K, et al. Extended comparison of quality of life between stable heart failure patients and heart transplant recipients. J Heart Lung Transplant 1994; 13(6):1109–1118.

34. Mussatto K, Frisbee SJ, Sachdeva RC, Pelech AN, Litwin SB, Tweddell JS. Subjects with surgically treated complex congenital heart disease report health related quality of life equal to healthy peers. J Am Coll Cardiol 2002; 39(5 suppl A):413A.

35. Torrance GW, Feeny DH, Furlong WJ, Barr RD, Zhang Y, Wang Q. Multiattribute utility function for a comprehensive health status classification system. Health Utilities Index Mark 2. Med Care 1996; 34(7):702–722.

36. Ware JE Jr, Gandek B. Overview of the SF-36 health survey and the International Quality of Life Assessment (IQOLA) project. J Clini Epidemiol 1998; 51(11):903–912.

37. Varni JW, Seid M, Knight TS, Uzark K, Szer IS. The PedsQL 4.0 Generic Core Scales: sensitivity, responsiveness, and impact on clinical decision-making. J Behav Med 2002; 25(2):175–193.

38. Dunbar-Masterson C, Wypij D, Bellinger DC, et al. General health status of children with D-transposition of the great arteries after the arterial switch operation. Circulation 2001; 104(12 suppl 1):I138–I142.

39. Moyen Laane K, Meberg A, Otterstad JE, et al. Quality of life in children with congenital heart defects. Acta Paediatr 1997; 86(9):975–980.

40. Uzark K, Jones K, Varni JW. Severity of illness and perceived quality of life in children with heart disease. Circulation 2001; 104(17); II-1–II-1088: p. 797.

41. Connolly D, Rutkowski M, Auslender M, Artman M. The New York University Pediatric Heart Failure Index: a new method of quantifying chronic heart failure severity in children [comment]. J Pediatr 2001; 138(5):644–648.

42. Lane DA, Lip GY, Millane TA. Quality of life in adults with congenital heart disease. Heart (British Cardiac Society) 2002; 88(1):71–75.

43. Saliba Z, Butera G, Bonnet D, et al. Quality of life and perceived health status in surviving adults with univentricular heart [comment]. Heart (British Cardiac Society) 2001; 86(1):69–73.

44. Williams DL, Gelijns AC, Moskowitz AJ, et al. Hypoplastic left heart syndrome: valuing the survival. J Thorac Cardiovasc Surg 2000; 119(4 Pt 1):720–731.

45. Gorkin L, Norvell NK, Rosen RC, et al. Assessment of quality of life as observed from the baseline data of the Studies of Left Ventricular Dysfunction (SOLVD) trial quality-of-life substudy. Am J Cardiol 1993; 71(12):1069–1073.

46. Putzke JD, Williams MA, Daniel JF, Foley BA, Kirklin JK, Boll TJ. Neuropsychological functioning among heart transplant candidates: a case control study. J Clin Exp Neuropsychol 2000; 22(1):95–103.

47. Almeida OP, Flicker L. The mind of a failing heart: a systematic review of the association between congestive heart failure and cognitive functioning. Intern Med J 2001; 31(5):290–295.
48. Wernovsky G, Newburger J. Neurologic and developmental morbidity in children with complex congenital heart disease [comment]. J Pediatr 2003; 142(1):6–8.
49. Majnemer A, Limperopoulos C. Developmental progress of children with congenital heart defects requiring open heart surgery. Semin Pediatr Neurol 1999; 6(1):12–19.
50. Ferry PC. Neurologic sequelae of cardiac surgery in children. Am J Dis Child 1987; 141(3):309–312.
51. Mahle WT, Wernovsky G. Long-term developmental outcome of children with complex congenital heart disease. Clin Perinatol 2001; 28(1):235–247.
52. Limperopoulos C, Majnemer A, Shevell MI, Rosenblatt B, Rohlicek C, Tchervenkov C. Neurodevelopmental status of newborns and infants with congenital heart defects before and after open heart surgery [comment]. J Pediatr 2000; 137(5):638–645.
53. Bellinger DC, Wypij D, Kuban KC, et al. Developmental and neurological status of children at 4 years of age after heart surgery with hypothermic circulatory arrest or low-flow cardiopulmonary bypass. Circulation 1999; 100(5):526–532.
54. Glauser TA, Rorke LB, Weinberg PM, Clancy RR. Congenital brain anomalies associated with the hypoplastic left heart syndrome. Pediatrics 1990; 85(6):984–990.
55. Goldmuntz E. The epidemiology and genetics of congenital heart disease. Clin Perinatol 2001; 28(1):1–10.
56. Limperopoulos C, Majnemer A, Shevell MI, Rosenblatt B, Rohlicek C, Tchervenkov C. Neurologic status of newborns with congenital heart defects before open heart surgery. Pediatrics 1999; 103(2):402–408.
57. Bellinger DC, Bernstein JH, Kirkwood MW, Rappaport LA, Newburger J. Visual-spatial skills in children after open-heart surgery. Dev Behav Pediatr 2003; 24(3):169–179.
58. Ikle L, Hale K, Fashaw L, Boucek M, Rosenberg AA. Developmental outcome of patients with hypoplastic left heart syndrome treated with heart transplantation [comment]. J Pediatr 2003; 142(1):20–25.
59. Kern JH, Hinton VJ, Nereo NE, Hayes CJ, Gersorty WM. Early developmental outcome after the Norwood procedure for hypoplastic left heart syndrome. Pediatrics 1998; 102(5):1148–1152.
60. Limperopoulos C, Majnemer A, Shevell MI, et al. Predictors of developmental disabilities after open heart surgery in young children with congenital heart defects. J Pediatr 2002; 141(1):51–58.
61. Limperopoulos C, Majnemer A, Shevell MI, et al. Functional limitations in young children with congenital heart defects after cardiac surgery. Pediatrics 2001; 108(6):1325–1331.

62. Morris RD, Krawiecki NS, Wright JA, Walter LW. Neuropsychological, academic, and adaptive functioning in children who survive in hospital cardiac arrest and resuscitation. J Learn Disabil 1993; 26(1):46–51.

63. Uzark K, Lincoln A, Lamberti JJ, Mainwaring RD, Spicer RL, Moore JW. Neurodevelopmental outcomes in children with Fontan repair of functional single ventricle. Pediatrics 1998; 101(4 Pt 1):630–633.

64. Wernovsky G, Stiles KM, Gauvreau K, et al. Cognitive development after the Fontan operation. Circulation 2000; 102(8):883–889.

65. Wray J, Pot-Mees C, Zeitlin H, Radley-Smith R, Yacoub M. Cognitive function and behavioural status in paediatric heart and heart–lung transplant recipients: the Harefield experience. BMJ 1994; 309(6958):837–841.

66. Mahle WT. Neurologic and cognitive outcomes in children with congenital heart disease. Curr Opin Pediatr 2001; 13(5):482–486.

67. Bellinger DC, Jonas RA, Rappaport LA, et al. Developmental and neurologic status of children after heart surgery with hypothermic circulatory arrest or low-flow cardiopulmonary bypass [comment]. N Engl J Med 1995; 332(9):549–555.

68. Bellinger DC, Rappaport LA, Wypij D, Wernovsky G, Newburger JW. Patterns of developmental dysfunction after surgery during infancy to correct transposition of the great arteries. J Dev Behav Pediatr 1997; 18(2):75–83.

69. Bellinger DC, Wypij D, Duplessis AJ, et al. Eight-year neurodevelopmental status: the Boston circulatory arrest study. Circulation 2000; 102(18 suppl II):497.

70. Freedom RM. Neurodevelopmental outcome after the Fontan procedure in children with the hypoplastic left heart syndrome and other forms of single ventricle pathology: challenges unresolved [comment]. J Pediatr 2000; 137(5):602–604.

71. Goldberg CS, Schwartz EM, Brunberg JA, et al. Neurodevelopmental outcome of patients after the Fontan operation: a comparison between children with hypoplastic left heart syndrome and other functional single ventricle lesions [comment]. J Pediatr 2000; 137(5):646–652.

72. Mahle WT, Clancy RR, Moss EM, Gerdes M, Jobes DR, Wernovsky G. Neurodevelopmental outcome and lifestyle assessment in school-aged and adolescent children with hypoplastic left heart syndrome. Pediatrics 2000; 105(5):1082–1089.

73. Todaro JF, Fennell EB, Sears SF, Rodrigue JR, Roche AK. Review: cognitive and psychological outcomes in pediatric heart transplantation. J Pediatr Psychol 2000; 25(8):567–576.

74. Suddaby EC, Samango-Sprouse C, Vaught DR, Custer DA. Neurodevelopmental outcome of infant cardiac transplant recipients. J Transplant Coordination 1996; 6(1):9–13.

75. Fleisher BE, Baum D, Brudos G, et al. Infant heart transplantation at Stanford: growth and neurodevelopmental outcome. Pediatrics 2002; 109(1):1–7.

76. MacMahon KM, Lip GY. Psychological factors in heart failure: a review of the literature. Arch Intern Med 2002; 162(5):509–516.

77. Denollet J, Brutsaert DL. Personality, disease severity, and the risk of long-term cardiac events in patients with a decreased ejection fraction after myocardial infarction [comment]. Circulation 1998; 97(2):167–173.

78. Ferketich AK, Schwartzbaum JA, Frid DJ, Moeschberger ML. Depression as an antecedent to heart disease among women and men in the NHANES I study. National Health and Nutrition Examination Survey [comment]. Arch Intern Med 2000; 160(9):1261–1268.

79. Frasure-Smith N, Lesperance F, Gravel G, et al. Social support, depression, and mortality during the first year after myocardial infarction. Circulation 2000; 101(16):1919–1924.

80. Krumholz HM, Butler J, Miller J, et al. Prognostic importance of emotional support for elderly patients hospitalized with heart failure. Circulation 1998; 97(10):958–964.

81. Borsody JM, Courtney M, Taylor K, Jairath N. Using self-efficacy to increase physical activity in patients with heart failure. Home Healthcare Nurse 1999; 17(2):113–118.

82. Tavazzi L, Zotti AM, Mazzuero G. Acute pulmonary edema provoked by psychologic stress. Report of two cases. Cardiology 1987; 74(3):229–235.

83. Chin MH, Goldman L. Correlates of early hospital readmission or death in patients with congestive heart failure. Am J Cardiol 1997; 79(12):1640–1644.

84. Murberg TA, Bru E. Social relationships and mortality in patients with congestive heart failure. J Psychosom Res 2001; 51(3):521–527.

85. Alden B, Gilljam T, Gillberg C. Long-term psychological outcome of children after surgery for transposition of the great arteries. Acta Paediatr 1998; 87(4):405–410.

86. Hovels-Gurich HH, Konrad K, Wiesner M, et al. Long term behavioural outcome after neonatal arterial switch operation for transposition of the great arteries. Arch Dis Child 2002; 87(6):506–510.

87. Janus M, Goldberg S. Treatment characteristics of congenital heart disease and behaviour problems of patients and healthy siblings. J Paediatr Child Health 1997; 33(3):219–225.

88. Utens EM, Verhulst FC, Duivenvoorden HJ, Meijboom FJ, Erdman RA, Hess J. Prediction of behavioural and emotional problems in children and adolescents with operated congenital heart disease. Eur Heart J 1998; 19(5):801–807.

89. Yildiz S, Savaser S, Tatlioglu GS. Evaluation of internal behaviors of children with congenital heart disease. J Pediatr Nurs 2001; 16(6):449–452.

90. Wray J, Sensky T. How does the intervention of cardiac surgery affect the self-perception of children with congenital heart disease? Child: Care Health Dev 1998; 24(1):57–72.

91. Gantt LT. Growing up heartsick: the experiences of young women with congenital heart disease. Health Care Women Int 1992; 13(3):241–248.

92. Gupta S, Mitchell I, Giuffre RM, Crawford S. Covert fears and anxiety in asthma and congenital heart disease. Child: Care Health Dev 2001; 27(4):335–348.

93. Spurkland I, Bjornstad PG, Lindberg H, Seem E. Mental health and psychosocial functioning in adolescents with congenital heart disease. A comparison between adolescents born with severe heart defect and atrial septal defect. Acta Paediatr 1993; 82(1):71–76.

94. Utens EM, Verhulst FC, Meijboom FJ, et al. Behavioural and emotional problems in children and adolescents with congenital heart disease. Psycholo Med 1993; 23(2):415–424.

95. Utens EM, Verhulst FC, Erdman RA, et al. Psychosocial functioning of young adults after surgical correction for congenital heart disease in childhood: a follow-up study. J Psychosom Res 1994; 38(7): 745–758.

96. Salzer-Muhar U, Herle M, Floquet P, et al. Self-concept in male and female adolescents with congenital heart disease. Clin Pediatr 2002; 41(1):17–24.

97. Lawoko S, Soares JJ. Distress and hopelessness among parents of children with congenital heart disease, parents of children with other diseases, and parents of healthy children. J Psychosom Res 2002; 52(4):193–208.

98. Gardner FV, Freeman NH, Black AM, Angelini GD. Disturbed mother–infant interaction in association with congenital heart disease [comment]. Heart 1996; 76(1):56–59.

99. Santacroce SJ. Measuring parental uncertainty during the diagnosis phase of serious illness in a child. J Pediatr Nurs 2001; 16(1):3–12.

100. Tak YR, McCubbin M. Family stress, perceived social support and coping following the diagnosis of a child's congenital heart disease. J Adv Nurs 2002; 39(2):190–198.

101. Schulz R, Quittner AL. Caregiving for children and adults with chronic conditions: introduction to the special issue. Health Psychol 1998; 17(2):107–111.

102. McCubbin MA, McCubbin HI. Family coping with health crisis: the resiliency model of family stress, adjustment and adaptation. In: Danielson C, Hamel-Bissell B, Winsted-Fry P, eds. Families Health and Illness. St. Louis: Mosby, 1993:21–63.

103. DeMaso DR, Campis LK, Wypij D, Bertram S, Lipshitz M, Freed M. The impact of maternal perceptions and medical severity on the adjustment of children with congenital eart disease. J Pediatr Psychol 1991; 16(2):137–149.

104. Carey LK, Nicholson BC, Fox RA. Maternal factors related to parenting young children with congenital heart disease. J Pediatr Nurs 2002; 17(3):174–183.

105. Sparacino PS, Tong EM, Messias DK, Foote D, Chesla CA, Gilliss CL. The dilemmas of parents of adolescents and young adults with congenital heart disease. Heart Lung: J Acute Critical Care 1997; 26(3):187–195.

106. Phipps L. Psychiatric evaluation and outcomes in candidates for heart transplantation. Clin Invest Med—Medecine Clinique et Experimentale 1997; 20(6):388–395.

107. Trumper A, Appleby L. Psychiatric morbidity in patients undergoing heart, heart and lung, or lung transplantation. J Psychosom Res 2001; 50(2):103–105.

108. Hanton LB. Caring for children awaiting heart transplantation: psychosocial implications. Pediatr Nurs 1998; 24(3):214–218.

109. Serrano-Ikkos E, Lask B, Whitehead B. Psychosocial morbidity in children, and their families, awaiting heart or heart–lung transplantation. J Psychosom Res 1997; 42(3):253–260.

110. Suddaby EC, Flattery MP, Luna M. Stress and coping among parents of children awaiting cardiac transplantation. J Transplant Coordination 1997; 7(1):36–40.

111. Serrano-Ikkos E, Lask B, Whitehead B, Rees P, Graham P. Heart or heart–lung transplantation: psychosocial outcome. Pediatr Transplant 1999; 3(4):301–308.

112. Uzark KC, Sauer SN, Lawrence KS, Miller J, Addonizio L, Crowley DC. The psychosocial impact of pediatric heart transplantation. J Heart Lung Transplant 1992; 11(6):1160–1167.

113. Wray J, Radley-Smith R, Yacoub M. Effect of cardiac or heart–lung transplantation on the quality of life of the paediatric patient. Qual Life Res 1992; 1(1):41–46.

114. DeMaso DR, Twente AW, Spratt EG, O'Brien P. Impact of psychologic functioning, medical severity, and family functioning in pediatric heart transplantation. J Heart Lung Transplant 1995; 14(6 Pt 1): 1102–1108.

115. Higgins SS, Kayser-Jones J. Factors influencing parent decision making about pediatric cardiac transplantation. J Pediatr Nurs 1996; 11(3):152–160.

116. Higgins SS, Kayser-Jones J, Savedra M. Parental understanding of the consequences of pediatric cardiac transplantation. Prog Cardiovasc Nurs 1996; 11(3):10–16.

117. Higgins SS. Parental role in decision making about pediatric cardiac transplantation: familial and ethical considerations. J Pediatr Nurs 2001; 16(5):332–337.

118. Rodrigue JR, MacNaughton K, Hoffmann RG III, et al. Perceptions of parenting stress and family relations by fathers of children evaluated for organ transplantation. Psychol Rep 1996; 79(3 Pt 1):723–727.

119. Young GS, Mintzer LL, Seacord D, Castaneda M, Mesrkhani V, Stuber ML. Symptoms of posttraumatic stress disorder in parents of transplant recipients: incidence, severity, and related factors. Pediatrics 2003; 111(6 Pt 1):e725–e731.
120. Weekes DP. Adolescents growing up chronically ill: a life-span developmental view. Fam Community Health 1995; 17(4):22–34.
121. Hinoki KW. Congenital heart disease: effects on the family. Neonatal Network—J Neonatal Nurs 1998; 17(5):7–10.
122. DeMaso DR, Gonzalez-Heydrich J, Erickson JD, Grimes VP, Strohecker C. The experience journal: a computer-based intervention for families facing congenital heart disease. J Am Acad Child Adolesc Psychiatry 2000; 39(6):727–734.

23

Heart Failure in the Adult with Congenital Heart Disease (ACHD)

MICHAEL J. LANDZBERG

Brigham and Women's Hospital,
Boston, Massachusetts, U.S.A.

Past assessment and review of the causes of heart failure in the adult with congenital heart disease largely focused on measures of ventricular systolic performance, typically emphasizing relationship with the "old baggage" of longstanding alterations of volume and anatomic loading conditions on ventricular function (1,2). These issues not withstanding, this chapter will focus on the multitude of additional potentials for heart failure specific to, varying in, or first recognized in the aging patient with congenital heart disease, with referenced literature geared to this population.

Almost nowhere else in medicine does the categorization of a patient with "heart failure" carry so many pathophysiologic potentials as in the adult patient with congenital heart disease. Classic clinical definition of "failure of the heart (in whatever form it may be) to keep up with the demands of the body" is demonstrated by what may be considered premature senescence and decrement of not only cardiac function, but potentially by abnormalities and increased demand of nearly every organ system (Table 1). Increased potential for

Table 1 "Noncardiac" Potential Etiologies for "Heart Failure" in the ACHD Patient

Endocrinologic/neurohormonal
   Hypothyroidism
   Diabetes
   Loss of adrenergic and vagal responsiveness
Pulmonary
   Restrictive lung disease
   Hypoventilation/obstructive sleep apnea
   Arterio-venous malformations
   Pulmonary vascular disease
   Chronic parenchymal infection
Liver
   Chronic hepatitis
   Portal hypertension
   Cirrhosis
Renal
   Altered glomeralar filtration
   Altered water handling
   Hyperuricemia
Hematologic
   Iron deficiency
   Erythrocytosis
   Lymphopenia
Skeletal
   Metabolically dependent poor muscle training
   Volitional/iatrogenic poor muscle training
   Kypho-scoliosis
Infectious
   Chronic infectious potential
Neurologic
   Cerebrovascular injury
Pregnancy

endocrinologic dysfunction, gas-exchanging and nonparenchymal lung disease, abnormalities of renal or hepatic function, and altered skeleton and muscle metabolism, highlight the multitude of extra-cardiac conditions contributing to abnormal functional capacity or performance.

The adult with congenital heart disease objectively may be profoundly limited in aerobic functional capacity compared to normal controls (3). Maximal achievable peak oxygen consumption (peak VO_2) may be < 50% normal controls, with important reductions seen even in patients after repair of simple atrial-level defects (Fig. 1). Restriction in ventilatory function (with respiratory volumes typically 75–85% normal predictions), whether due to developmental or acquired structural or physiologic changes, may contribute to fatigue and incapacity (Fig. 2) (3). Hepatitis-induced and "cardiac" cirrhosis, felt by many to be a disease of passing medical generations, have found recapitulation in a patient population plagued by higher central venous pressures, potential for low systemic

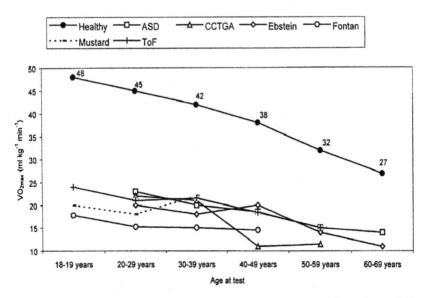

Figure 1 Impaired maximal oxygen consumption in adult patients with congenital heart disease. (From Ref. 3.)

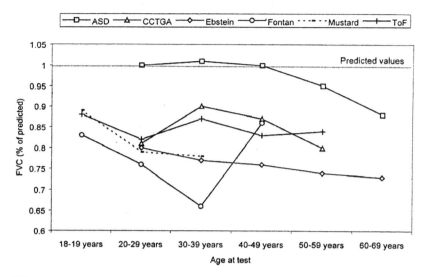

Figure 2 Impaired vital capacity as a marker of restrictive lung disease in adult patients with congenital heart disease. (From Ref. 3.)

cardiac index, and continued exposure to blood products. The neurohormonal activation caused by portal hypertension may be profound, and it exacerbates volume retention and curbs functional ability.

Compromise of effective circulation may result from intrinsic factors not typically considered within the cardiopulmonary tree (Table 2). For example, critical energy conservation within high-pressure nonpulsatile systemic venous inflow may be markedly diminished due to anatomic venous–atrial connections, jeopardizing forward output in atriopulmonary-type Fontari palliations (Fig. 3) (4). As well, impaired atrial–ventricular transport, due to intrinsic functional or anatomic baffle abnormalities, may be, in part, responsible for limits in stroke volume augmentation in patients with atrial-level repair for d-transposition of the great arteries (Fig. 4) (5). Pulmonary endothelial dysfunction, worse in nonpulsatile atriopulmonary connection-type repairs, increases nonanatomic pulmonary ventricular afterload, contributing to reduction in transpulmonary flow in patients with Fontan palliation (6).

Table 2 "Nonmyocardial" Potential Cardiopulmonary Etiologies for "Heart Failure" in the ACHD Patient

Alteration in
Systemic venous–atrial transport
Ventricular transport
Atrial–ventricular transport
Pulmonary vascular function
Systemic arterial conduit function
Pericardial constriction
Residual
Anatomic obstruction
Shunting
Outflow tract aneurysm
Semilunar valve regurgitation
Intracardiac/vascular thrombosis
Chronic arrhythmia

At the other end of the circuit, conduit arteries have the potential to act as a cushion, balancing the load of the systemic arterial bed on the systemic ventricle. In acquired congestive heart failure states, alterations in arterial stiffness, pulse pressure, wave characteristics, and velocities have been correlated with development of systemic ventricular hypertrophy, decrease in functional capacity, and worse survival outcomes (7). Demonstration of abnormal brachial arterial responsiveness to endothelium-dependent and -independent vasomediators in young adults after successful aortic coarctation repair led to investigation of conduit artery pulse wave velocity (PWV) as a marker of arterial stiffness in similar patients (8,9). Delay of conduit artery PWV correlated with alterations in vasodilation, pulse pressure, and development of increase in LV mass, as well as abnormal baroreflex sensitivity and reduced inhibition of sympathetic drive (10). Further investigation of similar pulse wave abnormalities in other congenital heart syndromes in the adult and their relationship to heart failure syndromes are thus far lacking.

Abnormalities in diastolic muscle function may correlate with functional capacity and survival. Most notable are those seen in patients after repair of tetralogy of Fallot, in whom early

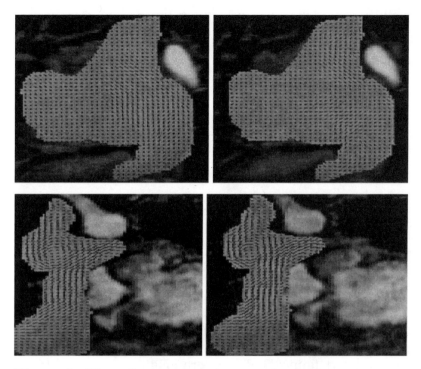

Figure 3 Magnetic resonance images of velocity vectors as a correlate of energy in atriopulmonary connection (top two panels) and total cavopulmonary anastomosis (bottom two panels)-type Fontan patients. Note diminution and alteration of direction of vectors in atriopulmonary Fontan patients. (From Ref. 4.)

postoperative echocardiographically demonstrable restrictive physiologic changes correlate with later similar restrictive markers, smaller chamber size, and narrower QRS duration (11,12). Such physiology appears to limit the effects of pulmonary regurgitation, possibly improving late survival. Regional changes in not only systolic but diastolic function, as well, in patients with tetralogy of Fallot have been shown using echocardiographic tissue Doppler analyses (Fig. 5) (13). Analysis of similar tissue Doppler characteristics has recently revealed regional variation and reduced early and late diastolic myocardial velocities, with prolonged isovolumic relaxation time and potential absence of A wave myocardial velocities, independent of systolic

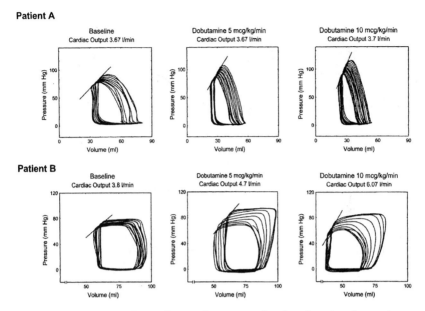

Figure 4 Flow volume loops during preload reduction in patients with (S, D, D) transposition of the great arteries following atrial level repair. Top panel: failure to increase cardiac output with dobutamine yet preservation of rise of contractile indices. Bottom panel: increase in both cardiac output as well as contractility is seen. In both patients, however, fall in stroke volume occurs. (From Ref. 5.)

abnormalities of the systemic right ventricle, in patients with d-transposition of the great arteries (Fig. 6) (14). These changes may reflect intrinsic muscle abnormalities, changes in electrical–mechanical coupling, or regional injury in affected patients (15).

Native and postoperative anatomic sequelae, aside from residual shunts and obstructions, can contribute to abnormalities in cardiac output, functional capacity, and survival. The presence of right ventricular outflow aneurysm in patients with tetralogy of Fallot correlates with magnetic resonance imaging-determined right ventricular dilation and hypertrophy, and lower RV and LV ejection fractions (Fig. 7) (16). The role of interventricular dependency for efficient systolic function is emphasized by these findings (Fig. 8). The

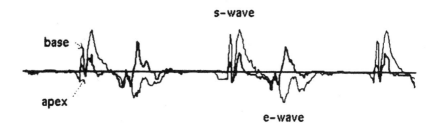

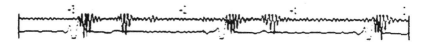

Figure 5 Tissue Doppler interrogation in a patient with tetralogy of Fallot. Arrow denotes abnormal diastolic regional movement. (From Ref. 13.)

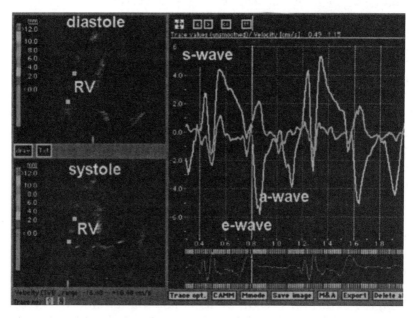

Figure 6 Tissue Doppler interrogation in a patient with d-transposition of the great arteries and abnormal diastolic regional motion. See text for details. (From Ref. 14.)

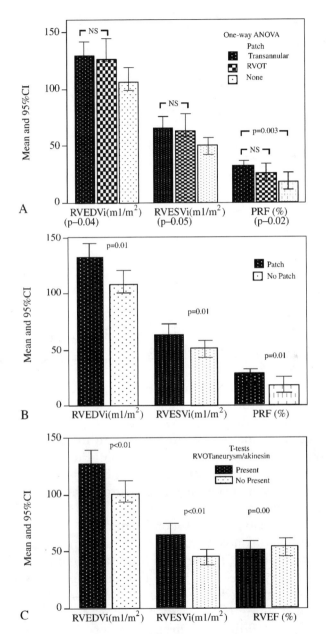

Figure 7 Correlation of patch outflow tract repair (panels A and B) and RV aneurysm (panel C) with increase in RV volumes and decrease in RV ejection fraction. RV = right ventricle; RVOT = right right ventricular outflow tract. (From Ref. 16.)

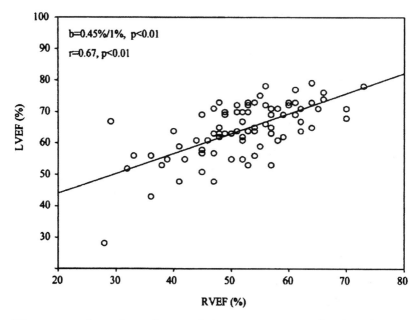

Figure 8 Interdependence of RV and LV systolic function, as demonstrated by ejection fraction. (From Ref. 16.)

presence of aortic regurgitation, caused in some patients by longstanding volume loading of the left ventricle and aortic root, may contribute, as well, to LV dysfunction (17). Progressive aortic dilatation or distortion can eventuate in obstruction to coronary arterial origins or dissection. Pulmonary arterial enlargement has been reported to encroach on the origins of the coronary arteries, causing acute ischemia or global myocardial hibernation.

Abnormalities of cardiac autonomic nervous activity (CANA) and elevations of neurohormones have been sought in the ACHD population due, in part, to recognized heart rate reduction after surgery, effects of prior thoracic operations, and subsequent surgery-mediated denervation, alterations in gas exchange, and aging (18,19). Such changes have been shown in chronic heart failure syndromes to correlate with degree of left ventricular dysfunction, functional capacity, and mortality, and have been incorporated into the definition of heart failure syndromes (20–23).

In children (primarily teenagers) who had undergone right ventricular outflow tract reconstruction, Ohuchi et al. (24) demonstrated that relatively severe postoperative sympathetic denervation of the ventricle was common (likely denervation rather than mediated via muscle dysfunction). They confirmed in this population that exercise-mediated changes in heart rate, much related to parasympathetic nervous tone, and postsynaptic β-adrenergic sensitivity (shown to correlate to functional ability) could be effected and was related to CANA. Parasympathetic activity early postsurgical repair appeared related to numbers of surgeries, significantly lowered with each, and had tendency to recover in the first year after operation (likely related to recovery of sinus node ischemia). Postoperative β-adrenergic sensitivity was maintained, allowing for adequacy of augmentation of heart rate. Augmentation of heart rate correlated with maximal oxygen consumption (peak VO_2) for postoperative patients without residual outflow tract stenosis, in contrast to patients with residual obstruction where it did not. As a model to other, more recent, study:

- Most recent hemodynamics were recorded along with radionuclear assessment of biventricular function.
- Neurohormones were directly measured (found to be higher in most noncontrol patients), and norepinephrine activity was assessed by direct measurement as well as metaiodobenzylguanidine (MIBG) heart and mediastinal scintigraphy (persisting abnormalities).
- Heart rate variability (low and high frequency domains) and R–R interval baroreflex sensitivity (BRS) to bolus phenylephrine (unrelated to restrictive ventilatory defects) were measured (lower than controls, BRS correlating with age at surgery and improving with time postsurgery).
- Parasympathetic nervous tone (PSNT) was assessed by postprandial atropine administration, both alone as well as altered by either isoproterenol (postsynaptic β-adrenergic sensitivity) or propranolol.

This study emphasized that surgically mediated changes in heart rate (PSNT, BRS) and their recovery were important determinants to functional ability. A relationship of abnormalities in CANA and arrhythmogenesis in the ACHD patient was theorized.

A follow-up assessment of CANA in mostly teenage patients after Fontan palliation of single ventricle physiology by this same group demonstrated similar global alterations in CANA, again excepting for preservation of postsynaptic β-adrenergic sensitivity, which was important for potential heart rate augmentation (25). CANA abnormalities correlated with reduction in augmentation of heart rate, and did not correlate to number of surgical procedures, age at time of Fontan operation, or length of follow-up. Similar to patients with residual RV outflow obstruction, HR augmentation in patients with Fontan physiology did not correlate with peak VO_2. The authors theorized that, taken together, these changes suggested that the Fontan circulation (with attendant higher central filling pressures, lower resting systemic cardiac index, and lower resting systemic arterial blood pressure) and surgery-related direct or subclinical damage, per se, rather than specific hemodynamic abnormalities, led to changes in CANA. In a relatively small subset of studied patients, nonspecific use of angiotensin-converting enzyme inhibition for an average 6-month period of time did not correlate with altered CANA abnormalities.

These findings, in part, were challenged by Davos et al. (26) who assessed CANA in 22 adult Fontan patients. Baroreflex sensitivity was assessed, and HRV was evaluated according to low and high frequency domains. Global depression of BRS and both domains of HRV were noted, with a greater reduction in the low frequency (reduction in sympathetic modulation) range. In contrast to the findings of Ohuchi et al. in younger patients: (1) reduction in low frequency HRV correlated with a marker of hemodynamic abnormality: increase in right atrial dimension, and (2) BRS was greater in patients with history of sustained atrial tachyarrhythmia.

Bolger et al. (27) measured resting neurohormones in 53 adults with a wide spectrum of congenital physiologies, and correlated findings with clinical patient variables, electrocardiographic indices, radiographic cardiothoracic ratio (CTR), and echocardiographic and exercise parameters. Regardless of NYHA functional class, neurohormones were elevated in all patients, and correlated stepwise with worsening subjective functional ability. ANP, BNP, endothelin-1, norepinephrine, and epinephrine all correlated well with each other and with increases in QT interval and CTR, all of which correlated with echocardiographically measured ventricular function and exercise peak VO_2. Aldosterone and renin correlated only with each other and with RA and LA volumes, suggesting control mechanisms other than central-pressure–volume relationships (instrumental in control of natriuretic peptides and catecholamines). The authors theorized a global "phenotype of congenital heart disease" aligned with the syndrome of congestive heart failure. Neurohormonal abnormalities could persist even decades after surgical repairs, though the authors suggested potential for variation in abnormalities based, in part, upon completeness of surgical correction. In a separate study, this same group showed elevation in circulating inflammatory cytokines, again correlating stepwise with patient functional class (Fig. 9) (28).

Ohuchi et al. (29) expanded on the results of Bolger et al., assessing both neurohormones as well as measures of CANA in 297 pediatric (75%) and adult (25%) patients with congenital heart disease. Stepwise increase in neurohormonal activation, correlating with subjective functional class regardless of asymptomatic state, was confirmed in pediatric and adult patients, with higher levels of natriuretic peptides seen in pediatric patients. Elevation of NE differentiated class II from III and IV adults, but not in children. Baroreflex sensitivity, heart rate variability, and vital capacity were related to functional capacity in NYHA I and II patients (but not class III and IV) of all ages, with adults having higher BRS and HRV. The authors suggest that measure of both neurohormones and CANA are useful in categorizing patients with CHD, with measures of PSA most helpful in the less symptomatic patients and neurohormones better in the more symptomatic patients (Fig. 10). Adults, with a greater vital capacity

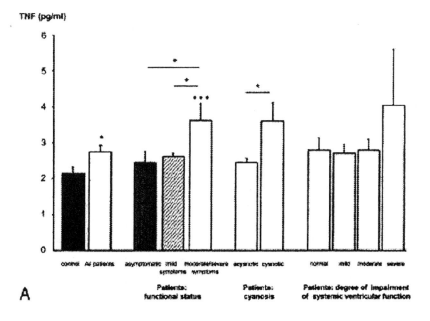

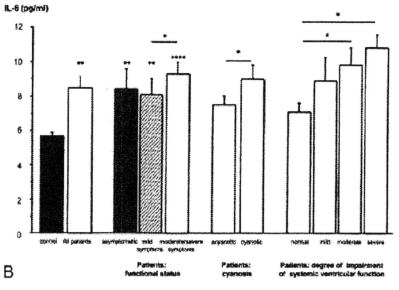

Figure 9 Elevation of inflammatory cytokines in adult patients with congenital heart disease correlates with functional capacity. (From Ref. 28.)

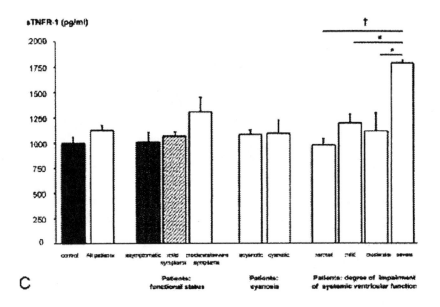

C

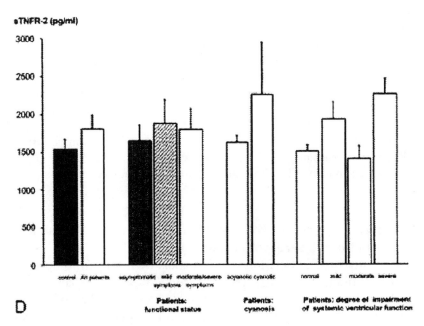

D

Figure 9 *(Continued)*

NYHA class

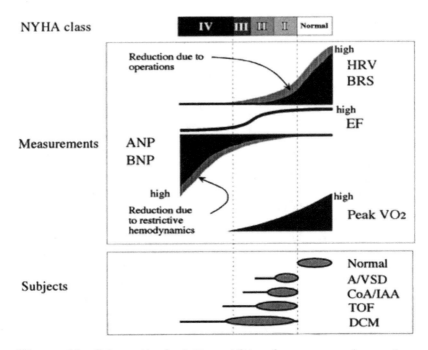

Figure 10 Schematic depicting utility of measures of neurohormonal activation (symptomatic end of spectrum) and CANA, in particular PSNT (asymptomatic end of spectrum) in adult patients with congenital heart disease. ANP, atrial natriuretic peptide; A/VSD, atrial or ventricular septal defect; BNP, B-type natriuretic peptide; BRS, baroreflex sensitivity; CoA/IAA, coarctation of the aorta or interrupted aortic arch; DCM, dilated cardiomyopathy; EF, ejection fraction; HRV, heart rate variability; NYHA, New York Heart Association; TOF, tetralogy of Fallot; VO₂, oxygen consumption. (From Ref. 29.)

(mitigating restrictive ventilatory reduction in HRV), had lesser reduction of parasympathetic activity (PSA) and a lesser rise in natriuretic hormones (with their own stimulatory ventilatory effects) than affected children. The authors theorized that exercise rehabilitation or other CANA- or neurohormonally targeted interventions might lead to decrease in HRV- and BRS-mediated arrhythmogenesis.

This decade has seen the rise in population of adults with congenital heart disease to numbers surpassing their pediatric counterparts. Patients with increasing anatomic complexity, greater numbers of operative and catheter-based surgeries, alterations in pulmonary and systemic arterial and venous function, neurohormonal activation, and abnormalities in rhythm, coupled with changes of myocardial, vascular, and multiorgan "premature" senescence, are alive, functioning, and demanding our protection and care for today and for their futures. The past number of years has seen an explosion in the understanding of heart failure syndromes in these patients, who, in their own existence, define a uniquely altered physiology. To date, single-center anecdotal investigations of therapies, each with limited meaning, have been rampant. It is only through continued insights, coupled with multicenter randomized clinical therapeutic trials utilizing tested outcomes measures in this growing population, that a future of optimal functioning can be best guaranteed for these patients.

REFERENCES

1. Graham TP. Ventricular performance in congenital heart disease. Circulation 1991; 84:2259–2274.
2. Perloff JK, Warnes CA. Challenges posed by adults with repaired congenital heart disease. Circulation 2001; 103:2637–2643.
3. Fredriksen PM, Veldtman G, Hechter S, et al. Aeorboic capacity in adults with various congenital heart diseases. Am J Cardiol 2001; 87:310–314.
4. Be'eri E, Maier SE, Landzberg MJ, et al. In vivo evaluation of Fontan pathway flow dynamics by multidimension phase-velocity magnetic resonance imaging. Circulation 1998; 98:2873–2882.
5. Derrick GP, Narang I, White PA, et al. Failure of stroke volume augmentation during exercise and dobutamine stress is unrelated to load-independent indexes of right ventricular performance after the Mustard operation. Circulation 2000; 102(suppl III):III154–III159.
6. Khambadkone S, Li J, de Leval MR, et al. Basal pulmonary vascular resistance and nitric oxide responsiveness late after Fontan-type operation. Circulation 2003; 107:3204–3208.
7. Bonapace S, Rossi A, Cicoira M, et al. Aortic distensibility independently affects exercise tolerance in patients with dilated cardiomyopathy. Circulation 2003; 107:16-3–1608.
8. Gardiner HM, Celermajer DS, Sorensen KE, et al. Arterial reactivity is significantly impaired in normotensive young adults after successful

repair of aortic coarctation in childhood. Circulation 1994; 89:1745–
1750.

9. de Devitiis M, Pilla C, Kattenhorn M, et al. Vascular dysfunction after
    repair of coarctation of the aorta. Circulation 2001; 104(suppl I):I165–
    I170.
10. de Devitiis M, Pilla C, Kattenhorn M, et al. Ambulatory blood pres-
    sure, left ventricular mass, and conduit artery function late after suc-
    cessful repair of coarctation of the aorta. J Am Coll Cardiol 2003;
    41:2259–2265.
11. Norgard G, Gatzoulis MA, Moraes F, et al. Relationship between type
    of outflow tract repair and postoperative right ventricular diastolic
    physiology in tetralogy of Fallot: implications for long term outcome.
    Circulation 1996; 94:3276–3280.
12. Norgard G, Gatzoulis MA, Josen M, Cullen S, Redington AN. Does
    restrictive right ventricular physiology in the postoperative period
    predict subsequent right ventricular restriction after repair of tetral-
    ogy of Fallot? Heart 1998; 79:481–484
13. Vogel M, Sporing J, Cullen S, Deanfield JE, Redington AN. Regional
    wall motion and abnormalities of electrical depolarization in patients
    after surgical repair of tetralogy of Fallot. Circulation 2001; 103:1660–
    1673.
14. Vogel M, Derrick G, White PA, et al. Systemic ventricular function in
    patients with transposition of the great arteries after atrial repair: a
    tissue Doppler and conductance catheter study. J Am Coll Cardiol
    2004; 43:100–106.
15. Chaturvedi RR, Shore DF, Lincoln C, et al. Acute right ventricular
    restrictive physiology after repair of tetralogy of Fallot. Association
    with myocardial injury and oxidative stress. Circulation 1999;
    100:1540–1547.
16. Davlouros PA, Kilner PJ, Hornung TS, et al. Right ventricular func-
    tion in adults with tetralogy of Fallot assessed with cardiovascular
    magnetic resonance imaging. Detrimental role of right ventricular
    outflow aneurysms or akinesia and adverse right-left ventricular
    interaction. J Am Coll Cardiol 2002; 40:2044–2052.
17. Niwa K, Siu SC, Webb GD, Gatzoulis MA. Progressive aortic root dila-
    tion in adults late after repair of tetralogy of Fallot. Circulation 2002;
    106:1374–1378.
18. Driscoll DJ, Danielson GK, Puga FJ, et al. Exercise tolerance and car-
    diorespiratory response to exercise after the Fontan operation for tri-
    cuspid atresia or functional single ventricle. J Am Coll Cardiol 1986;
    7:1087–1094.
19. Kondo C, Nazakawa M, Momma K, et al. Sympathetic denervation
    and reinnervation after arterial switch operation for complete
    transposition. Circulation 1998; 97: 2414–2419.

20. Cohn JN, Levine TB, Olivari MT, et al. Plasma norepinephrine as a guide to prognosis in patients with chronic congestive heart failure. N Engl J Med 1984; 311:819–823.
21. Gottlieb SS, Kukin ML, Ahern D, et al. Prognostic importance of atrial natriuretic peptide in patients with chronic heart failure. J Am Coll Cardiol 1989; 13:1534–1539.
22. Eichorn EJ. Prognosis determination in heart failure. Am J Med 2001; 110:14S–36S.
23. Remme WJ, Swedberg K, and the Task Force for the Diagnosis and Treatment of Chronic Heart Failure, and European Society of Cardiology. Guidelines for the diagnosis and treatment of chronic heart failure. Eur Heart J 2001; 22:1527–1560.
24. Ohuchi H, Suzuki H, Toyohara K, et al. Abnormal cardiac autonomic nervous activity after right ventricuclar outflow tract reconstruction. Circulation 2000; 102:2732–2738.
25. Ohuchi H, Hasegawa S, Yasuda K, et al. Severely impaired cardiac autonomic nervous activity after the Fontan operation. Circulation 2001; 104:1513–1518.
26. Davos CH, Francis DP, Leenarts MF, et al. Global impairment of cardiac autonomic nervous activity late after the Fontan operation. Circulation 2003; 108(suppl II):III80–II185.
27. Bolger AP, Sharma R, Li W, et al. Neurohormonal activation and the chronic heart failure syndrome in adults with congenital heart disease. Circulation 2002; 106:92–99.
28. Sharma R, Bolger AP, Li W, et al. Elevated circulating levels of inflammatory cytokines and bacterial endotoxin in adults with congenital heart disease. Am J Cardiol 2003; 92.
29. Ohuchi H, Takasugi H, Ohashi H, et al. Stratification of pediatric heart failure on the basis of neurohormonal and cardiac autonomic nervous activities in patients with congenital heart disease. Circulation 2003; 108:2368–2376.

Index